Kaplan's Clinical Hypertension

Norman M. Kaplan, MD

Clinical Professor of Medicine
Department of Internal Medicine
University of Texas Southwestern Medical School
Dallas, Texas

Ronald G. Victor, MD

Associate Director, Clinical Research
Director, Hypertension Center
The Heart Institute
Cedars-Sinai Medical Center
Los Angeles, California

With a Chapter by

Joseph T. Flynn, MD, MS

Professor of Pediatrics
Division of Nephrology
Seattle Children's Hospital
Seattle, Washington

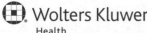 Wolters Kluwer | Lippincott Williams & Wilkins
Health

Philadelphia • Baltimore • New York • London
Buenos Aires • Hong Kong • Sydney • Tokyo

Acquisitions Editor: Frances R. DeStefano
Product Manager: Leanne McMillan
Production Manager: Alicia Jackson
Senior Manufacturing Manager: Benjamin Rivera
Marketing Manager: Kimberly Schonberger
Design Coordinator: Holly Reid McLaughlin
Production Service: SPi Technologies

©2010 by LIPPINCOTT WILLIAMS & WILKINS, a WOLTERS KLUWER business
530 Walnut Street
Philadelphia, PA 19106 USA
LWW.com

9th Edition, © 2006 Lippincott Williams & Wilkins
8th Edition, © 2000 Lippincott Williams & Wilkins
7th Edition, © 1998 Lippincott Williams & Wilkins
6th Edition, © 1994 Williams & Wilkins
5th Edition, © 1990 Williams & Wilkins
4th Edition, © 1986 Williams & Wilkins
3rd Edition, © 1982 Williams & Wilkins
2nd Edition, © 1978 Williams & Wilkins
1st Edition, © 1973 Williams & Wilkins

Printed in China

Library of Congress Cataloging-in-Publication Data
Kaplan's clinical hypertension / editors, Norman M. Kaplan, Ronald G. Victor; with a chapter
by Joseph T. Flynn. —10th ed.
    p. ; cm.
  Rev. ed. of: Kaplan's clinical hypertension / Norman M. Kaplan. 9th ed. c2006.
  Includes bibliographical references and index.
  ISBN-13: 978-1-60547-503-5
  ISBN-10: 1-60547-503-3
 1. Hypertension. I. Kaplan, Norman M., 1931- II. Victor, Ronald G. III. Kaplan, Norman M., 1931- Kaplan's clinical hypertension. IV. Title: Clinical hypertension.
  [DNLM: 1. Hypertension. WG 340 K171 2010]
  RC685.H8K35   2010
  616.1'32—dc22
                                                                              2009029663

To purchase additional copies of this book, call our customer service department at (800) 638–3030 or fax orders to (301) 223–2320. International customers should call (301) 223–2300.

Visit Lippincott Williams & Wilkins on the Internet: at LWW.com. Lippincott Williams & Wilkins customer service representatives are available from 8:30 am to 6 pm, EST.

10 9 8 7 6 5 4 3 2 1

CCS1009

To those such as
Goldblatt and Grollman,
Braun-Menéndez and Page,
Lever and Pickering,
Mancia, Brenner, and Laragh,
Julius, Hansson, and Freis,
and the many others, whose work has made it
possible for us to put
together what we hope will be a useful book on
clinical hypertension

H ypertension is increasingly being diagnosed worldwide, in developed and undeveloped societies, as populations become fatter and older. The literature on hypertension keeps pace with the increased prevalence of the disease. The ability required of a simple author to digest and organize this tremendous body of information into a relatively short book that is both current and inclusive has become almost impossible. Fortunately, Dr. Ronald Victor has been willing and able to join as a coauthor. After 10 years of close contact at the University of Texas Southwestern Medical School, I know him to be a clearheaded and open-minded clinician, teacher, and researcher. Despite his move to smoggy Los Angeles, he brings a fresh perspective that adds greatly to this book.

As noted in the previous edition, I am amazed at the tremendous amount of hypertension-related literature published over the past 4 years. A considerable amount of significant new information is included in this edition, presented in a manner that I hope enables the reader to grasp its significance and place it in perspective. Almost every page has been revised, using the same goals:

• Give more attention to the common problems; primary hypertension takes up almost half.

• Cover every form of hypertension at least briefly, providing references for those seeking more information. Additional coverage is provided on some topics that have recently assumed importance.
• Include the latest data, even if available only in abstract form.
• Provide enough pathophysiology to permit sound clinical judgment.
• Be objective and clearly identify biases, although my views may differ from those of others.

I have tried to give reasonable attention to those with whom I disagree.

Dr. Joseph T. Flynn, Professor of Pediatrics, Division of Nephrology, Seattle Children's Hospital, Seattle, Washington has contributed a chapter on hypertension in children and adolescents. I have been fortunate in being in an academic setting wherein such endeavors are nurtured and wish to thank all who have been responsible for establishing this environment and all of our colleagues who have helped us through the years.

Norman M. Kaplan, MD
Ronald G. Victor, MD

CONTENTS

CHAPTER 1

Hypertension in the Population at Large

Hypertension provides both despair and hope: despair because it is quantitatively the largest risk factor for cardiovascular diseases (CVD), it is growing in prevalence, and it is poorly controlled virtually everywhere; and hope because prevention is possible (though rarely achieved) and treatment can effectively control almost all patients, resulting in marked reductions in stroke and heart attack.

Although most of this book addresses hypertension in the United States and other developed countries, it should be noted that CVDs are the leading cause of death worldwide, more so in the economically developed countries, but also in the developing world. As Lawes et al. (2008) note: "Overall about 80% of the attributable burden (of hypertension) occurs in low-income and middle-income economies."

In turn, hypertension is, overall, the major contributor to the risks for CVDs. When the total global impact of known risk factors on the overall burden of disease is calculated, 54% of stroke and 47% of ischemic heart disease (IHD) are attributable to hypertension (Lawes et al., 2008). Of all the potentially modifiable risk factors for myocardial infarction in 52 countries, hypertension is exceeded only by smoking (Danaei et al., 2009).

The second contributor to our current despair is the growing prevalence of hypertension as seen in the ongoing survey of a representative sample of the U.S. population (Cutler et al., 2008; Lloyd-Jones et al., 2009). According to their analysis, the prevalence of hypertension in the United States has increased from 24.4% in 1990 to 28.9% in 2004. This increased prevalence primarily is a consequence of the population becoming older and more obese.

The striking impact of aging was seen among participants in the Framingham Heart Study: Among those who remained normotensive at either age 55 or 65 (providing two cohorts) over a 20-year follow-up, hypertension developed in almost 90% of those who were now aged 75 or 85 (Vasan et al., 2002).

The impact of aging and the accompanying increased prevalence of hypertension on both stroke and IHD mortality has been clearly portrayed in a meta-analysis of data from almost one million adults in 61 prospective studies by the Prospective Studies Collaboration (Lewington et al., 2002). As seen in Figure 1-1, the absolute risk for IHD mortality was increased at least twofold at every higher decade of age, with similar lines of progression for both systolic and diastolic pressure in every decade.

At the same time as populations are growing older, obesity has become epidemic in the United States (Hedley et al., 2004) and is rapidly increasing wherever urbanization is occurring (Yusuf et al., 2001). With weight gain, blood pressure (BP) usually increases and the increased prevalence of overweight is likely responsible for the significant increase in the BP of children and adolescents in the United States over the past 12 years (Ostchega et al., 2009).

The third contributor to our current despair is the inadequate control of hypertension virtually everywhere. According to similar surveys performed in the 1990s, with control defined at the 140/90 mm Hg threshold, control has been achieved in 29% of hypertensives in the United States, 17% in Canada, but in fewer than 10% in five European countries (England, Germany, Italy, Spain, and Sweden) (Wolf-Maier et al., 2004). Some improvement in the U.S. control rate has subsequently been found but the percentage has reached only 45% (Lloyd-Jones et al., 2009) (Table 1-1), whereas better control rates are reported from Canada (Mohan & Campbell, 2008), Cuba (Ordunez-Garcia et al., 2006), Denmark

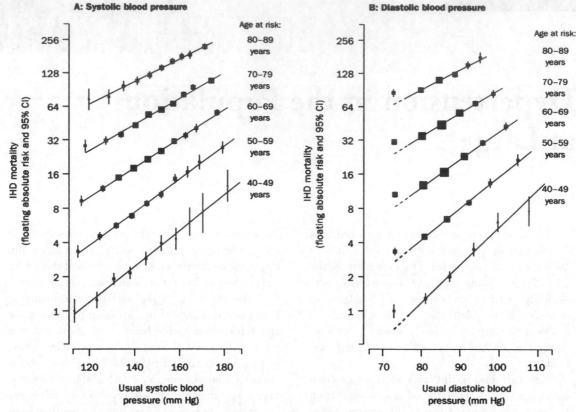

FIGURE 1-1   Ischemic heart disease (IHD) mortality rate in each decade of age plotted for the usual systolic **(left)** and diastolic **(right)** BPs at the start of that decade. Data from almost one million adults in 61 prospective studies. (Modified from Lewington S, Clarke R, Qizilbash N, et al. Age-specific relevance of usual blood pressure to vascular mortality: A meta-analysis of individual data for one million adults in 61 prospective studies. *Lancet* 2002;360:1903–1913.)

(Kronborg et al., 2009), and England (Falaschetti et al., 2009). As expected, even lower rates of control have been reported from less developed countries such as China (Dorjgochoo et al., 2009). Moreover, in the United States, control rates among the most commonly afflicted, the elderly, are significantly lower: only 29% of women 70 to 79 years of age are controlled (Lloyd-Jones et al., 2009). Furthermore, the relatively lower control rates among Hispanics and African Americans compared to whites remain unchanged (McWilliams et al., 2009). And of even greater concern, even when hypertensives are treated

TABLE 1.1   Trends in Awareness, Treatment, and Control of High Blood Pressure in U.S. Adults (Over Age 20) 1976–2004

	National Health and Nutrition Examination Survey (%)				
	1976–1980	1988–1991	1991–1994	2000–2004	2005–2006
Awareness	51	73	68	70	79
Treatment	31	55	54	59	61
Control	10	29	27	34	45

Percentage of adults aged 18 to 74 years with SBP of 140 mm Hg or greater, with DBP of 90 mm Hg or greater, or taking antihypertensive medication.
Adapted from Lloyd-Jones D, Adams R, Carnethon M, et al. Heart disease and stroke statistics-2009 update: A report from the American Heart Association statistics committee and stroke statistics subcommittee. *Circulation* 2009;119:e21–e181.

down to an optimal level, below 120/80 mm Hg, they continue to suffer a greater risk of stroke than normotensives with similar optimal BP levels (Asayama et al., 2009).

Despite all of these problems, there is hope, starting with impressive evidence of decreased mortality from CVDs, at least in the United States (Parikh et al., 2009) and England (Unal et al., 2004). However, as well as can be ascertained, control of hypertension has played only a relatively small role in the decreased mortality from coronary disease in the United States (Ford et al., 2007).

Nonetheless, there is also hope relative to hypertension. Primary prevention has been found to be possible (Whelton et al., 2002) but continues to be rarely achieved (Kotseva et al., 2009). Moreover, the rising number of the obese seriously questions the ability to implement the necessary lifestyle changes in today's world of faster foods and slower physical activity. Therefore, controlled trials of primary prevention of hypertension using antihypertensive drugs have begun (Julius et al., 2006).

On the other hand, the ability to provide protection against stroke and heart attack by antihypertensive therapy in those who have hypertension has been overwhelmingly documented (Blood Pressure Trialists, 2008). There is no longer any argument as to the benefits of lowering BP, though uncertainty persists as to the most cost-effective way to achieve the lower BP. Meanwhile, the unraveling of the human genome has given rise to the hope that gene manipulation or transfer can prevent hypertension. As of now, that hope seems extremely unlikely beyond the very small number of patients with monogenetic defects that have been discovered.

All in all, hope about hypertension seems overshadowed by despair. However, health care providers must, by nature, be optimistic, and there is an inherent value in considering the despairs about hypertension to be a challenge rather than an acceptance of defeat. As portrayed by Nolte and McKee (2008), the most realistic way to measure the health of nations is to analyze the mortality that is amenable to health care. By this criterion, the United States ranks 19th among the 19 developed countries analyzed. This sobering fact can be looked upon as a failure of the vastly wasteful, disorganized U.S. health care system. We prefer to look upon this poor rating as a challenge: current health care is inadequate, including, obviously, the management of hypertension, but the potential to improve has never been greater (Shih et al., 2008).

This book summarizes and analyses the works of thousands of clinicians and investigators worldwide who have advanced our knowledge about the mechanisms behind hypertension and who have provided increasingly effective therapies for its control. Despite their continued efforts, however, hypertension will almost certainly not ever be conquered totally, because it is one of those diseases that, in the words of a *Lancet* editorialist (Anonymous, 1993):

> …afflict us from middle age onwards [that] might simply represent "unfavorable" genes that have accumulated to express themselves in the second half of our lives. This could never be corrected by any evolutionary pressure, since such pressures act only on the first half of our lives: once we have reproduced, it does not greatly matter that we grow "sans teeth, sans eyes, sans taste, sans everything."

In this chapter, the overall problems of hypertension for the population at large are considered. We define the disease, quantify its prevalence and consequences, classify its types, and describe the current status of detection and control. In the remainder of the book, these generalities will be amplified into practical ways to evaluate and treat hypertension in its various presentations.

CONCEPTUAL DEFINITION OF HYPERTENSION

Although it has been more than 100 years since Mahomed clearly differentiated hypertension from Bright's renal disease, authorities still debate the level of BP that is considered abnormal (Task Force, 2007). Sir George Pickering challenged the wisdom of that debate and decried the search for an arbitrary dividing line between normal and high BP. In 1972, he restated his argument: "There is no dividing line. The relationship between arterial pressure and mortality is quantitative; the higher the pressure, the worse the prognosis." He viewed arterial pressure "as a quantity and the consequence numerically related to the size of that quantity" (Pickering, 1972).

However, as Pickering realized, physicians feel more secure when dealing with precise criteria, even if the criteria are basically arbitrary. To consider a BP of 138/88 mm Hg as normal and one of 140/90 mm Hg as high is obviously arbitrary, but medical practice requires that some criteria be used to determine the need for workup and therapy. The criteria should be established on some rational basis that includes the risks of disability and death associated with various levels of BP as well as the ability to reduce those risks by lowering the BP. As stated by Rose (1980): "The operational definition of hypertension is the level at which the benefits… of action exceed those of inaction."

Even this definition should be broadened, because action (i.e., making the diagnosis of hypertension at any level of BP) involves risks and costs as well as benefits, and inaction may provide benefits. These are summarized in Table 1-2. Therefore, the conceptual definition of hypertension should be that level of BP at which the benefits (minus the risks and costs) of action exceed the risks and costs (minus the benefits) of inaction.

Most elements of this conceptual definition are fairly obvious, although some, such as interference with lifestyle and risks from biochemical side effects of therapy, may not be. Let us turn first to the major consequence of inaction, the increased incidence of premature CVD, because that is the prime, if not the sole, basis for determining the level of BP that is considered abnormal and is called *hypertension*.

Risks of Inaction: Increased Risk of CVD

The risks of elevated BP have been determined from large-scale epidemiologic surveys. The Prospective Studies Collaboration (Lewington et al., 2002) obtained data on each of 958,074 participants in 61 prospective observational studies of BP and mortality. Over a mean time of 12 years, there were 11,960 deaths attributed to stroke, 32,283 attributed to IHD, 10,092 attributed to other vascular causes, and 60,797 attributed to nonvascular causes. Mortality during each decade of age at death was related to the estimated usual BP at the start of that decade. The relation between usual systolic and diastolic BP and the absolute risk for IHD mortality is shown in Figure 1-1. From ages 40 to 89, each increase of 20 mm Hg systolic BP or 10 mm Hg diastolic BP is associated with a twofold increase in mortality rates from IHD and more than a twofold increase in stroke mortality. These proportional differences in vascular mortality are about half as great in the 80 to 89 decade as it is in the 40 to 49 decade, but the annual absolute increases in risk are considerably greater in the elderly. As is evident from the straight lines in Figure 1-1, there is no evidence of a threshold wherein BP is not directly related to risk down to as low as 115/75 mm Hg.

As the authors conclude: "Not only do the present analyses confirm that there is a continuous relationship with risk throughout the normal range of usual blood pressure, but they demonstrate that within this range the usual blood pressure is even more strongly related to vascular mortality than had previously been supposed." They conclude that a 10 mm Hg higher than usual systolic BP or 5 mm Hg higher than usual diastolic BP would, in the long term, be associated with about a 40% higher risk of death from stroke and about a 30% higher risk of death from IHD.

These data clearly incriminate levels of BP below the level usually considered as indicative of

TABLE 1.2	Factors Involved in the Conceptual Definition of Hypertension	
Action	**Benefits**	**Risks and Costs**
Action	Reduce risk of CVD, debility, and death	Assume psychological burdens of "the hypertensive patient"
		Interfere with QOL
	Decrease monetary costs of catastrophic events	Require changes in lifestyle
		Add risks and side effects from therapy
		Add monetary costs of health care
Inaction	Preserve "nonpatient" role	
	Maintain current lifestyle and QOL	Increase risk of CVD, debility, and death
	Avoid risks and side effects of therapy	Increase monetary costs of catastrophic events
	Avoid monetary costs of health care	

hypertension, i.e., 140/90 mm Hg or higher. Data from the closely observed participants in the Framingham Heart Study confirm the increased risks of CVD with BP levels previously defined as *normal* (120 to 129/80 to 84 mm Hg) or *high-normal* (130 to 139/85 to 89 mm Hg) compared to those with *optimal* BP (<120/80 mm Hg) (Vasan et al., 2001) (Fig. 1-2). The data of Lewington et al. (2002) and Vasan et al. (2001) are the basis of a new classification of BP levels, as will be described later in this chapter.

A similar relation between the levels of BP and CVDs has been seen in 15 Asian Pacific countries, although the association is even stronger for stroke and somewhat less for coronary disease than seen in the western world (Martiniuk et al., 2007). Some of these differences in risk and BP levels can be explained by obvious factors such as socioeconomic differences and variable access to health care (Victor et al., 2008; Wilper et al., 2008).

Beyond the essential contribution of BP per se to cardiovascular risk, a number of other associations may influence the relationship.

Gender and Risk

Although some studies of women have shown that they tolerate hypertension better than do men and have lower coronary mortality rates with any level of hypertension (Barrett-Connor, 1997), the Prospective Studies Collaboration found the age-specific associations of IHD mortality with BP to be slightly greater for women than for men and concluded that "for vascular mortality as a whole, sex is of little relevance" (Lewington et al., 2002). In the United States, women have a higher prevalence

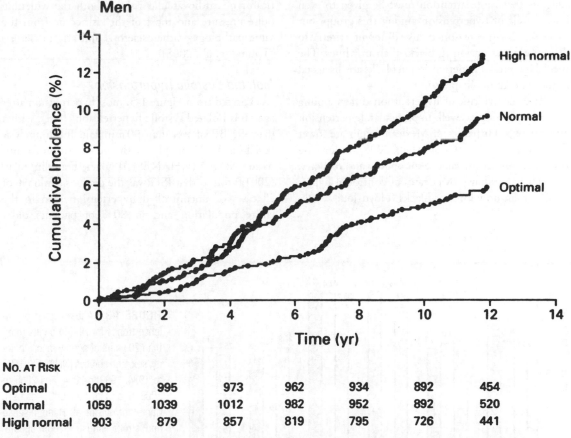

NO. AT RISK							
Optimal	1005	995	973	962	934	892	454
Normal	1059	1039	1012	982	952	892	520
High normal	903	879	857	819	795	726	441

FIGURE 1-2 The cumulative incidence of cardiovascular events in men enrolled in the Framingham Heart Study with initial BPs classified as optimal (below 120/80 mm Hg), normal (120 to 129/80 to 84 mm Hg), or high-normal (130 to 139/85 to 89 mm Hg) over a 12-year follow-up. (Modified from Vasan RS, Larson MG, Leip EP, et al. Impact of high-normal blood pressure on the risk of cardiovascular disease. *N Engl J Med* 2001;345:1291–1297.)

of uncontrolled hypertension than men (Ezzati et al., 2008).

Race and Risk

As shown in Figure 1-3, U.S. blacks tend to have higher rates of hypertension than do nonblacks (Lloyd-Jones et al., 2009), and overall hypertension-related mortality rates are higher among blacks (Hertz et al., 2005). In the Multiple Risk Factor Intervention Trial, which involved more than 23,000 black men and 325,000 white men who were followed up for 10 years, an interesting racial difference was confirmed: the mortality rate for coronary heart disease (CHD) was lower in black men with a diastolic pressure exceeding 90 mm Hg than in white men (relative risk, 0.84), but the mortality rate for cerebrovascular disease was higher (relative risk, 2.0) (Neaton et al., 1989).

The greater risk of hypertension among blacks suggests that more attention must be given to even lower levels of hypertension among this group, but there seems little reason to use different criteria to diagnose hypertension in blacks than in whites. The special features of hypertension in blacks are discussed in more detail in Chapter 4.

The relative risk of hypertension differs among other racial groups as well. In particular, hypertension rates in U.S. Hispanics of Mexican origin are lower than those in whites (Cutler et al., 2008). In keeping with their higher prevalence for obesity and diabetes, U.S. Hispanics have lower rates of control of hypertension than do whites or blacks (Lloyd-Jones et al., 2009).

Age and Risk: The Elderly

The number of people older than 65 years is rapidly increasing and, in fewer than 30 years, one of every five people in the United States will be over age 65. Systolic BP rises progressively with age (Lloyd-Jones et al., 2009) (Fig. 1-4), and elderly people with hypertension are at greater risk for CVD (Wong et al., 2007).

Pulse Pressure

As seen in Figure 1-5, systolic levels rise progressively with age, whereas diastolic levels typically start to fall beyond age 50 (Burt et al., 1995). Both of these changes reflect increased aortic stiffness and pulse-wave velocity with a more rapid return of the reflected pressure waves, as are described in more detail in Chapter 3. It therefore comes as no surprise that the progressively widening of pulse pressure is a prognosticator of cardiovascular risk, as both the widening pulse pressure and most of the risk come from the same pathology—atherosclerosis and arteriosclerosis (Thomas et al., 2008).

Isolated Systolic Hypertension

As expected from Figure 1-5, most hypertension after age 50 is isolated systolic hypertension (ISH), with a diastolic BP of less than 90 mm Hg. In an analysis based on the National Health and Nutrition Examination Survey (NHANES) III data, Franklin et al. (2001a) found that ISH was the diagnosis in 65% of all cases of uncontrolled hypertension seen in the entire population and in 80% of patients older

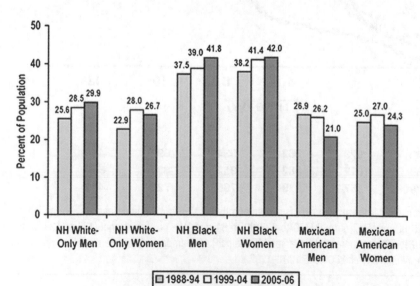

FIGURE 1-3 Age-adjusted prevalence trends for HBP in adults more than 20 years of age by race/ethnicity, sex, and surveys (NHANES: 1988 to 1994, 1999 to 2004, and 2005 to 2006). (From Lloyd-Jones D, Adams R, Carnethon M, et al. Heart disease and stroke statistics-2009 update: A report from the American Heart Association statistics committee and stroke statistics subcommittee. *Circulation* 2009;119:e21–e181, with permission.)

FIGURE 1-4 Prevalence of HBP in adults more than 20 years by age and sex (NHANES: 2005 to 2006). Adapted from NCHS and NHLBI. Hypertension is defined as SBP ≥ 140 mm Hg or DBP ≥ 90 mm Hg, taking antihypertensive medication, or being told twice by a physician or other professional that one has hypertension. (From Lloyd-Jones D, Adams R, Carnethon M, et al. Heart disease and stroke statistics-2009 update: A report from the American Heart Association statistics committee and stroke statistics subcommittee. *Circulation* 2009;119:e21–e181, with permission.)

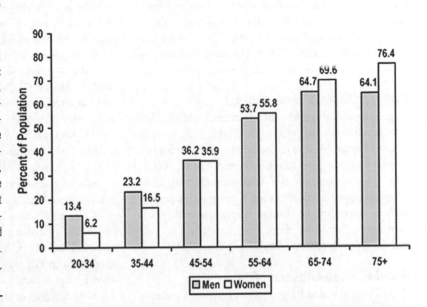

than 50. It should be noted that, unlike some reports that define ISH as a systolic BP of 160 mm Hg or greater, Franklin et al. (2001a) appropriately used 140 mm Hg or higher.

ISH is associated with increased morbidity and mortality from coronary disease and stroke in patients as old as 94 years (Lloyd-Jones et al., 2005). However, as older patients develop CVD and cardiac pump function deteriorates, systolic levels often fall and a U-shaped curve of cardiovascular mortality becomes obvious: Mortality increases both in those with systolic BP of less than 120 mm Hg and in those with

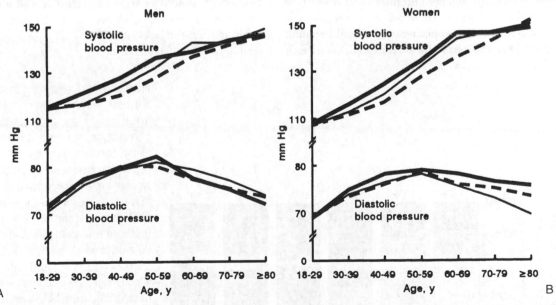

A   B

FIGURE 1-5 Mean systolic and diastolic BPs by age and race or ethnicity for men and women in the U.S. population 18 years of age or older. *Thick solid line*, non-Hispanic blacks; *dashed line*, non-Hispanic whites; *thin solid line*, Mexican Americans. Data from the NHANES III survey. (Modified from Burt VL, Whelton P, Roccella EJ, et al. Prevalence of hypertension in the U.S. adult population. Results from the Third National Health and Nutrition Examination Survey, 1988–1991. *Hypertension* 1995;25:305–313.)

systolic BP of more than 140 mm Hg. Similarly, mortality is higher in those 85 years of age or older if their systolic BP is lower than 140 mm Hg or their diastolic BP is lower than 70 mm Hg, both indicative of poor overall health (van Bemmel et al., 2006).

Isolated Diastolic Hypertension

In people under age 45, ISH is exceedingly rare but isolated diastolic hypertension (IDH), i.e., systolic below 140 mm Hg and diastolic 90 mm Hg or higher, may be found in 20% or more (Franklin et al., 2001a) (Fig. 1-6). Among the 346 such patients with IDH followed up for up to 32 years, no increase in cardiovascular mortality was found, whereas mortality was increased 2.7-fold in those with combined systolic and diastolic elevations (Strandberg et al., 2002).

Relative Versus Absolute Risk

The risks of elevated BP are often presented as relative to risks found with lower levels of BP. This way of looking at risk tends to exaggerate its degree, as is described in Chapter 5 where the benefits of therapy and the decision to treat are discussed. For now, a single example should suffice. As seen in Figure 1-7, when the associations among various levels of BP to the risk of having a stroke were examined in a total of 450,000 patients followed up for 5 to 30 years, there was a clear increase in stroke risk with increasing levels of diastolic BP (Prospective Studies Collaboration, 1995). In *relative* terms, the increase in risk was much

greater in the younger group (<45 years), going from 0.2 to 1.9, which is almost a 10-fold increase in relative risk compared to the less than twofold increase in the older group (10.0 to 18.4). But, it is obvious that the *absolute* risk is much greater in the elderly, with 8.4% (18.4 − 10.0) more having a stroke with the higher diastolic BP while only 1.7% (1.9 − 0.2) more of the younger were afflicted. The importance of this increased risk in the young with higher BP should not be ignored, but the use of the smaller change in absolute risk rather than the larger change in relative risk seems more appropriate when applying epidemiologic statistics to individual patients.

The distinction between the risks for the population and for the individual is important. For the population at large, risk clearly increases with every increment in BP, and levels of BP that are accompanied by significantly increased risks should be called *high*. As Stamler et al. (1993) note: "Among persons aged 35 years or more, most have BP above optimal (<120/<80 mm Hg); hence, they are at increased CVD risk, i.e., the BP problem involves most of the population, not only the substantial minority with clinical hypertension." However, for individual patients, the absolute risk from slightly elevated BP may be quite small. Therefore, more than just the level of BP should be used to determine risk and, even more importantly, to determine the need to institute therapy (Jackson, 2009). This issue is covered in detail in Chapter 5.

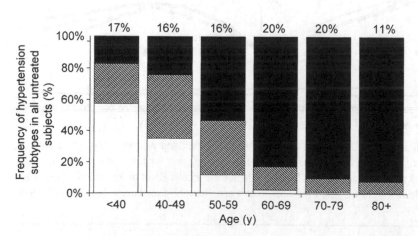

FIGURE 1-6 Frequency distribution of untreated hypertensive individuals by age and hypertension subtype. Numbers at the top of the bars represent the overall percentage distribution of all subtypes of untreated hypertension in that age group. Black bar = ISH (SBP 140 mm Hg and DBP ≥ 90 mm Hg); lined bar = SDH (SBP 140 mm Hg ≥ 90 mm Hg); open bar = IDH (SBP ≥ 140 mm Hg and DBP ≥ 90 mm Hg). (Reproduced from Franklin SS, Jacobs MJ, Wong ND, et al. Predominance of isolated systolic hypertension among middle-aged and elderly U.S. hypertensives. *Hypertension* 2001a;37: 869–874, with permission.)

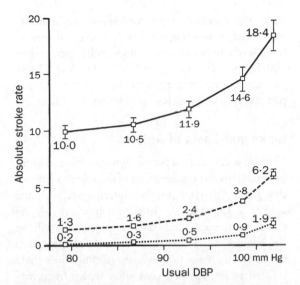

FIGURE 1-7 The absolute risks for stroke by age and usual diastolic BP in 45 prospective observational studies involving 450,000 individuals with 5 to 30 years of follow-up during which 13,397 participants had a stroke. *Dotted line,* less than 45 years old; *dashed line,* 45 to 65 years old; *solid line,* ≥65 years old. (Modified from Prospective Studies Collaboration. Cholesterol, diastolic blood pressure, and stroke: 13,000 strokes in 450,000 people in 45 prospective cohorts. *Lancet* 1995;346:1647–1653.)

Benefits of Action: Decreased Risk of CVD

We now turn to the major benefit listed in Table 1-2 that is involved in a conceptual definition of hypertension, the level at which it is possible to show the benefit of reducing CVD by lowering the BP. Inclusion of this factor is predicated on the assumption that it is of no benefit—and, as we shall see, is potentially harmful—to label a person hypertensive if nothing will be done to lower the BP.

Natural Versus Treatment-Induced BP

Before proceeding, one caveat is in order. As noted earlier, less CVD is seen in people with low BP, who are not receiving antihypertensive therapy. However, that fact cannot be used as evidence to support the benefits of therapy, because naturally low BP may offer a degree of protection not provided by a similarly low BP resulting from antihypertensive therapy (Asayama et al., 2009).

The available evidence supports that view: Morbidity and mortality rates, particularly those of coronary disease, continue to be higher in many patients at relatively low risk who are undergoing antihypertensive drug treatment than in untreated people with similar levels of BP. This has been shown for coronary disease in follow-up studies of multiple populations (Andersson et al., 1998; Clausen & Jensen, 1992; Thürmer et al., 1994) and in Japanese for strokes (Asayama et al., 2009). This issue, too, will be covered in more detail in Chapter 5, but one piece of the evidence will be acknowledged here.

An analysis of all-cause and cardiovascular mortality observed in seven randomized trials of middle-aged patients with diastolic BP from 90 to 114 mm Hg showed a reduction in mortality in the treated half in those trials wherein the population was at fairly high risk, as defined by an all-cause mortality rate of greater than 6 per 1,000 person-years in the untreated population (Hoes et al., 1995). However, in those studies involving patients who started at a lower degree of risk, those who were treated had *higher* mortality rates than were seen in the untreated groups.

These disquieting data should not be taken as evidence against the use of antihypertensive drug therapy. They do not, in any way, deny that protection against cardiovascular complications can be achieved by successful reduction of BP with drugs in patients at risk. They simply indicate that the protection may not be universal or uniform for one or more reasons, including the following: (i) only a partial reduction of BP may be achieved; (ii) irreversible hypertensive damage may be present; (iii) other risk factors that accompany hypertension may not be improved; and (iv) there are dangers inherent to the use of some drugs, in particular the high doses of diuretics used in the earlier trials covered by Hoes et al. (1995). Whatever the explanation, these data document a difference between the natural and the induced levels of BP.

In contrast to these data, considerable experimental, epidemiologic, and clinical evidences indicate that reducing elevated BP is beneficial, particularly in high-risk patients (Blood Pressure Trialists, 2008).

Rationale for Reducing Elevated BP

Table 1-3 presents the rationale for lowering elevated BP. The reduction in CVD and death (listed last in the table) has been measured to determine the BP level at which a benefit is derived from antihypertensive therapy. That level can be used as part of the operational definition of hypertension.

During the past 40 years, controlled therapeutic trials have included patients with diastolic BP levels

TABLE 1.3	Rationale for the Reduction of Elevated BP

1. Morbidity and mortality as a result of CVDs are directly related to the level of BP

2. BP rises most in those whose pressures are already high

3. In humans, there is less vascular damage where the BP is lower: beneath a coarctation, beyond a renovascular stenosis, and in the pulmonary circulation

4. In animal experiments, lowering the BP has been shown to protect the vascular system

5. Antihypertensive therapy reduces CVD and death

as low as 90 mm Hg. Detailed analyses of these trials are presented in Chapter 5. For now, it is enough to say that there is no question that protection against CVD has been documented for reduction of diastolic BP levels that start at or above 95 mm Hg, but there is continued disagreement about whether protection has been shown for those whose diastolic BP starts at or above 90 mm Hg who are otherwise at low risk. Similarly, protection for the elderly with ISH has been documented with a systolic BP ≥ 160 mm Hg or higher, but there are no data for the large elderly population between 140 and 160 mm Hg. Therefore, expert committees have disagreed about the minimum level of BP at which drug treatment should begin.

In particular, the British guidelines (Williams et al., 2004) are more conservative than those from the United States (Chobanian et al., 2003). Whereas the U.S. guidelines recommend drug therapy for all with sustained BP above 140/90 mm Hg, the British use 160/100 mm Hg as the level mandating drug therapy with the decision to be individualized for those with levels of 140 to 159/90 to 99 mm Hg.

These disagreements have highlighted the need to consider more than the level of BP in making that decision. As will be noted in Chapter 5, the consideration of other risk factors, target organ damage, and symptomatic CVD allows a more rational decision to be made about whom to treat.

Prevention of Progression of Hypertension

Another benefit of action is the prevention of progression of hypertension, which should be looked on as a surrogate for reducing the risk of CVD. Evidence of that benefit is strong, based on data from multiple, randomized, placebo-controlled clinical trials. In such

trials, the number of patients whose hypertension progressed from their initially less severe degree to more severe hypertension, defined as BP greater than 200/110 mm Hg, increased from only 95 of 13,389 patients on active treatment to 1,493 of 13,342 patients on placebo (Moser & Hebert, 1996).

Risks and Costs of Action

The decision to label a person hypertensive and begin treatment involves assumption of the role of a patient, changes in lifestyle, possible interference with the quality of life (QOL), risks from biochemical side effects of therapy, and financial costs. As will be emphasized in the next chapter, the diagnosis should not be based on one or only a few readings since there is often an initial white-coat effect which frequently dissipates after a few weeks, particularly when readings are taken out of the office.

Assumption of the Role of a Patient and Worsening QOL

Merely labeling a person hypertensive may cause negative effects as well as enough sympathetic nervous system activity to change hemodynamic measurements (Rostrup et al., 1991). People who know they are hypertensive may have considerable anxiety over the diagnosis of "the silent killer" and experience multiple symptoms as a consequence (Kaplan, 1997). The adverse effects of labeling were identified in an analysis of health-related QOL measures in hypertensives who participated in the 2001–2004 NHANES (Hayes et al., 2008). Those who knew they were hypertensive had significantly poorer QOL measures than did those who were hypertensive with similar levels of BP but were unaware of their condition. QOL measures did not differ by the status of hypertension control. Fortunately, hypertensive people who receive appropriate counseling and comply with modern-day therapy usually have no impairment and may have improvements in overall QOL measures (Degl'Innocenti et al., 2004; Grimm et al., 1997).

Risks from Biochemical Side Effects of Therapy

Biochemical risks are less likely to be perceived by the patient than the interferences with QOL, but they may actually be more hazardous. These risks are discussed in detail in Chapter 7. For now, only two will be mentioned: Hypokalemia, which develops in 5% to 20% of diuretic-treated patients, and elevations in blood triglyceride and glucose levels, which may accompany the use of β-blockers.

Overview of Risks and Benefits

Obviously, many issues are involved in determining the level of BP that poses enough risk to mandate the diagnosis of hypertension and to call for therapy, despite the potential risks that appropriate therapy entails. An analysis of issues relating to risk factor intervention by Brett (1984) clearly defines the problem:

> Risk factor intervention is usually undertaken in the hope of long-term gain in survival or quality of life. Unfortunately, there are sometimes trade-offs (such as inconvenience, expense, or side effects), and something immediate must be sacrificed. This tension between benefits and liabilities is not necessarily resolved by appealing to statements of medical fact, and it is highlighted by the fact that many persons at risk are asymptomatic. Particularly when proposing drug therapy, the physician cannot make an asymptomatic person feel any better, but might make him feel worse, since most drugs have some incidence of adverse effects. But how should side effects be quantitated on a balance sheet of net drug benefit? If a successful antihypertensive drug causes impotence in a patient, how many months or years of potentially increased survival make the side effect acceptable? There is obviously no dogmatic answer; accordingly, global statements such as "all patients with asymptomatic mild hypertension should be treated" are inappropriate, even if treatment were clearly shown to lower morbidity or mortality rates.

On the other hand, as noted in Figures 1-1 and 1-2, the risks related to BP are directly related to the level, progressively increasing with every increment of BP. Therefore, the argument has been made that, with currently available antihypertensive drugs, which have few, if any, side effects, therapy should be provided even at BP levels lower than 140/90 mm Hg to prevent both the progression of BP and target organ damages that occur at "high-normal" levels (Julius, 2000). Dr. Julius and coworkers have conducted a controlled trial of placebo versus active drug therapy in such patients to prove the principle that drug therapy can prevent or at least delay progression (Julius et al., 2006).

An even more audacious approach toward the prevention of cardiovascular consequences of hypertension has been proposed by the English epidemiologists Wald and Law (2003) and Law et al. (2009).

They recommend a "Polypill" composed of low doses of a statin, a diuretic, an ACEI, a β-blocker, folic acid (subsequently deleted), and aspirin to be given to all people from age 55 on and everyone with existing CVD, regardless of pretreatment levels of cholesterol or BP. Wald and Law concluded that the use of the Polypill in this manner would reduce IHD events by 88% and stroke by 80%, with one third of people benefiting and gaining an average 11 years of life free from IHD or stroke. They estimated side effects in 8% to 15% of people, depending on the exact formulation. In their more recent analysis, the use of their currently devised Polypill would provide a 46% reduction in CHD and a 62% reduction in stroke (Law et al., 2009).

The ability to reduce CVD in developing societies depends, in large part, on the costs of therapy (Lim et al., 2007). A polypill with generic components would meet this need. A pilot trial with such a polypill has been performed (Indian Polycap Study, 2009). The risk reductions from the observed effects of the Polycap were estimated to be a 62% reduction in CHD and 48% reduction in strokes. These effects were seen after only 12 weeks; greater benefits might be seen over a longer duration of therapy. Therapy with the Polycap was discontinued by 16% and a variety of side effects were seen in 3% to 9% of the subjects.

Both the investigators and a commentator (Cannon, 2009) call for additional, larger scale trials with hard end-points. Cannon (2009) predicts that it may be possible to "vastly broaden the number of patients who might benefit from drugs that have been proven in multiple trials to reduce cardiovascular disease and mortality." The adoption of such an inexpensive therapy will have to overcome numerous obstacles, not the least of which would be the billions of dollars that the pharmaceutical companies with patent-protected antihypertensive drugs will use to persuade the public, the FDA, and Congress that this shall not come to pass.

OPERATIONAL DEFINITIONS OF HYPERTENSION

Seventh Joint National Committee Criteria

In recognition of the data shown in Figures 1-1 and 1-2, the Seventh Joint National Committee report

TABLE 1.4	Changes in Blood Pressure Classification	
JNC 6 Category	**SBP/DBP**	**JNC 7 Category**
Optimal	<120/80	Normal
Normal	120–129/80–84	Prehypertension
Borderline	130–139/85–89	Prehypertension
Hypertension	≥140/90	Hypertension
Stage 1	140–159/90–99	Stage 1
Stage 2	160–179/100–109	Stage 2
Stage 3	≥180/110	Stage 2

The sixth report of the Joint National Committee on Prevention, Detection, Evaluation, and Treatment of high Blood Pressure. *Arch Intern Med* 1997;157:2413–246; The seventh report of the Joint National Committe on Prevention, Detection, Evaluation, and Treatment of High Blood Pressure. *JAMA* 2003;289:2560–2571.

(JNC-7) has introduced a new classification—prehypertension—for those whose BPs range from 120 to 139 mm Hg systolic and/or 80 to 89 mm Hg diastolic, as opposed to the JNC-6 classification of such levels as "normal" and "high-normal" (Chobanian et al., 2003) (Table 1.4). In addition, the former stages 2 and 3 have been combined into a single stage 2 category, since management of all patients with BP above 160/100 mm Hg is similar.

Classification of BP

Prehypertension

The JNC-7 report (Chobanian et al., 2003) states

> Prehypertension is not a disease category. Rather it is a designation chosen to identify individuals at high risk of developing hypertension, so that both patients and clinicians are alerted to this risk and encouraged to intervene and prevent or delay the disease from developing. Individuals who are prehypertensive are not candidates for drug therapy on the basis of their level of BP and should be firmly and unambiguously advised to practice lifestyle modification in order to reduce their risk of developing hypertension in the future.... Moreover, individuals with prehypertension who also have diabetes or kidney disease should be considered candidates for appropriate drug therapy if a trial of lifestyle modification fails to reduce their BP to 130/80 mm Hg or less.... The goal for individuals with prehypertension and no compelling indications is to lower BP to normal with lifestyle changes and prevent the progressive rise in BP using the recommended lifestyle modifications.

The guidelines from the European (Task Force, 2007), World Health Organization-International Society of Hypertension (WHO-ISH Writing Group, 2003), the British Hypertension Society (Williams et al., 2004), and the Latin American committee (Sanchez et al., 2009) continue to classify BP below 140/90 mm Hg, as did JNC-6, into normal and high-normal. However, the JNC-7 classification seems appropriate, recognizing the significantly increased risk for patients with above-optimal levels. Since for every increase in BP by 20/10 mm Hg the risk of CVD doubles, a level of 135/85 mm Hg, with a double degree of risk, is better called prehypertension than high-normal.

Not surprisingly, considering the bell-shaped curve of BP in the U.S. adult population (Fig. 1-8), the number of people with prehypertension is even greater than those with hypertension, 37% versus 29% of the adult population (Lloyd-Jones et al., 2009).

It should be remembered that—despite an unequivocal call for health-promoting lifestyle modifications and no antihypertensive drug for such prehypertensives (unless they have a compelling indication such as diabetes or renal insufficiency)—the labeling of prehypertension could cause anxiety and lead to the premature use of drugs which have not yet been shown to be protective at such low levels of elevated BP. Americans are pill happy and their doctors often acquiesce to their requests even when they

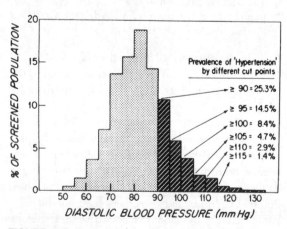

FIGURE 1-8 Frequency distribution of diastolic BP measured at home screening (*n* = 158,906, aged 30 to 69 years). (Reprinted from Hypertension Detection and Follow-up *Program* Cooperative Group. The hypertension Detection and Follow-up Program. A progress report. *Circ Res* 1977;40(Suppl. 1):I106–I109, with permission.)

know better. So, time will tell: Are Americans too quick or is the rest of the world too slow?

Systolic Hypertension in the Elderly

In view of the previously noted risks of isolated systolic elevations, JNC-7 recommends that, in the presence of a diastolic BP of less than 90 mm Hg, a systolic BP level of 140 mm Hg or higher is classified as ISH. Although risks of such elevations of systolic BP in the elderly have been clearly identified (Franklin et al., 2001b), the value of therapy to reduce systolic levels that are between 140 and 160 mm Hg in the elderly has not been well documented.

Hypertension in Children

For children, JNC-7 uses the definition from the *Report of the Second Task Force on Blood Pressure Control in Children* (National High Blood Pressure, 1996), which identifies *significant hypertension* as BP persistently equal to or greater than the ninety-fifth percentile for age and height and *severe hypertension* as BP persistently equal to or greater than the ninety-ninth percentile for age and height. Hypertension in children is covered in Chapter 16, wherein more recent guidelines are provided.

Labile Hypertension

As ambulatory readings have been recorded, the marked variability in virtually everyone's BP has become obvious (see Chapter 2). In view of the usual variability of BP, the term *labile* is neither useful nor meaningful.

Borderline Hypertension

The term *borderline* may be used to describe hypertension in which the BP only occasionally rises above 140/90 mm Hg. Persistently elevated BP is more likely to develop in such people than in those with consistently normal readings. However, this progression is by no means certain. In one study of a particularly fit, low-risk group of air cadets with borderline pressures, only 12% developed sustained hypertension over the subsequent 20 years (Madsen & Buch, 1971). Nonetheless, people with borderline pressures tend to have hemodynamic changes indicative of early hypertension and greater degrees of other cardiovascular risk factors, including greater body weight, dyslipidemia, and higher plasma insulin levels (Julius et al., 1990), and should, therefore, be followed up more closely and advised to modify their lifestyle.

PREVALENCE OF HYPERTENSION

As previously noted, the prevalence of hypertension is increasing worldwide, in developed countries because of increasing longevity with its burden of systolic hypertension and in developing countries because of increasing obesity related to urbanization.

Prevalence in the U.S. Adult Population

The best sources of data for the U.S. population are the previously noted NHANES surveys, which examine a large representative sample of the U.S. adult population aged 18 and older.

The presence of hypertension has been defined in the NHANES as having a measured systolic BP of 140 mm Hg or higher, a measured diastolic BP of 90 mm Hg or higher, or taking antihypertensive drug therapy. In the latest NHANES data, the mean of three BP readings taken in the clinic was used. Analysis of the 1999–2004 data shows a definite increase in the prevalence of hypertension in the United States to a total of 28.9%. As seen in Figure 1-4, the prevalence rises in both genders with age, more so in older women than older men. As seen in Figure 1-3, the prevalence among U.S. blacks is higher than in whites and Mexican Americans in both genders and at all ages. Compared to their proportion of the total population, U.S. whites constitute the same proportion of the hypertensive population whereas U.S. blacks constitute 21.2% more and Mexican Americans 33.8% less than expected (Fields et al., 2004). Part of the lower overall rates in Mexican Americans reflects their younger average age. With age adjustment, Mexican Americans had prevalence rates similar to U.S. whites.

These increases in prevalence over the past 10 years are attributed to a number of factors, including:

- An increased number of hypertensives who live longer as a result of improved lifestyles or more effective drug therapy.
- The increased number of older people: 81% of all U.S. hypertensive adults are 45 years of age or older, though this group constituted only 46% of the U.S. population (Fields et al., 2004).
- The increase in obesity; Hajjar and Kotchen (2003) calculate that more than half of the increased prevalence can be attributed to the increase in body mass index (BMI).

• An increased rate of new-onset hypertension not attributable to older age or obesity; the prevalence rates increased in all groups except those aged 18 to 29.

Populations Outside the United States

In national surveys performed in the 1990s using similar sampling and reporting techniques, significantly higher prevalences of hypertension were noted in six European countries (England, Finland, Germany, Italy, Spain, and Sweden) compared to the United States and Canada (Wolf-Maier et al., 2003). The age- and sex-adjusted prevalence of hypertension was 28% in the United States and Canada and 44% in the six European countries. The overall 60% higher prevalence of hypertension was closely correlated with stroke mortalities in the various countries, adding to the validity of the findings.

Rather marked differences in the prevalence of hypertension among similar populations that cannot be easily explained have also been noted. For example, Shaper et al. (1988) reported a threefold variation among 7,735 middle-aged men in 24 towns throughout Great Britain, with higher rates in northern England and Scotland. Some of the variation could be explained by such obvious factors as body weight or alcohol and sodium and potassium intake, but most of the variation remains unexplained (Bruce et al., 1993).

Equally striking are the major differences in mortality due to coronary disease as related to levels of BP in various countries (van den Hoogen et al., 2000). Rates of CHD mortality at any level of BP were more than three times higher in the United States and northern Europe than in Japan and southern Europe; however, the relative increase in CHD mortality for a given increase in BP is similar in all countries.

INCIDENCE OF HYPERTENSION

Much less is known about the incidence of newly developed hypertension than about its prevalence. The Framingham study provides one database (Parikh et al., 2008) and the National Health Epidemiologic Follow-up Study another (Cornoni-Huntley et al., 1989). In the latter study, 14,407 participants in NHANES I (1971 to 1975) were followed up for an average of 9.5 years. The incidence of hypertension in white men and women had about a 5% increase for each 10-year interval of age at baseline from age 25 to 64. The incidence among blacks was at least twice that among whites.

As seen in Figure 1-9, the incidence of hypertension in the Framingham cohort over 4 years was directly related to the prior level of BP, BMI, smoking, and hypertension in both parents (Parikh et al., 2008).

CAUSES OF HYPERTENSION

The list of causes of hypertension (Table 1-5) is quite long; however, the cause of about 90% of the cases of

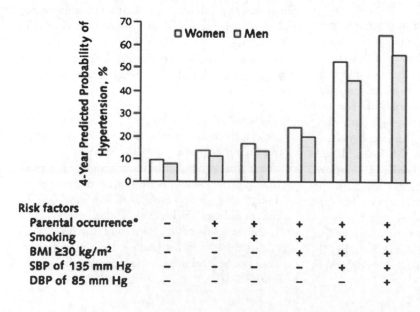

FIGURE 1-9 BP was 120/80 mm Hg, unless otherwise indicated. Plus and minus signs below the graph indicate the presence or absence of risk factors. *Both parents with hypertension. BMI, body mass index; DBP, diastolic blood pressure; SBP, systolic blood pressure. (Reproduced from Parikh NI, Pencina MJ, Wang TJ, et al. A risk score for predicting near-term incidence of hypertension: The Framingham Heart Study. *Ann Intern Med* 2008;148:102–110, with permission.)

hypertension is unknown, i.e., primary or essential. The proportion of cases secondary to some identifiable mechanism has been debated considerably, as more specific causes have been recognized. Claims that one cause or another is responsible for up to 20% of all cases of hypertension repeatedly appear from investigators who are particularly interested in a certain category of hypertension, and therefore see only a highly selected population.

Older data from surveys of various populations are available which report that more than 90% of patients had no discernable cause (Sinclair et al., 1987). However, improved diagnostic procedures are now available that almost certainly would increase the frequency of various identifiable (secondary) forms than those uncovered in these older surveys. In truth, the frequency of various forms in an otherwise unselected population of hypertensives is unknown.

TABLE 1.5 Types and Causes of Hypertension

Systolic and Diastolic Hypertension	Foods Containing Tyramine and Monoamine Oxidase Inhibitors
Primary, essential, or idiopathic	Coarctation of the aorta and aortitis
Identifiable causes	Pregnancy-induced
Renal	Neurological disorders
Renal parenchymal disease	Increased intracranial pressure
Acute glomerulonephritis	Central sleep apnea
Chronic nephritis	Quadriplegia
Polycystic disease	Acute porphyria
Diabetic nephropathy	Familial dysautonomia
Hydronephrosis	Lead poisoning
Renovascular disease	Guillain-Barré syndrome
Renal artery stenosis	Acute stress (including surgery)
Other causes of renal ischemia	Psychogenic hyperventilation
Renin-producing tumors	Hypoglycemia
Renoprival	Burns
Primary sodium retention: Liddle syndrome,	Alcohol withdrawal
Gordon syndrome	Sickle cell crisis
Endocrine	After resuscitation
Acromegaly	Perioperative
Hypothyroidism	Increased intravascular volume
Hyperthyroidism	Alcohol
Hypercalcemia (hyperparathyroidism)	Nicotine
Adrenal disorders	Cyclosporine, tacrolimus
Cortical disorders	Other agents (see Table 15-5)
Cushing syndrome	
Primary aldosteronism	**Systolic hypertension**
Congenital adrenal hyperplasia	Arterial rigidity
Medullary tumors: pheochromocytoma	Increased cardiac output
Extra-adrenal chromaffin tumors	Aortic valvular insufficiency
11-β-hydroxysteroid Dehydrogenase	Arteriovenous fistula, patent ductus
Deficiency or Inhibition (Licorice)	Thyrotoxicosis
Carcinoids	Paget disease of bone
Exogenous hormones	Beriberi
Estrogen	
Glucocorticoids	
Mineralocorticoids	
Sympathomimetics	
Erythropoietin	

POPULATION RISK FROM HYPERTENSION

Now that the definition of hypertension and its classification have been provided, along with various estimates of its prevalence, the impact of hypertension on the population at large can be considered. As noted, for the individual patient, the higher the level of BP, the greater the risk of morbidity and mortality. However, for the population at large, the greatest burden from hypertension occurs among people with only minimally elevated pressures, because there are so many of them. This burden can be seen in Figure 1-10, where 12-year cardiovascular mortality rates observed with each increment of BP are plotted against the distribution of the various levels of BP among the 350,000 35- to 57-year-old men screened for the Multiple Risk Factor Intervention Trial (National High Blood Pressure, 1993). Although the mortality rates climb progressively, most deaths occur in the much larger proportion of the population with minimally elevated pressures. By multiplying the percentage of men at any given level of BP by the relative risk for that level, it can be seen that more cardiovascular

mortality will occur in those with a diastolic BP of 80 to 84 mm Hg than among those with a diastolic BP of 95 mm Hg or greater.

Strategy for the Population

This disproportionate risk for the population at large from relatively mild hypertension bears strongly on the question of how to achieve the greatest reduction in the risks of hypertension. In the past, most effort has been directed at the group with the highest levels of BP. However, this "high-risk" strategy, as effective as it may be for those affected, does little to reduce total morbidity and mortality if the "low-risk" patients, who make up the largest share of the population at risk, are ignored (Rose, 1985).

Many more people with mild hypertension are now being treated actively and intensively with antihypertensive drugs. However, as emphasized by Rose (1992), a more effective strategy would be to lower the BP level of the entire population, as might be accomplished by reduction of sodium intake. Rose estimated that lowering the entire distribution of BP by only 2 to 3 mm Hg would be as effective in reducing

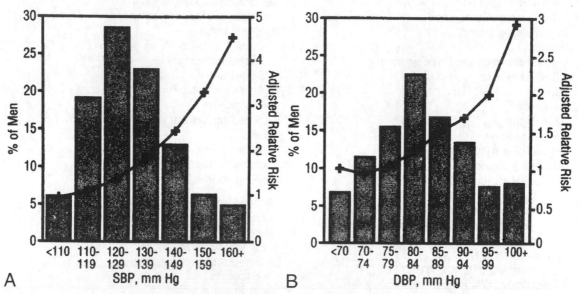

FIGURE 1-10   A: Percentage distribution of SBP for men screened for the MRFIT who were 35 to 57 years old and had no history of myocardial infarction (n = 347,978) (*bars*) and corresponding 12-year rates of cardiovascular mortality by SBP level adjusted for age, race, total serum cholesterol level, cigarettes smoked per day, reported use of medication for diabetes mellitus, and imputed household income (using census tract for residence) (*curve*). **B:** Same as part (**A**), showing the distribution of DBP (n = 356,222). (Modified from National High Blood Pressure Education Program Working Group. *Arch Intern Med* 1993;153:186–208.)

the overall risks of hypertension as prescribing current antihypertensive drug therapy for all people with definite hypertension.

This issue is eloquently addressed by Stamler (1998):

> The high-risk strategy of the last 25 years—involving detection, evaluation, and treatment (usually including drug therapy) of tens of millions of people with already established high BP—useful as it has been, has serious limitations: It is late, defensive, mainly reactive, time-consuming, associated with adverse effects (inevitable with drugs, however favorable the mix of benefit and risk), costly, only partially successful, and endless. It offers no possibility of ending the high BP epidemic.

> However, present knowledge enables pursuit of the additional goal of the primary prevention of high BP, the solution to the high BP epidemic. For decades, extensive concordant evidence has been amassed by all research disciplines showing that high salt intake, obesity, excess alcohol intake, inadequate potassium intake, and sedentary lifestyle all have adverse effects on population BP levels. This evidence is the solid scientific foundation for the expansion in the strategy to attempt primary prevention of high BP by improving lifestyles across entire populations.

PREVENTION

The broader approach is almost certainly correct on epidemiologic grounds. However, the needed changes in lifestyle cannot be achieved on an individual basis (Woolf, 2008). They require broad, societal changes. Health care providers can play a role, as described in Chapter 7. But the main tasks must be assumed by others, including:

• City planners to provide sidewalks and bicycle paths.
• School administrators to require physical activity in school time and to get rid of soft drinks and candy bars.
• Food processors and marketers to quit preparing and pushing high calorie, high fat, high salt products.
• Television programmers to quit assaulting young children with unhealthy choices.
• Parents to take responsibility for their children's welfare.
• Adults to forgo instant pleasures (Krispy Crèmes) for future benefits.

• Society to protect immature young adults—old enough to die in Iraq—who will surely continue to smoke, drink, and have unprotected sex. Ways to help include enforcing selling restrictions on cigarettes and alcohol, providing chaperones at student drinking parties, ensuring availability of condoms and morning-after pills. Adults may not like what hot-blooded young people do but "just saying no" is not enough.

Until (and if) such nirvana arrives, it may take active drug therapies, either in the slow, measured approach being taken by Julius et al. (2006) or the broad, unmeasured use of a Polypill as advocated by Yusuf (2002) and formulated by Wald and Law (2003) and Law et al. (2009). However it may be accomplished, we need to keep the goal of prevention in mind as we consider the overall problems of hypertension for the individual patient in the ensuing chapters.

REFERENCES

Andersson OK, Almgren T, Persson B, et al. Survival of treated hypertension. *Br Med J* 1998;317:167–171.

Anonymous. Rise and fall of diseases [Editorial]. *Lancet* 1993;341: 151–152.

Asayama K, Ohkubo T, Yoshida S, et al. Stroke risk and antihypertensive drug treatment in the general population: The Japan arteriosclerosis longitudinal study. *J Hypertens* 2009;27: 357–364.

Barrett-Connor E. Sex differences in coronary heart disease. *Circulation* 1997;95:252–264.

Blood Pressure Lowering Treatment Trialists' Collaboration. Effects of different regimens to lower blood pressure on major cardiovascular events in older and younger adults: Meta-analysis of randomised trials. *Br Med J* 2008;336:1121–1123.

Brett AS. Ethical issues in risk factor intervention. *Am J Med* 1984; 76:557–561.

Bruce NG, Wannamethee G, Shaper AG. Lifestyle factors associated with geographic blood pressure variations among men and women in the UK. *J Hum Hypertens* 1993;7:229–238.

Burt VL, Whelton P, Roccella EJ, et al. Prevalence of hypertension in the US adult population. Results from the Third National Health and Nutrition Examination Survey, 1988–91. *Hypertension* 1995;25:305–313.

Cannon CP. Can the polypill save the world from heart disease? *Lancet* 2009;373:1313–1314.

Chobanian AV, Bakris GL, Black HR, et al. Seventh report of the Joint National Committee on the Prevention, Detection, Evaluation, and Treatment of High Blood Pressure. *Hypertension* 2003;42:1206–1252.

Clausen J, Jensen G. Blood pressure and mortality: And epidemiological survey with 10 years follow-up. *J Hum Hypertens* 1992; 6:53–59.

Cornoni-Huntley J, LaCroix AZ, Havlik RJ. Race and sex differentials in the impact of hypertension in the United States. *Arch Intern Med* 1989;149:780–788.

Cutler JA, Sorlie PD, Wolz M, et al. Trends in hypertension prevalence, awareness, treatment, and control rates in United States adults between 1988–1994 and 1999–2004. *Hypertension* 2008;52:818–827.

Danaei G, Ding EL, Mozaffarian D, et al. The preventable cause of death in the United States: Comparative risk assessment of dietary, lifestyle, and metabolic risk factors. *PLOS Medicine* 2009;6:e1000058.

Degl'Innocenti A, Elmfeldt D, Hofman A, et al. Health-related quality of life during treatment of elderly patients with hypertension: Results from the Study on Cognition and Prognosis in the Elderly (SCOPE). *J Hum Hypertens* 2004;18: 239–245.

Dorjgochoo T, Shu XO, Zhang X, et al. Relation of blood pressure components and categories and all-cause, stroke and coronary heart disease mortality in urban Chinese women: A population-based prospective study. *Hypertension* 2009;27(3): 468–475.

Ezzati M, Oza S, Danaei G, et al. Trends and cardiovascular mortality effects of state-level blood pressure and uncontrolled hypertension in the United States. *Circulation* 2008;117: 905–914.

Falaschetti E, Chaudhury M, Mindell J, et al. Continued improvement in hypertension management in England: Results from the Health Survey for England 2006. *Hypertension* 2009;53: 480–486.

Fields LE, Burt VL, Cutler JA, et al. The burden of adult hypertension in the United States 1999 to 2000: A rising tide. *Hypertension* 2004;44:398–404.

Ford ES, Ajani UA, Croft JB, et al. Explaining the decrease in U.S. deaths from coronary disease, 1980–2000. *N Engl J Med* 2007; 356:2388–2398.

Franklin SS, Jacobs MJ, Wong ND, et al. Predominance of isolated systolic hypertension among middle-aged and elderly U.S. hypertensives. *Hypertension* 2001a;37:869–874.

Franklin SS, Larson MG, Khan SA, et al. Does the relation of blood pressure to coronary heart disease change with aging? *Circulation* 2001b;103:1245–1249.

Grimm RH Jr, Grandits GA, Cutler JA, et al. Relationships of quality-of-life measures to long-term lifestyle and drug treatment in the Treatment of Mild Hypertension Study. *Arch Intern Med* 1997;157:638–648.

Hajjar I, Kotchen TA. Trends in prevalence, awareness, treatment, and control of hypertension in the United States, 1988–1990. *JAMA* 2003;290:199–206.

Hayes DK, Denny CH, Keenan NL, et al. Health-related quality of life and hypertension status, awareness, treatment, and control: National Health and Nutrition Examination Survey, 2001–2004. *J Hypertens* 2008;26:641–647.

Hedley AA, Ogden CL, Johnson CL, et al. Prevalence of overweight and obesity among US children, adolescents, and adults, 1999–2002. *JAMA* 2004;291:2847–2850.

Hertz RP, Unger AN, Cornell JA, et al. Racial disparities in hypertension prevalence, awareness, and management. *Arch Intern Med* 2005;165:2098–2104.

Hoes AW, Grobbee DE, Lubsen J. Does drug treatment improve survival? Reconciling the trials in mild-to-moderate hypertension. *J Hypertens* 1995;13:805–811.

Indian Polycap Study (TIPS). Effects of polypill (Polycap) on risk factors in middle-aged individuals without cardiovascular disease (TIPS): A phase II, double-blind, randomized trial. *Lancet* 2009;373:1341–1351.

Jackson R. Attributing risk to hypertension: What does it mean? *Am J Hypertens.* 2009;22(3):237–238.

Julius S. Trials of antihypertensive treatment. *Am J Hypertens* 2000;13:11S–17S.

Julius S, Jamerson K, Mejia A, et al. The association of borderline hypertension with target organ changes and higher coronary risk. *JAMA* 1990;264:354–358.

Julius S, Nesbitt SD, Egan BM, et al. Feasibility of treating prehypertension with an angiotensin-receptor blocker. *N Engl J Med* 2006;354:1685–1697.

Kaplan NM. Anxiety-induced hyperventilation. *Arch Intern Med* 1997;157:945–948.

Kotseva K, Wood D, De BG, et al. Cardiovascular prevention guidelines in daily practice: A comparison of EUROASPIRE I, II, and III surveys in eight European countries. *Lancet* 2009; 373:929–940.

Kronborg CN, Hallas J, Jacobsen IA. Prevalence, awareness, and control of arterial hypertension Denmark. *J Am Soc Hypertens* 2009;3(1):19–24.

Law MR, Morris JK, Wald NJ. Use of blood pressure lowering drugs in the prevention of cardiovascular disease: Meta-analysis of 147 randomized trials in the context of expectations from prospective epidemiological studies. *Br Med J* 2009;338: b1665.

Lawes CM, Hoorn SV, Rodgers A. Global burden of blood-pressure-related disease, 2001. *Lancet* 2008;371:1513–1518.

Lewington S, Clarke R, Qizilbash N, et al. Age-specific relevance of usual blood pressure to vascular mortality: A meta-analysis of individual data for one million adults in 61 prospective studies. *Lancet* 2002;360:1903–1913.

Lim SS, Gaziano TA, Gakidou E, et al. Prevention of cardiovascular disease in high-risk individuals in low-income and middle-income countries: Health effects and costs. *Lancet* 2007;370: 2054–2062.

Lloyd-Jones D, Adams R, Carnethon M, et al. Heart disease and stroke statistics-2009 update: A report from the American Heart Association statistics committee and stroke statistics subcommittee. *Circulation* 2009;119:e21–e181.

Lloyd-Jones DM, Evans JC, Levy D. Hypertension in adults across the age spectrum: Current outcomes and control in the community. *JAMA* 2005;294:466–472.

Madsen RER, Buch J. Long-term prognosis of transient hypertension in young male adults. *Aerospace Med* 1971;42: 752–755.

Martiniuk AL, Lee CM, Lawes CM, et al. Hypertension: Its prevalence and population-attributable fraction for mortality from cardiovascular disease in the Asia-Pacific region. *J Hypertens* 2007;25:73–79.

McWilliams JM, Meara E, Zaslavsky AM, et al. Differences in control of cardiovascular disease and diabetes by race, ethnicity, and education: U.S. trends from 1999 to 2006 and effects of medicare coverage. *Ann Intern Med* 2009;150:505–515.

Mohan S, Campbell NR. Hypertension management in Canada: Good news, but important challenges remain. *CMAJ* 2008;178: 1458–1460.

Moser M, Hebert PR. Prevention of disease progression, left ventricular hypertrophy and congestive heart failure in hypertension treatment trials. *J Am Coll Cardiol* 1996;27:1214–1218.

National High Blood Pressure Education Program Working Group. National High Blood Pressure Education Program Working Group report on primary prevention of hypertension. *Arch Intern Med* 1993;153:186–208.

National High Blood Pressure Education Program Working Group. Update on the 1987 Task Force Report on high blood pressure in children and adolescents. *Pediatrics* 1996;98:649–658.

Neaton JD, Wentworth D, Sherwin R, et al. Comparison of 10 year coronary and cerebrovascular disease mortality rates by hypertensive status for black and non-black men screened in the Multiple Risk Factor Intervention Trial (MRFIT) [Abstract]. *Circulation* 1989;80(Suppl. 2):II-300.

Nolte E, McKee M. Measuring the health of nations: Updating an earlier analysis. *Health Affairs* 2008;27:58–71.

Ordunez-Garcia P, Munoz JL, Pedraza D, et al. Success in control of hypertension in a low-resource setting: The Cuban experience. *J Hypertens* 2006;24:845–849.

Ostchega Y, Carroll M, Prineas, et al. Trends of elevated blood pressure among children and adolescents: Data from the national health and nutrition examination survey 1988–2006. *Am J Hypertens* 2009;22:59–67.

Parikh NI, Gona P, Larson MG, et al. Long-term trends in myocardial infarction incidence and case fatality in the National Heart, Lung, and Blood Institute's Framingham Heart study. *Circulation* 2009;119:1203–1210.

Parikh NI, Pencina MJ, Wang TJ, et al. A risk score for predicting near-term incidence of hypertension: The Framingham Heart Study. *Ann Intern Med* 2008;148:102–110.

Pickering G. Hypertension: Definitions, natural histories and consequences. *Am J Med* 1972;52:570–583.

Prospective Studies Collaboration. Cholesterol, diastolic blood pressure, and stroke. *Lancet* 1995;346:1647–1653.

Rose G. Epidemiology. In: Marshall AJ, Barritt DW, eds. *The Hypertensive Patient*. Kent, UK: Pitman Medical; 1980:1–21.

Rose G. Sick individuals and sick populations. *Int J Epidemiol* 1985;14:32–38.

Rose G. *The Strategy of Preventive Medicine*. Oxford, UK: Oxford University Press; 1992.

Rostrup M, Mundal MH, Westheim A, et al. Awareness of high blood pressure increases arterial plasma catecholamines, platelet noradrenaline and adrenergic responses to mental stress. *J Hypertens* 1991;9:159–166.

Sanchez RA, Ayala M, Baglivo H, et al. Latin American guidelines on hypertension. *J Hypertens* 2009;27:905–922.

Shaper AG, Ashby D, Pocock SJ. Blood pressure and hypertension in middle-aged British men. *J Hypertens* 1988;6:367–374.

Shih A, Davis K, Schoenbaum S, et al. Organizing the U.S. health care delivery system for high performance. *The Commonwealth Fund*. 2008;98.

Sinclair AM, Isles CG, Brown I, et al. Secondary hypertension in a blood pressure clinic. *Arch Intern Med* 1987;147:1289–1293.

Stamler J. Setting the TONE for ending the hypertension epidemic. *JAMA* 1998;279:878–879.

Stamler J, Stamler R, Neaton JD. Blood pressure, systolic and diastolic, and cardiovascular risks. *Arch Intern Med* 1993;153:598–615.

Strandberg TE, Salomaa VV, Vanhanen HT, et al. Isolated diastolic hypertension, pulse pressure, and mean arterial pressure as predictors of mortality during a follow-up of up to 32 years. *J Hypertens* 2002;20:399–404.

Task Force. The Task Force for the Management of Arterial Hypertension of the European Society of Hypertension (ESH) and of the European Society of Cardiology (ESC). *J Hypertens* 2007; 25:1105–1187.

Thomas F, Blacher J, Benetos A, et al. Cardiovascular risk as defined in the 2003 European blood pressure classification: The assessment of an additional predictive value of pulse pressure on mortality. *J Hypertens* 2008;26:1072–1077.

Thürmer HL, Lund-Larsen PG, Tverdal A. Is blood pressure treatment as effective in a population setting as in controlled trials? Results from a prospective study. *J Hypertens* 1994;12: 481–490.

Unal B, Critchley JA, Capewell S. Explaining the decline in coronary heart disease mortality in England and Wales between 1981 and 2000. *Circulation* 2004;109:1101–1107.

van Bemmel T, Gussekloo J, Westendorp RG, et al. In a population-based prospective study, no association between high blood pressure and mortality after age 85 years. *J Hypertens* 2006;24: 287–292.

van den Hoogen PCW, Feskens EJM, Nagelkerke NJD, et al. The relation between blood pressure and mortality due to coronary heart disease among men in different parts of the world. *N Engl J Med* 2000;342:1–8.

Vasan RS, Beiser A, Seshadri S, et al. Residual lifetime risk for developing hypertension in middle-aged women and men: The Framingham Heart Study. *JAMA* 2002;287:1003–1010.

Vasan RS, Larson MG, Leip EP, et al. Impact of high-normal blood pressure on the risk of cardiovascular disease. *N Engl J Med* 2001;345:1291–1297.

Victor RG, Leonard D, Hess P, et al. Factors associated with hypertension awareness, treatment, and control in Dallas County, Texas. *Arch Intern Med* 2008;168:1285–1293.

Wald NJ, Law MR. A strategy to reduce cardiovascular disease by more than 80%. *Br Med J* 2003;326:1419–1423.

Whelton PK, He J, Appel LJ, et al. Primary prevention of hypertension: Clinical and public health advisory from the National High Blood Pressure Education Program. *JAMA* 2002;288: 1882–1888.

WHO/ISH Writing Group. World Health Organization (WHO) International Society of Hypertension (ISH) statement on management of hypertension. *J Hypertens* 2003;21:1983–1992.

Williams B, Poulter NR, Brown MJ, et al. Guidelines for management of hypertension: Report of the fourth working party of the British Hypertension Society, 2004—BHS IV. *J Hum Hypertens* 2004;18:139–185.

Wilper AP, Woolhandler S, Lasser KE, et al. A national study of chronic disease prevalence and access to care in uninsured U.S. adults. *Ann Intern Med* 2008;149:170–176.

Wolf-Maier K, Cooper RS, Banegas JR, et al. Hypertension prevalence and blood pressure levels in 6 European countries, Canada, and the United States. *JAMA* 2003;289:2363–2369.

Wolf-Maier K, Cooper RS, Kramer H, et al. Hypertension treatment and control in five European countries, Canada, and the United States. *Hypertension* 2004;43:10–17.

Wong ND, Lopez VA, L'Italien G, et al. Inadequate control of hypertension in US adults with cardiovascular disease comorbidities in 2003–2004. *Arch Intern Med* 2007;167:2431–2436.

Woolf SH. The power of prevention and what it requires. *JAMA* 2008;299:2437–2439.

Yusuf S. Two decades of progress in preventing vascular disease. *Lancet* 2002;360:2–3.

Yusuf S, Reddy S, Ôunpuu S, et al. Global burden of cardiovascular diseases. Part I: General considerations, the epidemiologic transition, risk factors, and impact of urbanization. *Circulation* 2001;104:2746–2753.

CHAPTER 2

Measurement of Blood Pressure

Now that some of the major issues about hypertension in the population at large have been addressed, we turn to the evaluation of the individual patient with hypertension. This chapter covers the measurement of blood pressure (BP), first considering many aspects of its variability. These, in turn, are involved in a number of special features that are of considerable clinical importance including the "white-coat" effect, nocturnal dipping, and the early morning surge in pressure.

BP is now recognized as a continuous variable, impossible to characterize accurately except by multiple readings under various conditions. Its measurement is often inaccurate (Keenan et al., 2009; Mitka, 2008) and in need of escaping the physician's office to be fully effective as a tool for the control of hypertension (Pickering, 2006). Multiple out-of-office measurements are essential for accurate diagnosis and management. Self-measurements at home are the logical alternative since, at least in the United States, ambulatory monitoring is not generally available.

An excellent review of these and other issues about BP measurements has been provided by a committee of experts (Pickering et al., 2008). At the same time, three experts in the field of hypertension have published a proposal that, though it first sounds radical, would likely improve the recognition and management of hypertension: In all people over age 50, do not measure or record the diastolic BP because, as they say, "systolic pressure is all that matters" (Williams et al., 2008). These authors partly are correct: Over age 50, most hypertension is predominately, or purely, systolic, and attention to the easier to reduce diastolic level may preclude adequate control of the systolic level. However the combination adds more predictive power.

Before going into particulars, a more general comment seems appropriate: self-monitoring of each patient's BP at home and work must be more widely implemented. The variability of BP covered in the next section is typical. Most patients have variable BP, poorly controlled on multiple medications. Practitioners in their office cannot solve the problem. In fact, the doctor's office is responsible for a good part of the problem (Ogedegbe et al., 2008).

The only solution is to have hypertensive patients (and their practitioners) take measurement of BP more seriously, as seriously as insulin-taking diabetics monitor their blood glucose and as seriously as breast cancer survivors take the need for careful follow-up. This may sound overly dramatic, but hypertension-related consequences maim and kill many more people than diabetes and cancer. We know the problem: hypertension usually does not hurt until it is too late.

One of the few ways proven to improve patients' adherence to therapy is home BP monitoring (HBPM) (Pickering et al., 2008). We believe every hypertensive must have a home BP device and must monitor their BP as carefully as a diabetic should monitor their blood glucose. All practitioners should realize how variable BP can be, how the morning surge is so difficult to minimize, and how the late afternoon can expose orthostatic symptoms from too tightly controlled hypertension the rest of the day.

The practitioner must take direct responsibility for the individual patient. We know of nothing more helpful in achieving good control of an individual patient's hypertension than the home monitoring of BP. In the best of worlds, the patient could alter his or her antihypertensive regimen based on his or her home BP readings just as diabetics are allowed to alter their insulin dosage based on their home glucose readings. Such self-modification may be too much to ask, but phones, faxes, and e-mails can easily send the readings to an office assistant or practitioner who can then provide appropriate advice.

For too long, practitioners have kept patients out of the loop, either too proud to give up some of their power or too suspicious of the ability of their patients to help themselves. We need to recognize the potential of home monitoring and use it to our patients' benefit. An appreciation of the variability of BP is a good place to start.

VARIABILITY OF BLOOD PRESSURE

In the absence of 24-hour ambulatory BP monitoring (ABPM), the variability of the BP is much greater than most practitioners realize (Keenan et al., 2009).

The adverse consequences of not recognizing and dealing with this variability are obvious: Individual patients may be falsely labeled as hypertensive or normotensive. If falsely labeled as normotensive, needed therapy may be denied. If falsely labeled as hypertensive, the label itself may provoke ill effects, as noted in Chapter 1, and unnecessary therapy will likely be given. Moreover, variability per se is

associated with greater degrees of target organ damage (Jankowski et al., 2008).

The typical variability of the BP through the 24-hour day is easily recognized by ABPM (Fig. 2-1). This printout of readings taken in a single patient every 15 minutes during the day and every 30 minutes at night displays the large differences in daytime readings, the typical dipping during sleep, and the abrupt increase on arising.

Sources of Variation

BP readings are often variable because of the problems involving the observer (measurement variation) or factors working within the patient (biologic variation).

Measurement Variations

An impressively long list of factors that can affect the immediate accuracy of office measurements has been compiled and referenced by Reeves (1995) (Table 2-1).

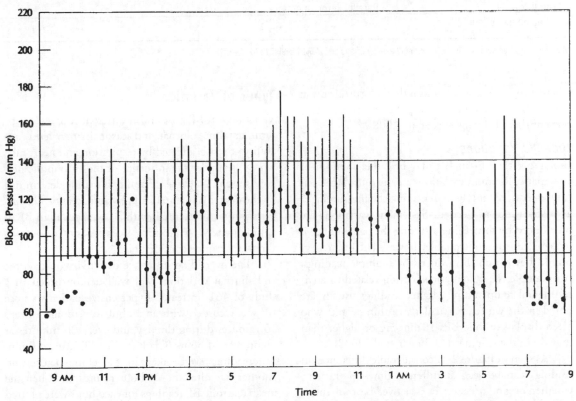

FIGURE 2-1 Computer printout of BPs obtained by ABPM over 24 hours, beginning at 9 a.m., in a 50-year-old man with hypertension receiving no therapy. The patient slept from midnight until 6 a.m. *Solid circles,* heart rate in beats per minute. (From Zachariah PK, Sheps SG, Smith RL. Defining the roles of home and ambulatory monitoring. *Diagnosis* 1988;10:39–50, with permission.)

TABLE 2.1   Factors Affecting the Immediate Accuracy of Office BP Measurements

Increases BP	Decreases BP	No Effect on BP
Examinee	Examinee	Examinee
Soft Korotkoff sounds	Soft Korotkoff sounds	Menstrual phase
Pseudohypertension	Recent meal	Chronic caffeine ingestion
White-coat reaction	Missed auscultatory gap	Cuff self-inflation
Paretic arm (due to stroke)	High stroke volume	Examinee and examiner
Pain, anxiety	Setting, equipment	Discordance in gender or race
Acute smoking	Noisy environs	Examination
Acute caffeine	Faulty aneroid device	Thin shirtsleeve under cuff
Acute ethanol ingestion	Low mercury level	Bell vs. diaphragm
Distended bladder	Leaky bulb	Cuff inflation per se
Talking, signing	Examiner	Hour of day (during work hours)
Setting, equipment	Reading to next lowest 5 or	
Cold environment	10 mm Hg, or expectation bias	
Leaky bulb valve	Impaired hearing	
Examination	Examination	
Cuff too narrow	Resting for too long	
Arm below heart level	Arm above heart level	
Too-short rest period	Too rapid deflation	
Arm, back unsupported	Excess bell pressure	
Parallax error	Parallax error (aneroid)	
Using phase IV (adult)		

Modified from Reeves RA. Does this patient have hypertension? *JAMA* 1995;273:1211–1218.

These errors are more common than most realize and regular, frequent retraining of personnel is needed to prevent them (Niyonsenga et al., 2008).

Biologic Variations

Biologic variations in BP may be either random or systematic. Random variations are uncontrollable but can be reduced simply by repeating the measurement as many times as needed. Systematic variations are introduced by something affecting the patient and, if recognized, are controllable; however, if not recognized, they cannot be reduced by multiple readings. An example is a systematic variation related to environmental temperature: Higher readings usually are noted in the winter, particularly in thin people, who often display systolic BPs 10 mm Hg or higher than they do in the summer (Al-Tamer et al., 2008).

As seen in Figure 2-1, considerable differences in readings can be seen at different times of the day, whether or not the subject is active. Beyond these, between-visit variations in BP can be substantial. Even after three office visits, the standard deviation of the difference in BP from one visit to another in 32 subjects was 10.4 mm Hg for systolic BP and 7.0 mm Hg for diastolic BP (Watson et al., 1987).

Types of Variation

Variability in BP arises from different sources: short-term, daytime, diurnal, and seasonal. *Short-term* variability at rest is affected by respiration and heart rate, which are under the influence of the autonomic nervous system. *Daytime* variability is mainly determined by the degree of mental and physical activity. *Diurnal* variability is substantial, with an average fall in BP of approximately 15% during sleep. As noted, *seasonal* variations can be considerable.

The overriding influence of activity on daytime and diurnal variations was well demonstrated in a study of 461 untreated hypertensive patients whose BP was recorded with an ambulatory monitor every 15 minutes during the day and every 30 minutes at night over 24 hours (Clark et al., 1987). In addition, five readings were taken in the clinic before and another five after the 24-hour recording. When the mean diastolic BP readings for each hour were plotted against each patient's mean clinic diastolic BP, considerable variations were noted, with the lowest BPs occurring during the night and the highest near midday (Fig. 2-2A). The patients recorded in a diary the location at which their BP was taken (e.g., at

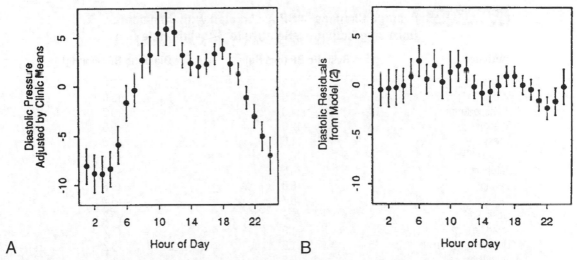

FIGURE 2-2   A: Plot of diastolic BP readings adjusted by individual clinic means. **B:** Plot of the diastolic BP hourly mean residuals after adjustments for various activities by a time-of-day model. The hourly means (*solid circles*) ± 2 standard errors of the mean (*vertical lines*) are plotted versus the corresponding time of day. (Modified from Clark LA, Denby L, Pregibon D, et al. A quantitative analysis of the effects of activity and time of day on the diurnal variations of blood pressure. *J Chronic Dis* 1987;40:671–679.)

home, work, or other location) and what they were doing at the time, selecting from 15 choices of activity. When the effects of the various combinations of location and activity on the BP were analyzed, variable effects relative to the BP recorded while relaxing were seen (Table 2-2). When the estimated effects of the various combinations of location and activity were subtracted from the individual readings obtained throughout the 24-hour period, little residual effect related to the time of day was found (Fig. 2-2B). To be sure, BP usually falls during sleep, and an abrupt morning surge is typical, but beyond these, there is no circadian rhythm of BP (Peixoto & White, 2007).

Additional Sources of Variation

Beyond the level of activity and the stresses related to the measurement, a number of other factors affect BP variability, including the sensitivity of barore-flexes and the level of BP, with more variability occurring with higher BPs (Ragot et al., 2001). This latter relationship probably is responsible for the wide-spread perception that the elderly have more variable BP. When younger and older hypertensives with comparable BP levels were studied, variability was

not consistently related to age (Brennan et al., 1986).

It is important to minimize the changes in BP that arise because of variations within the patient. Even little things can have an impact: both systolic BP and diastolic BP may rise 10 mm Hg or more with a distended urinary bladder (Faguis & Karhu-vaara, 1989) or during ordinary conversation (Le Pailleur et al., 1998). Just the presence of a medical student was found to increase the BP by an average of 6.4/2.4 mm Hg (Matthys et al., 2004). Those who are more anxious or elated tend to have higher levels (Ogedegbe et al., 2008). Particularly in the elderly, eating may lower the BP (Smith et al., 2003). Two common practices may exert significant pressor effects: smoking (Groppelli et al., 1992) or drinking caffeinated beverages (Hartley et al., 2004).

The BP may vary between the left and right arms, and it should be taken in both on initial exam, with the higher arm used in subsequent measurements. Although some find few significant differences and those few related to obstructive arterial disease (Eguchi et al., 2007), others find differences to be common and indicative of an increased all-cause mortality (Agarwal et al., 2008).

TABLE 2.2	Average Changes in BP Associated with Commonly Occurring Activities, Relative to BP while Relaxing	
Activity	**Systolic BP (mm Hg)**	**Diastolic BP (mm Hg)**
Meetings	+20.2	+15.0
Work	+16.0	+13.0
Transportation	+14.0	+9.2
Walking	+12.0	+5.5
Dressing	+11.5	+9.5
Chores	+10.7	+6.7
Telephone	+9.5	+7.2
Eating	+8.8	+9.6
Talking	+6.7	+6.7
Desk work	+5.9	+5.3
Reading	+1.9	+2.2
Business (at home)	+1.6	+3.2
Television	+0.3	+1.1
Relaxing	0.0	0.0
Sleeping	−10.0	−7.6

Data adapted from Clark LA, Denby L, Pregibon D, et al. A quantitative analysis of the effects of activity and time of day on the diurnal variations of blood pressure. *J Chronic Dis* 1987;40:671–679.

The greater the variability, usually measured by a weighted 24-hour standard deviation of readings taken by ABPM (Bilo et al., 2007), the greater the degree of both current target organ damage (Shintani et al., 2007; Tatasciore et al., 2007) and future cardiovascular risk (Jankowski et al., 2008). Therefore, damage induced by hypertension is related not only to the average BP level but also to the magnitude of its variability.

Blood Pressure During Sleep and on Awakening

Normal Pattern

The usual fall in BP at night is largely the result of sleep and inactivity rather than the time of day (Sayk et al., 2007). Whereas the nocturnal fall averages approximately 15% in those who are active during the day, it is only about 5% in those who remain in bed for the entire 24 hours (Casiglia et al., 1996). The usual falls in BP and heart rate that occur with sleep reflect a decrease in sympathetic nervous tone. In healthy young men, plasma catecholamine levels fell during rapid-eye-movement sleep, whereas awakening immediately increased epinephrine, and subsequent standing induced a marked increase in norepinephrine (Dodt et al., 1997).

The nocturnal dip in pressure is normally distributed with no evidence of bimodality in both normotensive and hypertensive people (Staessen et al., 1997). The separation between "dippers" and "nondippers" is, in a sense, artefactual. Therefore, to improve the diagnostic reliability of dipping status, some recommend at least two 24-hour ambulatory monitorings (Cuspidi et al., 2004); others define nondipping as the presence of a nocturnal BP that remains above 125/80 (White & Larocca, 2003); others as a less than 10% fall from average daytime levels (Henskens et al., 2008).

What appears to be nondipping may be simply a consequence of getting up to urinate (Perk et al., 2001) or a reflection of obstructive sleep apnea (Pelttari et al., 1998), or simply poor sleep quality (Matthews et al., 2008). Moreover, the degree of dipping during sleep is affected by the amount of dietary sodium in those who are salt sensitive: Sodium loading attenuates these individuals' dipping, whereas sodium reduction restores their dipping status (Uzu et al., 1999). Among 325 African French, those who excreted a large portion of urinary sodium during the day had more dipping at night (Bankir et al., 2008). Furthermore, dipping is more common among people who are more physically active during the day (Cavelaars et al., 2004).

Associations with Nondipping

A number of associations have been noted with a lesser fall than usual in nocturnal BP. These include:

- Older age (Staessen et al., 1997)
- Cognitive dysfunction (Van Boxtel et al., 1998)
- Diabetes (Björklund et al., 2002)
- Obesity (Kotsis et al., 2005)
- African Americans (Jehn et al., 2008) and Hispanics (Hyman et al., 2000)
- Impaired endothelium-dependent vasodilation (Higashi et al., 2002)
- Elevated levels of markers of cellular adhesion and inflammation (Von Känel et al., 2004)
- Left ventricular hypertrophy (Cuspidi et al., 2004)
- Intracranial hemorrhage (Tsivgoulis et al., 2005)
- Loss of renal function (Fukuda et al., 2004)
- Mortality from cardiovascular disease (Redon & Lurbe, 2008)

With concern over a greater risk in nondippers, Hermida et al. (2008) changed the prevalence of dipping from 16% to 57% by giving one of the three medications being taken by 250 resistant patients at bedtime.

Associations with Excessive Dipping

Just as a failure of the BP to fall during sleep may reflect or contribute to cardiovascular damage, there may also be danger from too great a fall in nocturnal BP. Floras (1988) suggested that nocturnal falls in BP could induce myocardial ischemia in hypertensives with left ventricular hypertrophy and impaired coronary vasodilator reserve, contributing to the J-curve of increased coronary events when diastolic BP is lowered below 85 mm Hg (see Chapter 5).

The first objective evidence for this threat from too much dipping was the finding by Kario et al. (1996) that more silent cerebrovascular disease (identified by brain magnetic resonance imaging) was found among extreme dippers who had a greater than 20% fall in nocturnal systolic BP. Subsequently, Kario et al. (2001), in a 41-month follow-up of 575 elderly hypertensives, found the lowest stroke risk to be at a sleep diastolic BP of 75 mm Hg, with an increased risk below 75 mm Hg that was associated with their intake of antihypertensive drugs. Similarly, in a smaller group of hypertensives with stable coronary artery disease, myocardial ischemia occurred during the night more frequently in untreated nondippers and in treated overdippers (Pierdomenico et al., 1998). Too great a fall in nocturnal pressure may also increase the risk of anterior ischemic optic neuropathy

and glaucoma (Pickering, 2008). These findings serve as a warning against late evening or bedtime dosing of drugs that have a substantial antihypertensive effect in the first few hours after intake.

Early Morning Surge

The BP abruptly rises, i.e., surges, upon arising from sleep, whether it be in the early morning (Gosse et al., 2004) or after a midafternoon siesta (Bursztyn et al., 1999), although the degree of surge may vary on repeated measurements (Wizner et al., 2008). As amply described, the early morning hours after 6 a.m. are accompanied by an increased prevalence of all cardiovascular catastrophes as compared to the remainder of the 24-hour period (Muller, 1999). Early morning increases have been noted for stroke (Foerch et al., 2008; Kario et al., 2003), cardiac arrest (Peckova et al., 1998; Soo et al., 2000), rupture of the abdominal aorta (Manfredini et al., 1999), and epistaxis (Manfredini et al., 2000), possibly by destabilizing atherosclerotic plaques (Marfella et al., 2007) within the thickened resistance arteries (Rizzoni et al., 2007).

These abrupt changes are likely mediated by heightened sympathetic activity after hours of relative quiescence (Dodt et al., 1997; Panza et al., 1991), which may be accentuated in subjects with a great deal of hostility (Pasic et al., 1998). The surge may be aggravated by increased physical activity (Leary et al., 2002), but simply arising from sleep may significantly raise BP even in patients with hypertension under apparently good control (Redon et al., 2002). As will be noted, home BP measurements are the only practical way to recognize and then modulate this surge, logically by using long-acting medications or adding a bedtime dose of an α-blocker (Kario et al., 2008).

White-Coat Effect

Measurement of the BP may invoke an alerting reaction, a reaction that is only transient in most patients but persistent in some. It usually is seen more often in people who have a greater rise in BP under psychological stress (Palatini et al., 2003), but the majority of people have higher office BP than out-of-office BP (O'Brien et al., 2003).

Environment

There is a hierarchy of alerting: least at home, more in the clinic or office, and most in the hospital. Measurements by the same physician were higher in the hospital than in a health center (Enström et al., 2000).

To reduce the alerting reaction, patients should relax in a quiet room and have multiple readings taken with an automatic device (Myers et al., 2009).

Measurer

Figure 2-3 demonstrates that the presence of a physician usually causes a rise in BP that is sometimes very impressive (Mancia et al., 1987). The data in Figure 2-3 were obtained from patients who had an intra-arterial recording. When the intra-arterial readings were stable, the BP was measured in the non-catheterized arm by both a male physician and a female nurse, half of the time by the physician first, the other half by the nurse first. The patients had not met the personnel but had been told that they would be coming. When the physician took the first readings, the BPs rose an average of 22/14 mm Hg

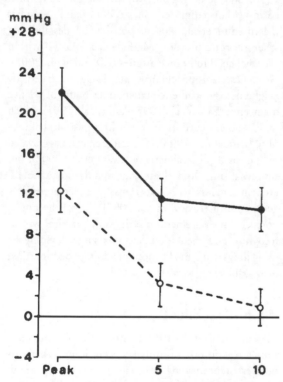

FIGURE 2-3 Comparison of maximum (or peak) rises in systolic BP in 30 subjects during visits with a physician (*solid line*) and a nurse (*dashed line*). The rises occurring at 5 and 10 minutes into the visits are shown. Data are expressed as mean (±standard error of the mean) changes from a control value taken 4 minutes before each visit. (Modified from Mancia G, Paroti G, Pomidossi G, et al. Alerting reaction and rise in blood pressure during measurement by physician and nurse. *Hypertension* 1987;9:209–215.)

and as much as 74 mm Hg systolic. The readings were approximately half that much above baseline at 5 and 10 minutes. Similar rises were seen during three subsequent visits. When the nurse took the first set of readings, the rises were only half as great as those noted by the physician, and the BP usually returned to near-baseline when measured again after 5 and 10 minutes. The rises were not related to patient age, gender, overall BP variability, or BP levels. These marked differences are not limited to handsome Italian doctors or their excitable patients. Similar nurse–physician differences have been repeatedly noted elsewhere (Little et al., 2002).

A large amount of data indicate a marked tendency in most patients for BP to fall after repeated measurements, regardless of the time interval between readings (Verberk et al., 2006a). They strongly suggest that nurses and not physicians should measure the BP and that at least three sets of readings should be taken before the patient is labeled hypertensive and the need for treatment is determined (Graves & Sheps, 2004).

White-Coat Hypertension

As will be noted, *white-coat hypertension* (WCH) has been variably defined. The most appropriate definition is an average of multiple daytime out-of-office BPs of less than 135/85 mm Hg in the presence of usual office readings above 140/90 mm Hg (O'Brien et al., 2003; Verdecchia et al., 2003).

Most patients have higher BP levels when taken in the office than when taken out of the office, as shown in a comparison between the systolic BPs obtained by a physician versus the average daytime systolic BPs obtained by ambulatory monitors (Pickering, 1996) (Fig. 2-4). In the figure, all the points above the diagonal line represent higher office readings than out-of-office readings, indicating that a majority of patients demonstrate the white-coat *effect*.

Whereas most patients exhibiting a white-coat effect also had elevated out-of-office readings, so that they are hypertensive in all settings (Fig. 2-4, group 2), a smaller but significant number of patients had normal readings outside the office—i.e., WCH (Fig. 2-4, group 1)—whereas another group had normal office readings but elevated outside readings (Fig. 2-4, group 4). As will be described, such *masked* hypertension has received increasing attention. Pickering et al. (1988) had previously found that among 292 untreated patients with persistently elevated

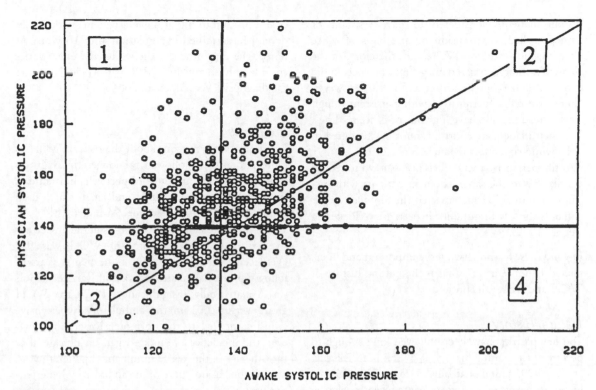

FIGURE 2-4   Plot of clinic systolic and daytime ambulatory BP readings in 573 patients. *1*, Patients with WCH; *2*, patients with sustained hypertension; *3*, patients with normal BP; *4*, patients whose clinic BP underestimates ambulatory BP. The majority of sustained hypertensives and normotensives had higher clinic pressures than awake ambulatory pressures. (Adapted from Pickering TG. Ambulatory monitoring and the definition of hypertension. *J Hypertens* 1992,10:401–409.)

office readings over an average of 6 years, the out-of-office readings recorded by a 24-hour ambulatory monitor were normal in 21%. Since that observation, the prevalence of WCH has been found to be approximately 15% in multiple groups of patients with office hypertension (Dolan et al., 2004). To ensure the diagnosis, more than one ABPM should be obtained (Cuspidi et al., 2007).

It is important to avoid confusion between the white-coat *effect* and WCH. As Pickering (1996) emphasized, "White coat hypertension is a measure of BP level, whereas the white coat effect is a measure of change. A large white coat effect is by no means confined to patients with white coat hypertension, and indeed is often more pronounced in patients with severe hypertension."

As interest in WCH has grown, a number of its features have become apparent, including:

• The prevalence depends largely on the definition of the upper limit of normal for daytime out-of-office readings; depending on the level chosen, the prevalence has been shown to vary from as low as 12% to as high as 53.2% (Verdecchia et al., 1995). A level of below 135/85 mm Hg has been generally accepted (Fagard & Cornelissen, 2007).

• The prevalence of WCH may be reduced if the office readings are based on at least five separate visits. The less the elevation in office BP, the greater the frequency of WCH (Verdecchia et al., 2001).

• Obviously, only daytime ambulatory readings should be used to define WCH, as nighttime readings are typically lower.

• Multiple self-obtained home readings are as good as ambulatory readings to document WCH (Den Hond et al., 2003).

• The prevalence rises with the age of the patient (Mansoor et al., 1996) and is particularly high in elderly patients with isolated systolic hypertension (Jumabay et al., 2005).

• Women are more likely to have WCH (Dolan et al., 2004).

- Some patients considered to have resistant or uncontrolled hypertension on the basis of office readings instead have WCH and, therefore, in the absence of target organ damage, may not need more intensive therapy (Redon et al., 1998). However, most treated hypertensives with persistently high office readings also have high out-of-office readings, so their inadequate control cannot be attributed to the white-coat effect (Mancia et al., 1997).
- Antihypertensive therapy has been shown to reduce office BP to the same extent in patients with sustained and WCH but lowered the ambulatory BP in only those with sustained hypertension (Pickering et al., 1999).

Beyond these features, two more important and inter-related issues remain: What is the natural history of WCH and what is its prognosis?

Natural History
Too few patients have been followed long enough to be sure of the natural history of WCH, but Pickering et al. (1999) found that only 10% to 30% become hypertensive over 3 to 5 years. More recently, Mancia et al. (2009) found that 43% of patients with WCH developed sustained hypertension after 10 years. As noted, the magnitude of the white-coat effect varies considerably, so multiple ABPMs are needed to ensure the diagnosis (Verberk et al., 2006b).

Prognosis
Less uncertainty remains about the risks of WCH as more patients are followed for longer times. In an analysis of data from four prospective cohort studies from the United States, Italy, and Japan which used comparable methodology for 24-hour ABPM in 1,549 normotensives and 4,406 essential hypertensive patients, the prevalence of WCH was 9% (Verdecchia et al., 2005). Over the first 6 years of follow-up, the risk of stroke in a multivariate analysis was a statistically insignificant 1.15 in the WCH group versus 2.01 in the ambulatory hypertensive group compared to the normotensive group. However, the incidence of stroke began to increase after the 6th year in the WCH group and, by the 9th year, crossed the hazard curve of the ambulatory hypertensive group.

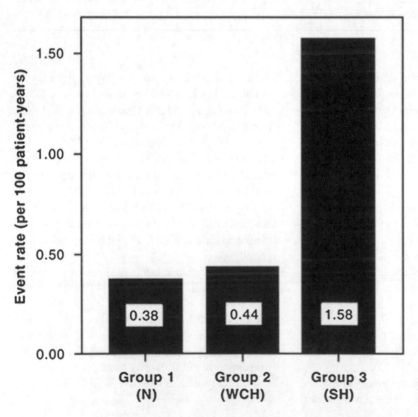

FIGURE 2-5 Event-free survival curve in patients with normotension, WCH, and sustained hypertension. (Reprinted from Pierdomenico SD, Lapenna D, Di Mascio R, et al. Short- and long-term risk of cardiovascular events in white-coat hypertension. *J Hum Hypertens* 2008; 22:408–414, with permission.)

Similar but less striking changes in all cardiovascular events have been noted in 14-year follow-ups (Ben-Dov et al., 2008; Pierdomenico et al., 2008). Pierdomenico et al. (2008) followed 305 people with normal BP (NT), 399 with WCH (defined as clin >140/90, ABPM <135/85 mm Hg), and 1,333 with sustained hypertension. By the end of the follow-up, antihypertensive therapy was being taken by 7% of the NTs, 47% of the WCHs, and 94% of the sustained hypertensives. As seen in Figure 2-5, event-free survival rates were the same in the NTs and WCHs until the 10th year when it fell among the WCHs but still remained much higher than seen in the sustained hypertensives through the 14th year. Similar data were reported by Ben-Dov et al. (2008) in an even larger group of treated WCHs compared to those with sustained hypertension.

Before clinical events are seen, WCHs have been found to have increased arterial stiffness (De Simone et al., 2007) and thickness (Puato et al., 2008). Obviously, close follow-up of patients carefully diagnosed with WCH is mandatory. At the least, they should be encouraged to modify their lifestyle in an appropriate manner and continue to monitor their BP status.

Masked Hypertension

As seen in the lower right portion of Figure 2-4, labeled as no. 4, some patients have normal office BP (<140/90) but elevated ambulatory readings (>135/85). These "masked" hypertensives may comprise a significant portion, 10% or more, of the general population (Cuspidi & Parati, 2007). Higher daytime ambulatory BPs than clinic readings were found in more than 20% of 713 elderly hypertensives (Wing et al., 2002) and in 13.8% of never-treated stage 1 hypertensives (Palatini et al., 2004). Such patients have increased rates of cardiovascular morbidity, almost as high as seen in those with both clinic and ambulatory hypertension (Ben-Dov et al., 2008; Bobrie et al., 2008).

Since by definition these patients have normal office BP readings, the only way to exclude masked hypertension is to obtain out-of-office readings on every patient. Though only a few home readings are usually needed (Mallion et al., 2004), most patients cannot get them. Therefore, the search should be narrowed to those more likely to be higher out of the office. These include patients with diabetes (Leitão et al., 2007), unexplained tachycardia (Grassi et al., 2007), left ventricular

hypertrophy (Lurbe et al., 2005), or obstructive sleep apnea (Baguet et al., 2008).

OFFICE MEASUREMENT OF BLOOD PRESSURE

In the everyday practice of medicine, office measurements of BP may be the least accurately performed procedure which, at the same time, have the greatest impact on patient care. Under the best of circumstances, all of the previously described causes of variability are difficult to control. Therefore, we must do what can be done to improve current practice. Use of the guidelines shown in Table 2-3 will prevent most measurement errors.

Patient and Arm Position

The patient should be seated comfortably with the arm supported and positioned at the level of the heart (Fig. 2-6). Measurements taken with the arm hanging at the patient's side averaged 10 mm Hg higher than those taken with the arm supported in a horizontal position at heart level (Netea et al., 2003). When sitting upright on a table without support, readings may be as much as 10 mm Hg higher because of the isometric exertion needed to support the body and arm. Systolic readings are approximately 8 mm Hg higher in the supine than in the seated position even when the arm is at the level of the right atrium (Netea et al., 2003).

Differences Between Arms

As noted earlier in this chapter, initially, the BP should be measured in both arms to ascertain the differences between them; if the reading is higher in one arm, that arm should be used for future measurements. Absolute differences greater than 10 mm Hg in systolic levels were found in 9% of subjects by Kimura et al. (2004) and in 20% by Lane et al. (2002). Lower BP in the left arm is seen in patients with subclavian steal caused by reversal of flow down a vertebral artery distal to an obstructed subclavian artery, as noted in 9% of 500 patients with asymptomatic neck bruits (Bornstein & Norris, 1986). The BP may be either higher or lower in the paretic arm of a stroke patient (Dewar et al., 1992).

Standing Pressure

Readings should be taken immediately on standing and after standing at least 2 minutes to check for spontaneous or drug-induced postural changes, particularly in

TABLE 2.3	Guidelines for Measurement of BP

Patient Conditions
  Posture
- Initially, particularly >65 years, with diabetes, or receiving antihypertensive therapy, check for postural changes by taking readings after 5 min supine, then immediately and 2 min after standing
- For routine follow-up, the patient should sit quietly with the arm bared and supported at the level of the heart and the back resting against a chair. The length of time before measurement is uncertain, but most guidelines recommend 5 min

  Circumstances
- No caffeine or smoking within 30 min preceding the reading
- A quiet, warm setting

Equipment
  Cuff size
- The bladder should encircle at least 80% of the circumference and cover two thirds of the length of the arm
- A too small bladder may cause falsely high readings

  Manometer
- Either a mercury, recently calibrated aneroid or validated electronic device

  Stethoscope
- The bell of the stethoscope should be used
- Avoid excess bell pressure

  Infants
- Use ultrasound (e.g., the Doppler method)

Technique
  Number of readings
- On each occasion, take at least two readings, separated by as much time as is practical; if readings vary >5 mm Hg, take additional readings until two are close
- For diagnosis, obtain three sets of readings at least 1 week apart
- Initially, take pressure in both arms; if the pressures differ, use the arm with the higher pressure
- If the arm pressure is elevated, take the pressure in one leg, particularly in patients <30 years old
  Performance
- Inflate the bladder quickly to a pressure 20 mm Hg above the systolic pressure, recognized by the disappearance of radial pulse, to avoid an auscultatory gap
- Deflate the bladder 3 mm Hg/s
- Record the Korotkoff phase I (appearance) and phase V (disappearance)
- If the Korotkoff sounds are weak, have the patient raise the arm and open and close the hand 5–10 times, then inflate the bladder quickly

  Recordings
- Note the pressure, patient position, the arm, and the cuff size (e.g., 140/90, seated, right arm, and large adult cuff, respectively)

---

the elderly and in diabetics. If no fall in BP is seen in patients with suggestive symptoms, the time of quiet standing should be prolonged to at least 5 minutes. In most people, systolic BP falls and diastolic BP rises by a few millimeters of mercury on changing from the supine to the standing position. In the elderly, significant postural falls of 20 mm Hg or more in systolic BP are more common, occurring in approximately 10% of ambulatory people older than 65 years and in more than half of frail nursing-home residents, particularly in those with elevated supine systolic BP (Gupta & Lipsitz, 2007).

Leg Pressure

If the arm reading is elevated, particularly in a patient younger than 30, the BP should be taken in one leg to rule out coarctation.

Sphygmomanometer

Independent evaluations of BP device accuracy and performance are available at www.dableducational. org, but there are no obligatory standards which must be met. Significant errors of both mercury and aneroid

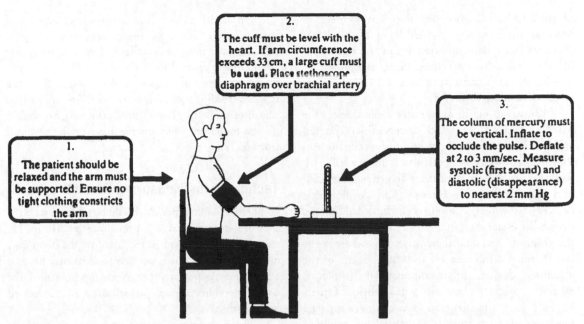

1.
The patient should be relaxed and the arm must be supported. Ensure no tight clothing constricts the arm

2.
The cuff must be level with the heart. If arm circumference exceeds 33 cm, a large cuff must be used. Place stethoscope diaphragm over brachial artery

3.
The column of mercury must be vertical. Inflate to occlude the pulse. Deflate at 2 to 3 mm/sec. Measure systolic (first sound) and diastolic (disappearance) to nearest 2 mm Hg

FIGURE 2-6 Technique of BP measurement recommended by the British Hypertension Society. (From British Hypertension Society. Standardization of blood pressure measurement. *J Hypertens* 1985;3:29–31. Reproduced with permission)

manometers were found in more than 5% of readings in physicians' offices (Niyonsenga et al., 2008).

As mercury manometers are being phased out because of the toxic potential of mercury spills and with the inaccuracies of aneroid manometers, automated electronic devices are increasingly being used, which should improve the accuracy of readings.

Bladder Size

The width of the bladder should be equal to approximately two thirds the distance from the axilla to the antecubital space; a 16-cm-wide bladder is adequate for most adults. The bladder should be long enough to encircle at least 80% of the arm. Erroneously high readings may occur with the use of a bladder that is too short (Aylett et al., 2001) and erroneously low readings with a bladder that is too wide (Bakx et al., 1997).

Most sphygmomanometers sold in the United States have a cuff with a bladder that is 12 cm wide and 22 cm long, which is too short for patients with an arm circumference greater than 26 cm, whether fat or muscular (Aylett et al., 2001). The British Hypertension Society (BHS) recommends longer cuff size (12 × 40 cm) for obese arms (O'Brien et al., 2003). The American Heart Association recommends progressively larger cuffs with larger arm circumference:

- Arm circumference 22 to 26 cm, 12 × 22 cm cuff (small adult)
- Arm circumference 27 to 34 cm, 16 × 30 cm cuff (adult)
- Arm circumference 35 to 44 cm, 16 × 36 cm cuff (large adult)
- Arm circumference 45 to 52 cm, 16 × 42 cm cuff (adult thigh)

Children require smaller cuffs depending on their size.

Cuff Position

If the bladder within the cuff does not completely encircle the arm, particular care should be taken to ensure that the bladder is placed over the brachial artery. The lower edge of the cuff should be approximately 2.5 cm above the antecubital space. In extremely obese people, a thigh cuff may be used with the wide bladder folded on itself if necessary, or the bladder may be placed on the forearm and the sounds heard over the radial artery.

Manometer

Electronic devices are rapidly taking over the home market and are becoming standard in offices and hospitals. Fortunately, their accuracy and reliability are improving, and more have passed the protocols of the U.S. Association for the Advancement of Medical Instrumentation (AAMI) and the BHS. Websites (www.dableducational.com and bhsec.org/blood_pressure.list.stm) have been established to provide all of the available information needed about the devices being marketed.

Almost all of the newer electronic devices are based on oscillometry, which detects initial (systolic) and maximal (mean arterial pressure) oscillations in the brachial artery and calculates the diastolic BP based on proprietary algorithms. In general, the readings obtained by auscultatory and oscillometric devices are closely correlated. The oscillometric devices are easier and faster to use, and they minimize the common terminal digit preference wherein the last number is rounded off to 0 or 5. Some of the electronic devices inflate automatically, which is especially useful for patients with arthritis. Others have a printer attached, and some can have the data downloaded after storing a number of readings. Devices are available for automatic transmission of data to a central location (Møller et al., 2003). An adequate device can be purchased for less than $40. To ensure its proper use and accuracy, the electronic device should be checked by having the patient use it on one arm while the pressure is simultaneously taken in the office with a sphygmomanometer on the other arm.

Wrist and Finger Devices

Wrist oscillometric devices are particularly useful for obese people whose upper arm is too large for accurate readings. They must be kept at the level of the heart. At least one, the Visocor HM 40, has been approved (Dorigatti et al., 2009).

Finger devices measure the pressure in the finger by volume-clamp plethysmography. The Finapres finger cuff may be used for continuous BP monitoring under carefully controlled conditions (Silke & McAuley, 1998), but it is not suitable for intermittent readings. Home finger units are not recommended for self-monitoring (Pickering et al., 2008).

Automated Devices

The automated oscillometric devices increasingly used in offices, emergency rooms, and hospitals often overestimate the BP by 10/5 mm Hg (Park et al., 2001). Nonetheless, these and other automated devices usually provide readings that are satisfactory for most clinical settings (www.dableducational.org).

On the other hand, community-based automated machines may be more inaccurate, particularly in patients with arm sizes smaller or larger than average (Van Durme et al., 2000). For those who cannot use more accurate (and more easily validated) home devices, readings obtained by such an automated machine are better than nothing, but patients should not be managed solely on the basis of the readings from such machines.

Technique for Measuring Blood Pressure

As noted in Table 2-3, care should be taken to raise the pressure in the bladder approximately 20 mm Hg above the systolic level, as indicated by the disappearance of the radial pulse, because patients may have an auscultatory gap (a temporary disappearance of the sound after it first appears), which is related to increased arterial stiffness.

The measurement may be repeated after as little a span as 15 seconds without significantly affecting accuracy. The cuff should be deflated at a rate of 2 to 4 mm Hg per second; either a slower or faster rate may cause falsely higher readings (Bos et al., 1992).

By auscultation, disappearance of the sound (phase V) is a more sensitive and reproducible end point than muffling (phase IV) (De Mey, 1995). In some patients with a hyperkinetic circulation, e.g., anemia or pregnancy, the sounds do not disappear, and the muffled sound is heard well below the expected diastolic BP, sometimes near zero. This phenomenon can also be caused by pressing the stethoscope too firmly against the artery. If arrhythmias are present, additional readings with either auscultatory or oscillometric devices may be required to estimate the average systolic and diastolic BP (Lip et al., 2001).

Pseudohypertension

In some elderly patients with very rigid, calcified arteries, the bladder may not be able to collapse the brachial artery, giving rise to falsely high readings, or pseudohypertension (Spence, 1997). The possibility of pseudohypertension should be suspected in elderly people whose vessels feel rigid; who have little vascular damage in the retina or elsewhere, despite markedly high BP readings; and who suffer inordinate postural symptoms despite cautious therapy.

If one is suspicious, automatic oscillometric devices are usually more accurate (Zweifler & Shahab, 1993), but a direct intra-arterial reading may rarely be needed.

Ways to Amplify the Sounds

With auscultation, the loudness and sharpness of the Korotkoff sounds depend in part on the pressure differential between the arteries in the forearm and those beneath the bladder. To increase the differential and thereby increase the loudness of the sounds, either the amount of blood in the forearm can be decreased or the capacity of the vascular bed can be increased. The amount of blood can be decreased by rapidly inflating the bladder, thereby shortening the time when venous outflow is prevented but arterial inflow continues, or by raising the arm for a few seconds to drain venous blood before inflating the bladder. The vascular bed capacity can be increased by inducing vasodilation through muscular exercise, specifically by having the patient open and close the hand ten times before the observer inflates the bladder. If the sounds are not heard well, the balloon should be emptied and reinflated; otherwise, the vessels will have been partially refilled and the sounds thereby muffled.

Taking Blood Pressure in the Thigh

A large (thigh) cuff should be used to avoid factitiously elevated readings. With the patient lying prone and the leg bent and cradled by the observer, the observer listens with the stethoscope for the Korotkoff sounds in the popliteal fossa. This should be done as part of the initial workup of every young hypertensive, in whom coarctation is more common. Normally, the systolic BP is higher and the diastolic BP a little lower at the knee than in the arm because of the contour of the pulse wave (Hugue et al., 1988).

Taking Blood Pressure in Children

If the child is calm, the same technique that is used with adults should be followed; however, smaller, narrower cuffs must be used (see Chapter 16). If the child is upset, the best procedure may be simply to determine the systolic BP by palpating the radial pulse as the cuff is deflated. In infants, ultrasound is usually used.

Recording of Findings

Regardless of which method is used to measure BP, notation should be made of the conditions so that others can compare the findings or interpret them properly. This is particularly critical in scientific reports, yet many articles about hypertension fail to provide this information.

Blood Pressure during Exercise

An exaggerated response of BP during or immediately after graded exercise, stress testing has been found to predict the development of hypertension in normotensives (Miyai et al., 2000) and their subsequent morbidity or mortality from cardiovascular disease (Laukkanen et al., 2004). Different upper limits for a normal response to exercise have been used in various series, but an exaggerated response to a systolic level above 200 mm Hg at a 100 W workload increases the likelihood of the onset of hypertension from twofold to fourfold over the subsequent 5 to 10 years as compared with that seen with nonexaggerated responses.

Despite the increased likelihood of the development of hypertension with an exaggerated rise in BP during stress testing, follow-up over a mean of 6.6 years of 6,145 men who had symptom-limited exercise stress testing found a significantly increased cardiovascular mortality in the half whose systolic rise was 43 mm Hg or lower (13.7%) compared to the half with a rise of 44 mm Hg or higher (8.2%) (Gupta et al., 2007).

Importance of Office Blood Pressures

Even if all the guidelines listed in Table 2-3 are followed, routine office measurements of BP by sphygmomanometry will continue to show considerable variability. However, before discounting even single casual BP readings, recall that almost all the data on the risks of hypertension described in Chapter 1 are based on only one or a few office readings taken in large groups of people. There is no denying that such data have epidemiologic value, but a few casual office readings are usually not sufficient to determine the status of an individual patient. Two actions minimize variability. First, at least two readings should be taken at every visit, as many as needed to obtain a stable level with less than a 5-mm Hg difference; second, at least three and, preferably, more sets of readings, weeks apart, should be taken unless the initial value is so high, e.g., greater than 180/120 mm Hg, that immediate therapy is needed.

Although multiple carefully taken office readings may be as reliable as those taken by ambulatory monitors, out-of-office readings provide additional data, both to confirm the diagnosis and, more important, to document the adequacy of therapy.

HOME MEASUREMENTS

From the preceding, it is clear that BPs recorded in the hospital or office often are affected by both acute and chronic alerting reactions that tend to accentuate variability and raise the BP, giving rise to a significant white-coat effect. Two techniques—home measurements and ABPM—minimize these problems. Whereas ABPM will likely continue to have more limited applications, the use of home measurements will continue to expand (Pickering et al., 2008).

Two statements authored by multiple experts in the area of BP monitoring have been published (Parati et al., 2008a; Pickering et al., 2008). We can do no better than to quote the abstract of the U.S. document while recommending that every reader obtain a full copy from the American Society of Hypertension (website, www.ash-us.org) or call 800-242-8721 (in the United States only) or write to the American Heart Association, 7272 Greenville Ave., Dallas, Texas 75231-4596, asking for reprint No. 71-0443. The European guidelines are closely in agreement with the U.S. guidelines.

> There is rapidly growing literature showing that measurements taken by patients at home are often lower than readings taken in the office and closer to the average BP recorded by 24-hour ambulatory monitors, which is the BP that best predicts cardiovascular risk. Because of the larger numbers of readings that can be taken by HBPM than in the office and the elimination of the white-coat effect (the increase of BP during an office visit), home readings are more reproducible than office readings and show better correlations with measures of target organ damage. In addition, prospective studies that have used multiple home readings to express the true BP have found that home BP predicts risk better than office BP.

These recommendations are made:

- HBPM should become a routine component of BP measurement in the majority of patients with known or suspected hypertension.
- Patients should be advised to purchase oscillometric monitors that measure BP on the upper arm with an appropriate cuff size and that have been shown to be accurate according to the standard international protocols. They should be shown how to use them by their health care providers.
- Two to three readings should be taken while the subject is resting in the seated position, both in the

morning and at night, over a period of 1 week. A total of ≥12 readings are recommended for making clinical decisions.
- HBPM is indicated in patients with newly diagnosed or suspected hypertension, in whom it may distinguish between white-coat and sustained hypertension. In patients with prehypertension, HBPM may be useful for detecting masked hypertension.
- HBPM is recommended for evaluating the response to any type of antihypertensive treatment and may improve adherence.
- The target HBPM goal for treatment is less than 135/85 mm Hg or less than 130/80 mm Hg in high-risk patients.
- HBPM is useful in the elderly, in whom both BP variability and the white-coat effect are increased; in patients with diabetes, in whom tight BP control is of paramount importance; and in pregnant women, children, and patients with kidney disease.
- HPBM has the potential to improve the quality of care while reducing costs and should be reimbursed (Pickering et al., 2008).

This statement includes a table amplifying the recommendations. Many of these are found in Table 2-3, all of which are also applicable to home monitoring. Some points particular to home monitoring are listed in Table 2-4.

These references provide the evidence for the usefulness of home monitoring:

- *Diagnosis*: Kawabe and Saits (2007), Padfield and Parati (2007), Stergiou and Parati, (2007), and Verberk et al. (2006a)
- *Prognosis*: Asayama et al. (2004) and Bobrie et al. (2004)
- *Treatment*: Green et al. (2008), Obara et al. (2008), Cuspidi and Sala (2008), Staessen et al. (2004), and Verberk et al. (2007)
- *Cost-effectiveness*: Fukunaga et al. (2008)
- *Telematic connection*: Bobrie et al. (2007) and Palmas et al. (2008)

A few patients cannot overcome their anxiety over measuring their own BP, a continuing alerting reaction. Others become overly concerned, despite prior advice, over a significantly high reading. For a few, the stress is beyond the value, and they should be advised to give the device to a relative or sell it to a neighbor.

TABLE 2.4	**Additional Recommendations for Home BP Monitoring**

Equipment
- Use a fully automated battery-operated device that has been validated (access www. dableducational.org)
- Use an upper arm cuff that is appropriate to the size of the arm. Most commercially available home devices include only a small adult cuff but provide access to a larger cuff if needed

Measurement
- *Initial measurements*: Use a 7-day measurement period with two to three measurements each morning and two to three measurements in the evening at prestipulated times (an average of 12 morning and 12 evening measurements). Exclude the first-day measurements from the analyses to remove the alerting reaction. If any symptoms of postural hypotension are noted, take readings after 5 min supine, immediately, and 2 min after unsupported standing
- *Dose-titration phase* (*titration of initial dose and adjustment of therapy*): All measurements should be made under identical conditions and at the same times of day as the initial values. HBPM data should be ascertained before medication taken in the early morning to evaluate the morning surge and again at night to ensure persistence of control. Use the average of BPs measured after 2–4 weeks to assess the effect of treatment
- *Long-term observation*: For stable normotensive (controlled) patients, patients should conduct HBPM a minimum of 1 week per quarter (an average of 12 morning and evening measurements under conditions described above). Measurements should be made more frequently in patients with poor compliance

Target blood pressure
- Most readings at or below 135/85 mm Hg for uncomplicated hypertension
- If diabetes, chronic renal disease, or coronary heart disease, most readings should be at or below 130/80 mm Hg
- If multiple readings are above 140/90 mm Hg, contact the health care provider
- If multiple readings are below 110/70 mm Hg or if symptoms of postural hypertension are noted, contact the health care provider

AMBULATORY MONITORING

ABPM has been available for over 30 years and was shown to have prognostic value in 1983 (Perloff et al., 1983). A steadily growing literature has attested to its value, the lead position taken by O'Brien (2008). He concludes his 2008 paper thusly:

> Every patient suspected of having hypertension should have ABPM to confirm or refute the diagnosis, and every patient with uncontrolled hypertension should have ABPM repeated as necessary until 24-hour control of BP is achieved.

O'Brien is not alone in his enthusiasm. Floras (2007) stated: "Blood pressure measurement is one of the few areas of medical practice where patients in the twenty-first century are assessed almost universally using a methodology developed in the nineteenth." O'Brien (2008) provides a detailed comparison of the qualities of the three techniques of BP measurement which has been extensively shrunken into Table 2-5. As is obvious, ABPM is as good as or better than office and home techniques except in cost. That quality has played a major role in restricting the use of ABPM in the United States. Despite (or because of) the extravagantly expensive cost of health care in the United States, third party payers will not cover the actual expense of ABPM, much less provide a profit to those who use it.

Though many espouse its greater use—even making it routine—Palatini (2008) has provided a much-needed reality check, stating:

> When a new diagnostic procedure becomes available, the most efficient match between the new technology and the patients' needs must be determined. Given the relatively high cost of routine ABPM application, advocating screening requires cost-effectiveness studies, which are largely missing. No trial has been designed to investigate whether a strategy based on ABPM is more cost-effective than a strategy based on multiple OBP and home BP readings.

TABLE 2.5	Relative Qualities of BP Measuring Techniques		
	Office	Home	Ambulatory
Cost	+	++	–
Need for training	–	+	+
Accuracy	–	+	++
Identification of WCH	–	+	+
Identification of masked HT	–	+	+
Nocturnal readings	–	–	++
Prognostic ability	+	++	++
Recognition of control	–	+	+
Nocturnal	–	–	+
Morning surge	–	+	+
Excessive lowering	–	+	+
Resistance	–	+	+
Improve adherence	–	+	?

–, less favorable; +, favorable; ++, greatly favorable.
Modified from O'Brien E. Ambulatory blood pressure measurement: the case for implementation in primary care. *Hypertension* 2008; 51:1435–1441.

The one clear advantage of ABPM is its unique ability to measure nocturnal BP, the measure reported to be most accurate for prognosis (Boggia et al., 2007; Fagard et al., 2008) (Table 2.6). Unfortunately, the diagnostic thresholds for optimal, normal, and high BP with ABPM remain in question (Hansen et al., 2008) (Table 2.7). The use of appropriate mathematical models may improve the value of ABPM (Parati et al., 2008b).

All in all, the debate seems increasingly irrelevant. With the costs of health care exploding, even in countries with a national system, the wider application of a more costly technology which lacks unique qualities seems unlikely. The algorithm provided by Pickering et al (2008) (Fig. 2-7) places ABPM at the bottom of the scheme for evaluating the need for therapy, which is one of the major uses of all BP measurements.

Despite issues about its wider use in clinical practice, ABPM is unquestionably the best way to evaluate the efficacy of new antihypertensive agents (Mancia & Parati, 2004).

Schema for Evaluating Need for Treatment

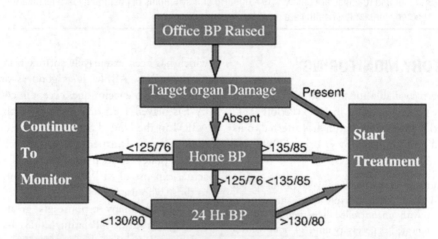

FIGURE 2-7   Schema for evaluating BP status of hypertensive patients, which can be used in patients in whom the decision to start treatment may be uncertain on the basis of the office BP, which may be just above or below the cutoff point defining adequate control. HBPM may be used to aid the diagnosis if necessary in conjunction with ABPM. (Modified from Pickering TG, Miller NH, Ogedegbe G, et al. Call to Action on use and reimbursement for home blood pressure monitoring: A joint scientific statement from the American Heart Association, American Society of Hypertension, and Preventive Cardiovascular Nurses Association. *Hypertension* 2008;52:10–29.) (Reprinted with permission.)

TABLE 2.6	Situations where ABPM is Helpful

Excluding WCH in patients with office hypertension but no
    target organ damage
Deciding on treatment of elderly patients
Identifying nocturnal hypertension (dipping status)
Assessing apparent resistance to therapy
Assuring efficacy of treatment over entire 24 h
Managing hypertension during pregnancy
Evaluating hypotension and episodic hypertension

TABLE 2.7	Recommended Thresholds for ABPM in Adults		
	Optimal	**Normal**	**Abnormal**
Awake	<130/80	<135/85	>140/90
Asleep	<115/65	<120/70	>125/75

Adapted from O'Brien E, Asmar R, Beilin L, et al. European Society of Hypertension recommendations for conventional, ambulatory, and home blood pressure measurement. *J Hypertens* 2003;21:821–848.

CENTRAL BLOOD PRESSURE

Beyond ABPM, a newer technique may be moving from investigation into clinical practice: Measurement of central BP, noninvasively, using a number of commercially available devices (Agabiti-Rosei et al., 2007). Most recent studies have utilized a high-fidelity micromanometer to record radial artery waveforms, using a generalized transfer function to generate a corresponding central (ascending aortic) pressure waveform (Fig. 2-8). The Sphygmocor device was used in clinical studies which first documented better prognostic accuracy (Roman et al., 2007) and the reason for differing therapeutic response (Williams et al., 2006) with central BP over peripheral measurement.

A detailed description of pulse wave reflections and velocity, arterial stiffness, and much more about this emerging area of hypertension is provided in Chapter 3. For now, measurement of central BP will remain an interesting investigative tool but will likely not move into clinical practice since much of the information it provides is provided by pulse pressure and other measures of arterial stiffness (Waldstein et al., 2008). Nonetheless, as the cost of the equipment (now about $15,000) comes down and proof of its superiority over peripheral (brachial) measurements becomes even more persuasive (Franklin, 2008; Najjar et al., 2008; Pini et al., 2008), measurement of central BP may be the next advance in clinical hypertension.

Heart Rate

With all the deserved attention to BP measurements, the heart rate and its variability have been shown to add to the assessment of cardiovascular risk (Palatini et al., 2008).

CONCLUSION

Despite all the reasons that home and ambulatory measurements are better than office readings, for now office sphygmomanometry will continue to be the primary tool for diagnosing and monitoring hypertension. Home readings are being more widely used, both to confirm the diagnosis and to provide better assurance of appropriate therapy. Ambulatory monitoring should be increasingly used to look for WCH, to evaluate the apparent resistance to therapy, and to determine the adequacy of therapy, particularly during sleep and the early morning hours. Central BP measurement may become the next major advance.

We next turn to the mechanisms responsible for elevated BP in 90% of those with hypertension, i.e., those with primary (essential) hypertension.

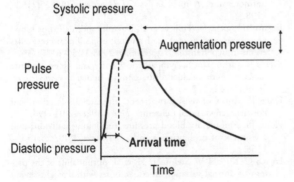

FIGURE 2-8 Central pressure waveform. The height of the late systolic peak above the inflection defines the augmented pressure, and the ratio of augmented pressure to PP defines the augmentation index (in percentage). (Reprinted from Agabiti-Rosei E, Mancia G, O'Rourke MF, et al. Central blood pressure measurements and antihypertensive therapy: A consensus document. *Hypertension* 2007;50:154–160, with permission.)

REFERENCES

Agabiti-Rosei E, Mancia G, O'Rourke MF, et al. Central blood pressure measurements and antihypertensive therapy: A consensus document. *Hypertension* 2007;50:154–160.

Agarwal R, Bunaye Z, Bekele DM. Prognostic significance between-arm blood pressure differences. *Hypertension* 2008; 51:657–662.

Al-Tamer YY, Al-Hayali JMT, Al-Ramadhan EAH. Seasonality of hypertension. *J Clin Hypertens (Greenwich)* 2008;10:125–129.

Asayama K, Ohkubo T, Kikuya M, et al. Prediction of stroke by self-measurement of blood pressure at home versus casual screening blood pressure measurement in relation to the joint national committee 7 classification: The Ohasaha study. *Stroke* 2004;35:2356–2361.

Aylett M, Marples G, Jones K, et al. Evaluation of normal and large sphygmomanometer cuffs using the Omron 705CP. *J Hum Hypertens* 2001;15:131–134.

Baguet J-P, Levy P, Barone-Rochette G, et al. Masked hypertension in obstructive sleep apnea syndrome. *J Hypertens* 2008;26: 885–892.

Bakx C, Oeriemans G, van den Hoogen H, et al. The influence of cuff size on blood pressure measurement. *J Hum Hypertens* 1997;11(7):439–445.

Bankir L, Bochud M, Maillard M, et al. Nighttime blood pressure and nocturnal dipping are associated with daytime urinary sodium excretion in African subjects. *Hypertension* 2008; 51:891–898.

Ben-Dov IZ, Kark JD, Mekler J, et al. The white coat phenomenon is benign in referred treated patients: A 14-year ambulatory blood pressure mortality study. *J Hypertens* 2008;26: 699–705.

Bilo G, Giglio A, Styczkiewicz K, et al. A new method for assessing 24-h blood pressure variability after excluding the contribution of nocturnal blood pressure fall. *J Hypertens* 2007;25:2058–2066.

Björklund K, Lind L, Andren B, et al. The majority of nondipping men do not have increased cardiovascular risk: A population-based study. *J Hypertens* 2002;20:1501–1506.

Bobrie G, Clerson P, Ménard J, et al. Masked hypertension: A systematic review. *J Hypertens* 2008;26:1715–1725.

Bobrie T, Postel-Vinay N, Delonca J, et al. Self-measurement and self-titration in hypertension: A pilot telemedicine study. *Am J Hypertens* 2007;20:1314–1320.

Boggia J, Li Y, Thijs L, et al. Prognostic accuracy of day versus night ambulatory blood pressure: A cohort study. *Lancet* 2007;370:1219–1229.

Bornstein NM, Norris JW. Subclavian steal: A harmless haemodynamic phenomenon? *Lancet* 1986;2:303–305.

Bos WJW, van Goudoever J, van Montfrans GA, et al. Influence of short-term blood pressure variability on blood pressure determinations. *Hypertension* 1992;19:606–609.

Brennan M, O'Brien E, O'Malley K. The effect of age on blood pressure and heart rate variability in hypertension. *J Hypertens* 1986;4(Suppl. 6):S269–S272.

Bursztyn M, Ginsberg, G, Hammerman-Rozenberg R, et al. The siesta in the elderly: Risk factor for mortality? *Arch Intern Med* 1999;159:1582–1586.

Casiglia E, Palatini P, Colangeli G, et al. 24 h rhythm of blood pressure and forearm peripheral resistance in normotensive and hypertensive subjects confined to bed. *J Hypertens* 1996;14: 47–52.

Cavelaars M, Tulen JHM, van Bemmel JH, et al. Physical activity, dipping and haemodynamics. *J Hypertens* 2004;22:2303–2309.

Clark LA, Denby L, Pregibon D, et al. A quantitative analysis of the effects of activity and time of day on the diurnal variations of blood pressure. *J Chronic Dis* 1987;40:671–679.

Cuspidi C, Parati G. Masked hypertension: An independent predictor of organ damage. *J Hypertens* 2007;25:275–279.

Cuspidi C, Sala C. Home blood pressure measurement: A means for improving blood pressure control? *J Hum Hypertens* 2008; 22:159–162.

Cuspidi C, Meani S, Sala C, et al. How reliable is isolated clinical hypertension defined by a single 24-h ambulatory blood pressure monitoring? *J Hypertens* 2007;25:315–320.

Cuspidi C, Meani S, Salerno M, et al. Cardiovascular target organ damage in essential hypertensives with or without reproducible nocturnal fall in blood pressure. *J Hypertens* 2004;22: 273–280.

De Mey C. Method specificity of the auscultatory estimates of the inodilatory reduction of diastolic blood pressure based on Korotkoff IV and V criteria. *Br J Clin Pharmacol* 1995;39: 485–490.

De Simone G, Schillaci G, Chinali M, et al. Estimate of white-coat effect and arterial stiffness. *J Hypertens* 2007;25:827–831.

Den Hond E, Celis H, Fagard R, et al. Self-measured versus ambulatory blood pressure in the diagnosis of hypertension. *J Hypertens* 2003;21:717–722.

Dewar R, Sykes D, Mulkerrin E, et al. The effect of hemiplegia on blood pressure measurement in the elderly. *Postgrad Med J* 1992;68:888–891.

Dodt C, Breckling U, Derad I, et al. Plasma epinephrine and norepinephrine concentrations of healthy humans associated with nighttime sleep and morning arousal. *Hypertension* 1997;30:71–76.

Dolan E, Stanton A, Atkins N, et al. Determinanats of white-coat hypertension. *Blood Press Monit* 2004;9:307–309.

Dorigatti F, Bonso E, Saladini F, et al. Validation of the visocor HM40 wrist blood pressure measuring devise according to the International Protocol. *Blood Press Monit* 2009;14:83–86.

Eguchi K, Yacoub M, Jhalani J, et al. Consistency of blood pressure differences between the left and right arms. *Arch Intern Med* 2007;167:388–393.

Enström I, Pennert K, Lindholm LH. Difference in blood pressure, but not in heart rate, between measurements performed at a health centre and at a hospital by one and the same physician. *J Hum Hypertens* 2000;14:355–358.

Fagard RH, Cornelissen VA. Incidence of cardiovascular events in white-coat, masked and sustained hypertension versus true normotension: A meta-analysis. *J Hypertens* 2007;25:2193–2198.

Fagard RH, Celis H, Thijs L, et al. Daytime and nighttime blood pressure as predictors of death and cause-specific cardiovascular events in hypertension. *Hypertension* 2008;51:55–61.

Faguis J, Karhuvaara S. Sympathetic activity and blood pressure increases with bladder distension in humans. *Hypertension* 1989;14:511–517.

Floras JS. Antihypertensive treatment, myocardial infarction, and nocturnal myocardial ischaemia. *Lancet* 1988;2:994–996.

Floras JS. Ambulatory blood pressure: Facilitating individualized assessment of cardiovascular risk. *J Hypertens* 2007;25:1565–1568.

Foerch C, Korf H-W, Steinmetz H, et al. Abrupt shift of the pattern of diurnal variation in stroke onset with daylight saving time transitions. *Circulation* 2008;118:284–290.

Franklin SS. Beyond blood pressure: Arterial stiffness as a new biomarker of cardiovascular disease. *J Am Soc Hypertens* 2008;2(3): 140–151.

Fukuda M, Munemura M, Usami T, et al. Nocturnal blood pressure is elevated with natriuresis and proteinuria as renal function deteriorates in nephropathy. *Kidney Int* 2004;65: 621–625.

Fukunaga H, Ohkubo T, Kobayashi M, et al. Cost-effectiveness of the introduction of home blood pressure measurement in patients with office hypertension. *J Hypertens* 2008;26:685–690.

Gosse P, Lasserre R, Minifié C, et al. Blood pressure surge on rising. *J Hypertens* 2004;22:1113–1118.

Grassi G, Seravalle G, Trevano FQ, et al. Neurogenic abnormalities in masked hypertension. *Hypertension* 2007;50:537–542.

Graves JW, Sheps SG. Does evidence-based medicine suggest that physicians should not be measuring blood pressure in the hypertensive patient? *Am J Hypertens* 2004;17:354–360.

Green BB, Cook AJ, Ralston JD, et al. Effectiveness of home blood pressure monitoring, web communication, and pharmacist care on hypertension control: A randomized controlled trial. *JAMA* 2008;299(24):2857–2867.

Groppelli A, Giorgi DMA, Omboni S, et al. Persistent blood pressure increase induced by heavy smoking. *J Hypertens* 1992; 10:495–499.

Gupta V, Lipsitz LA. Orthostatic hypotension in the elderly: Diagnosis and treatment. *Am J Med* 2007;120:841–847.

Gupta MP, Polena S, Coplan N, et al. Prognostic significance of systolic blood pressure increases in men during exercised stress testing. *Am J Cardiol* 2007;100:1609–1613.

Hansen TW, Kikuya M, Thijs L, et al. Diagnostic thresholds for ambulatory blood pressure moving lower: A review based on a meta-analysis—clinical implications. *J Clin Hypertens (Greenwich)* 2008;10:377–381.

Hartley TR, Lovallo WR, Whitsett TL. Cardiovascular effects of caffeine in men and women. *Am J Cardiol* 2004;93:1022–1026.

Henskens LH, Kroon AA, van Oostenbrugge RJ, et al. Different classifications of nocturnal blood pressure dipping affect the prevalence of dippers and nondippers and the relation with target-organ damage. *J Hypertens* 2008;26:691–698.

Hermida RC, Ayala DE, Fernandez JR, et al. Chronotherapy improves blood pressure control and reverts the nondipper pattern in patients with resistant hypertension. *Hypertension* 2008;51:69–76.

Higashi Y, Nakagawa K, Kimura M, et al. Circadian variation of blood pressure and endothelial function in patients with essential hypertension: A comparison of dippers and non-dippers. *J Am Coll Cardiol* 2002;40:2039–2043.

Hugue CJ, Safar ME, Aliefierakis MC, et al. The ratio between ankle and brachial systolic pressure in patients with sustained uncomplicated essential hypertension. *Clin Sci* 1988;74: 179–182.

Hyman DJ, Ogbonnaya K, Taylor AA, et al. Ethnic differences in nocturnal blood pressure decline in treated hypertensives. *Am J Hypertens* 2000;13:884–891.

Jankowski P, Kawecka-Jaszcz K, Czarnecka D, et al. Pulsatile but not steady component of blood pressure predicts cardiovascular events in coronary patients. *Hypertension* 2008;51: 848–855.

Jehn ML, Brotman DJ, Appel LJ. Racial differences in diurnal blood pressure and heart rate patterns: Results from the dietary approaches to stop hypertension (DASH) trial. *Arch Intern Med* 2008;168(9):996–1002.

Jumabay M, Ozawa Y, Kawamura H, et al. White coat hypertension in centenarians. *Am J Hypertens* 2005;18:1040–1045.

Kario K, Matsuo T, Kobayashi H, et al. Nocturnal fall of blood pressure and silent cerebrovascular damage in elderly hypertensive patients. *Hypertension* 1996;27:130–135.

Kario K, Matsui Y, Shibasaki S, et al. An α-adrenergic blocker titrated by self-measured blood pressure recordings lowered blood pressure and microalbumineria in patients with morning hypertension: the Japan morning surge-1 study. *J Hypertens* 2008;26:1257–1265.

Kario K, Pickering TG, Umeda Y, et al. Morning surge in blood pressure as a predictor of silent and clinical cerebrovascular disease in elderly hypertensives: A prospective study. *Circulation* 2003;107:1401–1406.

Kario K, Shimada K, Schwartz JE, et al. Silent and clinically overt stroke in older Japanese subjects with white-coat and sustained hypertension. *J Am Coll Cardiol* 2001;38:238–245.

Kawabe H, Saito I. Which measurement of home blood pressure should be used for clinical evaluation when multiple measurements are made? *J Hypertens* 2007;25:1369–1374.

Keenan K, Haven A, Neal BC, et al. Long term monitoring in patients receiving treatment to low blood pressure: Analysis of data from placebo controlled randomised controlled trial. *BMJ* 2009;338:b1492.

Kimura A, Hashimoto J, Watabe D, et al. Patient characteristics and factors associated with inter-arm difference of blood pressure measurements in a general population in Ohasama, Japan. *J Hypertens* 2004;22:2277–2283.

Kotsis V, Stabouli S, Bouldin M, et al. Impact of obesity on 24-hour ambulatory blood pressure and hypertension. *Hypertension* 2005;45:602–607.

Lane D, Beevers M, Barnes N, et al. Inter-arm differences in blood pressure: When are they clinically significant? *J Hypertens* 2002;20:1089–1095.

Laukkanen JA, Kurl S, Salonen R, et al. Systolic blood pressure during recovery from exercise and the risk of acute myocardial infarction in middle-aged men. *Hypertension* 2004;44: 820–825.

Le Pailleur C, Helft G, Landais P, et al. The effects of talking, reading, and silence on the "white coat" phenomenon in hypertensive patients. *Am J Hypertens* 1998;11:203–207.

Leary AC, Struthers AD, Donnan PT, et al. The morning surge in blood pressure and heart rate is dependent on levels of physical activity after waking. *J Hypertens* 2002;20:865–870.

Leitão CB, Canani LH, Kramer CK, et al. Masked hypertension, urinary albumin excretion rate, and echocardiographic parameters in putatively normotensive type 2 diabetic patients. *Diabetes Care* 2007;30:1255–1260.

Lip GYH, Zarifis J, Beevers DG. Blood pressure monitoring in atrial fibrillation using electronic devices. *Arch Intern Med* 2001;161:294.

Little P, Barnett J, Barnsley L, et al. Comparison of agreement between different measures of blood pressure in primary care and daytime ambulatory blood pressure. *Br Med J* 2002; 325:254–257.

Lurbe E, Torro I, Alvarez V, et al. Prevalence, persistence, and clinical significance of masked hypertension in youth. *Hypertension* 2005;45:493–498.

Mallion JM, Genes N, Vaur L, et al. Detection of masked hypertension by home blood pressure measurement: Is the number of measurements an important issue? *Blood Press Monit* 2004;9:301–305.

Mancia G, Parati G. Office compared with ambulatory blood pressure in assessing response to antihypertensive treatment: A meta-analysis. *J Hypertens* 2004;22:435–445.

Mancia G, Bombelli M, Facchetti R, et al. Long-term risk of sustained hypertension in white-coat or masked hypertension. *J Hypertens* 2009;54:226–232.

Mancia G, Parati G, Pomidossi G, et al. Alerting reaction and rise in blood pressure during measurement by physician and nurse. *Hypertension* 1987;9:209–215.

Mancia G, Sega R, Milesi C, et al. Blood pressure control in the hypertensive population. *Lancet* 1997;349:454–457.

Manfredini R, Portaluppi F, Salmi R, et al. Circadian variation in onset of epistaxis. *Br Med J* 2000;321:11–12.

Manfredini R, Portaluppi F, Zamboni P, et al. Circadian variation in spontaneous rupture of abdominal aorta. *Lancet* 1999; 353:643–644.

Mansoor GA, McCabe EJ, White WB. Determinants of the white-coat effect in hypertensive subjects. *J Hum Hypertens* 1996; 10:87–92.

Marfella R, Siniscalchi M, Portoghese M, et al. Morning blood pressure surge as a destabilizing factor of atherosclerotic plaque: Role of ubiquitin—proteasome activity. *Hypertension* 2007; 49:784–791.

Matthews KA, Kamarck TW, Hall MH, et al. Blood pressure dipping and sleep disturbance in African-American and Caucasian men and women. *Am J Hypertens* 2008;21:826–831.

Matthys J, De Meyere M, Mervielde I, et al. Influence of the presence of doctors-in-training on the blood pressure of patients: A randomised controlled trial in 22 teaching practices. *J Hum Hypertens* 2004;18:769–773.

Mitka M. Many physician practices fall short on accurate blood pressure measurement. *JAMA* 2008;299(24):2842–2843.

Miyai N, Arita M, Morioka I, et al. Exercise BP response in subjects with high-normal BP. *J Am Coll Cardiol* 2000;36:1626–1631.

Møller DS, Dideriksen A, Sørensen S, et al. Accuracy of telemedical home blood pressure measurement in the diagnosis of hypertension. *J Hum Hypertens* 2003;17:549–554.

Muller JE. Circadian variation in cardiovascular events. *Am J Hypertens* 1999;12:35S–42S.

Myers MG, Valdivieso M, Kiss A. Use of automated office blood pressure measurement to reduce the white coat response. *J Hypertens* 2009;27:280–286.

Najjar SS, Scuteri A, Shetty V, et al. Pulse wave velocity is an independent predictor of the longitudinal increase in systolic blood pressure and of incident hypertension in the Baltimore Longitudinal Study of Aging. *J Am Coll Cardiol* 2008;51:1377–1383.

Netea RT, Lenders JW, Smits P, et al. Influence of body and arm position on blood pressure readings: An overview. *J Hypertens* 2003;21:237–241.

Niyonsenga T, Vanasse A, Courteau J, et al. Impact of terminal digit preference by family physicians and sphygmomanometer calibration errors on blood pressure value: Implication for hypertension screening. *J Clin Hypertens (Greenwich)* 2008;10:341–347.

O'Brien E. Ambulatory blood pressure measurement: the case for implementation in primary care. *Hypertension* 2008;51:1435–1441.

O'Brien E, Asmar R, Beilin L, et al. European Society of Hypertension recommendations for conventional, ambulatory and home blood pressure measurement. *J Hypertens* 2003;21:821–848.

Obara T, Ohkubo T, Asayama K, et al. Home blood pressure measurements associated with better blood pressure control: The J-HOME study. *J Hum Hypertens* 2008;22:197–204.

Ogedegbe G, Pickering TG, Clemow L, et al. The misdiagnosis of hypertension: The role of patient anxiety. *Arch Intern Med* 2008;168:2459–2465.

Padfield PL, Parati G. Home blood pressure monitoring in clinical practice: How many measurements and when? *J Hypertens* 2007;25:1337–1339.

Palatini P. Ambulatory blood pressure monitoring in clinical practice: Is being superior good enough? *J Hypertens* 2008;26:1300–1302.

Palatini P, Palomba D, Bertolo O, et al. The white-coat effect is unrelated to the difference between clinic and daytime blood pressure and is associated with greater reactivity to public speaking. *J Hypertens* 2003;21:545–553.

Palatini P, Parati G, Julius S. Office and out of office heart rate measurements: Which clinical value? *J Hypertens* 2008;26:1540–1545.

Palatini P, Winnicki M, Santonastaso M, et al. Prevalence and clinical significance of isolated ambulatory hypertension in young subjects screened for stage 1 hypertension. *Hypertension* 2004;44:170–174.

Palmas W, Pickering TG, Teresi J, et al. Telemedicine home blood pressure measurements and progression of albuminuria in elderly people with diabetes. *Hypertension* 2008;1282–1288.

Panza JA, Epstein SE, Quyyumi AA. Circadian variation in vascular tone and its relation to alpha-sympathetic vasoconstrictor activity. *N Engl J Med* 1991;325:986–990.

Parati G, Mancia G. Hypertension staging through ambulatory blood pressure monitoring. *Hypertension* 2002;40:792–794.

Parati G, Stergiou GS, Asmar R, et al. European society of hypertension guidelines for blood pressure monitoring at home: A summary report of the Second International Consensus Conference on home blood pressure monitoring. *J Hypertens* 2008a;26:1505–1530.

Parati G, Vrijens B, Vincze G. Analysis and interpretation of 24-h blood pressure profiles: Appropriate mathematical models may yield deeper understanding. *Am J Hypertens* 2008b;21(2):123–125.

Park MK, Menard SW, Yuan C. Comparison of auscultatory and oscillometric blood pressures. *Arch Pediatr Adolesc Med* 2001;155:50–53.

Pasic J, Shapiro D, Motivala S, et al. Blood pressure morning surge and hostility. *Am J Hypertens* 1998;11:245–250.

Peckova M, Fahrenbruch CE, Cobb LA, et al. Circadian variations in the occurrence of cardiac arrests. *Circulation* 1998;98:31–39.

Peixoto AJ, White WB. Circadian blood pressure: Clinical implications based on the pathophysiology of its variability. *Kidney Int* 2007;71:855–860.

Pelttari LH, Hietanen EK, Salo TT, et al. Little effect of ordinary antihypertensive therapy on nocturnal high blood pressure in patients with sleep disordered breathing. *Am J Hypertens* 1998;11:272–279.

Perk G, Ben-Arie L, Mekler J, et al. Dipping status may be determined by nocturnal urination. *Hypertension* 2001;37:749–752.

Perloff D, Sokolow M, Cowan R. The prognostic value of ambulatory blood pressure. *JAMA* 1983;249(20):2792–2798.

Pickering TG. White coat hypertension. *Curr Opin Nephrol Hypertens* 1996;5:192–198.

Pickering TG. Should doctors still measure blood pressure? *J Clin Hypertens* 2006;8(6):394–396.

Pickering TG. Ambulatory blood pressure and diseases of the eye: Can low nocturnal blood pressure be harmful? *J Clin Hypertens* 2008;10(5):411–414.

Pickering TG, Coats A, Mallion JM, et al. White-coat hypertension. *Blood Press Monit* 1999;4:333–341.

Pickering TG, James GD, Boddie C, et al. How common is white coat hypertension? *JAMA* 1988;259:225–228.

Pickering TG, Miller NH, Ogedegbe G, et al. Call to action on use and reimbursement for home blood pressure monitoring: A joint scientific statement from the American Heart Association, American Society of Hypertension, and Preventive Cardiovascular Nurses Association. *Hypertension* 2008;52:10–29.

Pierdomenico SD, Bucci A, Costantini F, et al. Circadian blood pressure changes and myocardial ischemia in hypertensive patients with coronary artery disease. *J Am Coll Cardiol* 1998;31:1627–1634.

Pierdomenico SD, Lapenna D, Di Mascio R, et al. Short- and long-term risk of cardiovascular events in white-coat hypertension. *J Hum Hypertens* 2008;22:408–414.

Pini R, Cavallini MC, Palmieri V, et al. Central but not brachial blood pressure predicts cardiovascular events in an unselected geriatric population. *J Am Coll Cardiol* 2008;51:2432–2439.

Puato M, Palatini P, Zanardo M, et al. Increase in carotid intima-media thickness in grade I hypertensive subjects: White-coat versus sustained hypertension. *Hypertension* 2008;51:1300–1305.

Ragot S, Herpin D, Siché JP, et al. Relationship between short-term and long-term blood pressure variabilities in essential hypertensives. *J Hum Hypertens* 2001;15:41–48.

Redon J, Lurbe E. Nocturnal blood pressure versus nondipping pattern: What do they mean? *Hypertension* 2008;51:41–42.

Redon J, Campos C, Narciso ML, et al. Prognostic value of ambulatory blood pressure monitoring in refractory hypertension. *Hypertension* 1998;31:712–718.

Redon J, Roca-Cusachs A, Mora-Macia J. Uncontrolled early morning blood pressure in medicated patients: The ACAMPA study. *Blood Press Monit* 2002;7:111–116.

Reeves RA. Does this patient have hypertension? *JAMA* 1995; 273:1211–1218.

Rizzoni D, Porteri E, Platto C, et al. Morning rise of blood pressure and subcutaneous small resistance artery structure. *J Hypertens* 2007;25:1698–1703.

Roman MJ, Devereux RB, Kizer JR, et al. Central pressure more strongly relates to vascular disease and outcome than does brachial pressure: the strong heart study. *Hypertension* 2007; 50:197–203.

Sayk F, Becker C, Teckentrup C, et al. To dip or not to dip: On the physiology of blood pressure decrease during nocturnal sleep in healthy humans. *Hypertension* 2007;49:1070–1076.

Shintani Y, Kikuya M, Hara A, et al. Ambulatory blood pressure, blood pressure variability and the prevalence of carotid artery alteration: The Ohasama study. *J Hypertens* 2007;25:1704–1710.

Silke B, McAuley D. Accuracy and precision of blood pressure determination with the Finapres. *J Hum Hypertens* 1998;12:403–409.

Smith NL, Psaty BM, Rutan GH, et al. The association between time since last meal and blood pressure in older adults: The cardiovascular health study. *J Am Geriatr Soc* 2003;51:824–828.

Soo LH, Gray D, Young T, et al. Circadian variation in witnessed out of hospital cardiac arrest. *Heart* 2000;84:370–376.

Spence JD. Pseudo-hypertension in the elderly. *J Hum Hypertens* 1997;11:621–623.

Staessen JA, Bieniaszewski L, O'Brien E, et al. Nocturnal blood pressure fall on ambulatory monitoring in a large international database. *Hypertension* 1997;29:30–39.

Staessen JA, Hond ED, Celis H, et al. Antihypertensive treatment based on blood pressure measurement at home or in the physician's office: A randomized controlled trial. *JAMA* 2004; 291:955–964.

Stergiou GS, Parati G. The optimal schedule for self-monitoring of blood pressure by patients at home. *J Hypertens* 2007;25:1992–1997.

Tatasciore A, Renda G, Zimarino M, et al. Awake systolic blood pressure variability correlates with target-organ damage in hypertensive subjects. *Hypertension* 2007;50:325–332.

Tsivgoulis G, Vemmos KN, Zakopoulos N, et al. Asssociation of blunted nocturnal blood pressure dip with intracerebral hemorrhage. *Blood Press Monit* 2005;10:189–195.

Uzu T, Fujii T, Nishimura M, et al. Determinants in circadian blood pressure rhythm in essential hypertension. *Am J Hypertens* 1999;12:35–39.

Van Boxtel MPJ, Gaillard C, Houx PJ, et al. Is nondipping in 24 h ambulatory blood pressure related to cognitive dysfunction? *J Hypertens* 1998;16:1425–1432.

Van Durme DJ, Goldstein M, Pal N, et al. The accuracy of community-based automated blood pressure machines. *J Fam Pract* 2000;49:449–452.

Verberk WJ, Kroon AA, Kessels AGH, et al. The optimal scheme of self blood pressure measurement as determined from ambulatory blood pressure recordings. *J Hypertens* 2006a;24:1541–1548.

Verberk WJ, Kroon AA, Lenders JWM, et al. Self-measurement of blood pressure at home reduces the need for antihypertensive drugs: a randomized, controlled trial. *Hypertension* 2007;50:1019–1025.

Verberk WJ, Kroon AA, Thien T, et al. Prevalence of the white-coat effect at multiple visits before and during treatment. *J Hypertens* 2006b;24:2457–2463.

Verdecchia P, O'Brien E, Pickering T, et al. When can the practicing physician suspect white coat hypertension? Statement from the Working Group on Blood Pressure Monitoring of the European Society of Hypertension. *Am J Hypertens* 2003; 16:87–91.

Verdecchia P, Palatini P, Schillaci G, et al. Independent predictors of isolated clinic ("white-coat") hypertension. *J Hypertens* 2001; 19:1015–1020.

Verdecchia P, Reboldi GP, Angeli F, et al. Short- and long-term incidence of stroke in white-coat hypertension. *Hypertension* 2005;45:203–208.

Verdecchia P, Schillaci G, Borgioni C, et al. White coat hypertension and white coat effect. *Am J Hypertens* 1995;8:790–798.

Von Känel R, Jain S, Mills PJ, et al. Relation of nocturnal blood pressure dipping to cellular adhesion, inflammation and hemostasis. *J Hypertens* 2004;22:2087–2093.

Waldstein SR, Rice SC, Thayer JF, et al. Pulse pressure and pulse wave velocity are related to cognitive decline in the Baltimore longitudinal study of aging. *Hypertension* 2008;51:99–104.

Watson RDS, Lumb R, Young MA, et al. Variation in cuff blood pressure in untreated outpatients with mild hypertension—Implications for initiating antihypertensive treatment. *J Hypertens* 1987;5:207–211.

White WB, Larocca GM. Improving the utility of the nocturnal hypertension definition by using absolute sleep blood pressure rather than the "dipping" proportion. *Am J Cardiol* 2003; 92:1439–1441.

Williams B, Lacy PS, Thom SM, et al. Differential impact of blood pressure-lowering drugs on central aortic pressure and clinical outcomes: principal results of the Conduit Artery Function Evaluation (CAFÉ) study. *Circulation* 2006;113:1213–1225.

Williams B, Lindholm LH, Sever P. Systolic pressure is all that matters. *Lancet* 2008;371:2219–2221.

Wing LM, Brown MA, Beilin LJ, et al. 'Reverse white-coat hypertension' in older hypertensives. Second Australian National Blood Pressure Study. *J Hypertens* 2002;20:639–644.

Wizner B, Dechering DG, Thijs L, et al. Short-term and long-term repeatability of the morning blood pressure in older patients with isolated systolic hypertension. *J Hypertens* 2008;26:1328–1335.

Zweifler AJ, Shahab ST. Pseudohypertension. *J Hypertens* 1993; 11:1–6.

Primary Hypertension: Pathogenesis

D espite decades of research and debate, we still have no unifying mechanism—and thus no single therapeutic target—for primary human hypertension. A strong case can be made that neural, renal, hormonal, and vascular mechanisms are all involved and conspire in a myriad of ways to produce hypertension. In the past 4 years since the last edition of this book, significant progress has been made in each of these areas. But the new mechanistic insights have yet to alter the clinical approach to the diagnosis, treatment, and prevention of hypertension. As a result, antihypertensive drug therapy remains empirical. As will be discussed in Chapters 6 and 7, most patients will need multiple antihypertensive drugs of different classes—and ideally multiple lifestyle modifications—to counteract the multiple mechanisms suspected of causing their hypertension.

GENERAL CONSIDERATIONS

Before diving into specific theories and data, some general considerations are in order. In particular, the pathogenesis of primary hypertension has been difficult to unravel for several reasons:

• The relevance of rodent models to clinical hypertension is uncertain and methods are limited for testing mechanistic hypotheses in humans.
• The dichotomy between normotension and hypertension is arbitrary because BP is a quantitative trait, showing a continuous positive relation with cardiovascular risk (Lewington et al., 2002). Thus, many experts—beginning with Sir Thomas Pickering (Pickering, 1964) and including members of the American Society of Hypertension Working Group (Giles et al., 2005)—have argued that high BP per se is not even a disease. The same argument can be made for high serum cholesterol levels and

yet we know much more about the molecular mechanisms of hyperlipidemia than hypertension. The search for causation is not necessarily futile but it is difficult.
• The difficulty begins with taking an accurate snapshot of a person's "usual" BP. As discussed in Chapter 2, a person's BP varies more from moment to moment and from day to day than any other routine measurement in clinical medicine. The within-subject variability further blurs the distinction between normal and abnormal, between normotension and hypertension.
• BP is a complex trait influenced by both environmental factors, which are well characterized, and genetic factors, which are poorly characterized. After initial excitement over the Human Genome Project, hypertension has been far more resistant to genetic dissection than dyslipidemia and atherosclerosis. After expenditure of hundreds of millions of research dollars, many negative studies and many false-positive association studies engendered a sense of futility. But lately, a few leads have emerged, some withstanding the scrutiny of independent replication in multiple study samples.
• All clinical research designs have their limitations. Cross-sectional case-control studies of normotensives versus hypertensives have a hard time distinguishing causal mechanisms from compensatory adjustments. Once BP is even mildly elevated, other cardiovascular risk factors are also present and considerable remodeling has occurred throughout the cardiovascular system (Nesbitt et al., 2005). The horse already is out of the barn. Normotensive children of hypertensive parents offer one approach to identify pathogenic factors that precede the onset of hypertension and thus may be causal. However, these studies require large samples to detect small effects. Clinic-based studies suffer from recruitment bias for health care–seeking

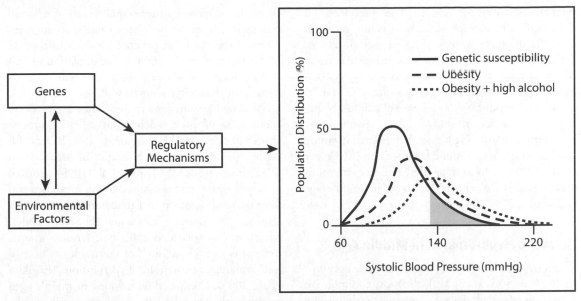

FIGURE 3-1   Interaction among genetic and environmental factors in the development of hypertension. The **left side** of the figure shows that genes and environment interact to affect multiple hypertensive mechanisms. The **right side** of the figure depicts schematically the cumulative effects of genetic and environmental factors on population-level BP, which is normally distributed. *The solid line* shows the theoretic BP distribution caused by genetic susceptibility alone; the *shaded area* indicates systolic BP in the hypertensive range. *Broken lines* and *dotted lines* indicate populations in which one (obesity) or two (obesity plus high alcohol intake) environmental factors have been added. (Modified from Carretero OA, Oparil S. Essential hypertension. *Circulation* 2000;101:329–335.)

individuals who do not reflect the greater disease burden in the general population, especially minority populations who have been underrepresented in clinical research (Victor et al., 2004). Epidemiological studies are observational by nature and do not prove causation. Too often mechanistic inferences are derived from post hoc analyses of randomized controlled drug trials that were not designed to interrogate disease mechanisms and where the sponsor had a financial or economic interest in the outcome.

• Primary hypertension can no longer be considered a single entity but rather can be subdivided into several different hemodynamic subsets, including diastolic hypertension in mainly middle-age persons and isolated systolic hypertension in mainly older persons. Obesity-related hypertension seems to be a different entity from hypertension in lean persons. More rigorously defined phenotypes hopefully will pave the way to a better mechanistic understanding of the genesis and progression of hypertension in specific segments of the population and identify individuals who can benefit from personalized medicine.

It is not possible to describe the contributions of so many past and present investigators in the confines of a single chapter. The ensuing discussion will explain basic concepts in broad strokes and, wherever possible, emphasize recent data from translational studies in human subjects. We will begin with systemic hemodynamics and then discuss disease mechanisms, human genetics, and environmental modifiers (Fig. 3-1).

HEMODYNAMIC SUBTYPES

Mounting evidence from the Framingham Heart Study investigators and others indicates that human hypertension can be divided into at least three separate hemodynamic subtypes that vary by age.

Systolic Hypertension in Young Adults

At one end of the age spectrum is isolated systolic hypertension in young adults (typically 17 to 25 years of age). The key hemodynamic abnormalities are increased cardiac output and a stiff aorta (McEniery et al., 2005), both presumably reflecting an overactive sympathetic nervous system. The prevalence is estimated to be as high as 25% in young men but only 2% in young women (McEniery et al., 2005). This may be an overestimate because brachial artery BP overestimates central aortic pressure by approximately 20 mm Hg in young adults due to peripheral pulse wave amplification (Hulsen et al., 2006). Nonetheless, in the largest study to date, central aortic pressure was 20 mm Hg higher than normal in young adults with isolated systolic hypertension (McEniery et al., 2005). A hyperdynamic circulation in youth may precede diastolic hypertension in middle age (Julius et al., 1991).

Diastolic Hypertension in Middle Age

When hypertension is diagnosed in middle age (typically 30 to 50 years of age), the most common BP pattern is elevated diastolic pressure with systolic pressure being either normal (isolated diastolic hypertension) or elevated (combined systolic/diastolic hypertension) (Franklin et al., 2005). This is classic "essential hypertension." Isolated diastolic hypertension is more common in men and often associated with middle-age weight gain (Franklin et al., 2005) and the metabolic syndrome (Franklin et al., 2006). Without treatment, isolated diastolic hypertension often progresses to combined systolic/diastolic hypertension.

The fundamental hemodynamic fault is an elevated systemic vascular resistance coupled with an inappropriately "normal" cardiac output (Staessen et al., 2003). Vasoconstriction at the level of the resistance arterioles (100 to 200 μm in diameter) results from increased neurohormonal drive and an autoregulatory reaction of vascular smooth muscle to an expanded plasma volume, the latter due to impairment in the kidneys' ability to excrete sodium (Staessen et al., 2003).

Isolated Systolic Hypertension in Older Adults

After age 55, isolated systolic hypertension (systolic BP > 140 mm Hg and diastolic BP < 90 mm Hg) is the most common form (Franklin, 2006). In developed countries, systolic pressure rises steadily with age; by contrast, diastolic pressure rises until about age 55 and then falls progressively thereafter (Burt et al., 1995). The resultant widening of pulse pressure (PP) indicates stiffening of the central aorta, reduced

aortic diameter, and a more rapid return of reflected pulse waves from the periphery, causing an augmentation of systolic aortic pressure (Agabiti-Rosei et al., 2007; Mitchell et al., 2008a). Accumulation of collagen (which is poorly distensible) adversely increases its ratio to elastin in the aortic wall.

Isolated systolic hypertension may represent an acceleration of this age-dependent stiffening process (Mitchell et al., 2007), although systolic BP and PP do not rise with age in the absence of urbanization (e.g., cloistered nuns) (Timio et al., 1999). Isolated systolic hypertension is more common in women and is a major risk factor for diastolic heart failure, which also is more common in women (Franklin, 2006). Most cases of isolated systolic hypertension arise de novo after age 60 and are not the result of "burned out" middle-age diastolic hypertension (Franklin et al., 2005). Compared with young or middle-aged adults with optimal BP, those with BP in the prehypertensive range are more likely to develop isolated systolic hypertension after age 60 (Franklin et al., 2005).

A multitude of neurohormonal, renal, and vascular mechanisms interact to varying degrees in driving these different hemodynamic patterns of hypertension.

NEURAL MECHANISMS

Overactivity of the sympathetic nervous system plays an important role in the early pathogenesis of several frequently used rat models of hypertension (Guyenet, 2006). Pioneering work by Julius et al. (1991) and others indicate that hypertension is often initiated by adrenergically driven increases in cardiac output (a "hyperdynamic" circulation), but sustained by subsequent vasoconstriction, vascular remodeling and autoregulation—leading to increased vasoconstriction with an inappropriately normal cardiac output.

Until recently, interest in sympathetic neural mechanisms of human hypertension has waned. One reason is that, compared with the renin-angiotensin-aldosterone system (RAAS), the activity of the sympathetic nervous system is harder to measure. In addition, compared with RAAS blockers, central sympatholytics and adrenergic blockers have less favorable side-effect profiles due to multiple sites of action within the central nervous system. In recent cardiovascular outcomes trials, α-blockers and β-blockers have not performed as well as other classes of antihypertensives; they are no longer considered first line therapy for uncomplicated hypertension by many experts (Chapter 7).

Yet at the cell and molecular level, norepinephrine (NE) is just as potent as angiotensin II (Ang II) in causing hypertrophy of vascular smooth muscle and cardiac muscle (Victor & Shafiq, 2008). Furthermore, sympathetic activation stimulates renin release and renal sodium retention, contributing to hypertension in numerous animal models (Guyenet, 2006). Sustained sympathetic activation has been demonstrated in several forms of human hypertension, but large gaps remain in our understanding of the precise mechanisms driving this activity and its contribution to the development and progression of hypertension. A better understanding of sympathetic neural mechanisms of human hypertension may identify more specific therapeutic targets.

Over the past few years, significant progress has been made in several areas, including: (i) primary hypertension, (ii) renal parenchymal hypertension, and (iii) obesity-related hypertension. There is increasing evidence that these hypertensive states are accompanied by sympathetic overactivity but with differences in mechanisms and patterns of sympathetic activation and in sympathetic responsiveness to specific countermeasures. Moreover, the emergence of invasive procedures for lowering sympathetic nerve activity (SNA) and BP in patients with refractory hypertension has rekindled excitement about neural mechanisms even before these procedures have been approved by the FDA. These invasive procedures are an implantable carotid sinus pacemaker (Mohaupt et al., 2007) and catheter-based radiofrequency ablation of the renal sympathetic nerves (Krum et al., 2009).

Renal parenchymal hypertension will be covered in Chapter 9. Obesity-related hypertension has become such an important topic that it merits a separate discussion later in this chapter. But first we will review the neural control of BP.

Overview of the Sympathetic Nervous System

As shown in Figure 3-2, multiple central and reflex mechanisms are involved in the neural control of BP.

Baroreceptors

The major inhibitory reflexes arise in the (i) high pressure arterial baroreceptors of the carotid sinus and aortic arch and (ii) low pressure cardiopulmonary baroreceptors of the heart and great veins. The activation of these baroreceptors, by increased BP or increased cardiac filling pressure, respectively, sends inhibitory signals to the central nervous system via the nucleus tractus solitarius (NTS) and evokes reflex increases in efferent parasympathetic and decreases in efferent sympathetic activity, causing bradycardia and peripheral vasodilation which buffer the increases in BP (Guyenet, 2006).

In primary hypertension, the baroreceptors reset to defend a higher BP level (Guyenet, 2006). Surgically implanted carotid baroreceptor pacemakers produce sustained BP reductions in dog models of hypertension (Lohmeier et al., 2007), and possibly in patients with medically refractory hypertension (Mohaupt et al., 2007). Complete baroreflex failure is a rare cause of labile hypertension most often seen in throat cancer survivors as a late complication of radiation therapy, which causes a gradual destruction of the baroreceptor nerves (Heusser et al., 2005). By contrast, partial baroreceptor dysfunction is very common in elderly hypertensives and typically presents with a combination of orthostatic and postprandial hypotension, with supine hypertension (Vloet et al., 2005).

Excitatory Neural Reflexes

The major excitatory reflexes are those arising in carotid body chemoreceptors, the kidneys, and skeletal muscles. Activation of carotid body chemoreceptors by hypoxia evokes reflex sympathetic activation. Repeated activation of this excitatory chemoreflex has been implicated in the pathogenesis of hypertension with sleep apnea. The kidneys are richly innervated with sensory afferents that project centrally to the NTS and can evoke reflex sympathetic excitation. Activation of excitatory renal afferents by ischemic metabolites (e.g., adenosine) has been implicated in the pathogenesis of renovascular hypertension. Activation of these afferents by ischemic or uremic metabolites (e.g., urea) has been implicated in the pathogenesis of hypertension in chronic kidney disease. The skeletal muscles also are innervated with sensory afferents that signal the brain of local mechanical and chemical changes occurring during muscle contraction. During exercise, muscle afferents evoke reflex increases in BP and cardiac output that increase muscle perfusion. This reflex mechanism may be augmented in hypertension and lead to an exaggerated rise in BP during exercise (Leal et al., 2008).

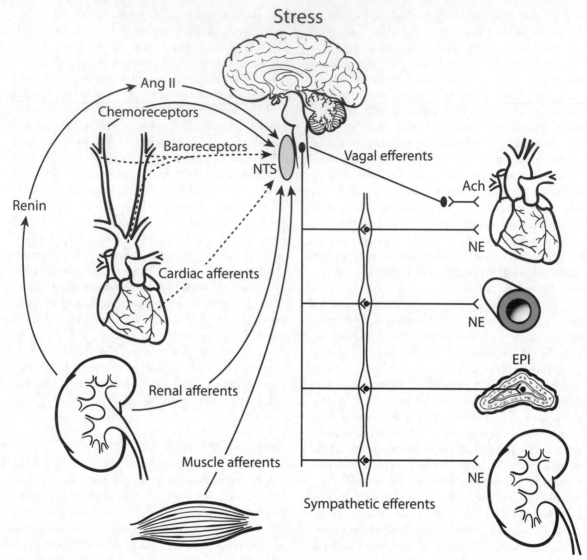

FIGURE 3-2   Central and reflex mechanisms involved in the neural control of BP. Dotted arrows represent inhibitory neural influences and solid arrows represent excitatory neural influences on sympathetic outflow. EPI, epinephrine; NTS, nucleus tractus solitarius; NE, norepinephrine; Ach, acetyl choline; Ang II, angiotensin II. (Modified from Victor RG, Shafiq M. Sympathetic neural mechanisms in human hypertension. *Curr Hypertens Rep* 2008;10:241–247.)

Central Sympathetic Outflow

Excitatory and inhibitory synaptic inputs from the NTS project centrally to neurons in the rostral ventrolateral medulla (RVLM), the site of origin of sympathetic outflow from the brainstem (Guyenet, 2006). From there, preganglionic sympathetic fibers synapse in the adrenal medulla (to release epinephrine [EPI]) and in the paravertebral sympathetic chain ganglia. The postganglionic fibers, which release NE, innervate the heart, blood vessels, and kidney.

Adrenergic Receptors

Cathecholamines induce their effects via G protein–coupled α- and β-adrenergic receptors. The α_1-adrenoreceptors are most abundant on resistance vessels and mediate most of the vasoconstriction caused by neurally released NE. There are three subtypes of α_2-adrenoreceptors which vary in location and function (Knaus et al., 2007). Studies in genetically engineered mice indicate that α_{2A} are located in the RVLM and tonically suppress sympathetic outflow. They mediate the hypotensive effect of clonidine and related central sympatholytics. Both α_{2A} and α_{2C} subtypes are located on sympathetic nerve terminals and cause feedback inhibition of NE release. By contrast, α_{2B} subtypes are located on resistance vessels. But, unlike α_1 receptors, they are not part of the neuroeffector junction but rather mediate vasoconstriction from circulating catecholamines. Their response also explains the paradoxical hypertension seen when patients with autonomic failure are treated with clonidine, which stimulates all three α_2-adrenergic receptor subtypes.

β-adrenergic stimulation of the heart increases ventricular contractility and heart rate, thereby increasing cardiac output. α adrenergic stimulation of the peripheral vasculature causes vasoconstriction and, over time, promotes vascular remodeling and hypertrophy (Bleeke et al., 2004).

The renal sympathetic nerves are thought to be involved in the pathogenesis of hypertension (DiBona,

2005). The renal nerves cause renal vasoconstriction (and hypertrophy) via α_1 receptors, stimulate renin release via β_1 receptors, and enhance renal sodium and water reabsorption via α_1 receptors (Fig. 3-3).

Cortical Influences

Cortical influences are particularly evident in the normal nocturnal dip in BP, the morning surge in BP, during physical and emotional stress (especially panic disorder), and with the white-coat reaction (see Chapter 2).

Long-term Sympathetic Regulation of BP

As noted above, the sympathetic nervous system is well known to regulate short-term changes in BP such as transient pressor responses during physical and emotional stress. In addition, sustained activation of the renal sympathetic nerves may contribute to long-term BP regulation by promoting sodium

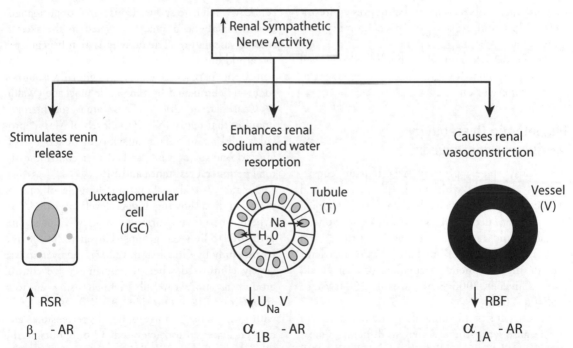

FIGURE 3-3 Effects of increased renal sympathetic nerve activity on the three renal neuroeffectors: the juxtaglomerular granular cells (JGC) with increased renin secretion rate (RSR) via stimulation of the β_1-adrenoceptors (AR), the renal tubular epithelial cells (T) with increased renal tubular sodium reabsorption and decreased urinary sodium excretion ($U_{Na}V$) via stimulation of α_{1B} AR, and the renal vasculature (V) with decreased renal blood flow (RBF) via stimulation of α_{1A} AR. (From DiBona GF. Physiology in perspective: The wisdom of the body. Neural control of the kidney. *Am J Physiol Regul Integr Comp Physiol* 2005;289:R633–R641, with permission.)

retention (DiBona, 2005). Moreover, NE's action on α_1-adrenoreceptors constitutes a trophic stimulus to cardiac and vascular smooth muscle hypertrophy (Bleeke et al., 2004). In patients with hypertension and left ventricular hypertrophy (LVH), SNA is increased and may predispose to the hypertrophy and sudden cardiac death (Burns et al., 2007; Schlaich et al., 2003).

Sustained sympathetic overactivity has been demonstrated not only in early primary hypertension but also in several other forms of established human hypertension. These include hypertension associated with obesity, sleep apnea, early type 2 diabetes mellitus and prediabetes, chronic kidney disease, heart failure, and immunosuppressive therapy with calcineurin inhibitors such as cyclosporine A (Victor & Shafiq, 2008). In these conditions, central sympathetic outflow can be driven by deactivation of inhibitory neural inputs (e.g., baroreceptors), activation of excitatory neural inputs (e.g., carotid body chemoreceptors, renal afferents), or by circulating Ang II, which activates pools of excitatory brainstem neurons that are devoid of a blood-brain barrier (Fig. 3-2). On the other hand, SNA seems to be suppressed in primary aldosteronism and in pheochromocytoma (Grassi et al., 2008a).

With this background in mind, we now will review the evidence for a neurogenic component to primary hypertension.

Sympathetic Overactivity in Primary Hypertension

In its early stages, primary hypertension consistently is associated with increased heart rate and cardiac output, plasma and urinary NE, regional NE spillover, decreased NE reuptake, peripheral postganglionic sympathetic nerve firing, and α-adrenergic receptor–mediated vasoconstrictor tone in the peripheral circulation (Grassi et al., 2008a; Guyenet, 2006; Schlaich et al., 2004; Victor & Shafiq, 2008)

These effects are difficult to demonstrate, in part because sympathetic activity is difficult to measure especially in the clinical setting. Plasma NE levels are an insensitive measure. Although easily performed and noninvasive, frequency analysis of heart rate variability simply is not a valid measure of sympathetic activity (Taylor & Studinger, 2006). The two state-of-the-art techniques to quantify sympathetic activity in humans are radiotracer measurements of regional NE spillover and microneurography (microelectrode measurements of SNA) (Schlaich et al., 2004; Wallin & Charkoudian, 2007). The former is invasive and requires arterial cannulation. The latter is minimally invasive but requires specialized training.

Regional NE Spillover

Considerable work by Esler, Lambert and coworkers shows that Stage 1 primary hypertension is characterized by sympathetic activation targeted to the kidney, heart, and skeletal muscle vasculature (Esler et al., 2006; Schlaich et al., 2004).

Direct Measurements of Sympathetic Nerve Activity

As shown in Figure 3-4, microneurography provides direct measurements of postganglionic SNA—the proximate neural stimulus to NE release (Guyenet, 2006). This is a powerful clinical research tool (Wallin & Charkoudian, 2007) but too technically demanding for routine diagnostic testing.

Muscle sympathetic nerve activity (*muscle SNA* or *MSNA*) refers to spontaneous bursts of postganglionic sympathetic discharge targeted to the skeletal muscle vasculature. The activity is tightly regulated by carotid sinus and aortic arch baroreceptors, accompanied by parallel changes in regional vasomotor tone, and eliminated by ganglionic blockade (Wallin & Charkoudian, 2007). These are vasoconstrictor impulses that release NE. Basal levels of MSNA provide a valid measure of resting sympathetic activity—at least to one major vascular bed that contributes to total peripheral resistance and BP.

Figure 3-4 also shows an example of one of many studies showing higher levels of MSNA in hypertensive than normotensive individuals, but with overlap between groups (Guyenet, 2006). In a recent study by Grassi et al. (2007), the overlap was largely eliminated when the normotensive control group was more carefully defined using 24-hour ambulatory BP monitoring (ABPM). When those with white-coat (office-only) hypertension and masked hypertension (elevated BP only outside the physician's office) were eliminated from the normotensive control group, mean values of MSNA were 70% higher in the persistent hypertensives compared to true normotensives. When measured under experimental circumstances, the MSNA was higher than normal in individuals with either white-coat or masked hypertension.

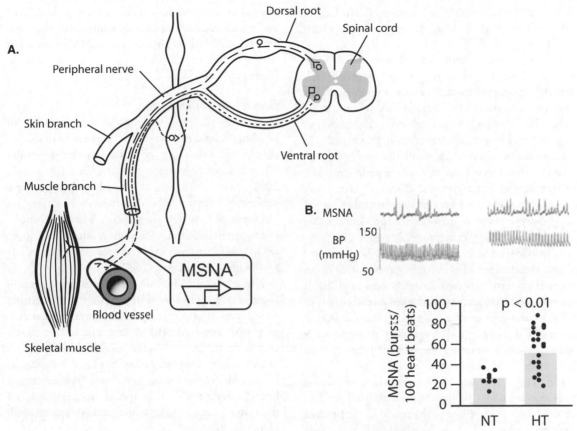

FIGURE 3-4 Microneurographic measurements of muscle sympathetic nerve activity (MSNA) in normotensive and hypertensive humans. **A:** Schematic diagram showing site of insertion of the recording microelectrode into a peripheral sympathetic nerve bundle innervating blood vessels in human skeletal muscle. **B:** Multi-unit recordings of MSNA and BP from two illustrative human subjects (**top panel**) and summary data (**bottom panel**) showing higher mean levels of nerve firing in hypertensive (HT) than normotensive (NT) humans. (**Panel A** modified from Guyenet PG. The sympathetic control of blood pressure. *Nat Rev Neurosci* 2006;7:335–346, with permission; **Panel B** adapted from Schlaich MP, Lambert E, Kaye DM, et al. Sympathetic augmentation in hypertension: Role of nerve firing, norepinephrine reuptake, and angiotensin neuromodulation. *Hypertension* 2004;43:169–175, with permission.)

Potential Mechanisms

Several mechanisms have been implicated in driving the sympathetic nervous system in hypertension.

Emotional and Physical Stress

Sympathoadrenal activation increases BP and heart rate transiently during episodes of physical and emotional stress, but the issue remains: can it cause chronic hypertension?

Guyton viewed the nervous system as only a short-term controller, adjusting beat-to-beat and minute-to-minute changes in BP, but playing a trivial role in chronic hypertension (Guyton, 1991). By contrast, the Swedish physiologist Bjorn Folkow hypothesized that repeated adrenergic spikes in BP eventually will damage the blood vessels producing sustained hypertension (Folkow, 2004).

Despite a vast literature, there still is no conclusive proof for Folkow's hypothesis (Carroll et al., 2001; Flaa et al., 2008; Matthews et al., 2004). Psychological stress is hard to quantify and standard semiquantitative laboratory stressors are often weak sympathetic stimuli that do not mirror real-life stress. The acute rise in BP during the cold pressor test (hand in ice water) is an indirect index of increased

MSNA and α-adrenergic vasoreactivity (Carroll et al., 2001; Chen et al., 2008a; Flaa et al., 2008; Victor et al., 1987).

The pattern of hemodynamic response to more realistic stresses in a laboratory setting may predict real-life BP measured by ambulatory monitoring. For example, in a study of 150 normotensive and prehypertensive young adults, an enhanced cardiac output response to a frustrating mirror-tracing task predicted elevated daytime and nocturnal BP but only in subjects who also showed evidence of impaired peripheral vasodilator capacity (Ottaviani et al., 2006). The latter may be associated with markers of vascular inflammation and a slower recovery of stress-induced pressor responses (Ottaviani et al., 2007; Steptoe & Marmot, 2005).

In the study by Grassi et al. (2007) mentioned above, the elevated MSNA in the patients with documented primary hypertension were indistinguishable from those in patients with masked hypertension or white-coat hypertension—presumably reflecting an exaggerated adrenergic BP reactivity to either daily life or the medical setting, respectively. Job stress may be a cause of hypertension (Pickering, 2006; Uno & Kario, 2006). Among minorities, perceived racism may be associated with higher nocturnal BP (Brondolo et al., 2008). NE spillover is increased in the brain of patients with primary hypertension and in those with panic disorder (Esler et al., 2008a).

Baroreceptor Resetting
Although the baroreceptors are reset to defend a higher BP, this does not explain sympathetic overactivity in human hypertension (Schlaich et al., 2004). Baroreflex control of heart rate is impaired even in mild hypertension but baroreflex control of SNA, vascular resistance, and BP is well preserved (Guo et al., 1983). Even baroreflex failure after bilateral carotid body tumor resection does not cause sustained hypertension (Timmers et al., 2004).

Central Effects of Angiotensin II
In rodent models, Ang II can enter the brainstem via unique neuronal pools that lack a blood-brain barrier—*the circumventricular organs*—and increase central sympathetic outflow via an AT_1 receptor mechanism (Guyenet, 2006). In the spontaneously hypertensive rat (SHR)—a common model of genetically programmed hypertension—inhibition of the brain RAAS in the pregnant mother will eliminate hypertension in her offspring (Wu & Berecek, 1993). If the RAAS blocker is given systemically to the rat

pups after delivery, the hypertension will be delayed and attenuated but not entirely eliminated. However, oral RAAS blockers do not lower MSNA in adult patients with uncomplicated primary hypertension (Esler et al., 2006).

Brainstem Compression
Jannetta et al., neurosurgeons at the University of Pittsburgh, hold that pulsatile compression of the left RVLM by a looping posterior inferior cerebellar artery can cause neurogenic hypertension (Levy et al., 2001). After developing an animal model, they have performed microvascular decompression surgery on hundreds of hypertensive patients. However, uncertainty persists due to inconsistent results from uncontrolled observations in small samples with short follow-up (Tan & Chan, 2007).

In a recent study from an independent group in Germany, 14 patients with primary hypertension were followed sequentially for 24 months after surgery with repeated ABPM and microneurography (Frank et al., 2009). Neurovascular decompression provided only temporary relief from hypertension, as BP and MSNA fell for the first 6 months after surgery but then returned steadily toward preoperative levels thereafter. Larger long-term studies are needed. Hypertension may be the cause rather than the result of vascular tortuosity.

When Does Increased MSNA Cause Hypertension?

Increased MSNA alone does not cause hypertension when it is accompanied by compensatory decreases in cardiac output and α-adrenergic receptor sensitivity to NE (Joyner et al., 2008). Presumably, sympathetic overactivity leads to hypertension only when these compensations fail.

Increased MSNA may cause hypertension only when accompanied by one or more of the following additional mechanisms:

- Inappropriately "normal" cardiac output (Charkoudian et al., 2005). This may be less of a factor in women than men (Hart et al., 2009).
- Increased α-adrenoreceptor sensitivity to NE (Charkoudian et al., 2005)
- Impaired NE reuptake by sympathetic nerve terminals (Esler et al., 2008b)
- Co-release of EPI from sympathetic nerve terminals (Berecek & Brody, 1982; Floras et al., 1988; Rumantir et al., 2000).

Emergence of Invasive Procedures for Lowering SNA and BP in Patients with Severe Refractory Hypertension

Two invasive strategies for lowering SNA are in early stages of clinical evaluation for the treatment of severe, medically refractory hypertension:

- Implantation of a carotid sinus pacemaker device, which has been the subject of preclinical studies (Lohmeier et al., 2007) and a clinical case report (Mohaupt, 2007); and
- Catheter-based radiofrequency ablation of the renal nerves, which has undergone an uncontrolled phase 1 clinical trial (Krum, 2009).

Observed reductions in BP, if confirmed and graded to reductions in SNA and NE, will strengthen the case for an important neurogenic component, at least in the most severe cases of primary hypertension.

Summary

Despite abundant documentation of sympathetic overactivity in uncomplicated primary hypertension, we still cannot quantify this neurogenic contribution. Most of the clinical research is correlational, cross-sectional, and based on intraneural recordings of SNA to the skeletal muscle bed and does not always reflect SNA to the kidney which presumably is more important in hypertension. With that caveat, we now will turn to renal mechanisms.

RENAL MECHANISMS

The kidneys are considered to be both the culprit and the victim in hypertension. Renal parenchymal hypertension will be discussed in Chapter 9 and renovascular hypertension in Chapter 10.

In the mid-19th century, Richard Bright linked hypertensive heart disease with small shrunken kidneys. In the 1930s, seminal work by Harry Goldblatt proved that the kidneys can cause hypertension. Beginning with the work of Guyton and his trainees in the 1960s, many believe that renal dysfunction is the sine qua non for hypertension.

According to this view, the fundamental defect in all hypertension is the kidneys' inability to excrete the excessive sodium load imposed by a high-salt diet (He & MacGregor, 2007).

Excess Sodium Intake as a Major Cause of Hypertension

The basis for the generally accepted—but not in itself sufficient—role of dietary sodium excess is as follows. Because our prehistoric ancestors consumed less than 0.5 g of NaCl (<10 mmol of Na) per day, our kidneys evolved efficient transport mechanisms to retain filtered sodium, which benefits survival during salt and water deprivation but contributes to hypertension when dietary salt is plentiful (He & MacGregor, 2007). For only the past few hundred years—a very short period in human evolution—daily NaCl consumption in developed countries has increased by orders of magnitude to 10 to 12 g per day, which overwhelms the capacity of the human kidney to maintain Na balance (He & MacGregor, 2007; Johnson et al., 2008). The residual excess total body Na—the main extracellular cation—expands plasma volume, increases cardiac output, and triggers autoregulatory responses that increase systemic vascular resistance. The sodium ion also augments the smooth muscle contraction evoked by multiple endogenous vasoconstrictor substances.

Most of the excess sodium in our diets does not come from the saltshaker but from modern food processing, which both adds sodium and removes potassium. Table 3-1 shows that our herbivorous ancestors probably consumed less than 10 mmol of sodium per day, whereas our carnivorous ancestors might have eaten 30 mmol per day (Eaton et al., 1996). Human physiology evolved in a low-sodium/high-potassium environment, and we seem ill equipped to handle the current exposure to high sodium and low potassium (Adrogue & Madias, 2007). Our current preference for salt likely is an acquired taste, developing early in childhood (Zinner et al., 2002).

The evidence linking dietary salt to hypertension is overwhelming and comes from multiple lines of investigation:

Epidemiological Studies

- In undeveloped countries, people who eat little sodium have little or no hypertension, and their BP does not rise with age, as it does in all developed and developing countries (Denton et al., 1995; Page et al., 1981). For example, the Yanomamo Indians of northern Brazil, who excrete only 1 mmol of sodium per day, have an average BP of 107/67 mm Hg

TABLE 3.1   **Estimated Diet of Late Paleolithic Humans Versus that of Contemporary Americans**

Nutrient	Late Paleolithic Diet (Assuming 35% Meat)	Current American Diet
Total dietary energy, %		
Protein	30	12
Carbohydrate	45–50	46
Fat	20–25	42
Polyunsaturated:saturated fat ratio	1.41	0.44
Fiber, g/day	86	10–20
Sodium, mg	604	3,400
Potassium, mg	6,970	2,400
Potassium:sodium ratio	12:1	0.7:1
Calcium, mg	1,520	740

Data from Eaton SB, Eaton SM III, Konner MJ, and Shostak M. An evolutionary perspective enhances understanding of human nutritional requirements. *J Nutr* 1996;126:1732–1740.

among men and 98/62 mm Hg among women aged 40 to 49 (Oliver et al., 1975).

- The lack of hypertension may be attributable to other differences in lifestyle, but comparisons made in groups living under similar conditions relate the BP most directly to the level of dietary sodium intake (Page et al., 1981). In developing countries, urbanization—which includes increased salt consumption—brings hypertension (Lawes et al., 2008). Even without urbanization, hypertension occurs in undeveloped tribes who consume a high-salt diet (Page et al., 1981).

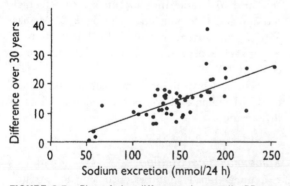

FIGURE 3-5   Plot of the difference in systolic BP over 30 years (age 55 minus age 25) in relation to median urinary sodium excretion across 52 populations. (Modified from Stamler J, Elliott P, Dyer AR, et al. Commentary: Sodium and blood pressure in the Intersalt study and other studies. *Br Med J* 1996;312:1285–1287.)

- Significant correlations between salt intake and hypertension development have been found in most large populations (Chien et al., 2008; Khaw et al., 2004; Zhou et al., 2003) but not in all (Smith et al., 1988). The seminal data come from the Intersalt study, which measured 24-hour urine electrolytes and BP in 10,079 men and women aged 20 to 59 years in 52 places around the world (Intersalt Cooperative Research Group, 1988; Elliott et al., 1996). For all 52 centers, there was a positive correlation between urine sodium excretion and both systolic and diastolic BP but an even more significant association between sodium excretion and the changes in BP with age (Fig. 3-5). Few populations were found whose levels of sodium intake were in the 50- to 100-mmol per day range (3 g NaCl), wherein the threshold for the sodium effect on BP likely resides (Fig. 3-6).

Migration Studies

Migration of people from a low-salt rural environment to a high-salt urban environment is accompanied by increased BP (He et al., 1991; Poulter et al., 1990).

Population-Level Dietary Interventions

It is very difficult to reduce salt intake at the population level with dietary counseling alone. When this has been successful, population-level BPs have fallen (Forte et al., 1989; Takahashi et al., 2006).

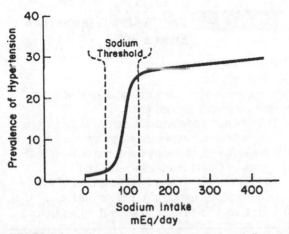

FIGURE 3-6 Probable association between usual dietary sodium intake and the prevalence of hypertension in large populations. (Modified from Kaplan NM. Dietary salt intake and blood pressure. *JAMA* 1984;251:1429–1430; Copyright 1984, American Medical Association.)

• In a randomized trial of tailored dietary education in 224 healthy volunteers in one rural community of northern Japan compared with 224 volunteers from a control community, a fall in urine NaCl excretion of only 2 g per day in the intervention group was accompanied by a 3 mm Hg fall in systolic BP (Takahashi et al., 2006).

• Over the past 30 years in Finland, a successful comprehensive nationwide campaign to lower salt intake by one third has been accompanied by a 10 mm Hg fall in population-average systolic and diastolic BP as well as a 75% to 80% fall in stroke and CHD mortality (Karppanen & Mervaala, 2006). Canada is following suit (Campbell & Spence, 2008). Larger effects will require societal and governmental regulation of the food industry, as 75% to 80% of dietary salt comes from food processing.

Feeding Trials

When hypertensives are sodium restricted, their BP falls. Dramatic falls in BP may follow rigid sodium restriction (Kempner, 1948), whereas less rigid restriction to a level of 100 mEq per day (5 to 6 g of NaCl) has been found to lower BP modestly—by 5/3 mm Hg on average (He & MacGregor, 2007)—as will be described further in Chapter 6.

• When prehypertensive individuals moderately restrict their sodium intake, progression to full-blown hypertension is reduced (Stamler et al., 1989; Whelton et al., 1998).

• Long-term intervention studies that start with infants and children to confirm that sodium restriction can prevent hypertension or that sodium excess can cause it are not feasible, but a recent meta-analysis showed short-term benefits (He & MacGregor, 2006). In ten trials involving 966 children and adolescents, BP fell by an average of 1.1/1.2 mm Hg after salt intake had been reduced by 42% for an average of 4 weeks. In three trials involving 551 infants, systolic BP fell by 2.5 mm Hg after salt intake had been reduced by 54% for an average of 8 weeks.

Non-Human Primate Studies

As seen in Figure 3-7, the most impressive evidence for salt-induced hypertension comes from a study on free-living chimpanzees, half of whom were given progressively increasing amounts of sodium in their food, while the other half remained on their usual low-sodium diet (Denton et al., 1995). During the 89 weeks in which the chimps received extra sodium, the BP rose an average of 33/10 mm Hg, returning to baseline after 20 weeks without added sodium. In keeping with varying sodium sensitivity, the BP rose in only seven of ten chimpanzees on the added sodium. An important point is that the chimpanzees' salt intake varied from 0.5 g per day (equivalent to that of our predecessors) to 10 to 15 g per day (equivalent to our modern high-salt diet).

Human Genetic Studies

Impaired renal sodium excretion is the final common pathway mediating almost all of the rare monogenic causes of human hypertension (Lifton et al., 2001), as discussed later in this section.

Salt as a Cause of Target Organ Damage Beyond BP

Most clinical studies but not all (Geleijnse et al., 2007) find that a high-salt diet, beyond raising BP, is an independent risk factor for target organ damage leading to fatal and nonfatal cardiovascular events including stroke (Perry & Beevers, 1992), aortic stiffness (du Cailar et al., 2004), cardiac hypertrophy and diastolic dysfunction (Frohlich, 2008; Pimenta & Calhoun, 2007), and renal failure (Pimenta & Calhoun, 2007). As if these damages were not enough, a high-salt diet also increases the risk of fatal stomach

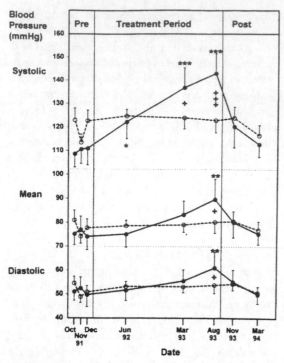

FIGURE 3-7 A group of 22 chimpanzees maintained in small, long-term, stable social groups and fed a vegetable-fruit diet with the addition of infant formula were studied. The 12 control animals (*open circles, dotted line*) experienced no change in conditions over 2.4 years and no significant change of systolic, diastolic, or mean BP (mean ± standard error of the mean). For the ten experimental animals (*solid circles, solid line*), 5 g per day NaCl was added to the infant formula for 19 weeks, 10 g per day for 3 weeks, and 15 g per day for 67 weeks. A 20-week period without salt addition followed. Significance values of the increase in BP relative to the mean of the three baseline determinations were as follows: *$p < 0.05$, **$p < 0.0021$; significance values of the difference between the experimental and control groups: *$p < 0.05$, ***$p < 0.001$. (Modified from Denton D, Weisinger R, Mundy NI, et al. The effect of increased salt intake on blood pressure of chimpanzees. *Nat Med* 1995;1:1009–1016.)

---

cancer (Joossens et al., 1996) and cataracts (Cumming et al., 2000).

How Does Salt Raise BP?

Despite all this evidence, there is no one simple explanation of how salt gluttony raises BP. There are multiple possibilities: salt promotes vasoconstriction,

---

TABLE 3.2	How Sodium Retention Can Elevate BP

Volume-dependent mechanisms
  Autoregulation
  Production of endogenous ouabain-like steroids[a]
Volume-independent mechanisms
  Angiotensin-mediated central nervous system effects
  Increase in sympathetic nervous system activity
  Hypertrophy in cardiac myoblasts and contractility of vascular smooth muscle cells
  Increase in production of nuclear factor-κB
  Increase in expression of AT_1R in renal tissue
  Increase in transforming growth factor β production

[a]Extracellular volume expansion induces the production of ouabain-like steroids with impairment of the sodium, potassium-adenosinetriphosphatase pump and increase in intracellular sodium. Sodium/calcium exchanger activity causes an increment in cytosolic calcium, which results in vasoconstriction and increased peripheral vascular resistance.
AT_1R, Angiotensin II type 1 receptor.
Adapted from Rodriguez-Iturbe B, Romero F, Johnson RJ. Pathophysiological mechanisms of salt-dependent hypertension. *Am J Kidney Dis* 2007a;50:655–672.

vascular remodeling, and hypertension by both volume-dependent and volume-independent mechanisms (Rodriguez-Iturbe et al., 2007a) (Table 3-2).

Volume-Dependent Mechanisms

Sodium, the principal extracellular cation, is the primary determinant of extracellular fluid volume, which in turn drives cardiac preload and cardiac output. Increased cardiac output may initiate hypertension, but either small-vessel vasoconstriction or large-vessel stiffness seems needed to sustain it.

Two theories—autoregulation and endogenous ouabain-like compounds—have been at the heart of the volume-dependent mechanism.

Autoregulation

The process of autoregulation was first described by Borst and Borst-De Geus (1963), and demonstrated experimentally by Guyton and Coleman (1969). According to this view, net renal sodium retention is the inciting event in all hypertensive states. The expanded blood volume increases cardiac preload and thus cardiac output, which increases perfusion of peripheral tissues. As tissue perfusion exceeds metabolic demands, the resistance arteries constrict thereby stopping overperfusion but at the "expense" of increases in

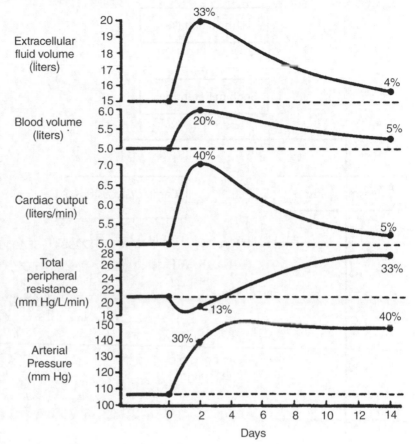

FIGURE 3-8 Progressive changes in important circulatory system variables during the first weeks in volume-loading hypertension. The initial rise in cardiac output is the basic cause of the hypertension. Subsequently, the autoregulation mechanism returns the cardiac output to almost normal and at the same time causes a secondary increase in total peripheral resistance. (Modified from Guyton AC. Kidneys and fluids in pressure regulation. *Hypertension* 1992;19(Suppl. 1):12–18.)

systemic vascular resistance and BP. The resultant increase in cardiac afterload returns cardiac output to normal. The term *autoregulation* implies that the vasoconstrictor response is an intrinsic property of vascular smooth muscle and does not require hormonal or neural inputs.

Guyton first showed conversion from high cardiac output to high systemic vascular resistance with inappropriately normal cardiac output during several days of volume infusion in dogs with reduced renal mass (Guyton, 1992) (Fig. 3-8). His concept has been supported by human studies indicating conversion over one or two decades from an initially high cardiac output to a later increased systemic vascular resistance (Julius et al., 1991).

Autoregulation is a property of small arteries and thus may have little to do with isolated systolic hypertension in the elderly, which involves mainly large conduit arteries (Franklin, 2005). It may play a larger role in the volume-dependence of diastolic hypertension

and of renal parenchymal hypertension, which is discussed in Chapter 9.

Endogenous Oubain-like Compounds

Haddy and Overbeck (1976) and Blaustein (1977) pioneered the theory that endogenous ouabain-like inhibitors (EOs) of Na-K-ATPase mediate peripheral vasoconstriction in salt hypertension. According to this theory which has evolved over 40 years (Fig. 3-9), salt retention can stimulate the adrenal glomerulosa cells to release EOs (cardiac glycosides) which inhibit Na/K-ATPase in vascular smooth muscle and cardiac muscle; the resultant increase in Na flux drives the Na-Ca-exchanger (NCX) to increase cytosolic Ca^{2+}, enhancing vasoconstriction and cardiac contractility as well as Ca^{2+}-dependent cardiac and vascular hypertrophy (Iwamoto, 2007).

Specific NCX inhibitors steeply reduce BP in multiple rat models of salt-sensitive hypertension but have no effect on BP in normotensive rats or those

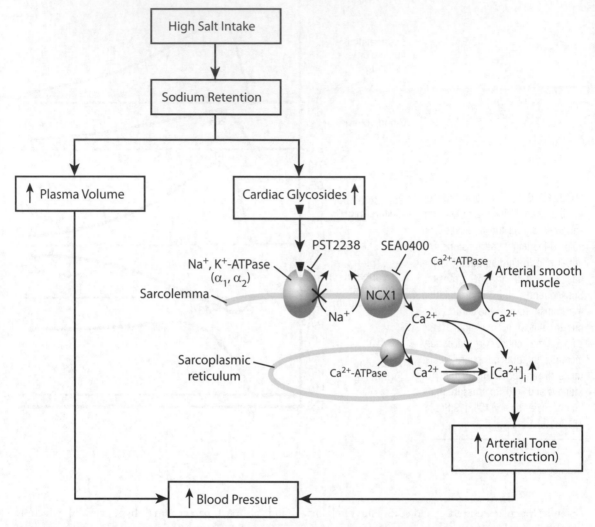

FIGURE 3-9 Proposed pathway by which Na^+/Ca^{2+} exchange mediates salt-sensitive hypertension. High salt intake increases plasma levels of endogenous cardiac glycosides that inhibit Na^+/K^+-ATPase. This increases subplasma membrane $[Na^+]$ in arterial smooth muscle, which elevates cytosolic $[Ca^{2+}]$ via the Na^+/Ca^{2+} exchanger (NCX1) and thus enhances arterial tone and contributes to hypertension. SEA0400, an inhibitor of NCX1, and PST2238, an ouabain antagonist, block Ca^{2+} entry and lower BP in experimental models of salt-sensitive hypertension. (Modified from Iwamoto T. Na^+/Ca^{2+} exchange as a drug target—insights from molecular pharmacology and genetic engineering. *Ann NY Acad Sci* 2007;1099:516–528, with permission.)

with hypertension that is not salt sensitive (Iwamoto, 2007). Thus, these and ouabain inhibitors may hold promise as new drugs specifically for salt-sensitive hypertension in patients.

Volume-Independent Mechanisms

Recent work has stressed several of the volume-independent mechanisms of salt-induced hypertension listed in Table 3-2:

- Small increases in serum Na may increase central sympathetic outflow (de Wardener et al., 2004). Small increases in Na in the CSF are sensed by Na channels in the subfornical organs (Orlov & Mongin, 2007).
- Extracellular sodium stimulates renal release of NF-κB and other proinflammatory cytokines that produce a chronic state of renal inflammation (Rodriguez-Iturbe et al., 2007b).

- Extracellular sodium stimulates production of transforming growth factor-β, TGF-β, a profibrotic cytokine that promotes vascular remodeling and hypertension. Mice lacking Emilin-1, the endogenous inhibitor of TGF-β, develop salt-sensitive hypertension (Zacchigna et al., 2006).
- Extracellular sodium increases expression of the Ang II type 1 receptors in the kidney (Gu et al., 1998).
- Aldosterone does not cause trouble when dietary sodium is restricted but becomes a cardiac, vascular, and renal toxin—promoting inflammation and fibrosis—when dietary sodium is plentiful (Pimenta & Calhoun, 2006).

Salt Sensitivity and Salt Resistance

Most adults have eaten a high-sodium diet since childhood but only a portion will have developed hypertension by age 55, suggesting a variable degree of BP sensitivity to sodium (Rodriguez-Iturbe et al., 2007a).

In the rat model developed by Lewis K. Dahl, inbred salt-sensitive rats remain normotensive on a low-salt diet but develop hypertension on a high-salt diet, whereas salt-resistant rats remain normotensive even on high salt (Dahl & Heine, 1975). Thus, salt-sensitive hypertension is often viewed as a classic example of a gene-environment interaction. But, in humans, salt sensitivity also can be acquired—for example, from weight gain, from low dietary potassium, from nonspecific renal injury, or from progressive renal injury caused by uncontrolled hypertension.

Salt sensitivity—and salt resistance—may be caused by mechanisms that are both intrinsic and extrinsic to the kidney (Table 3-3).

Monogenic Human Hypertension and Hypotension

The study of rare Mendelian traits by Richard Lifton's group and others has identified 20 genes in which homozygous mutations cause severe familial forms of hypotension or hypertension (Lifton et al., 2001). Remarkably, every one of these different mutations affects BP mainly by altering the kidney's ability to excrete sodium as illustrated in Figure 3-10.

To maintain salt and water balance, the kidneys normally reabsorb more than 99% of the filtered sodium load as follows: 60% of the filtered sodium is reabsorbed in the proximal tubule by Na^+/H^+

exchange, the target of acetazolamide; 30% in the thick ascending limb of the loop of Henle by the Na-K-2Cl transporter, the target of the "loop" diuretics; 7% in the distal convoluted tubule by the Na-Cl cotransporter, the target of the thiazide diuretics; and 2% in the cortical collecting duct by the epithelial sodium channel (ENaC), which is activated by aldosterone (as part of the effector arm of the RAAS) and the target of the aldosterone antagonists.

In the familial hypotensive disorders, exemplified by Bartter and Gitleman syndromes, the disease-causing mutations impair the diuretic-sensitive transporters, leading to salt-wasting and hypovolemic hypotension (Lifton et al., 2001). They typically present in the neonatal period or early childhood.

In the familial hypertensive disorders, the disease-causing mutations all increase ENaC activity either directly as in Liddle syndrome or indirectly due to overproduction of mineralocorticoids as in glucocorticoid-remediable aldosteronism or dysregulation of the mineralocorticoid receptor as pregnancy-exacerbated hypertension (Lifton et al., 2001). The net result is severe salt-sensitive hypertension typically presenting in the first two decades of life. Targeted diuretic therapy is the cornerstone of treatment.

Whether these or other mutations are involved in common primary hypertension in the general population will be discussed later in this chapter. Here, suffice it to say, that these are extreme *experiments of nature*, proving that altered renal sodium handling can have dramatic effects on human BP.

However, as described next, defining more moderate degrees of sodium resistance and sodium sensitivity in human subjects requires strict clinical research methodology, which is generally too cumbersome for routine clinical use.

Clinical Research Methodology

Since Luft and Weinberger (1997) and Kawasaki (1978) described varying responses of BP to short periods of low and high sodium intake, numerous protocols have been used to determine sodium sensitivity with variable results (de la Sierra et al., 2002).

Weinberger et al. (1986) defined sodium sensitivity as a 10-mm Hg or greater decrease in mean BP from the level measured after a 4-hour infusion of 2 L normal saline as compared to the level measured the morning after 1 day of a 10-mmol sodium diet, during which three oral doses of furosemide were given at 10 a.m., 2 p.m., and 6 p.m. Using this criterion,

TABLE 3.3   Pathophysiological Mechanisms Resulting in a Sustained Tendency to Sodium Retention by the Kidneys

Genetic defects
  Genetic variants and polymorphisms[a]
  Genetic mutations of renal sodium channels/transporters[b]
Systemic mechanisms
  Increased sympathetic tone
  Insufficient suppression of the rennin-angiotensin-aldosterone system
  Decreased atrial natriuretic peptide activity
  Decreased γ-melanocyte-stimulating hormone
    Insulin, metabolic syndrome
  Hyperuricemia
Renal mechanisms
  Specific defects
    Endothelin (A) receptor overactivity
    Impairment of endothelin 1 and endothelin (B) action on collecting duct
    Decreased dopamine activity (uncoupling)
  Nonspecific defects
    Decreased number of nephron units
    Sodium-driven renal TGF-β overproduction (progression of CKD)
    Decreased activity of kallikrenin-kinin system
    Impaired 20-HETE synthesis and decreased epoxygenase levels
    Renal-induced increase in sympathetic nervous system activity
    Intrarenal oxidative stress
    Increased intrarenal Ang II
    Tubulointerstitial inflammation

[a]Glucocorticoid-remediable aldosteronism, the p.Gly460Trp variant of the α-adducin gene, the p.Gly40Ser variant of the glucagon gene, mutations of glucocorticoid-regulated kinase, gene families involved in the metabolism of arachidonic acid (SS [homozygous for a small number of repeats] genotype of the human prostacyclin synthase gene), angiotensinogen polymorphisms.
[b]Mutations in the β and γ subunits of amiloride-sensitive ENaC (Liddle syndrome), sodium-chloride contransport (Gitelman syndrome), sodium-potassium-chloride cotransport, potassium and chloride channels (Bartter syndrome), WNK1 and WNK4 kinases (Gordon syndrome), aldosterone synthase/11β hydroxylase (glucocorticoid-remediable aldosteronism), 11β hydroxylase/11 α hydroxylase (adrenal hyperplasia), mineralo-corticoid receptor, 11β hydroxysteroid dehydrogenase (apparent mineralocorticoid excess), mineralocorticoid receptor (progesterone-induced hypertension), pseudohypoaldosteronism.
TGF-β, transforming growth factor β; CKD, chronic kidney disease; 20-HETE, 20-hydroxyarachidonic acid.
AT_1R, Angiotensin II type 1 receptor.
Adapted from Rodriguez-Iturbe B, Romero F, Johnson RJ. Pathophysiological mechanisms of salt-dependent hypertension. *Am J Kidney Dis* 2007a;50:655–672.

these researchers found that 51% of hypertensives and 26% of normotensives were sodium sensitive. Most studies find BP to be more salt sensitive among persons who are older, overweight, hypertensive, or of African descent (Luft & Weinberger, 1997).

Heightened BP-reactivity to cold pressor testing may be an easier way to identify individuals with sodium-sensitive BP (Chen et al., 2008a). A high dietary intake of sodium (relative to potassium) may act both centrally to augment the sympathetic reactivity to many stimuli such as cold stress and peripherally to augment vascular reactivity to neurally released NE.

Importance of Pressure-Natriuresis

In normotensive people, when BP rises, renal excretion of sodium and water increases, shrinking fluid volume and returning the BP to normal—the phenomenon of *pressure-natriuresis*. On the basis of animal experiments and computer models, Guyton (1961;1992) considered the regulation of body fluid volume by the kidneys to be the dominant mechanism for the long-term control of BP—the only one of many regulatory controls to have sustained and infinite power. Therefore, if hypertension develops, he reasoned that something must be amiss with

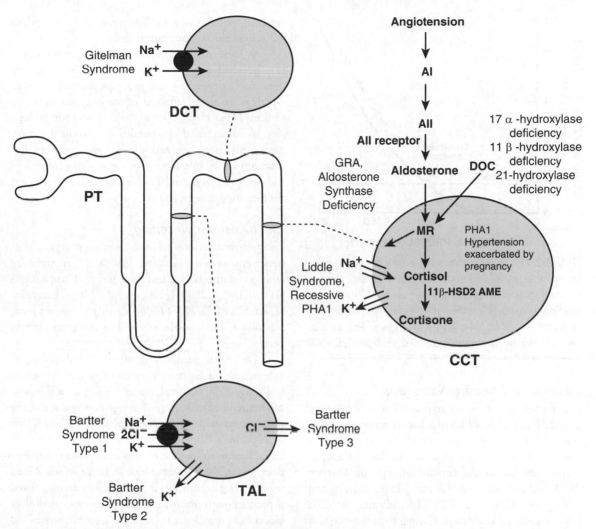

FIGURE 3-10 Mutations altering BP in humans—A diagram of nephron, the filtering unit of the kidney, is shown. The molecular pathways mediating NaCl reabsorption in individual renal cells in the thick ascending limb of the loop of Henle (TAL), distal convoluted tubule (DCT), and the cortical collecting tubule (CCT) are indicated, along with the pathway of the renin-angiotensin system, the major regulator of renal salt reabsorption. Inherited diseases affecting these pathways are indicated, with hypertensive disorders underlined. AI, angiotensin I; ACE, angiotensin converting enzyme; AII, angiotensin II; MR, mineralocorticoid receptor; GRA, glucocorticoid-remediable aldosteronism; PHA1, pseudohypoaldosteronism, type-1; AME, apparent mineralocorticoid excess; 11 β-HSD2, 11β-hydroxysteriod dehydrogenase-2; DOC, deoxycorticosterone; PT, proximal tubule. *(Adapted from Lifton RP, Gharavi AG, Geller DS. Molecular mechanisms of human hypertension. *Cell* 2001;104:545–556.)

pressure-natriuresis; otherwise, the BP would return to normal.

Experimental Support

The concept has a solid foundation: when BP is raised, the normal kidney excretes more salt and water—that is, pressure-natriuresis occurs (Selkurt, 1951). The curve relating BP to sodium excretion is steep (Fig. 3-11). A small change in renal perfusion pressure causes a large change in the rate of sodium and water excretion, acting as a powerful negative-feedback stabilizer of BP. As BP rises, increased renal perfusion pressure leads to a decrease in sodium reabsorption—particularly in the medulla in the thick ascending limb of the loop of Henle (Cowley 2008; Dickhout et al., 2002). As a result, body fluid volumes shrink enough to lower BP back to its previous normal level.

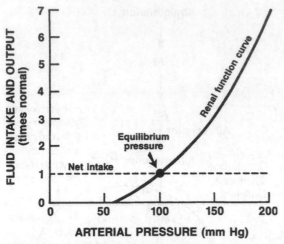

FIGURE 3-11   Graphic analysis of arterial pressure regulation by the kidney-fluid volume pressure control system. Pressure continually approaches the point at which the renal function curve intersects the net intake line (i.e., equilibrium pressure). (Modified from Guyton AC. Kidneys and fluids in pressure regulation. *Hypertension* 1992;19(Suppl. 1):I2–I8.)

Resetting of Pressure-Natriuresis

In patients with primary hypertension—as in every genetic form of experimental hypertension—a resetting of the pressure-sodium excretion curve prevents the return of BP to normal so that fluid balance is maintained but at the expense of high BP (Mayer, 2008). Much work by Guyton, Hall, Brands and colleagues (Hall et al., 1996b) indicates that the resetting plays a key role in causing hypertension and is not merely an adaptation to increased BP. This resetting explains why sodium retention occurs when BP is lowered by nondiuretic drugs.

As seen in Figure 3-12, either the entire curve can be shifted to the right or the slope can be depressed, depending on the type of renal insult, which is, in turn, reflected by varying sensitivity to sodium (Hall et al., 1996a). Salt-resistant hypertension is characterized by a parallel shift in the pressure-natriuresis curve, whereas salt-sensitive hypertension is accompanied by a change in slope—an exaggerated increase or decrease in BP with increased or decreased sodium intake, respectively.

Mechanisms of Resetting

Pressure-natriuresis—and the resetting that occurs in hypertension—is mediated first and foremost by changes in tubular sodium transport with unchanged GFR (Cowley, 2008; Johnson et al., 2008). Extensive rat studies of Cowley (2008) identify the outer renal medulla as the key site in which pressure-natriuresis occurs.

The renal medulla is uniquely vulnerable to ischemic insult for several reasons. Oxygen extraction is already near maximal under resting conditions to maintain the basal activity of energy-dependent sodium transporters, which are highly concentrated in this part of the kidney. With a sudden increase in BP, medullary blood flow must increase to match the increased energy demands of these transporters. In other words, blood flow to the renal medulla must be poorly autoregulated if pressure-natriuresis is to occur. Impaired medullary blood flow regulation impairs pressure-natriuresis and is evident in virtually all rat models of hypertension.

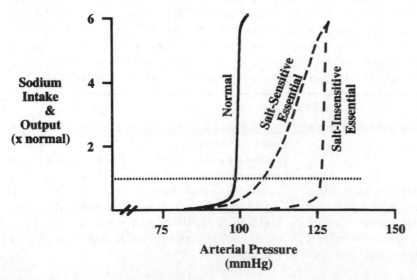

FIGURE 3-12   Schematic showing resetting of pressure-natriuresis in hypertension. Steady-state relationships between arterial pressures and sodium excretion (equal to intake) are shown for both salt-sensitive and salt-insensitive essential hypertension. (Modified from Hall JE, Brands MW, Henegar JR. Angiotensin II and long-term arterial pressure regulation. *J Am Soc Nephrol* 1999;10:S258–S265.)

Table 3-3 is a partial list of the many explanatory mechanisms that underlay a rightward shift in the pressure-natriuresis curve. These include augmented medullary vasoconstrictor mechanisms or impaired medullary vasodilator mechanisms—both autocrine mechanisms that are intrinsic to the kidney and extra-renal neurohormonal mechanisms.

Intrarenal Mechanisms

The best evidence—albeit in rodents—is for an imbalance between an overactive RAAS, which reduces renal medullary blood flow, and a defective nitric oxide pathway, which normally maintains med-ullary blood flow and protects against hypertension (Dickhout et al., 2002).

Intrarenal RAAS

The RAAS is a key mechanism regulating renal sodium handling, producing most of its biological effects via

AT_1 receptors. In the kidney, AT_1 receptors stimulate renal medullary vasoconstriction and increase sodium reabsorption. Renal cross-transplantation experiments between mice with and without targeted disruption of the AT_1 receptor gene by Crowley and Coffman (2008) emphasize the importance of the renal AT_1 receptors in the normal regulation of BP and in the genesis of Ang II–dependent hypertension. In addi-tion, AT_1 receptors in the brain regulate salt appetite, thirst, and modulate vasopressin release. Adrenal AT_1 receptors enhance secretion of aldosterone, the main mineralocorticoid.

Ang II has been shown repeatedly to cause a right-ward shift in the pressure-natriuresis curve (Hall et al., 1996b). The effect is potent because sodium retention is greatly augmented at Ang II concentrations far below those needed to cause vasoconstriction.

As illustrated in Figure 3-13, in the rat medulla, Ang II normally triggers a coordinated calcium signal

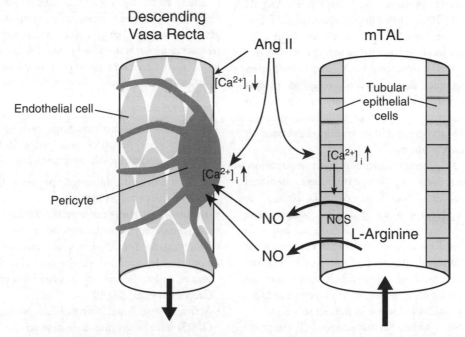

FIGURE 3-13 Model summarizing the observed actions of angiotensin II (Ang II) on the med-ullary thick ascending limb (mTAL) and the adjacent descending vasa recta. Ang II increases $[Ca^{2+}]_i$ in pericytes of the descending vasa recta and reduces it in endothelium of the descending vasa recta. Ang II increases nitric oxide (NO) in the pericytes of the descending vasa recta but only when these cells are in proximity to the tubules surrounding the mTAL. Ang II increases $[Ca^{2+}]_i$ and $[NO]_i$ in mTALs even when these tubules were observed in isolation. This indicates that Ang II exerts a constrictor effect on the descending vasa recta by its action on pericytes, and this constrictor action is buffered by NO diffusing from mTALs to the pericytes of the descending vasa recta. (From Dickhout JG, Mori T, Cowley AW Jr. Tubulovascular nitric oxide crosstalk: Buffering of angiotensin II–induced medullary vasoconstriction. *Circ Res* 2002;91:487–493.)

in the pericytes of the descending vasa recta—promoting vasoconstriction—and the tubular epithelial cells of the thick ascending limb—causing release of nitric oxide (NO), a potent vasodilator which diffuses to the adjacent vasa recta and offsets Ang II-dependent vasoconstriction (Dickhout et al., 2002). The balance between vasoconstrictor and vasodilator factors is termed "tubulovascular crosstalk." Other associated vasoconstrictor factors include reactive oxygen species (both superoxide and hydrogen peroxide); associated vasodilator factors include cyclooxygenase (COX-2) and prostaglandins (PGE2) (Cowley, 2008). Any imbalance can cause medullary ischemia, impaired pressure-natriuresis, and salt-induced hypertension.

One reason the RAAS is so important in renal sodium handling may be that Ang II is selectively concentrated in the kidney. Navar et al. have shown that intrarenal concentrations of Ang II are several-fold higher than circulating blood levels because the kidney actively produces and sequesters Ang II (Kobori et al., 2007). In multiple experimental forms of hypertension, renal Ang II levels are high even when plasma levels are normal or low. Thus, selective overactivity of the intrarenal RAAS may drive hypertension even when extrarenal blood tests (i.e., plasma renin activity [PRA] levels) indicate, as they do in most cases of primary human hypertension, that systemic RAAS activity is either frankly suppressed or "inappropriately normal."

While AT_1 receptors promote sodium retention, AT_2 receptors seem to promote natriuresis, mediated in part by release of NO (Carey & Padia, 2008). The angiotensin receptor blockers (ARBs), which cause selective AT_1 receptor blockade, induce natriuresis in rodents by unmasking and activating AT_2 receptors in the proximal tubule (Carey & Padia, 2008). Despite abundant experimental support, this theory remains untested in patients as selective AT_2 receptor antagonists are not available for use in human subjects.

Two more systems that may counter AT_1 receptor–mediated sodium retention deserve mention.

Renal Dopaminergic System

Dopamine evokes natriuresis in rodents and humans by stimulation of dopamine (D_1) receptors. The renal proximal tubular cells are able to synthesize dopamine locally from L-dopa and studies in dopamine receptor knockout mice suggest that the intrarenal dopaminergic system can explain half the renal sodium excretion seen with salt loading (Wang et al., 2008e). Renal dopamine

receptors are uncoupled in genetic rat models of hypertension (Rodriguez-Iturbe et al., 2007b) and during oxidative stress (Banday et al., 2008).

Renal Medullary Endothelin System

Endothelin, discovered as a potent endothelium-derived vasoconstrictor, also is plentiful in the renal medulla where it causes vasodilation and natriuresis, thus reducing BP and protecting against salt-induced hypertension (Kohan, 2006). These effects are mediated by the endothelin B (ETB) receptor, whereas the vasoconstrictor and prohypertensive actions of endothelin are mediated by the endothelin A (ETA) receptor.

A high-salt diet drives endothelin expression in the kidney, increasing renal medullary blood flow via PGE2 and nitric oxide (Schneider et al., 2008) and inhibiting the antinatriuretic effect of vasopressin. Genetically engineered mice and rats that cannot produce endothelin or the ETB receptor in the renal medulla develop salt-dependent hypertension (Gariepy et al., 2000; Kohan, 2006). Thus, the ETB receptor is a potential new antihypertensive drug target. *However, the first generation of clinical endothelin receptor antagonists inhibited both ETA and ETB receptors, which likely explains their disappointingly small effect on BP.*

Extrarenal Mechanisms

The following systemic mechanisms also have been shown to reset pressure-natriuresis and have been implicated in causing salt-sensitive hypertension:

- Dysfunction of the natriuretic peptides (Dries et al., 2005; Oliver et al., 1998)
- Insulin (Rodriguez-Iturbe et al., 2007a)
- α-Melanocyte stimulating hormone (α-MSH), which causes or exacerbates salt-sensitive hypertension in rodent models via the central melanocortin system and activation of SNA (da Silva et al., 2008; Greenfield et al., 2009).
- Activation of Renal Sympathetic Nerves. DiBona (2005) has shown that activation of the renal sympathetic nerves shifts the pressure-natriuresis curve and contributes to salt-sensitive hypertension in rats. Conversely, renal denervation prevents the development, attenuates the magnitude, or delays the onset of hypertension in multiple animal models (DiBona, 2005) and may lower BP in hypertensive patients (Krum et al., 2009). Campese et al. showed that even a mild renal parenchymal injury—with a single injection of phenol into the lower pole of one kidney in an otherwise normal rat—will produce

sustained salt-sensitive hypertension mediated in part by activation of renal afferents that reflexly increase renal SNA and in part by reduced NO production (decreased [nitric oxide synthase] NOS expression) by the injured kidney (Bai et al., 2007)—i.e., by both extrarenal and intrarenal mechanisms.

Importance of Renal Inflammation

Rodent studies point to renal inflammation as both a cause and a consequence of renal medullary ischemia (Majid & Kopkan, 2007; Rodriguez-Iturbe et al., 2007a). Renal inflammation—whether the chicken or the egg—is a hallmark of both the initiation and progression of experimental salt-sensitive hypertension. Eventually, ongoing renal ischemia will kill enough nephrons to decrease GFR.

Nocturia

Nocturia may be a clinical sign of abnormal pressure-natriuresis and a clue to uncontrolled salt-sensitive hypertension related to aging, hypertension, and particularly a blunted or reversed nocturnal dipping pattern in BP (Bankir et al., 2008). In normotensives, nocturnal urine flow accounts for 53% of urine output in 60- to 80-year-olds as compared to 25% in 25- to 35-year-olds (McKeigue & Reynard, 2000). Hypertensives have even more nocturia, presumably reflecting the resetting of the pressure-natriuresis relationship (Fukuda et al., 2006). Fluid retained peripherally during the day leads to central volume expansion at night, with elevated nocturnal BP driving pressure-natriuresis (Bankir et al., 2008).

Salt sensitivity of BP may be inherited or acquired—in utero, during early postnatal life, or during adult life as a result of a low-potassium diet or uncontrolled hypertension.

Inherited Renal Defects in Sodium Excretion

Using rats bred to be either sensitive or resistant to the hypertensive action of dietary sodium, Dahl and Heine (1975) demonstrated the primacy of the kidney in the development of hypertension by a series of transplant experiments. The BP follows the kidney: When a kidney from a normotensive donor was transplanted to a hypertensive host, the BP of the recipient fell to normal. Conversely, when a hypertensive kidney was transplanted into a normotensive host, the BP rose. Moreover, transplantation of a kidney from a hypertensive rat that has been briefly made

normotensive with an angiotensin-converting enzyme inhibitor (ACEI) causes the BP to normalize in a hypertensive host (Smallegange et al., 2004).

Curtis et al. (1983) observed long-term remission of hypertension after renal transplantation in six black men who likely developed renal failure solely as a consequence of primary hypertension. Because five of these patients had remained hypertensive after removal of their native kidneys, their hypertension was presumably not of renal pressor origin. The most likely explanation for the reversal of hypertension in these patients was the implantation of normal renal tissue, which provided control of body fluid volume, something their original kidneys had been unable to manage. Moreover, hypertension develops more frequently in recipients of renal transplants from hypertensive donors than in recipients from normotensive donors (Guidi et al., 1996).

As noted earlier, impaired renal sodium excretion is the final common pathway for most of the known monogenic forms of human hypertension (Lifton et al., 2001).

Perinatal Origin of Adult Salt-Sensitive Hypertension: Reduced Nephron Number

Low birth weight with reduced nephrogenesis increases the risk of developing adult salt-dependent hypertension. Adult hypertensives have fewer glomeruli per kidney but very few obsolescent glomeruli, suggesting that nephron dropout and decreased total filtration surface area are a cause and not the consequence of hypertension (Keller et al., 2003). This is one of the strongest areas of mechanistic clinical research on primary hypertension.

Brenner and Chertow (1994) first proposed that hypertension may arise from a congenital reduction in the number of nephrons or in the filtration surface area per glomerulus, thereby limiting the ability to excrete sodium, raising the BP, and setting off a vicious circle whereby systemic hypertension begets glomerular hypertension, which begets more systemic hypertension (Fig. 3-14).

The first major affirmation of the Brenner hypothesis came from a postmortem analysis of total nephron numbers in kidneys from ten previously hypertensive patients and ten previously normotensive people, all of whom having died from accidents (Keller et al., 2003). The two groups were matched for age, gender, height, and weight. The median number of glomeruli in the hypertensives was less

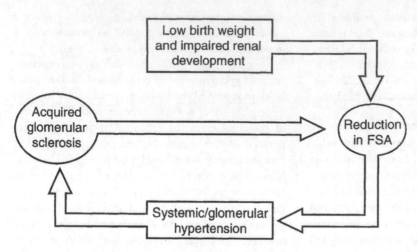

FIGURE 3-14 A diagram of the hypothesis that the risks of developing primary hypertension and progressive renal injury in adult life are increased as a result of congenital oligonephropathy, or an inborn deficit of filtration surface area (FSA), caused by impaired renal development. (Modified from Brenner BM, Chertow GM. Congenital oligonephropathy and the etiology of adult hypertension and progressive renal injury. *Am J Kidney Dis* 1994;23: 171–175.)

than half of the number in the normotensives. Moreover, the glomerular volume in the hypertensives was greater, suggesting that they were hyperfiltering. The likelihood that the lower number of glomeruli in the hypertensives was from birth was supported by the absence of adolescent glomeruli as would be seen if they had been present but dropped out.

Congenital Oligonephropathy

The Brenner hypothesis invokes a reduced number of nephrons from congenital oligonephropathy, i.e., fewer nephons as a result of intrauterine growth retardation (Mackenzie & Brenner, 1995). As first reported by Dr David Barker and colleagues on the basis of epidemiological studies, infants born small for gestational age, i.e., low birth weight, are at increased risk for development of hypertension, diabetes, and cardiovascular diseases later in life (Barker et al., 1989). The concept of "perinatal programming" has focused on maternal protein restriction (Woods et al., 2004) as responsible for the shunting of necessary fuels to the developing brain at the expense of less vital organs including the kidneys and pancreas, a hypothesis described as "thrifty-phenotype" (Hales & Barker, 2001).

The presence of congenital oligonephropathy in human babies born with intrauterine growth retardation was first shown by Hinchliffe et al. (1992) and confirmed by several groups (Hughson et al., 2008; Konje et al., 1996; Manalich et al., 2000), with an average of 260,000 fewer nephrons with each kilogram of decrease in birth weight. The reduced number of nephrons at birth in low-birth-weight

babies cannot be replenished later by excellent postnatal nutrition since most nephrons are formed in the first part of the last trimester and no further nephrogenesis occurs after 34 to 36 weeks of gestation (Lucas & Morley, 1994).

The subsequent scenario has been described by Mackenzie and Brenner (1995):

> Deficiencies in the total nephron supply, by limiting total renal excretory capacity and thereby influencing the point at which steady-state conditions between BP and sodium excretion are achieved, could profoundly affect long-term BP regulation. When renal mass is greatly reduced, as in the case of extensive experimental ablation of the kidney in rodents, BP increases in the systemic arterial circulation and in the glomerular capillaries, thus increasing glomerular filtration rate and promoting fluid excretion. However, sustained elevations in glomerular capillary hydraulic pressure are associated with the development of focal and segmental glomerular sclerosis leading to further loss of nephrons and a self-perpetuating vicious cycle of hypertension and progressive glomerular injury.... Given the association between low birth weight and fewer nephrons... it is naturally tempting to speculate that the origins of hypertension in adults who were of low birth weight lie in a deficient endowment of nephrons secondary to intrauterine growth retardation.

Recent evidence supporting the Barker/Brenner hypothesis includes the following:

• A registry study of 16,265 Swedish twins confirms the association of decreased birth weight with an increased risk of hypertension (at least as assessed by self-report) and indicates that this association is independent of shared genes, shared postnatal environment, and adult risk factors for hypertension including BMI (Bergvall et al., 2007).

- A case-control study involving a total of 332 young adults, aged 18 to 27 years, shows more insulin resistance and glucose intolerance, as well as higher BP, among those who have very low birth weight due to preterm delivery than those born at term (Hovi et al., 2007).

- Two groups have shown that low birth weight in whites is associated with salt sensitivity of BP in healthy young adults (de Boer et al., 2008) and in preadolescents and adolescents (Simonetti et al., 2008).

- Two large epidemiologic studies show that low birth weight is associated with retinal artery narrowing both in adults (Liew et al., 2008) and in 6-year-old children (Mitchell et al., 2008b). Arteriopathy may be both a cause and consequence of increased BP and is associated with increased risk of stroke (Norman, 2008).

- A retrospective chart review of 66 patients at one pediatric renal center finds that 50% of children with a congenital solitary kidney have developed hypertension and/or microalbuminuria by 9 years of age (Schreuder et al., 2008).

Postnatal Weight Gain

Despite all of the evidence supporting a role of low birth weight with adult hypertension, its contribution may be quantitatively small (Falkner et al., 1998; Huxley et al., 2002). An even greater contribution has been shown for the rapid postnatal "catch-up" in body weight (Singhal & Lucas, 2004). Shingal et al. (2004) have summarized a great deal of their own and others' convincing evidence for a critical period—the first 2 weeks after birth—where overfeeding programs the infant for later obesity, insulin resistance, and endothelial dysfunction which, in turn, result in diabetes, hypertension, and coronary disease.

Their evidence includes multiple observations on the benefits of feeding with breast milk (with lower caloric content and lower initial volume) rather than formula milk (with higher caloric content and larger volume) on subsequent adult health (Lawlor et al., 2004; Martin et al., 2004).

Along these lines, additional analyses of 2,003 Finnish people in the Helsinki birth cohort led Barker et al. (2007) to propose two different pathways by

which low birth weight predisposes to hypertension. In the first, low birth weight results from fetal under-nutrition and a small placenta, making the child vulnerable to poor postnatal living conditions such as a fast-food high-salt diet. Low birth weight during infancy is followed by rapid growth leading to overweight by age 11. As adults, they become obese and develop insulin resistance, severe hypertension, and coronary disease. In the second path, maternal rickets or even a lesser degree of vitamin C deficiency causes the mother to have a small diameter bony pelvis. The low-birth-weight infants remain short and thin throughout childhood, possibly due to protein malnutrition. As adults, they develop mild hypertension, atherogenic lipid profiles, and stroke.

In addition, mothers who smoke or have higher BP before pregnancy are more likely to have babies who are small for gestational age (Romundstad et al., 2007).

The public health implications seem obvious. Recent cutbacks in support for teenage contraception, maternal nutrition, and postnatal care in the United States suggest that we will continue to pay billions for the eventual care of hypertension-related end-stage renal disease, strokes, and heart attacks instead of millions for preventive care of the disadvantaged.

Limitations

These theories have been tested in mainly white European populations. They have not been shown to explain the excessive hypertension in African Americans. For example, a recent autopsy study of 59 African Americans and 32 whites found no evidence that the greater hypertensive disease in African Americans is associated with lower birth weight or fewer glomeruli (Hughson et al., 2008). In a large biracial cohort involving 55,908 pregnancies at 12 medical centers across the United States, children who were small for gestational age were not at increased risk for high BP at age 7 unless they showed rapid weight gain in early childhood, with the risk being 50% greater for white children than for black children (Hemachandra et al., 2007).

Summary

While there may be more evidence for renal mechanisms than for any other in primary hypertension, additional mechanisms are involved.

VASCULAR MECHANISMS

Alterations in the structure and function of both small and large arteries also play a pivotal role in the origin and progression of hypertension (Harrison, 2007). In most cases of human hypertension, peripheral vascular resistance is increased while cardiac output is normal. By Pouiselle's law, BP is directly related to the first power of cardiac output but inversely relating to the fourth power of blood vessel radius. Thus, small changes in blood vessel diameter have enormous effects on BP.

Cellular Mechanisms of Vasoconstriction

As shown in Figure 3-15, an increase in cytosolic calcium is the final common pathway mediating contraction of vascular smooth muscle (Harrison, 2007). Most potent antihypertensive drugs are vasodilators, as

discussed in Chapter 7. BP is elevated in genetically altered mice with increased vascular resistance, showing that blood vessel constriction alone, without renal involvement, can cause hypertension (Harrison, 2007).

Endothelial Cell Dysfunction and the Nitric Oxide (NO) Pathway

The endothelial lining of blood vessels is critical to vascular health and constitutes a major defense against atherosclerosis and hypertension (Munzel et al., 2008). Dysfunctional endothelium, a hallmark of hypertension and other cardiovascular risk factors, is characterized by impaired release of endothelial-derived relaxing factors (NO, endothelial-derived hyperpolarizing factor) and enhanced release of endothelial-derived constricting, proinflammatory,

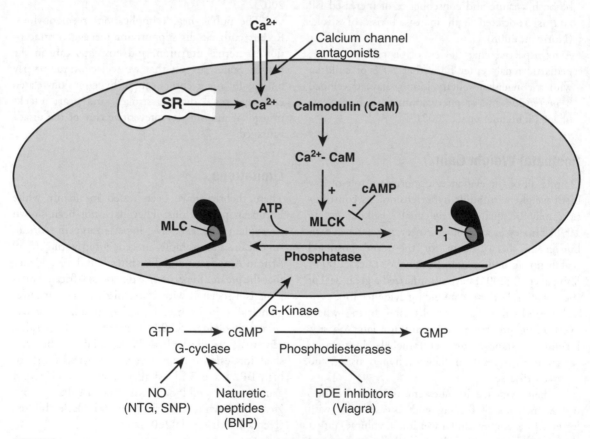

FIGURE 3-15   Mechanisms of vascular smooth muscle contraction. (From Harrison DG. Vascular mediators of hypertension in Clinical Hypertension Review Course Syllabus, American Society of Hypertension, Inc, New York, New York, 2007, pp. 107–125.) MLCK, myosin light chain kinase; MLC, myosin light chain; Pi, inorganic phosphorus; GTP, guanylyl triphosphate; GMP, guanylyl monophosphate; NO, nitric oxide; NTG, nitroclycerin; SNP, sodium nitroprusside; BNP, brain naturetic peptide; PDE, phosphodiesterase.

prothrombotic, and growth factors. The latter include endothelin, thromboxane, and TGF-β (August & Suthanthiran, 2006). Growing evidence indicates that blood vessels are inflamed in hypertension and that smoldering vascular inflammation plays a central role in the genesis and complications of high BP (Marchesi et al., 2008; Paravicini & Touyz, 2006).

The endothelium of all blood vessels expresses the enzyme NOS which can be activated by bradykinin or acetylcholine or by the cyclic laminar shear stress that accompanies hypertension (Thomas et al., 2001). Once activated, NOS converts L-arginine to citrulline, an inert substance, and NO, a volatile gas that diffuses to the adjacent vascular smooth muscle and activates a series of G-kinases that culminate in vasodilation (Fig. 3-16). Thus, the NO pathway is thought to be one of the most important regulatory mechanisms that protects against hypertension, and NO deficiency is thought to contribute to hypertension.

One of the principal mechanisms of endothelial cell dysfunction in hypertension is the production of superoxide anion and other reactive oxygen species that quench NO, thereby reducing its bioavailability. The term "oxidative stress" refers to chronic elevations in reactive oxygen species, which are associated with hypertension, atherosclerosis, and diabetes (Paravicini & Touyz, 2008).

The two main reactive oxygen species are superoxide radical (O_2) and hydrogen peroxide (H_2O_2) (Fig. 3-17). Overproduction of superoxide radial and H_2O_2 can activate signaling molecules that lead to cell growth, fibrosis, inflammation, and eventually vascular remodeling (Fig. 3-18).

Enzymatic Sources of Superoxide

There are four main enzymatic sources of vascular superoxide: (i) NADPH oxidases, which are universally expressed in all vascular cell types and are activated by circulating Ang II and other factors,

Endothelial Function Testing

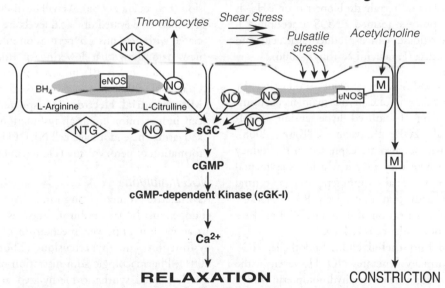

FIGURE 3-16 Regulation of vascular tone by the endothelium. The eNOS by a two-step oxidation of the amino acid L-arginine thereby leading to the formation of L-citruline. NO is released into the bloodstream thereby inhibiting platelet aggregation and the release of vasoconstricting factors such as serotonin and thromboxane. NO diffuses also into the media and activates the soluble guanylate cyclase (sGC). The resulting second messenger cGMP in turn activates the cGMP-dependent kinase, which mediates decreases in intracellular Ca^{2+} concentrations thereby causing vasorelaxation. The physiological stimuli to release NO are shear stress and pulsatile stretch. Muscarinic acetylcholine receptor (M), nitroglycerin (NTG). (From Munzel T, Sinning C, Post F, et al. Pathophysiology, diagnosis and prognostic implications of endothelial dysfunction. *Ann Med* 2008;40:180–196.)

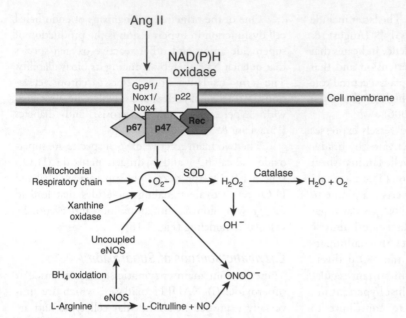

FIGURE 3-17 Generation of O_2 and H_2O_2 from O_2 in vascular cells. Many enzyme systems, including NAD(P)H oxidase, xanthine oxidase, and uncoupled NOS among others, have the potential to generate reactive oxygen species. NAD(P)H oxidase is a multi-subunit enzyme, comprising Gp91phox (or its homologues, Nox1 and Nox4), p22phox, p47phox, p67phox, and p40phox, that is regulated by many stimuli, including vasoactive agents, such as Ang II, superoxide dismutase (SOD), tetrahydrobiopterin (BH_4). (From Paravicini TM, Touyz RM. Redox signaling in hypertension. *Cardiovasc Res* 2006;71:247–258.)

(ii) NOS, which produces superoxide only when an important cofactor (tetrahydrobiopterin or BH_4) is deficient (a process termed "NOS uncoupling"), (iii) xanthine oxidase, which produces uric acid, and (iv) mitochondria (Paravicini & Touyz, 2006).

- **NADPH Oxidases.** Superoxide production by NADPH oxidase is one of the main mechanisms mediating Ang II–induced hypertension (Landmesser et al., 2002; Paravicini & Touyz, 2008). NADPH oxidases also are expressed in the kidney and brain where they play a role in experimental hypertension via renal sodium retention and central sympathetic activation, respectively. RAAS blockers should inhibit activation of these NADPH oxidases in patients but evidence is lacking.
- **Uncoupled Endothelial NOS.** Endothelial NOS (eNOS) normally generates NO. However, in the absence of ʟ-arginine or tetrahydrobiopterin (BH_4), NOS stops producing NO and instead starts using oxygen as a substrate for producing superoxide (Mueller et al., 2005) (Fig. 3-17). In experimental models, ROS generated by NADPH oxidase oxidizes BH4 and uncouples NOS; oxidative stress begets oxidative stress. Oral BH4 may improve endothelial function and lower BP in patients (Porkert et al., 2008).
- **Xanthine Oxidase.** Generation of reactive oxygen species by xanthine oxidase (XO) may account for the association between elevated serum uric acid

levels with endothelial dysfunction and hypertension (Feig et al., 2008a). As will be discussed later in the chapter, elevated uric acid levels are closely associated with new-onset hypertension in children and new data show that lowering of uric acid with allopurinol lowers BP in some pediatric patients (Feig et al., 2008b).
- **Mitochondrial Electron Transport.** Ang II also can induce mitochondrial dysfunction in vitro by activating the endothelial cell NADPH oxidase and formation of peroxynitrite (Doughan et al., 2008).

NOS Inhibition

Asymmetric dimethyl arginine (ADMA) is an endogenous NOS inhibitor, and, as such, is an attractive but unproven mechanism of endothelial dysfunction and hypertension (Thomas et al., 2001). Pharmacologic administration of ADMA or closely-related synthetic methylated arginines will sharply elevate BP in normotensive rats (Sander et al., 1997) and normotensive human subjects (Achan et al., 2003; Sander et al., 1999). Plasma ADMA levels are increased in patients with end-stage renal disease (ESRD) (Vallance et al., 1992) and are associated with reduced endothelial function in young overtly healthy adults with or without hypercholesterolemia (Ardigo et al., 2007; Boger et al., 1998) and in healthy black Africans compared with healthy white Europeans (Melikian et al., 2007). Plasma ADMA is an independent but weak

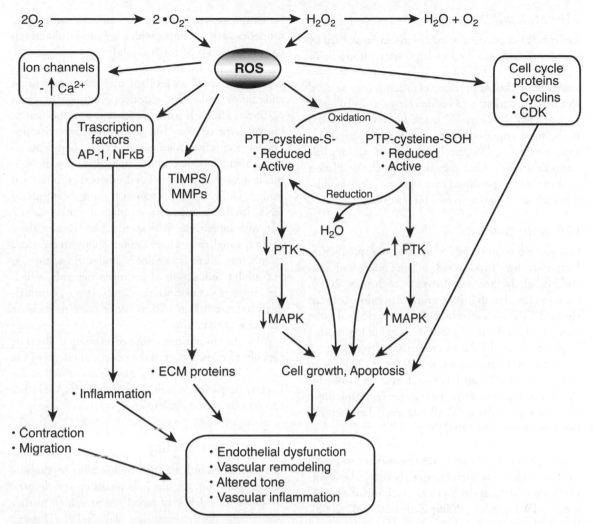

$$2O_2 \longrightarrow 2 \cdot O_2^- \longrightarrow H_2O_2 \longrightarrow H_2O + O_2$$

FIGURE 3-18   Redox-dependent signaling pathways in vascular smooth muscle cells. Intracellular reactive oxygen species (ROS) modify the activity of protein tyrosine kinases (PTK), such as Sre, Ras, JAK2, Pyk2, P13K, and EGFR, as well as mitogen-activated protein kinases (MAPK), particularly p38MAPK, JNK, and ERK5. These processes probably occur through oxidation/reduction of protein tyrosine phosphatases (PTP), which are susceptible to oxidation and inactivation by ROS. ROS also influence gene and protein expression by activating transcription factors, such as NF-κB, activator protein-1 (AP-1) and hypoxia-inducible factor-1 (HIF-1). ROS stimulate ion channels, such as plasma membrane Ca^{2+} and K^+ channels, leading to changes in cation concentration. Activation of these redox-sensitive pathways results in numerous cellular responses which, if uncontrolled, could contribute to hypertensive vascular damage. ECM, extracellular matrix; MMPs, matrix metalloproteinases; TIMP, tissue inhibitor of matrix metalloproteinase. (From Paravicini TM, Touyz RM. Redox signaling in hypertension. *Cardiovasc Res* 2006;71:247–258.)

predictor of all-cause mortality at the population level (Boger et al., 2009). Surprisingly, it is unknown whether plasma ADMA levels are associated with primary hypertension or predict its onset. Moreover, plasma levels of L-arginine (the endogenous substate for NOS) are more than two orders of magnitude higher than plasma ADMA levels (Boger et al.,

2009), which would seem too low to competitively inhibit NOS in vivo.

Measurement of Endothelial Dysfunction in Humans

There are several means of assessing endothelial function in humans (Munzel et al., 2008). They all have limitations.

Flow-Mediated Dilation

Endothelial-dependent vasodilation can be assessed by measuring increases in the large artery (forearm or coronary) diameter following either intra-arterial infusion of acetylcholine or release of ischemia (e.g., arrested forearm circulation) or a sudden elevation in BP (cold pressor test). Noninvasive brachial artery ultrasound is the most commonly used technique. Competitive inhibitors of NOS specifically block endothelial-dependent dilation but they do not block the dilation of these arteries produced by exogenous nitrovasodilators such as nitroglycerin and nitroprusside.

C-Reactive Protein

C-reactive protein (CRP) is an easily measured serum biomarker for blood vessel inflammation and thus endothelial dysfunction (Savoia & Schiffrin, 2006). Cross-sectional studies show strong correlations between elevated CRP with arterial stiffness and elevated pulse pressure (Lakoski et al., 2005). Longitudinal studies implicate elevated CRP as a risk marker/risk factor for new onset of hypertension (Niskanen et al., 2004; Sesso et al., 2003). CRP may be more than a risk marker for future development of hypertension: Transgenic mice that express human CRP develop hypertension (Vongpatanasin et al., 2007).

There has been controversy over whether the measurement of CRP and other biomarkers improves cardiovascular risk stratification beyond the traditional Framingham risk factors, which include hypertension (Wang et al., 2006; Zethelius et al., 2008). Statin therapy reduces the risk of cardiovascular events in patients with high CRPs despite an average baseline LDL cholesterol of 108 mg/dL and an average BP in the high-normal range (134/80 mm Hg) (Ridker et al., 2008).

Other Approaches

Oxidative stress also can be assessed indirectly by measuring urinary levels of isoproteins (Ashfaq et al., 2008) or directly by measuring levels of NADPH oxidase in acutely dissociated human endothelial cells (Donato et al., 2007).

Why Don't Antioxidant Vitamins Lower BP in Humans?

As shown in Figure 3-17, the cellular enzyme superoxide dismutase (SOD) converts superoxide to hydrogen peroxide which is then converted by catalase to water and oxygen. In rats and mice, hypertension can

be eliminated by treating the animals with SOD mimetics such as tempol which are powerful antioxidants (Paravicini & Touyz, 2008).

Given the wealth of the experimental data, the negative results of antioxidant trials for hypertension and cardiovascular disease are disappointing (Paravicini & Touyz, 2008). If oxidative stress is so important in human hypertension, why are antioxidants vitamins not more effective in lowering BP? The best explanation is that vitamins C and E are weak antioxidants—much weaker than tempol and others used in animal studies. Unlike tempol, vitamin E cannot continually renew itself and stops working after an initial interaction with superoxide. With standard oral dosing, these vitamin supplements have limited ability to cross cell membranes where superoxide is produced and they do not inhibit production of hydrogen peroxide, which itself impairs vascular health. Clearly, stronger antioxidants are needed, as well as better ways to measure oxidative stress in vivo.

In the meantime, reduced oxidative stress is thought to explain part of the beneficial effects of the RAAS blockers (Chapter 7) and statins as well as the Dietary Approach to stop Hypertension (DASH) diet and regular exercise (Chapter 6).

Vascular Remodeling

Over time, endothelial cell dysfunction, neurohormonal activation, vascular inflammation, and elevated BP cause remodeling of blood vessels, which further perpetuates the hypertension (Fig. 3-19) (Duprez, 2006). An increase in the medial thickness relative to lumen diameter (increased *media-to-lumen ratio*) is the hallmark of hypertensive remodeling in both small and large arteries.

Mechanisms

Small artery remodeling is initiated by vasoconstriction, which normalizes wall stress and avoids a trophic response (Duprez, 2006). Normal smooth muscle cells rearrange themselves around a smaller lumen, a process termed *inward eutrophic remodeling*. Media-to-lumen ratio increases but medial cross-sectional area is unchanged. In other words, inward eutrophic remodeling describes a decrease in lumen diameter without a change in the composition or amount of vessel wall material. By decreasing lumen diameter in the peripheral circulation, inward eutrophic remodeling increases systemic vascular resistance, the hemodynamic hallmark of diastolic hypertension.

FIGURE 3-19 Vascular remodeling of small and larger arteries in hypertension. Diagrams represent arteries in cross sections showing the tunica adventitia, tunica media, and tunica intima. (Modified from Duprez DA. Role of the renin-angiotensin-aldosterone system in vascular remodeling and inflammation: A clinical review. *J Hypertens* 2006;24:983–991.)

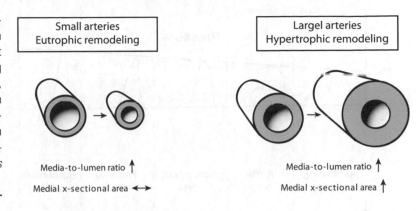

The RAAS seems to be the dominant mechanism in this form of remodeling (Duprez, 2006). Ang II drives this process by generating ROS, activating receptor tyrosine kinases, and negating protective effects of the peroxisome proliferator-activated receptor PPARγ.

By contrast, large artery remodeling is characterized by the expression of hypertrophic genes, triggering increases in medial thickness as well as media-to-lumen ratio (Duprez, 2006). Such *hypertrophic remodeling* involves not only an increase in the size of vascular smooth muscle cells but also an accumulation of extracellular matrix proteins such as collagen and fibronectin due to activation of TGF-β. The resultant large artery stiffness is the hemodynamic hallmark of isolated systolic hypertension.

Intravascular pressure (i.e., shear stress), sympathetic nerves, and Ang II–induced generation of reactive oxygen species—especially H_2O_2—seem to be the key mediators of hypertrophic remodeling.

Assessment of Vascular Remodeling in Human Hypertension

Several approaches are being used to study the remodeling of human arteries in hypertension:

Gluteal Biopsy

Resistance arteries can be isolated from subcutaneous tissue obtained by gluteal biopsy. Direct measurements of intra-arterial pressure, vessel wall dimensions, and receptor density show that small artery remodeling in hypertension can be reversed by oral treatment with RAAS blockers but not β-blockers (despite comparable levels of BP reduction), implicating a specific role for Ang II in the remodeling process (Touyz & Schiffrin, 2008). Arterial smooth muscle from hypertensive patients generates increased

amounts of superoxide when exposed to Ang II (Touyz & Schiffrin, 2008). Vascular AT_2 receptors are upregulated when hypertensive diabetic patients are treated with an ARB (but not with a β-blocker) (Savoia et al., 2007).

Noninvasive Assessment of Central Aortic Pressure

Vascular remodeling can be monitored noninvasively in patients by derivation of central aortic pressure waveforms via radial artery applanation tonography. Central aortic pressure—though measured indirectly—is superior to brachial artery BP as an index of the hemodynamic stress on the cerebral, coronary, and renal blood vessels (Agabiti-Rosei et al., 2007).

Contours of Central Versus Peripheral Pressure Waves

The arterial pressure waveform changes as it travels from the central aorta to the peripheral arteries. The key concepts are summarized in the consensus document from the American Heart Association (Agabiti-Rosei et al., 2007):

> The pressure wave generated by the left ventricle travels down the arterial tree and then is reflected at multiple peripheral sites, mainly at resistance arteries (small muscular arteries and arterioles). Consequently, the pressure waveform recorded at any site of the arterial tree is the sum of the forward traveling waveform generated by left ventricular ejection and the backward traveling wave, the "echo" of the incident wave reflected at peripheral sites. When the large conduit arteries are healthy and compliant, the reflected wave merges with the incident wave during diastole, thereby augmenting the diastolic BP and aiding coronary perfusion. In contrast, when the arteries are stiff, pulse wave velocity increases, accelerating the incident and reflected waves; thus, the reflected wave merges with the incident wave in systole and augments

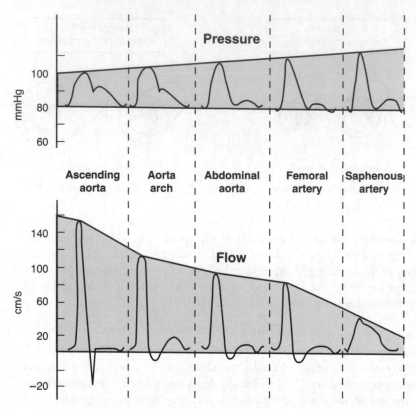

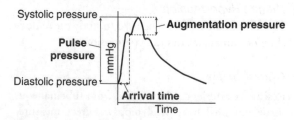

FIGURE 3-20 Change in contours in pressure wave (**top**) and flow wave (**bottom**) between the ascending aorta and the saphenous artery. (From Agabiti-Rosei E, Mancia G, O'Rourke MF, et al. Central blood pressure measurements and antihypertensive therapy: A consensus document. *Hypertension* 2007;50: 154–160.)

aortic systolic rather than diastolic pressure. As a result, left ventricular afterload increases, and normal ventricular relaxation and coronary filling are compromised.... Another important consideration is "pressure wave amplification." Typically, the diastolic and mean pressures change little across the arterial tree. However, systolic BP is amplified when moving from the aorta to periphery (Fig. 3-20).... In general, brachial systolic and pulse pressure tend to overestimate central systolic and pulse pressure, both in younger subjects and in older people.

COMMERICAL DEVICES Of the commercially available devices, SphygmoCor (AtCor Medical, Houston, TX) is the one most widely used in clinical studies. It uses standard cuff measurements of brachial artery BP and a validated generalized transfer function (proprietary software) to convert the radial or carotid artery waveform—measured by applanation tonography—to a derived central aortic BP waveform (Fig. 3-21) (Agabiti-Rosei et al., 2007). The derived values for aortic pulse pressure, the augmentation index, and the pulse wave velocity all are indices of vascular remodeling, in particular aortic stiffness. Typically, in hypertension, pulse pressure is widened, augmentation index is increased, pulse wave velocity is increased, and the dicrotic notch is absent.

AMBULATORY AORTIC STIFFNESS An index of aortic stiffness from standard ABPM can also be derived by plotting systolic pressure as a function of diastolic pressure (Dechering et al., 2008). The theory is simple: For a given rise in diastolic BP, systolic BP should rise more if the large arteries are stiff rather than compliant. The ambulatory arterial stiffness index (AASI) is calculated by plotting 1 minus the regression slope for individual values for systolic and diastolic BP

FIGURE 3-21 Central pressure waveform. The height of the late systolic peak above the inflection defines the augmented pressure, and the ratio of augmented pressure to PP defines the augmentation index (in percentage). (From Agabiti-Rosei E, Mancia G, O'Rourke MF, et al. Central blood pressure measurements and antihypertensive therapy: A consensus document. *Hypertension* 2007;50:154–160.)

downloaded from the ambulatory BP monitor. However, there are conflicting data over the reproducibility of AASI and its correlation with pulse wave velocity and other more established measures of arterial stiffness (Dechering et al., 2008; Gosse et al., 2007; Schillaci & Parati, 2008).

Small-Vessel Rarefaction and Impaired Tissue Perfusion

Both experimental and human hypertension are commonly accompanied by *microvascular rarefaction*—reduced number or combined length of small vessels in a given volume of tissue (Levy et al., 2008). Reactive oxygen species can cause both constriction of precapillary vessels with functional rarefaction (decreased capillary recruitment during metabolic demand) and apoptosis with anatomic rarefaction (vascular smooth muscle cell death with vessel dropout).

Microvascular rarefaction involves reduced skin capillary recruitment and reduced reactive hyperemia in forearm and coronary circulations even in the absence of coronary atherosclerosis (Levy et al., 2008). Microvascular rarefaction/ischemia is an attractive mechanism explaining the frequent coexistence of hypertension and diabetes (in particular, impaired insulin-mediated glucose uptake in skeletal muscle) and for the accelerated target organ damage in patients with both conditions.

Summary

Remodeling of large and small arteries may begin early in the hypertensive process and may be a cause as well as a consequence of high BP. Antihypertensive therapy may not provide optimal cardiovascular protection unless vascular remodeling is prevented or reversed by normalizing hemodynamic load, restoring normal endothelial cell function, quenching vascular inflammation, and eliminating adverse neurohormonal activation (Duprez, 2006).

HORMONAL MECHANISMS: THE RENIN-ANGIOTENSIN-ALDOSTERONE SYSTEM

As noted, activation of the RAAS is one of the most important mechanisms contributing to renal sodium retention, endothelial cell dysfunction, vascular inflammation and remodeling, and eventual hypertension (Fig. 3-22) (Duprez, 2006; Marchesi et al., 2008).

Overview

Beginning with the discovery of renin in 1898 by the Finnish physiologist Robert Tigerstedt and his medical student Bergman, work by multiple research groups has brought us to our current understanding, which continues to evolve (Luft, 2008).

Renin, a protease produced solely by the renal juxtaglomerular cells, cleaves angiotensinogen (renin substrate produced by the liver) to angiotensin I which is converted by angiotensin-converting enzyme (ACE) to angiotensin II (Ang II) (Fig. 3-22). ACE is most abundant in the lungs but also is present in the heart and systemic vasculature (*tissue ACE*). Chymase, a serine protease in the heart and systemic arteries, provides an alternative pathway for conversion of Ang I to Ang II. The interaction of Ang II with G protein–coupled AT_1 receptors activates numerous cellular processes that contribute to hypertension and accelerate hypertensive end-organ damage. These include vasoconstriction, generation of reactive oxygen species, vascular inflammation, vascular and cardiac remodeling, and production of aldosterone. There is increasing evidence that aldosterone, Ang II, and even renin and prorenin activate multiple signaling pathways that can damage vascular health and cause hypertension. Other metabolites of Ang I, including Ang 1–7, may protect against hypertension but the clinical evidence is less well developed.

Aldosterone and Epithelial Sodium Channel Regulation

RAAS activation constitutes a short-term defense mechanism against hypovolemic hypotension (as with hemorrhage or salt deprivation). Interaction of aldosterone with cytosolic mineralocorticoid receptors in the renal collecting duct cells recruits sodium channels from the cytosol to the surface of the renal epithelium. The ENaCs so recruited increase sodium reabsorption, thereby re-expanding plasma volume.

Conversely, modern high-salt diets should engender continual feedback inhibition of the RAAS. Suppression of serum aldosterone should cause endocytosis and destruction of ENaC (via dephosphorylation and thus activation of the unbiquitin ligase Nedd4-2) and increased renal sodium excretion,

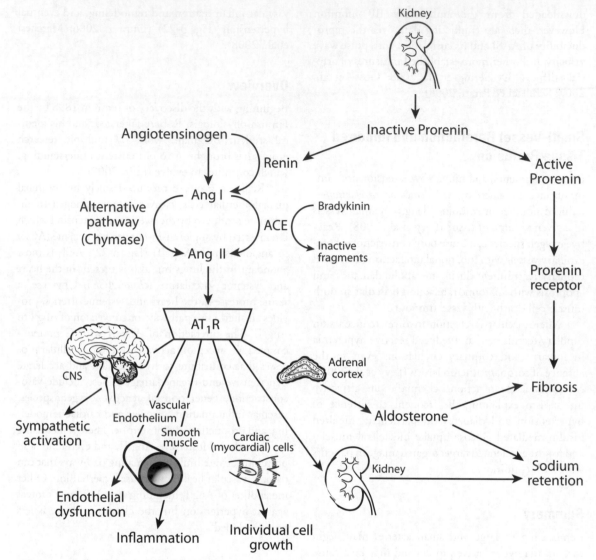

FIGURE 3-22   The renin-angiotensin-aldosterone system. Ang I, angiotensin 1; Ang II, angiotensin II, ACE, angiotensin converting enzyme; AT₁R, type 1 angiotensin receptor.

thereby shrinking plasma volume and defending against salt hypertension (Victor, 2007).

In the setting of high dietary sodium and elevated BP, the RAAS should be completely suppressed and any degree of RAAS activity is inappropriate (Victor, 2007). However, in normotensive individuals, the risk of developing hypertension increases with increasing levels of serum aldosterone within the "normal" range (Vasan et al., 2004). In Afro-Caribbean hypertensives, serum aldosterone levels are higher than in white hypertensives despite lower plasma renins (Stewart et al., 2006), implicating abnormal aldosterone

production by renin-independent mechanisms—a forme fruste of primary aldosteronism.

Mineralocorticoid receptors are widely expressed outside the kidney so that aldosterone can impair vascular health by multiple extrarenal mechanisms (Schiffrin, 2006). Aldosterone amplifies Ang II– induced vascular inflammation and remodeling (Duprez, 2006). By stimulating mineralocorticoid receptors in the heart and kidney, circulating aldosterone promotes cardiac and renal fibrosis in hypertension (Schiffrin, 2006). By stimulating mineralocorticoid receptors in the brainstem circumventricular organs, aldosterone may contribute to sympathetic overactivity. However, aldosterone only seems to cause trouble in the presence of a high-sodium diet (Williams et al., 2005a).

Receptor-Mediated Actions of Ang II

Ang II is the main effector peptide of the RAAS. Two main types of G protein–coupled angiotensin receptors are known. AT_1 receptors are widely expressed in the vasculature, kidneys, adrenals, heart, liver, and brain. AT_1 receptor activation explains most of the hypertensive actions of Ang II. As noted, stimulation of AT_1 receptors by Ang II is the best studied mechanism for the activation of vascular NADPH oxidase and thus, reactive oxygen species in the vasculature, in the kidneys, and in the brain.

Furthermore, enhanced AT_1 receptor-mediated signaling provides a common mechanistic explanation for the frequent coexistance of elevated BP with insulin resistance and atherosclerosis and constitutes a major therapeutic target for interrupting every step in cardiovascular disease progression from vascular remodeling and formation of atherosclerotic plaque to stroke, myocardial infarction (MI), and death (Fig. 3-23).

By contrast, AT_1 receptors are widely distributed in the fetus but in adults are found only in the adrenal medulla, uterus, ovary, vascular endothelium, and distinct brain regions. In rodents, AT_2 receptor activation opposes most (but perhaps not all) of the deleterious effects of AT_1 receptors by promoting endothelial-dependent vasodilation by bradykinin and nitric oxide pathways. However, other animal data suggest that AT_2 receptors can be profibrotic and the role of AT_2 receptors in human hypertension remains speculative.

The finding of several angiotensin metabolites has added to the complexity of the RAAS (Fig. 3-24).

Receptor-Mediated Actions of Renin and Prorenin

In the traditional view of the RAAS, prorenin has been considered to be the inactive precursor of renin, which functions solely to generate Ang I by enzymatic

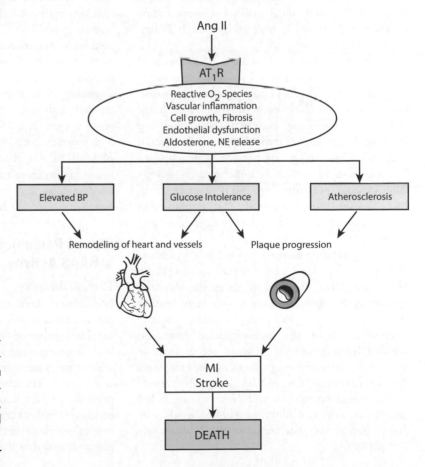

FIGURE 3-23 Central mechanistic role of Ang II type I receptor-mediated signaling in hypertension and cardiovascular disease progression. NE, norepinephrine; BP, blood pressure; MI, myocardial infarction.

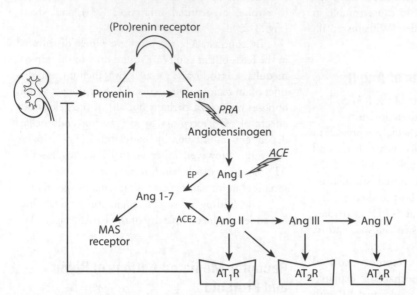

FIGURE 3-24 Increasing complexity in the understanding of the renin-angiotensin system. Ang 1–7 interacts with a specific G protein–coupled Mas receptor and generally opposes the vasoconstrictor and proliferative actions of Ang II. PRA, plasma renin activity; ACE, angiotensin converting enzyme; ACE2, type 2 angiotensin converting enzyme; EP, endopeptidase Ang I, angiotensin I; Ang II, angiotensin II; Ang III, angiotensin III; Ang IV, angiotensin IV; Ang 1–7; angiotensin one-through-seven; AT_1R, type 1 angiotensin receptor; AT_2R, type 2 angiotensin receptor; AT_4R, type 4 angiotensin receptor.

cleavage of angiotensinogen. New concepts are rapidly evolving as data implicate prorenin and renin as direct cardiac and renal toxins—a notion first advanced and vigorously pursued by Laragh, Sealey, and coworkers (Laragh, 2001).

Prorenin is inactive because a 43-amino acid hinge is closed and prevents it from binding to angiotensinogen. In the kidneys, inactive prorenin is converted to active renin when this inhibitory hinge region is enzymatically cleaved. When circulating prorenin binds to a newly discovered (pro)renin receptor in the heart and kidneys, the hinge is opened (but not cleaved) and this nonenzymatic process fully activates prorenin (Fig. 3-25) (Huang et al., 2006; Danser, 2006). As a result, TGF-β production is accelerated, leading to collagen deposition and fibrosis.

This receptor-mediated process is independent of Ang II generation and therefore unaffected by ACEIs and ARBs. While these are excellent antihypertensives (Chapter 7), they trigger large reactive increases in prorenin and renin production that may counter some of the cardiovascular protection afforded by reduced AT_1 receptor activation. The reactive increases are even greater with the new direct renin inhibitor aliskiren, which reduces renin's ability to cleave angiotensinogen and generate Ang I, but nevertheless does not inhibit profibrotic signaling by the pro(renin) receptor (Feldt et al., 2008; Schefe et al., 2008).

As prorenin blood levels typically are 100-fold higher than renin levels, pro(renin) receptor activation may turn out to be an important mechanism of human hypertension. Its recent discovery has rekindled interest in older, and largely forgotten, observations. Sealy and Laragh (1975) found prorenin in human plasma. Twenty years later, Wilson and Luetscher (Wilson & Luetscher, 1990) found that children with type 1 diabetes have high levels of prorenin despite their low PRA; moreover, those with high prorenin levels developed diabetic complications of renal failure, blindness, and neuropathy. Thus, prorenin may be a "new" biomarker, particularly for microvascular and macrovascular complications of hypertension and diabetes.

Plasma Renin Activity as a Clinical Index of RAAS Activity

Clinical Assays

Both plasma renin activity (PRA) and plasma renin concentration (PRC) can be measured. PRA is measured by incubating a patient's plasma, which contains both angiotensinogen and renin, to generate Ang I, which then is measured by radioimmunoassay (Sealey et al., 2005). The amount of Ang I generated is proportional to the amount of renin present. Care must be taken to prevent cryoactivation of prorenin, leading to spurious elevations in PRA (Sealey et al., 2005). If plasma is cooled to 4°C, the prosegment hinge unfolds

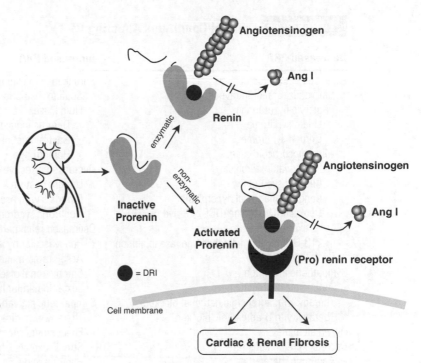

FIGURE 3-25 Inhibition of both enzymatic and nonenzymatic activation of prorenin. Ang, Angiotensin; DRI, direct renin inhibitor. (Modified from Danser AH, Deinum J. Renin, prorenin and the putative (pro)renin receptor. *Hypertension* 2005;46:1069–1076, with permission.)

and is subsequently cleaved by plasma proteases (Fig. 3-25). To avoid prorenin cryoactivation, plasma samples should be processed at room temperature.

PRA can be measured by many commercial clinical laboratories. By contrast, PRC and prorenin levels are measured mainly for research purposes. As yet, there is no clear clinical advantage of PRC over PRA, as both assays require rigorous laboratory standards and avoidance of cryoactivation.

PRA Levels

The multiple factors that can alter renin secretion include those shown in Table 3-4, with changes in pressure within the afferent arterioles (intrarenal baroreceptors), sodium concentration in the macula densa, and renal SNA (via β_1-adrenoceptors [ARs]) likely playing the most important roles.

Considering all the factors affecting PRA, the agreement noted in the literature is rather surprising: Almost all patients with primary aldosteronism have suppressed values, most patients with renovascular or accelerated malignant hypertension have elevated levels, and the prevalence of suppressed values among patients with primary hypertension is surprisingly similar in different series (Fig. 3-26). Specific information about the use of PRA assays in the evaluation of various identifiable forms of hypertension is provided in subsequent chapters.

The listing in Table 3-4 is not intended to cover every known condition and disease in which a renin assay has been performed, but the more clinically important ones are listed in an attempt to categorize them by mechanism. Some conditions could fit in two or more categories; for example, upright posture may involve a decreased effective plasma volume and sympathetic activation and decreased renal perfusion.

Role in Primary Hypertension

Elevated BP itself—particularly volume-expanded salt-sensitive hypertension—should cause complete feedback suppression of PRA. In fact, patients with primary hypertension tend to have lower PRA levels than do age- and gender-matched normotensives (Helmer, 1964; Meade et al., 1993). However, most patients with primary hypertension do not have suppressed PRA, stimulating much clinical research to explain the "inappropriately" normal or even elevated PRA levels (Fig. 3-26).

The following explanations have been proposed: Sealey et al. (1988) proposed the theory of nephron heterogeneity—a subpopulation of ischemic nephrons contributing excess renin. Esler et al. (1977) proposed that high renin primary hypertension is neurogenic—high renal SNA. Hollenberg, Williams and coworkers (Williams et al., 1992) proposed the concept of

TABLE 3.4	Clinical Conditions Affecting PRA

Decreased PRA	Increased PRA
Expanded fluid volume	Shrunken fluid volume
Salt loads, oral or intravenous	Sodium restriction
Primary salt retention	Fluid losses
Liddle syndrome	Diuretic induced
Gordon syndrome	Gastrointestinal losses
Mineralocorticoid excess	Hemorrhage
Primary aldosteronism	Decreased effective plasma volume
Cushing syndrome	Upright posture
Congenital adrenal hyperplasia	Cirrhosis with ascites
Deoxycorticosterone (DOC), 18-hydroxy-DOC excess	Nephrotic syndrome
11β-Hydroxysteroid dehydrogenase inhibition (licorice)	Decreased renal perfusion pressure
Sympathetic inhibition	Renovascular hypertension
Autonomic dysfunction	Accelerated-malignant hypertension
Therapy with adrenergic neuronal blockers	Chronic renal disease (renin dependent)
Therapy with β-adrenergic blockers	Juxtaglomerular hyperplasia
Hyperkalemia	Sympathetic activation
Decreased renin substrate (?)	Therapy with direct vasodilators
Androgen therapy	Pheochromocytoma
Decrease in renal tissue	Stress: exercise, hypoglycemia
Hyporeninemic hypoaldosteronism	Hyperthyroidism
Chronic renal disease (volume dependent)	Sympathomimetic agents (caffeine)
Anephric	Hypokalemia
Increasing age	Increased renin substrate
Unknown	Pregnancy
Low renin primary hypertension	Estrogen therapy
Black race	Autonomous renin hypersecretion
	Renin-secreting tumors
	Acute damage to juxtaglomerular cells
	Acute glomerulonephritis
	Decreased feedback inhibition
	Low AII levels (ACEI therapy)
	Unknown
	High renin primary hypertension

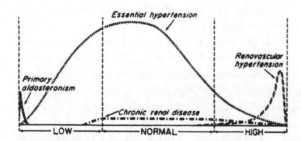

FIGURE 3-26 Schematic representation of PRA in various hypertensive diseases. The approximate number of patients with each type of hypertension is indicated along with their proportion of low, normal, or high renin levels. (Modified from Kaplan NM. Renin profiles. *JAMA* 1977;238:611–613; Copyright 1977, American Medical Association.)

nonmodulation—defective feedback regulation of RAAS within the kidneys and adrenal glands.

Primary Hypertension with Low Renin

Clearly, there are numerous possible explanations for normal levels of renin in hypertension, which is the usual finding. Although low renin levels are expected in the absence of one or another of the previously described circumstances, a great deal of work has been done to uncover special mechanisms, prognoses, and therapy for hypertensives with low renin, in particular for the twofold greater prevalence of low renin in blacks than in nonblacks (Sagnella, 2001).

MECHANISMS One of the possible mechanisms for low-renin hypertension is volume expansion with or without mineralocorticoid excess, but the majority of careful analyses fail to indicate volume expansion (Sagnella, 2001) or increased levels of mineralocorticoids (Pratt et al., 1999). In keeping with normal levels of aldosterone despite the low renin levels, low-renin hypertensives showed a lesser rise in aldosterone secretion on a low-sodium diet (Fisher et al., 1999).

Genetically determined impairment of renal sodium excretion has been associated with low-renin hypertension (Lifton et al., 2001). As described in Chapters 13 and 14, new forms of low-renin hypertension have recently been recognized, one with increased amounts of 18-hydroxylated steroids, the other with high levels of cortisol from inhibition of the 11β-hydroxysteroid dehydrogenase enzyme. Not surprisingly, subtle degrees of these defects have been looked for in low-renin hypertensives, with only equivocal results (Carvajal et al., 2005; Rossi et al., 2001; Soro et al., 1995; Williams et al., 2005b).

PROGNOSIS A retrospective analysis over a 7-year interval showed that patients with low-renin hypertension had no strokes or heart attacks, whereas 11% of normal-renin and 14% of high-renin patients had experienced one of these cardiovascular complications (Brunner et al., 1972). In a prospective study of 1,717 hypertensive subjects followed up for as long as 8 years while being treated, the incidence of MI was 14.7 per 1,000 person-years in the 12% with high renin levels, 5.6 per 1,000 person-years in the 56% with a normal level, and 2.8 per 1,000 person-years in the 32% with a low renin level (Alderman et al., 1991). The incidence of stroke was not correlated with renin status. In an expanded population followed up for as long as 3.6 years, the relation between PRA levels and MI remained independent and direct, but only in those with an initial BP above 95 mm Hg (Alderman et al., 1997).

Conversely, Meade et al. (1993) found no association between PRA levels and ischemic heart disease in a 20-year follow-up of 803 white, normotensive men. No increase in carotid artery disease was found among high-renin patients (Rossi et al., 2000). Some have noted direct relation between renin levels and LVH (Aronow et al., 1997; Koga et al., 1998).

THERAPY Laragh (1973) and Laragh and Sealey (2003) attach a great deal of significance to the various PRA levels found in patients with primary hypertension. According to their view, the levels of renin can identify the relative contributions of vasoconstriction and body fluid volume expansion to the pathogenesis of hypertension. According to the "bipolar vasoconstriction-volume analysis," arteriolar vasoconstriction by Ang II is predominantly responsible for the hypertension in patients with high renin, whereas volume expansion is predominantly responsible in those with low renin.

In keeping with their presumed but unproved volume excess, patients with low-renin primary hypertension have been found by some investigators (Vaughan et al., 1973; Preston et al., 1998) but not by others (Ferguson et al., 1977; Holland et al., 1979; Hunyor et al., 1975) to experience a greater fall in BP when given diuretics than do normal-renin patients. Age and race were found to be better predictors of response to various drugs (Preston et al., 1998) in some studies, and, in other studies, the renin status simply did not reflect the response at all (Weir & Saunders, 1998).

Recently, short-term studies find that a low PRA generally predicts a larger initial fall in BP with a thiazide diuretic, whereas a high PRA generally predicts a larger initial fall in BP with an ACE inhibitor or an ARB; however, the effect is small compared with the large degree of inter- and intra-subject variability in these responses. These studies are summarized as follows:

• In a study of 203 African American and 236 white hypertensives, pretreatment PRA was positively associated with the BP response to an ARB, with PRA accounting for 15% of the between-subject variation in the response (Canzanello et al., 2008).
• In a prospective study of 208 Finnish men with moderate hypertension, pretreatment PRA was positively correlated with the BP response to an ARB or a β-blocker and negatively correlated with the BP response to a thiazide diuretic; however, PRA accounted for only 4% of the overall variability in responses between patients (Suonsyrja et al., 2008).
• Similarly, PRA accounted for only 4% of the between-subject variability to 1-month of hydrochlorothiazide (HCTZ) monotherapy in another study of 197 African Americans and 190 whites with hypertension (Turner et al., 2001); moreover, the responses of individual subjects were not predictable among those who repeated the protocol.

In general clinical practice, most physicians do not find routine renin profiling to be necessary for establishing prognosis or determining therapy. However, as will be noted in subsequent chapters, renin profiling is often used in the diagnosis of low- and high-renin secondary forms of medically refractory hypertension.

T Cells and Ang II–Induced Hypertension: A Novel Unifying Hypothesis

Mouse studies seem to suggest that Ang II–induced hypertension can be caused by selective activation of NADPH oxidase only in blood vessels (Landmesser et al., 2002), only in the kidney (Dickhout et al., 2002), and only in the brain subfornical organ (Zimmerman et al., 2002). In trying to reconcile these confusing findings, Harrison et al. (2008) searched for a circulating blood-borne signal as a unifying hypothesis and have provided data that T cells—which also express AT_1 receptors

and NADPH oxidase—play a central role in the genesis of hypertension—at least in mice and possibly in humans.

According to this new theory which is illustrated in Figure 3-27, Ang II activates NADPH oxidase and increases reactive oxygen species in the subfornical organ, which triggers SNA to the spleen and lymph nodes causing additional T cells to be released into the circulation. At the same time, Ang II activates T cell NADPH oxidase causing T cell activation and increases expression of chemokines and cell surface receptors honing activated T cells to the adipose tissue encasing the blood vessels and the kidney.

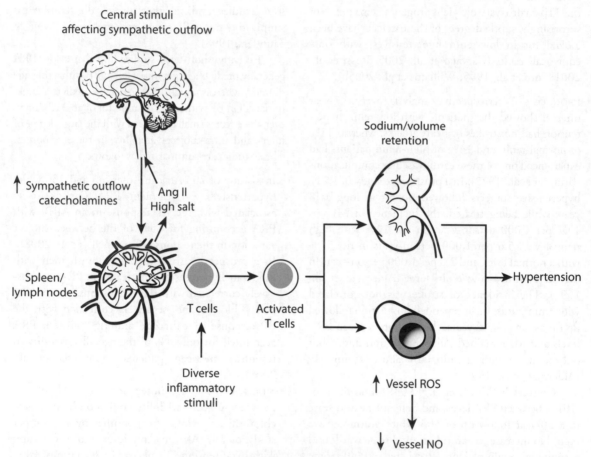

FIGURE 3-27 Proposed mechanism for the role of adaptive immunity in hypertension. Hypertensive stimuli such as Ang II can participate in T cell activation by directly acting on T cells and also via central nervous system activation. CNS activation leads to increased sympathetic outflow which also promotes T cell activation and enhances chemokine production in the perivascular fat and the perinephric adipose tissue, promoting T cell accumulation at these sites. Diverse inflammatory stimuli also promote hypertension by activating T cells. Activated T cells enter the perivascular fat, activating the vascular production of reactive oxygen species (ROS) and reducing NO production, thus causing vasoconstriction. T cells also affect renal sodium and volume handling. These actions on the kidney and vasculature lead to hypertension. (From Harrison DG, Guzik TJ, Goronzy J, et al. Is hypertension an immunologic disease? *Curr Cardiol Rep* 2008;10:464–469.)

These sequestered T cells release tumor necrosis factor (TNFα) and other cytokines that activate vascular and renal NADPH oxidase, continuously driving local production of reactive oxygen species. Thus, sequestration of activated T cells in perivascular fat promotes vasoconstriction and vascular remodeling. Sequestration of activated T cells in perinephric fat promotes renal dysfunction and sodium retention.

Experimental Evidence

The growing experimental evidence for activated T cells in hypertension includes the following:

• Neonatal thymectomy delays the development of hypertension in rodent models (Khraibi et al., 1987).
• The T cell–selective immunosuppressant mycophenolate mofetil (CellCept) lowers BP and lessens renal injury in Dahl salt-sensitive rats fed a high-salt diet (Tian et al., 2007) and in rats with salt-sensitive hypertension induced by acute renal ischemia (Pechman et al., 2008).
• Mice lacking the recombinase activating gene (RAG1-/- mice) lack both T and B cells, and have a blunted hypertensive response to challenge with either Ang II or DOCA-salt (Guzik et al., 2007). Adoptive transfer of T cells—but not B cells—fully restores the hypertension.
• The TNFα antagonist intercept blocks the generation of vascular reactive oxygen species and normalizes BP in mouse models of Ang II–induced hypertension and mineralocorticoid-induced hypertension (Guzik et al., 2007).

Translational Evidence

The translational evidence, though appealing, is as yet circumstantial:

• In patients with AIDS, BP is low before treatment and increases as T cell counts rise with highly effective antiretroviral therapy (Seaberg et al., 2005). Confounding effects of body weight and general health cannot be excluded in this large study of 5,578 men.
• Patients with rheumatoid arthritis, psoriasis, and other inflammatory collagen-vascular diseases have very high rates of hypertension (Panoulas et al., 2008). Although the risk of hypertension increases with increasing severity of the inflammatory disease (Neimann et al., 2006), steroid therapy also contributes (Panoulas et al., 2007).
• Preliminary data suggest that mycophenolate mofetil may benefit hypertension in patients with collagen-vascular disease (Herrera et al., 2006). In this uncontrolled study of eight patients with psoriasis or rheumatoid arthritis and uncomplicated stage 1 hypertension, average clinic BP fell from 152/92 to 137/83 mm Hg after 3 months of mycophenolate mofetil and then returned to pretreatment levels after therapy was stopped. Changes in BP mirrored changes in urinary excretion of TNFα. A proper trial is needed to draw mechanistic conclusions.

Implicating T cell activation as a cause of primary hypertension may seem counterintuitive because many other anti-inflammatory agents—including NSAIDs, prednisone, and cyclosporine—often cause hypertension as will be discussed in Chapter 14. In standard pharmacologic doses, these agents cause renal sodium retention and vasoconstriction by multiple other mechanisms.

T cell activation may be particularly important in obesity-related hypertension, which will be discussed next, followed by consideration of some clinical conditions that also are associated with a higher incidence of hypertension.

HYPERTENSION RELATED TO OBESITY, THE METABOLIC SYNDROME, AND TYPE 2 DIABETES

The first and foremost of these clinical conditions is the triad of obesity, the metabolic syndrome, and type 2 diabetes. Hypertension is part of the obesity epidemic which is escalating at a phenomenal rate especially in young people (Barlow, 2007). Before discussing mechanisms of obesity-related hypertension, a few introductory comments are in order.

The Obesity Epidemic

The past two decades have seen drastic increase in rates of obesity and type 2 diabetes in both developed and developing countries. Here are some startling statistics:

• Two thirds of the US adult population is overweight (BMI > 25) with about 32% being obese (BMI > 30); among the latter, 5% are extremely obese (BMI > 40) (Grundy, 2008).
• Among US children, the prevalence of obesity (defined as BMI > 95 percentile) has increased from 5% in 1970 to 17% in 2004 (Barlow, 2007).

• Obesity is associated with a shortened lifespan both in rodent models and in humans. Among nonsmokers, obesity will shorten life expectancy by 5.8 years in men and by 7.1 years in women (Peters et al., 2003). Conversely, in rhesus monkeys caloric restriction increases longevity and reduces the incidence of age-related diseases including diabetes, cardiovascular disease, brain atrophy, and cancer (Colman et al., 2009).

The Obesity Epidemic as a Gene-Environment Interaction

The recent obesity epidemic is attributed to our modern culture of fast food and sedentary lifestyle. In the words of Esler (2008), the escalation in childhood obesity is due to "potato chips and computer chips." Thus, lifestyle modification with diet and exercise is considered the cornerstone of treatment (Harsha & Bray, 2008). However, recidivism is nearly universal and, according to Mark (2008), "dietary therapy for obesity is an emperor with no clothes."

Both genetic and biological factors contribute to the universal difficulty in maintaining a low-calorie diet (Mark, 2008). On the one hand, weight loss activates powerful compensatory mechanisms that stimulate appetite and slow metabolism. On the other hand, twin and adoptive studies show that BMI is a highly heritable trait and that individuals vary greatly in their genetic propensity or resistance to gain weight in our toxic modern environment.

Association with Hypertension

Across populations, hypertension prevalence tracks with average BMI as illustrated among the African diaspora: Despite common ancestral genes, hypertension is present in only 10% of Africans living in rural Cameroon where average BMI is 22, 25% in Jamaicans with an average BMI 25, but 40% in African Americans in Illinois with an average BMI of 35 (Fig. 3-28) (Cooper et al., 1997). Weight gain, even to levels not considered to be a problem, increases the incidence of hypertension. The Framingham Heart Study investigators estimate that 70% of hypertension in men and 61% in women are directly attributable to excess adiposity; a 4.5-mm Hg average increase in systolic BP was seen with every 10-lb weight gain (Kannel et al., 1993).

Moreover, obesity is accompanied by an increased incidence of hypertension-related outcomes, including stroke (Jood et al., 2004), coronary disease (Widlansky et al., 2004), heart failure (Kenchaiah et al., 2002), and cardiomyopathy (Pilz et al., 2004).

Mechanisms of Obesity-Related Hypertension

The hemodynamic pattern of obesity-related hypertension is volume expansion, increased cardiac output, and systemic vascular resistance that fails to fall enough to balance the higher cardiac output (Esler et al., 2006).

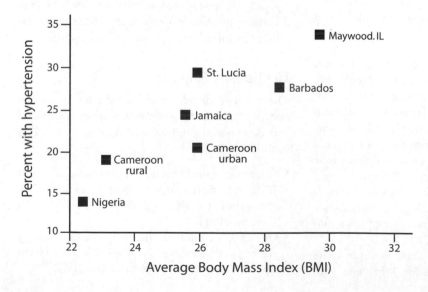

FIGURE 3-28 Age- and sex-adjusted prevalence of hypertension among seven populations of West African origin. (Modified from Cooper R, Rotimi C, Ataman S, et al. The prevalence of hypertension in seven populations of west African origin. *Am J Public Health* 1997;87:160–168, with permission.)

A large number of mechanisms are supported by data from animal and human observations. A partial list includes the following:

- Sympathetic overactivity (Esler et al., 2006)
- Selective leptin resistance (Correia & Haynes, 2004; Yang & Barouch, 2007)
- Adipokines including leptin, free fatty acids, Ang II (Katagiri et al., 2007)
- RAAS overactivity, reactive oxygen species and nitric oxide deficiency (Katagiri et al., 2007) with T cell activation (Wu et al., 2007)
- Overactivity of the endocannabinoid pathway (Grassi et al., 2008b)

As illustrated in Figure 3-29, visceral adipose tissue seems to link obesity with hypertension and atherosclerosis. Adipose tissue is no longer considered merely a passive energy storage depot. Fat cells produce large numbers of biologically active substances termed *adipokines* (Katagiri et al., 2007). Many of these have been implicated as prohypertensive, including leptin, angiotensinogen, resistin, retinol binding protein (RBP4), plasminogen activator inhibitor-1 (PAI-1), tumor necrosis factor (TNFα), fatty acids, sex steroids, and growth factors. Others such as adiponectin are considered antihypertensive. The prohypertensive/proatherosclerotic adipokines are thought to compromise

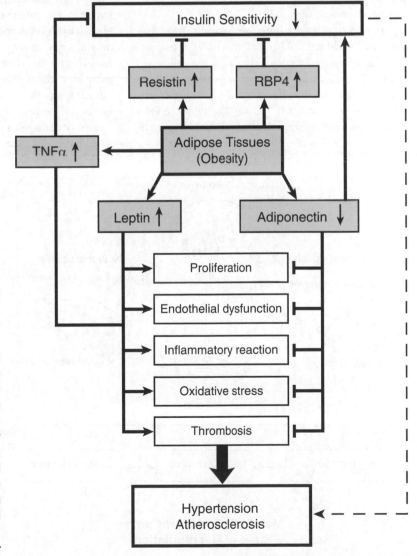

FIGURE 3-29 Adipocytokines interact in a complex way to regulate vascular function and ultimately the development of cardiovascular diseases. RBP4, retinol binding protein; TNFα, tumor necrosis factor. (From Katagiri H, Yamada T, Oka Y. Adiposity and cardiovascular disorders: Disturbance of the regulatory system consisting of humoral and neuronal signals. *Circ Res* 2007;101:27–39.)

vascular health by multiple mechanisms including proliferation of vascular smooth muscle, inflammation, oxidative stress, endothelial dysfunction, and thrombosis.

Neural Mechanisms of Obesity-Related Hypertension

Sympathetic overactivity is one of the most important mechanisms—perhaps the most important mechanism—linking obesity to hypertension and hypertensive target-organ damage (Mancia et al., 2007). The MSNA is higher in normotensive obese subjects than in normotensive lean subjects and higher still in obese hypertensives (Lambert et al., 2007). With weight gain, increased SNA is thought to be a compensatory mechanism to burn fat—but at the expense of sympathetic activation in tissues regulating BP—kidney and vascular smooth muscle (Fig. 3-30).

However, this appealing teleological theory, proposed by Landsberg (2006), has been called into question: Ganglionic blockade causes a greater fall in BP in obese than in lean hypertensive patients but surprisingly has a smaller effect on resting energy expenditure (Shibao et al., 2007). Thus, the evidence for a sympathetic contribution to obesity-related hypertension is strong but a complete picture is missing.

Several factors can activate the sympathetic nervous system in obese individuals: (i) obstructive sleep apnea, which causes recurrent hypoxia and activates the carotid body chemoreceptors that reflexively increase sympathetic activity (Biaggioni, 2007; Esler et al., 2006), (ii) accumulation of liver fat, which activates hepatic sensory afferents that reflexively increase SNA (Katagiri et al., 2007), and (iii) overfed fat cells, which release adipokines that cross the blood-brain barrier and activate SNA centrally (Katagiri et al., 2007).

Obstructive Sleep Apnea as a Cause of Neurogenic Hypertension

Obstructive sleep apnea, as will be discussed in Chapter 14, is common in obese persons and is considered an important cause of hypertension and hypertensive heart disease (Biaggioni, 2007). In obstructive sleep apnea, repeated episodes of arterial desaturation during sleep trigger large swings in MSNA and BP (Narkiewicz et al., 2005). Furthermore, the chemoreflex seems to reset, causing sustained sympathetic activation even during waking hours.

In patients with obstructive sleep apnea, the elevated levels of plasma and urine catecholamines may

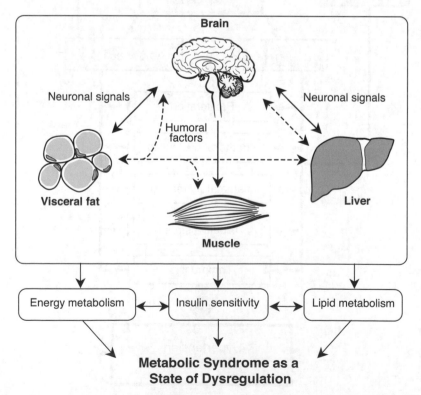

FIGURE 3-30 Proposed communications among organs/tissues via humoral and neuronal pathways involved in the metabolic syndrome. (From Katagiri H, Yamada T, Oka Y. Adiposity and cardiovascular disorders: Disturbance of the regulatory system consisting of humoral and neuronal signals. *Circ Res* 2007;101:27–39.)

mimic those seen with pheochromocytoma, as discussed in Chapter 12.

If obstructive sleep apnea is a common cause of neurogenic hypertension, why is continuous positive airway pressure (CPAP)—the best available treatment for obstructive sleep apnea—so underwhelming as an antihypertensive therapy? Three recent meta-analyses show that CPAP lowers BP by only 2/1 mm Hg on average (Alajmi et al., 2007; Bazzano et al., 2007; Haentjens et al., 2007). However, the meta-analyses indicate considerable interindividual variation in BP reduction with CPAP, the greatest effect being in patients with heart failure where daytime systolic BP falls by 15 mm Hg—and daytime MSNA by 17% (Usui et al., 2005). Moreover, short-term withdrawal of CPAP increases urinary NE (Phillips et al., 2007). Adequately powered long-term randomized controlled trials of CPAP for obstructive sleep apnea-related hypertension are needed.

Obstructive sleep apnea is not only a hyperadrenergic state but also a state of hyperaldosteronism (Calhoun et al., 2004; Pimenta & Calhoun, 2007; Pratt-Ubunama et al., 2007). Excessive stimulation of mineralocorticoid receptors in the brainstem has been shown to increase SNA in animals (Pimenta & Calhoun, 2007). Mineralocorticoid receptor antagonists can ameliorate obstructive sleep apnea–induced hypertension, but further clinical studies are needed to determine if this is a robust effect and mediated at least in part by reduced SNA (Pimenta & Calhoun, 2007).

Obesity-Related Hypertension as a Neurogenic Hypertension Variant

In the absence of obstructive sleep apnea, obesity-related hypertension is accompanied by a highly characteristic pattern of sympathetic activation—one that differs qualitatively from that in lean hypertensive individuals.

In both obese and nonobese hypertensive patients, sympathetic activation is targeted to the kidneys and skeletal muscle (Esler et al., 2006). In nonobese hypertensive patients, the sympathetic activation also is targeted to the heart, presumably contributing to LVH and ventricular arrhythmias. However, in obese patients with hypertension, the heart somehow is spared this sympathetic activation (Esler et al., 2006). Thus, the work by Esler, Lambert, and coworkers implicates the cardiac sympathetic nerves in pressure-overload cardiac hypertrophy (i.e., hypertension-related LVH) but not in obesity-related cardiac remodeling and hypertrophy.

Moreover, Lambert et al. (2007) find that hypertension in nonobese patients is associated with an increased firing rate of single axons that already were active. By contrast, obesity increases MSNA by recruiting previously silent fibers, with no increase in firing rate. The central neural circuits driving postganglionic MSNA may be frequency modulated in lean hypertensives but amplitude modulated in obesity-related hypertension—as though their brains were tuned to "FM" or "AM."

As illustrated in Figure 3-30 (Katagiri et al., 2007), additional neurohormonal mechanisms for obesity-related hypertension include (i) afferent neural signals from the liver and (ii) adipokines, i.e., hormonal signals from fat cells.

Afferent Neural Signals from the Liver

In rodent models, raising portal vein levels of glucose or free fatty acids increases the discharge of sensory afferents that project centrally via the vagus nerve and trigger reflex sympathetic activation (Katagiri et al., 2007). In obesity, fat accumulation in the liver may thereby signal the brain of excess energy storage and evoke reflex increases in SNA that increase energy expenditure and lipolysis but contribute to hypertension (Katagiri et al., 2007). This revised version of the Landsberg hypothesis has not been tested directly in humans. By contrast, much recent work has implicated adipokines in linking obesity—especially abdominal obesity—with hypertension, atherosclerosis, and type 2 diabetes.

Adipokines

Work has focused most on two adipokines—leptin, which increases with BMI and is thought to contribute to obesity-related hypertension, and adiponectin, which falls with increasing BMI and is thought to be protective.

LEPTIN Leptin, a 16 kDa protein mainly derived from adipocytes, acts on the hypothalamus and regulates energy metabolism by decreasing appetite and increasing energy expenditure via sympathetic stimulation of numerous tissues. In rodent models of obesity, leptin loses its ability to suppress appetite but retains its ability to increase SNA (particularly to the kidney), termed "selective leptin resistance" (Mark et al., 2004).

Leptin also may contribute to obesity hypertension by inducing smooth muscle cell proliferation, inflammation, and oxidative stress (Katagiri et al.,

2007). Leptin can stimulate NO release and cause endothelial-dependent vasodilation, a protective mechanism that may be lost with obesity—a state of inflammation and oxidative stress.

ADIPONECTIN Adiponectin is the protein most abundantly produced by adipocytes. Plasma levels are normally high (3 to 30 mg/mL) and correlate inversely with BMI (Katagiri et al., 2007). The inverse correlation is stronger with visceral than with subcutaneous adipose tissue. Adiponectin levels are normal in "healthy" obese subjects who do not have hypertension or diabetes (Aguilar-Salinas et al., 2008). Obese individuals with normal adiponectin levels may be protected against endothelial dysfunction, vascular remodeling, and atherosclerosis. The presence of hypertension is associated with lower plasma adiponectin levels (Shankar et al., 2008).

RAAS Overactivity and T Cell Activation in Adipose Tissue

Despite volume overload, which normally would suppress the RAAS, all components of the RAAS typically are increased in obese patients (Engeli et al., 2005) and more so when obesity is accompanied by hypertension (Dall'Asta et al., 2009). Obesity-related hypertension is high-renin hypertension (Umemura et al., 1997). Logically, renal SNA may be driving renin production by the juxtaglomerular granular (JG) cells.

In mouse models of Ang II–induced hypertension, the perivascular fat—but not the vascular smooth muscle per se—becomes infested with activated T cells, demonstrating selective honing to adipocytes (Guzik et al., 2007). Visceral adipose tissue also becomes infested with activated T cells in diet-induced obesity in both mice and humans (Wu et al., 2007). In obese patients, activation of the sympathetics, the RAAS, inflammatory cytokines, and T cells may be a perfect storm for hypertension (Harrison et al., 2008).

The Metabolic Syndrome

Abdominal (upper body) obesity is worse than subcutaneous (lower body) obesity from both a metabolic and cardiovascular standpoint. This difference was observed by Jean Vague (1956) (actually in 1947 but in a French paper that received little attention) and has been so well confirmed that an increased

waist circumference is a principal component of the metabolic syndrome (Grundy, 2008).

The diagnosis of metabolic syndrome requires three or more of the five components listed in Table 3-5. Associated conditions include fatty liver disease, cholesterol gallstones, gout, depression, obstructive sleep apnea, and polycystic ovarian syndrome (PCOS). The metabolic syndrome carries a twofold risk of atherosclerotic cardiovascular disease and a fivefold risk of type 2 diabetes. It increases the risks for coronary disease, stroke, and cardiovascular mortality beyond those seen with individual components of the syndrome such as hypertension.

The metabolic syndrome is a worldwide pandemic, affecting 20% to 30% of adults in most Western countries including the United States (Grundy, 2008).

Mechanisms

As shown in Figure 3-31, excess body fat is the main driver of the metabolic syndrome, with susceptibility factors—both genetic and environmental—being required for its full expression (Grundy, 2007). The full-blown syndrome is a proinflammatory, prothrombotic state leading to endothelial dysfunction, glucose intolerance, hypertension, and atherosclerosis. Pathogenetic mechanisms include adipokines, adhesion molecules, inflammatory mediators, overactivity of the RAAS and the sympathetic nervous system, as well as overactivity of the endocannaboid system.

Diabetes

Prevalence

The obesity epidemic is accompanied by a parallel epidemic of type 2 diabetes mellitus. Over 19 million Americans have type 2 diabetes, which is undiagnosed

TABLE 3.5	Diagnostic Criteria for the Metabolic Syndrome

Three or more of the following five features
1. Waist circumference, ≥102 cm in men or ≥88 cm in women
2. Triglycerides, ≥150 mg/dL
3. HDL-C, <40 mg/dL in men or <50 mg/dL in women
4. BP, ≥130/85 mm Hg
5. Fasting glucose, ≥100 mg/dL (including diabetes)

Modified from Grundy SM. Metabolic syndrome pandemic. *Arterioscler Thrombo Vasc Biol* 2008;28:629–636.

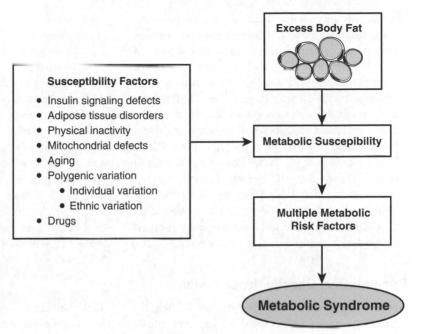

FIGURE 3-31 Proposed scheme for pathogenesis of the metabolic syndrome (MetS). For multiple metabolic risk factors, which compose the MetS that develops, an excess of body fat must be combined with a metabolic susceptibility. This susceptibility is often manifest by insulin resistance. Multiple adverse influences contribute to metabolic susceptibility. (From Grundy SM. Metabolic syndrome: A multiplex cardiovascular risk factor. *J Clin Endocrinol Metab* 2007;92:399–404.)

in one third of these cases and another 54 million adults have impaired glucose tolerance (Norris et al., 2008). Type 2 diabetes is a coronary risk equivalent and has become the number one cause of end-stage renal disease (Almdal et al., 2004). The lifetime risk of developing diabetes for people in the United States born in 2000 is 32.8% for men and 38.5% for women (Narayan et al., 2003). If diagnosed at age 40, diabetic men will lose 11.6 years of life and women, 14.3 years. By the year 2030, it is estimated that 366 million people worldwide will have diabetes (Wild et al., 2004).

Association with Hypertension

Diabetes and hypertension frequently coexist—much more commonly than is predicted by chance. Because diabetes is so prevalent in the hypertensive population and accelerates target organ damage, all patients with hypertension should be screened for diabetes (Norris et al., 2008).

Mechanisms

The same pathogenetic mechanisms underlying the metabolic syndrome are thought to explain the association of hypertension and diabetes.

The consequences of the coexistence of diabetes and hypertension are covered in Chapter 4 and the treatment of the diabetic hypertensive in Chapter 7. The special problems of diabetic nephropathy are described in Chapter 9.

Shortcomings of Current Theories and Unexplained Observations

There are some breaks in the chain linking hypertension with obesity and other components of the metabolic syndrome. Current theories do not fully explain some clinically important observations:

- *The metabolic syndrome varies by race/ethnicity.* In African Americans, hypertension predominates but serum triglyceride levels are lower than in nonblacks and the risk of hepatic steatosis is low (Browning et al., 2004; Ong et al., 2007). In Mexican Americans, diabetes predominates; the risk of hepatic steatosis is excessive but the risk of hypertension is disproportionately low for the high rates of obesity (Browning et al., 2004; Ong et al., 2007). Similarly, Native Americans have high rates of obesity-related diabetes and gallstones but low rates of hypertension and coronary disease (Saad et al., 1991). Levels of MSNA do not track with BMI in either Pima Indians (Spraul et al., 1993) or in African American men (Abate et al., 2001). These different susceptibilities are related in part to ancestral genes (Romeo et al., 2008).
- *Weight loss—whether by diet, drugs, or surgery—often causes proportionally smaller improvements in BP than in glucose tolerance, serum triglycerides, and other components of the metabolic syndrome.* The effects of bariatric surgery are particularly unbalanced (Mark, 2008). As the only effective treatment

for significant obesity, bariatric surgery produces sustained weight loss but, inexplicably, has a much greater long-term effect on diabetes and dyslipidemia than hypertension. The largest prospective study of bariatric surgery followed 1,700 patients, most of whom were 20 kg lighter 10 years later. Despite large and sustained benefits on glucose tolerance, triglycerides, and incident diabetes, the benefits on BP and hypertension risk were small and short-lived (Mark, 2008; Sjostrom et al., 2000; Sjostrom et al., 2004) (Fig. 3-32). By 8 to 10 years after bariatric surgery, there were no detectable effects on BP or incident hypertension. Perhaps body weight is overestimated as a driver of BP, or sustained surgically induced weight loss activates offsetting pressor mechanisms.

Prevention of Obesity Hypertension

The lifestyle changes and drug therapy of obesity-related hypertension are covered in Chapters 6 and 7, respectively. However, in view of its importance, a

few comments about the need and the possible methods for prevention of obesity seem appropriate.

The problem, as noted earlier in this chapter, starts in infancy and childhood. Particular demographic groups are disproportionately affected: 24% of African American girls and 22% of Mexican American boys are obese (Barlow, 2007). Obesity also is increasing rapidly among Native American and Asian American children. In general, obesity is more common among low-income inner city minorities who lack sufficient access to healthy food choices and safe playgrounds. Obese children are more likely than normal weight children to become obese adults and to develop hypertension, diabetes, and coronary disease. Prevention needs to begin in infancy and childhood.

Given the low success of individual behavior therapy, global societal changes will be needed (Table 3-6) (Ebbeling et al., 2002). The same aggressive, multifaceted strategies used against tobacco will likely be needed to force the large multinational

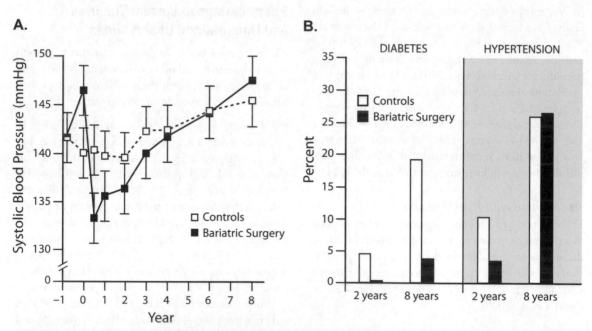

FIGURE 3-32   Data from the Swedish Obesity Study showing a differential long-term effect of bariatric surgery on diabetes and hypertension. BP decreased initially after bariatric surgery, but returned to control levels after 6 to 8 years despite persistent substantial decreases in body weight (**Panel A**). In addition, although bariatric surgery was accompanied by a persistent decrease in the incidence and severity of diabetes and dyslipidemia, the 8- to 10-year incidence of hypertension did not differ between the surgical and control groups (**Panel B**, *right*). (From Mark AL. Dietary therapy for obesity: An emperor with no clothes. *Hypertension* 2008;51:1426–1434; Adapted from Sjostrom L, Lindroos AK, Peltonen M, et al. Lifestyle, diabetes, and cardiovascular risk factors 10 years after bariatric surgery. *N Engl J Med* 2004;351:2683–2693; and Sjostrom CD, Peltonen M, Wedel H, et al. Differentiated long-term effects of intentional weight loss on diabetes and hypertension. *Hypertension* 2000;36:20–25.)

TABLE 3.6	A Common Sense Approach to Prevention and Treatment of Childhood Obesity
Home	Set aside time for
	Healthy meals
	Physical activity
	Limit television viewing and computer gaming
School	Fund mandatory physical education
	Establish stricter standards for school lunch programs
	Eliminate unhealthy foods—e.g., soft drinks and candy—from vending machines
	Provide healthy snacks through concession stands and vending machines
Urban design	Protect open spaces
	Build pavements (sidewalks), bike paths, parks, playgrounds, and pedestrian zones
Health care	Improve insurance coverage for effective obesity treatment
Marketing and media	Consider a tax on fast food and soft drinks
	Subsidies nutritious foods—e.g., fruits and vegetables
	Require nutrition labels on fast-food packaging
	Prohibit food advertisement and marketing directed at children
	Increase funding for public-health campaigns for obesity prevention
Politics	Regulate political contributions from the food industry

Modified from Ebbeling CB, Pawlak DB, and Ludwig DS. Childhood obesity: Public-health crisis, common sense cure. *Lancet* 2002;360:473–482.

companies that are responsible for pushing energy-dense foods on a willing public, particularly children. Until or if that campaign works, just increasing peoples' daily level of physical activity can make a major impact on the prevention of obesity and its adverse metabolic consequences (Blair & Church, 2004). Perhaps we can walk up that flight of stairs, just as an example to our patients.

URIC ACID AND HYPERTENSION

The steadily growing evidence for a causal role of uric acid and xanthine oxidase in primary hypertension is impressive. Yet it falls short of being conclusive or supporting the use of the xanthine oxidase inhibitor allopurinol to reduce the risk of developing hypertension in people with asymptomatic hyperuricemia (Trachtman, 2007).

Evidence

The growing appreciation of uric acid's potential role in causing hypertension appears largely due to the persistent work of Richard Johnson, Daniel Feig, and coworkers (Feig et al., 2008a). Their evidence includes:

- The initial description of an association between uric acid and hypertension by Mahomed in 1879 was followed by many similar observations over the next 100+ years (Feig et al., 2008a).
- The induction of hypertension in rats made hyperuricemic (Feig et al., 2008a).
- The continued publication of studies (over a dozen in all) showing that an increased uric acid level predicts the development of hypertension (Feig et al., 2008a). These include data from the Bogalusa Heart Study wherein childhood uric acid levels predicted hypertension over an average 12-year follow-up (Alper Jr et al., 2005) and from the Framingham Study wherein uric acid level was an independent—albeit modest—predictor of hypertension (Sundstrom et al., 2005).
- Recognition of impaired endothelial function with hyperuricemia that was improved when uric acid levels were reduced (Mercuro et al., 2004; Kato et al., 2005).
- Recognition of an elevated uric acid level as a strong predictor of cardiovascular mortality and chronic

kidney disease independent of BP and other traditional risk factors (Fang & Alderman, 2000; Meisinger et al., 2008; Weiner et al., 2008).

• Publication of the first carefully controlled trial showing that allopurinol lowers BP in primary hypertension (Feig et al., 2008b). In a randomized double-blind placebo-controlled crossover trial of 30 adolescents with hyperuricemia and recently diagnosed hypertension, 1-month treatment with allopurinol lowered 24-hour ambulatory BP by 7/5 mm Hg, achieving normotension in two thirds of subjects. This is a short-term study and it is unknown whether the impressive results are due to decreased uric acid or some other property of allopurinol—in particular reduced xanthine oxidase activity and thus reduced production of superoxide.

Potential Mechanisms

Mean uric acid levels have doubled in the past century, as Americans consume more meat, fructose, and total calories (Feig et al., 2008a). Hyperuricemia can be caused by overproduction (as in the metabolic syndrome) or decreased renal transport (as with excessive alcohol consumption or diuretic therapy).

Uric acid levels are higher in humans and monkeys than other mammals due to a missense mutation in the gene encoding hepatic uricase, which converts uric acid, an insoluble organic anion, to allantoin which is more soluble and thus more easily excreted in the urine (Mene & Punzo, 2008).

In humans, superoxide rather than uric acid may be the xanthine oxidase product that is the real culprit. Polymorphisms in the uric acid renal transporter have been associated with hyperuricemia and gout but not hypertension (Vitart et al., 2008).

GENDER DIFFERENCES AND SEX HORMONES

Before age 50, women have less hypertension than men but quickly catch up after menopause and have more hypertension thereafter (Ong et al., 2007). However, we know little about the mechanisms mediating these gender differences in hypertension. Are they linked to protective effects of estrogen, prohypertensive effects of androgens, or both?

Androgens

The role of androgens in the genesis of primary hypertension is controversial but evidence is mounting (Kienitz & Quinkler, 2008; Qiao et al., 2008). In almost all rodent models of hypertension, males have much higher BPs than females before but not after castration (Kienitz & Quinkler, 2008). Testosterone measurements may not tell the whole story because testosterone production can fall acutely with stress and androgens other than the testosterone may be involved.

In women with PCOS, higher BPs associate with hyperandrogenemia independent of age, insulin resistance, and obesity (Chen et al., 2007). Long-term administration of testosterone to female-to-male transsexuals increases BP—sometimes markedly (Mueller et al., 2007). Androgens may contribute to vasoconstriction and hypertension by up-regulation of thromboxane A2 expression, NE, Ang II expression, and endothelia action (Kienitz & Quinkler, 2008).

Estrogen

In physiological concentrations, estrogen's effects on BP are less clear than testosterone's (Qiao et al., 2008). Exogenous estrogen—as the contraceptive pill in premenopausal women or as hormone replacement therapy in postmenopausal women—can raise BP and contribute to hypertension, as will be discussed in Chapter 15.

Factors Associated with Hypertension in Women

There are no major gender differences in the factors predisposing to hypertension. In the Women's Health Initiative—a well-characterized cohort of 98,705 women ages 50 to 79 years—hypertension was more common in those who were overweight than lean (48% vs. 29%), physical inactive versus physically fit (45% vs. 31%), and nondrinkers and heavy drinkers than moderate drinkers (46% vs. 36% vs. 32%) (Oparil, 2006).

Other Associations

Lee (2002) has summarized the association of various hemorheological factors associated with hypertension. These factors may be associated with vascular inflammation and include the following: T cell activation (Harrison et al., 2008), increased hematocrit (Smith et al., 1994), elevated plasma fibrinogen levels (Landin et al., 1990), decreased fibrinolytic activity reflected by increased levels of plasminogen activator inhibitor and tissue plasminogen activator antigen (Poli et al., 2000), and increased whole-blood viscosity (Devereux et al., 2000). Increased blood viscosity along with increased hematocrits and thrombogenic factors may be involved in the greater threats of thrombotic rather than hemorrhagic complications in hypertensive patients.

A number of other diseases in which accompanying hypertension frequently is noted are described in Chapter 14.

GENES AND ENVIRONMENT

Family History

Hypertension runs in families. A parental history of hypertension increases the lifetime risk of developing hypertension, especially if both parents were hypertensive (Wang et al., 2008b). Large studies of biological and adopted siblings used ABPM estimate that approximately 60% of the familial association of BP is caused by shared genes and approximately 40% by shared environment (Kupper et al., 2005). We know much more about the environmental factors than the genetic ones.

Genetic Determinants of Primary Hypertension

General Comments

The complex regulation of BP has thwarted the genetic dissection of human hypertension either with candidate genes, genome-wide scans, intermediate phenotypes, gene expression studies, and comparative genomics in rodent models. The enthusiasm released by the elucidation of the human genome has been quickly dampened by the reality, as Sir George Pickering warned over 40 years ago (1964) that "elevated blood pressure is not a function of one gene, but rather a host of genes, each contributing a small effect." The seemingly weak genetic "signals," the strong environmental determinants of BP, the large amount of unrelated genetic information, and the large "noise" in BP measurement all increase the risk of both false-positive and false-negative studies.

In the words of Dr. Joseph Loscalzo (2007), editor-in-chief of *Circulation*,

> Whereas I and many others believe that understanding the genome in precise molecular detail will ultimately give us truly unique insight into disease risk and pathogenesis, my review of the growing body of genome-wide association studies does not convince me that this goal is likely to be realized soon...Because of the extraordinary number of comparisons made between two often large populations (e.g., 500,000 SNPs [single nucleotide polymorphisms] in the human genome of 17,000 subjects in a recent genome-side association study, modest differences in prevalence can achieve startling high statistical significance, even after adjustment for multiple comparisons.... Remember that although 500,000 SNPs may seem like a large number, there are 3.2 billion base pairs in the human genome, indicating that less than 0.02% of the genome is specifically assessed with this marker panel.... Genetic epidemiologists address this issue by noting the statistical association among groups of SNPs (i.e. haplotypes).

Genome-wide SNP Association Studies

The Wellcome Trust Case Control Consortium (Wellcome Trust Case Control Consortium, 2007) conducted a landmark genome-wide association study of 14,000 cases of seven common diseases (including 2,000 cases of primary hypertension) and 3,000 controls in the United Kingdom; analysis of 500,000 single nucleotide polymorphisms (SNPs) in each subject confirmed several previously defined SNPs and identified new SNPs associated with coronary disease and diabetes, but failed to identify any associated with hypertension at the predefined statistical significance level. However, six SNPs showed an association with a less stringent corrected P value, thus meriting future study.

Subsequently, only one of these six SNPs showed a potential association with hypertension in a study of 11,433 subjects in the United States conducted by the Family Blood Pressure Program (Ehret et al., 2008). Strangely, the association was positive for Americans of European origin, negative for those of Hispanic origin, with no association being found among African Americans. This SNP (rs1937506) is located in a gene "desert" on chromosome 13q21 where the two closest flanking genes have never been associated with hypertension.

Given these negative findings, positive reports from smaller SNP-association studies should be taken with a "grain of salt."

Other Gene Association Studies: Candidate and Newly Discovered SNPs

Nonetheless, we should note a few examples of recent positive findings from gene-association studies, including some that have been replicated in independent study samples.

- *Corin gene minor allele, hypertension, and LVH in blacks.* Corin is a serine protease that enzymatically converts pro-ANP and pro-BNP, which are inactive prohormones, into smaller biologically active natriuretic peptides. In the Dallas Heart Study—a large multiethnic population-based sample—a minor (less common) allele defined by two missense mutations in the corin gene is carried by 12% of blacks but by almost no whites and is associated with a greater prevalence of hypertension and higher systolic BP (4 mm Hg at the population level); these findings are confirmed in two more large independent population samples (Dries et al., 2005). When coexpressed in various cells, these SNPs reduce corin's enzymatic activity in vitro although neither one alone had any effect (Wang et al., 2008d). We still do not know if they reduce corin function in patients. If so, this would indicate that natriuretic peptides normally defend against hypertension and genetic impairments in this defense mechanism could explain ≥10% of hypertension and hypertensive heart disease in US blacks.

- *Adrenergic receptor polymorphisms.* In the same Dallas Heart Study, there is no association between candidate α_{2A} or α_{2C} alleles, alone or in combination, with hypertension, untreated BP, or LV mass (Li et al., 2006) and no association between several candidate β-adrenergic receptor alleles alone or in combination with α_{2C} alleles and LVH (Canham et al., 2007). On the other hand, O'Connor et al in San Diego find several associations between hypertension and indices (albeit indirect) of sympathetic reactivity to laboratory stressors with novel variants in genes regulating the synthesis and exocytotic release of catecholamines (Fung et al., 2008; O'Connor et al., 2008; Rao et al., 2007a; 2007b; Shih & O'Connor, 2008; Zhang et al., 2007). A concise picture is yet to emerge from this work, as some associations are specific for only diastolic BP; some are seen only in men, but others only in women. The implication is that individual variability in BP reactivity to environmental stressors is in part genetically predetermined.

- *Common Variants (SNPs) in Genes Underlying Monogenic Hypertension and Hypotension in the General Population.* In a study of 2,037 adults from 520 families in the United Kingdom (Tobin et al., 2008), 298 candidate SNPs were identified in regions of genes where deletions, copies, or substitutions of comparatively large chromosomal regions cause the rare monogenic forms of hypertension or hypotension described earlier in this chapter. Five polymorphisms in the gene encoding the ROMK potassium channel (involved in a form of Bartter syndrome) show negative associations with BP by 24-hour monitoring. The strongest effect is with one allele on chromosome 11, present in 16% of the population, which is associated with a lower systolic BP of 1.5 mm Hg and lower EKG-voltage (Tobin et al., 2008), a finding which awaits independent confirmation.

Carriers of Bartter and Gitleman Syndrome Mutations in the General Population

As stated earlier in the chapter, major mutations (not SNPs) in 20 salt-handling genes cause the ultra-rare monogenic forms of severe early onset hypotension and hypertension. But the applicability of this work to primary hypertension previously was unknown. New data from the Framingham Heart Study now show that gene mutations underlying the pediatric salt-wasting syndromes (Bartter's and Gitelman's) in the homozygous state are present in 1% to 2% of the general adult population in the heterozygous state and may confer resistance against primary hypertension (Ji et al., 2008). As many as one in 64 of these subjects carry one of three functional mutations of genes encoding the NCCT, the NKCC2, or ROMK. Among those between ages 51 to 60 years, hypertension is present in only 19% of the carriers compared with 42% of the noncarriers (Fig. 3-33).

Thus, normotensive young adults lacking these (and other) protective mutations may be at increased risk for developing salt-sensitive hypertension in middle age and may benefit from preemptive therapy with a low-dose diuretic or at least a low-sodium diet. The carriers presumably have salt-resistant BP and need not worry about eating too much salt.

Racial and Ethnic Aspects of Hypertension

Among US adults, approximately 40% of non-Hispanic blacks have hypertension compared with

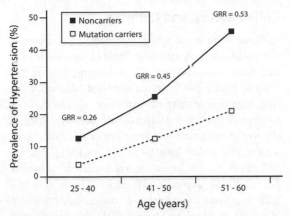

FIGURE 3-33 Reduced prevalence of hypertension among mutation carriers. Prevalence of hypertension at the last exam within ages 25 to 40, 41 to 50, and 51 to 60 years for mutation carriers and noncarriers of genes causing Bartter and Gitelman syndromes. The genotype relative risk (GRR) for mutation carriers is shown. (From Ji W, Foo JN, O'Roak BJ, et al. Rare independent mutations in renal salt handling genes contribute to blood pressure variation. *Nat Genet* 2008;40:592–599.)

approximately 28% of non-Hispanic whites or Hispanics (Ong et al., 2007). It is surprising that hypertension is not more common among Hispanics given the high rates of obesity and type 2 diabetes (Hertz et al., 2006). Even more surprising is that hypertension is more common in Mexico than among Mexican immigrants to the United States, suggesting the importance of environmental factors other than obesity (Barquera et al., 2008).

In US blacks, hypertension is not only more prevalent than in other racial and ethnic groups but also starts at a younger age, is more severe, and causes more target organ damage, premature disability, and death (Stewart et al., 2006). The high prevalence of hypertension in US blacks has been attributed to selection pressure of sub-Saharan African origin populations to develop augmented renal sodium absorption (Chun et al., 2008). Recent evidence from clinical research center studies includes the following: Compared to normotensive white individuals, normotensive black individuals tend to have a lower urine volume and a more concentrated urine (Bankir et al., 2007; Chun et al., 2008), possibly due to higher vasopressin levels (Bankir et al., 2007) or a more active furosemide-sensitive Na-K-2Cl transporter or both (Aviv et al., 2004; Chun et al., 2008). Blunted daytime urine sodium excretion is associated with blunted nocturnal dipping in BP, which is more often seen in black than white individuals (Bankir et al., 2008).

However, clinical research center studies generally are not designed to consider effects of socioeconomic disadvantage and other factors related to racial prejudice (Victor et al., 2004). Observed black-white differences in urine electrolytes may have more to do with a lifetime of a low income, low-potassium diet than with ancestral genes (Ganguli et al., 1997).

Although US blacks are often assumed to have the highest rates hypertension in the world, this is not so (Cooper et al., 2005). Hypertension is more prevalent in several predominately white European countries than in US blacks and is relatively uncommon among blacks living in Africa (Fig. 3-34). These

FIGURE 3-34 Age-adjusted hypertension prevalence in populations of African and European descent. (Modified from Cooper RS, Wolf-Maier K, Luke A, et al. An international comparative study of blood pressure in populations of European vs. African descent. *BMC Med* 2005;3:1–8.)

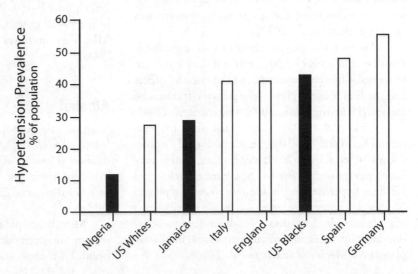

international data underscore the importance of environment in human BP variation and question the premise of searching for African ancestral genes that predispose to hypertension.

By contrast, as will be explained in Chapter 4, ancestral gene analysis has produced a major breakthrough in understanding the genetic underpinning of nondiabetic chronic kidney disease, which disproportionately affects African-origin populations. However, the same type of ancestral gene analysis has not produced a breatkthrough for hypertension.

ENVIRONMENTAL DETERMINANTS

For primary hypertension, the most important and best studied exposures—fetal environment, postnatal weight gain, adult obesity—were covered earlier in this chapter. Many other exposures may work to initiate hypertension, aggravate it, or counteract antihypertensive therapy.

Tobacco

The nicotine in cigarette smoke acutely raises BP mainly by stimulating release of NE from sympathetic nerve terminals (Grassi et al., 1994)—an effect that is augmented when baroreceptor reflexes are impaired as often the case in older patients with coronary disease (Shinozaki et al., 2008). No tolerance develops, so BP rises with each cigarette—by 7/4 mm Hg on average but twice as much in many patients (Verdecchia et al., 1995). Cigars and smokeless tobacco also raise BP (Bolinder & de Fu, 1998), but nicotine replacement therapy (even high dose) does not (Hatsukami et al., 2007).

However, the pressor effect of each cigarette is transient and is over by 30 minutes; if the BP is taken in a smoke-free environment, as in physicians' offices and medical research clinics, the pressor effect may be missed (Pickering et al., 2007; Verberk et al., 2008; Verdecchia et al., 1995). Thus, casual clinic BP measurements used in large epidemiological studies (Bowman et al., 2007; Halperin et al., 2008) may have underestimated the risk of cigarette smoking on incident hypertension. In addition to raising plasma NE levels, cigarette smoke also may contribute to hypertension by impairing NO-dependent vasodilation both by increasing oxidative stress and increasing plasma ADMA levels (Zhang et al., 2006).

Coffee, Colas, and Caffeine

Caffeine—the most widely consumed stimulant in the world—acutely raises BP by blocking vasodilatory adenosine receptors and by increasing plasma NE (Bonita et al., 2007). In a controlled laboratory setting, ingestion of caffeine, equivalent to that in—two to three cups of coffee will raise BP acutely; however, the size of the pressor response varies widely between studies and individuals from 3/4 to 15/13 mm Hg and tends to be larger in hypertensives (Mort & Kruse, 2008). Typically, BP peaks 1 hour after caffeine ingestion and returns to baseline after 4 hours. However, as stated by Myers (2004): "despite numerous studies…, it is still uncertain if caffeine increases BP only under ideal laboratory conditions or if it causes a clinically important pressor response with regular use during usual daily activities." In particular, do frequent coffee drinks show habituation to the acute pressor effect of caffeine throughout the day and are they at increased risk of developing chronic hypertension?

In the Nurses' Health Study, a woman's risk of developing hypertension did not vary with coffee consumption but increased steeply when caffeine was consumed in soft drinks (even with sugar-free diet colas) (Winkelmayer et al., 2005), presumably because coffee contains protective antioxidants (polyphenols) not present in colas (Vinson, 2006). The polyphenols in coffee also may confer some protection against developing diabetes, whereas soft drinks increase the risk of developing all components of the metabolic syndrome including hypertension (Dhingra et al., 2007).

Caffeine is metabolized mainly in the liver by cytochrome P-450. People carrying a polymorphism of the P-450 gene (CYP12A) are at risk of having an MI if they are heavy coffee drinkers (Cornelis et al., 2006).

Alcohol

A drink of alcohol sometimes raises BP due to increased SNA and sometimes lowers BP due to vasodilation (Chen et al., 2008b; Randin et al., 1995). Ethically, there can be no prospective randomized controlled trials of chronic ethanol consumption on BP levels.

Most large epidemiological studies find that the relation between alcohol consumption and many health outcomes—including BP levels, hypertension risk, stroke risk, and total mortality—is *J-shaped* (Fig. 3-35) (Kloner & Rezkalla, 2007; O'Keefe et al., 2007). The risk is higher in teetotalers than moderate drinkers—those who have one or two drinks per day—but then increases progressively with heavy drinking. The risk of developing hypertension seems to be highest in binge drinkers due to sympathetic activation with each intervening miniperiod of alcohol withdrawal (Kloner & Rezkalla, 2007).

However, a recent clever genetic approach from Japan calls this *J-shaped relation* into question (Chen et al., 2008b). Oriental persons with a loss-of-function mutation in the gene encoding alcohol dehydrogenase (*ALDH2*) become flushed and nauseated after drinking and thus drink little or no alcohol. A meta-analysis of ten published studies of mainly Japanese men found a linear gene-dose effect, with no evidence of an initial *J-limb*. Men with the *1*1 genotype (highest alcohol tolerance/intake) and those with the *1*2 genotype (intermediate alcohol tolerance/intake) were 2.4 and 1.7 times more likely to have hypertension than men with the *2*2 genotype (least alcohol tolerance/intake). Systolic BP was 7 mm Hg higher in men with the *1*1 genotype and 4 mm Hg higher in those with the *1*2 genotype than in those with the *2*2 genotype. By

contrast, no association was found between *ALDH2* genotype and hypertension or BP levels in Japanese women who drink very little alcohol for cultural reasons regardless of genotype.

Temperature and Altitude

BP tends to be higher in colder weather (Modesti et al., 2006), which may play a role in the increase in MI and sudden cardiac death during the winter months (Gerber et al., 2006). Similarly, ascent to higher altitude may raise the BP (Wolfel et al., 1994)—sometimes dramatically—and more hypertension may be seen among those who live at higher altitudes (Khalid et al., 1994).

Sympathetic activation likely underlies these effects. Cold exposure increases MSNA and BP (Victor et al., 1987). Lower partial pressures of oxygen activate the carotid body chemoreceptors (Hainsworth et al., 2007), with increased SNA lasting for at least 4 weeks after ascent to altitude (Hansen & Sander, 2003).

On the other hand, the largest study of ambient temperature and BP—based on ABPM in 6,404 patients—found that hot weather was associated not only with lower clinic and daytime ambulatory BPs but surprisingly with higher nighttime BPs especially in the elderly (Modesti et al., 2006). The lower daytime BP is likely due to vasodilation. The higher sleeping BP could be due to lower thermostats and more air-conditioning at night.

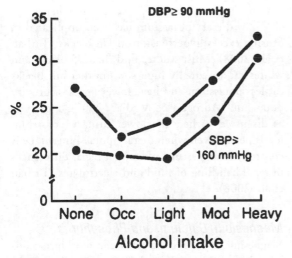

FIGURE 3-35 Age-adjusted prevalence rates (%) of measured systolic and diastolic hypertension by levels of alcohol intake in drinks. DBP, diastolic blood pressure; Occ, occasional drinking; Light, one or two drinks daily; Mod, moderate (three to six drinks daily); Heavy, more than six drinks daily; SBP, systolic blood pressure. (Modified from Shaper AG, Wannamethee G, Whincup P. Alcohol and blood pressure in middle-aged British men. *J Hum Hypertens* 1988;2:71S–78S.)

Vitamin D

Increasing evidence, albeit indirect, makes a case for mild vitamin D deficiency as a cause of hypertension. The evidence includes the following:

• In the Intersalt Study, hypertension was increasingly prevalent in populations that are further from the equator (Rostand, 1997).

• BP tends to be higher in winter than summer (Richart et al., 2007). This and the relation to latitude noted above may be related both to cold temperature and less sun exposure.

• Reduced absorption of vitamin D by dark skin has been suggested as one potential explanation for higher BP in blacks, who have lower vitamin D blood levels (Scragg et al., 2007)

• In prospective cohort studies, low blood levels of 25-hydroxy-vitamin D_2 have been independently associated with an increased risk of hypertension

(Forman et al., 2007; 2008; Wang et al., 2008a), cardiovascular events (Giovannucci et al., 2008; Wang et al., 2008c), and death (Melamed et al., 2008). In the Nurses' Health Study, normotensive women who took vitamin D supplements were less likely to develop hypertension two decades later (Forman et al., 2007).

About 80% of vitamin D comes from sunlight, specifically UVB light, absorbed through the skin and 20% from the dietary sources absorbed through the gut (Richart et al., 2007). Vitamin D3 is converted to 25-hydroxy-vitamin D_2, an inactive metabolite that is converted by a hydroxylase enzyme to 1,25-hydroxy D_2 which is the active form. The enzyme is abundantly expressed not only in the kidney but also in vascular smooth muscle and other tissues involved in BP regulation (Richart et al., 2007). Because human blood tests assay only for the inactive 25-hydroxy-vitamin D2, the epidemiological data—though positive—may underestimate the strength of association. Vitamin D receptor knockout mice develop high-renin hypertension, because vitamin D regulates the calcium signal that normally suppresses renin release from the JG cells (Bouillon et al., 2008).

However, enthusiasm for this hypothesis is dampened by negative results of a large randomized trial of over 36,000 postmenopausal women in whom calcium and vitamin D supplements had no effect on BP or on the risk of developing hypertension (Margolis et al., 2008). This and earlier clinical studies on this topic will be discussed further in Chapter 6.

Nutrients

INTERMAP (Stamler et al., 2003)—a major epidemiological study of 4,680 men and women ages 40 to 59 from 17 populations around the world—is providing new data about associations of macronutrients and micronutrients with BP, which was measured carefully (rather than by subjective recall as in other large studies such as the Nurses' Health Study). Diet recall can both underestimate and overestimate the levels in 24-hour urine collection (Leiba et al., 2005).

INTERMAP and other databases provide updated information about nutrient deficiencies as potential causes of hypertension:

BP is 7/7 mm Hg higher in INTERMAP participants from northern versus southern China, which is related to higher intake of calories and salt and lower intake of potassium, magnesium, and phosphorus (Zhao et al., 2004).

Analysis of individual nutrients may underestimate the full impact of diet on BP due to interactions, as between dietary sodium excess and dietary potassium deficiency (Adrogue & Madias, 2007).

Potassium

A low-potassium diet is a risk factor for hypertension (Adrogue & Madias, 2007) and stroke (Khaw & Barrett-Connor, 1987; Tobian et al., 1985). As reviewed by Androgue and Madias (2007), the evidence includes population surveys showing an inverse relation between dietary potassium intake and BP. However, two recent large studies found little or no association of low dietary/urinary potassium with stroke (Geleijnse et al., 2007; Larsson et al., 2008).

Skeletal muscle potassium (a better indicator of total body potassium stores) is decreased in untreated hypertensives (Ericsson, 1984). As noted in Chapter 6, potassium depletion will raise BP, whereas potassium supplementation may lower the BP. The overall potassium intake of modern people has certainly been reduced below that of our ancestors (Table 3-1), so there are logical reasons to advocate a return to a more "natural" higher-potassium/lower-sodium diet.

Low dietary potassium has been implicated in causing excess hypertension in US blacks (Turban et al., 2008). Most studies find that US blacks and whites eat an equally high sodium diet but blacks eat less potassium and have lower levels of urinary potassium (Adrogue & Madias, 2007). However, as discussed earlier, the lower urinary potassium levels persist even when dietary potassium intake is controlled, suggesting additional racial differences in renal handling of fluid and electrolytes (Turban et al., 2008).

Magnesium, Calcium, and Phosphorus

Magnesium is the second most common intracellular cation next to calcium. As most cations enter cells through voltage-gated calcium channels, magnesium can be viewed as an endogenous calcium channel blocker (Sontia & Touyz, 2007). Many epidemiological studies, including INTERMAP, show a statistically significant but often weak association between reduced magnesium intake and increased BP (Champagne, 2008; Elliott et al., 2008). Other association studies have been negative and interventional studies suggest little if any effect of magnesium supplements on BP (Champagne, 2008). Magnesium deficiency is particularly common in patients with type 2 diabetes and may play a role linking hypertension with diabetes (Barbagallo et al., 2007; Pham et al., 2007).

In INTERMAP, dietary calcium and phosphorus vary with magnesium, showing an inverse but weak association with increased BP (Elliott et al., 2008). Low magnesium intake has been associated with increased risk of stroke in high-risk individuals (Larsson et al., 2008).

Citrate

A low level of 24-hour urine excretion of citrate is associated with self-reported hypertension in the Nurses' Health Study and the Health Professionals Follow-up Study (Taylor et al., 2006). The hypocitruria could be due to dietary deficiency in citrus fruits or to acidic urine (from high meat consumption) which alters renal citrate transport. Low urinary citrate constitutes a putative common mechanism of a modestly increased risk of renal stones in patients with hypertension (Taylor et al., 2006). Potassium-magnesium-citrate is effective in dissolving renal stones (Pak, 2008) but has not yet been evaluated in the treatment or prevention of hypertension.

Toxic Exposures

Lead

Heavy occupational lead exposure has been shown to cause renal damage and thus hypertension (Vaziri, 2008). Whether low levels of environmental lead exposure cause hypertension is more controversial. However, even relatively low blood lead levels have been associated with increased cardiovascular and total mortality (Menke et al., 2006).

Most population studies indicate a positive but modest association between blood lead levels with BP and incident hypertension (Navas-Acien et al., 2007). However, blood levels reflect acute lead exposure and the association with chronic hypertension may be somewhat stronger on the basis of X-ray measurements of tibial bone lead, which better reflect cumulative exposure (Navas-Acien et al., 2007; Perlstein et al., 2007). Lead may play an even greater role in isolated systolic hypertension in the elderly, perhaps due to greater lead exposure in the past and to deposition of lead in the arterial wall contributing to arterial stiffness (Martin et al., 2006; O'Rourke & Hashimoto, 2007; Perlstein et al., 2007).

Air Pollution

Under experimental conditions, short-term exposure to air pollution rapidly increases BP (mainly diastolic BP) in normotensive subjects (Urch et al., 2005). Whether long-term exposure contributes to chronic hypertension remains to be seen (Brook, 2008). In the lungs, the particulate matter can activate excitatory neural reflexes that increase SNA, while the smallest particles can enter the systemic circulation, causing oxidative stress and vascular inflammation (Bhatnagar, 2006; Brook, 2008; Sun et al., 2005).

In postmenopausal women, long-term exposure to air pollution is associated with increased risk of cardiovascular disease and death (Miller et al., 2007). Thus, air pollution seems more likely to be involved in the progression rather than the genesis of hypertension, and mainly in susceptible individuals.

CONCLUSION

The preceding coverage does not exhaust the possible mechanisms for primary hypertension, but it at least touches on all that have received serious attention to date. It should be reemphasized that multiple defects likely are involved, and some of the initiating factors may no longer be discernible, having been dampened as hypertension develops. Without specific genetic markers, it is impossible to know whether a normotensive person, even with a strongly positive family history, will definitely develop hypertension, so that long-term prospective studies are difficult to design and perform.

In the absence of certainty about the pathogenesis of hypertension, it will be difficult to convince many patients that preventive measures should be undertaken. However, there seems no possible harm and a great deal of potential good to be gained from moderation in intake of sodium, calories, and alcohol; maintenance of good physical condition; and avoidance of unnecessary stress. As is described in Chapter 6, the value of these preventive measures has been demonstrated.

Now that the possible causes of primary hypertension have been examined, we turn to the natural history and clinical consequences of the disease. Regardless of cause, its consequences must be addressed.

REFERENCES

Abate NI, Mansour YH, Tuncel M, et al. Overweight and sympathetic overactivity in black Americans. *Hypertension* 2001;38: 379–383.

Achan V, Broadhead M, Malaki M, et al. Asymmetric dimethylarginine causes hypertension and cardiac dysfunction in humans and is actively metabolized by dimethylarginine dimethylaminohydrolase. *Arterioscler Thromb Vasc Biol* 2003;23: 1455–1459.

Adrogue HJ, Madias NE. Sodium and potassium in the pathogenesis of hypertension. *N Engl J Med* 2007;356:1966–1978.

Agabiti-Rosei E, Mancia G, O'Rourke MF, et al. Central blood pressure measurements and antihypertensive therapy: A consensus document. *Hypertension* 2007;50:154–160.

Aguilar-Salinas CA, Garcia EG, Robles L, et al. High adiponectin concentrations are associated with the metabolically healthy obese phenotype. *J Clin Endocrinol Metab* 2008;93:4075–4079.

Alajmi M, Mulgrew AT, Fox J, et al. Impact of continuous positive airway pressure therapy on blood pressure in patients with obstructive sleep apnea hypopnea: A meta-analysis of randomized controlled trials. *Lung* 2007;185:67–72.

Alderman MH, Madhavan S, Ooi WL, et al. Association of the renin-sodium profile with the risk of myocardial infarction in patients with hypertension. *N Engl J Med* 1991;324:1098–1104.

Alderman MH, Ooi WL, Cohen H, et al. Plasma renin activity: A risk factor for myocardial infarction in hypertensive patients 312. *Am J Hypertens* 1997;10:1–8.

Almdal T, Scharling H, Jensen JS, et al. The independent effect of type 2 diabetes mellitus on ischemic heart disease, stroke, and death: A population-based study of 13,000 men and women with 20 years of follow-up. *Arch Intern Med* 2004;164:1422–1426.

Alper AB Jr, Chen W, Yau L, et al. Childhood uric acid predicts adult blood pressure: The Bogalusa Heart Study. *Hypertension* 2005;45:34–38.

Ardigo D, Stuehlinger M, Franzini L, et al. ADMA is independently related to flow-mediated vasodilation in subjects at low cardiovascular risk. *Eur J Clin Invest* 2007;37:263–269.

Aronow WS, Ahn C, Kronzon I, et al. Association of plasma renin activity and echocardiographic left ventricular hypertrophy with frequency of new coronary events and new atherothrombotic brain infarction in older persons with systemic hypertension. *Am J Cardiol* 1997;79:1543–1545.

Ashfaq S, Abramson JL, Jones DP, et al. Endothelial function and aminothiol biomarkers of oxidative stress in healthy adults. *Hypertension* 2008;52:80–85.

August P, Suthanthiran M. Transforming growth factor beta signaling, vascular remodeling, and hypertension. *N Engl J Med* 2006;354:2721–2723.

Aviv A, Hollenberg NK, Weder A. Urinary potassium excretion and sodium sensitivity in blacks. *Hypertension* 2004;43:707–713.

Bai Y, Ye S, Mortazavi R, et al. Effect of renal injury-induced neurogenic hypertension on NO synthase, caveolin-1, AKt, calmodulin and soluble guanylate cyclase expressions in the kidney. *Am J Physiol Renal Physiol* 2007;292:F974–F980.

Banday AA, Lau YS, Lokhandwala MF. Oxidative stress causes renal dopamine D1 receptor dysfunction and salt-sensitive hypertension in Sprague-Dawley rats. *Hypertension* 2008;51: 367–375.

Bankir L, Perucca J, Weinberger MH. Ethnic differences in urine concentration: Possible relationship to blood pressure. *Clin J Am Soc Nephrol* 2007;2:304–312.

Bankir L, Bochud M, Maillard M, et al. Nighttime blood pressure and nocturnal dipping are associated with daytime urinary sodium excretion in African subjects. *Hypertension* 2008;51: 891–898.

Barbagallo M, Dominguez LJ, Resnick LM. Magnesium metabolism in hypertension and type 2 diabetes mellitus. *Am J Ther* 2007;14:375–385.

Barker DJ, Osmond C, Forsen TJ, et al. Maternal and social origins of hypertension. *Hypertension* 2007;50:565–571.

Barker DJ, Osmond C, Golding J, et al. Growth in utero, blood pressure in childhood and adult life, and mortality from cardiovascular disease. *Br Med J* 1989;298:564–567.

Barlow SE. Expert committee recommendations regarding the prevention, assessment, and treatment of child and adolescent overweight and obesity: Summary report. *Pediatrics* 2007;120 (Suppl. 4):S164–S192.

Barquera S, Durazo-Arvizu RA, Luke A, et al. Hypertension in Mexico and among Mexican Americans: Prevalence and treatment patterns. *J Hum Hypertens* 2008;22:617–626.

Bazzano LA, Khan Z, Reynolds K, et al. Effect of nocturnal nasal continuous positive airway pressure on blood pressure in obstructive sleep apnea. *Hypertension* 2007;50:417–423.

Berecek KH, Brody MJ. Evidence for a neurotransmitter role for epinephrine derived from the adrenal medulla. *Am J Physiol* 1982;242:H593–H601.

Bergvall N, Iliadou A, Johansson S, et al. Genetic and shared environmental factors do not confound the association between birth weight and hypertension: A study among Swedish twins. *Circulation* 2007;115:2931–2938.

Bhatnagar A. Environmental cardiology: Studying mechanistic links between pollution and heart disease. *Circ Res* 2006;99: 692–705.

Biaggioni I. Should we target the sympathetic nervous system in the treatment of obesity-associated hypertension? *Hypertension* 2007;49:27–33.

Blair SN, Church TS. The fitness, obesity, and health equation: Is physical activity the common denominator? *JAMA* 2004;292: 1232–1234.

Blaustein MP. Sodium ions, calcium ions, blood pressure regulation, and hypertension: A reassessment and a hypothesis. *Am J Physiol* 1977;232:C165–C173.

Bleeke T, Zhang H, Madamanchi N, et al. Catecholamine-induced vascular wall growth is dependent on generation of reactive oxygen species. *Circ Res* 2004;94:37–45.

Boger RH, Bode-Boger SM, Szuba A, et al. Asymmetric dimethylarginine (ADMA): A novel risk factor for endothelial dysfunction: Its role in hypercholesterolemia. *Circulation* 1998;98:1842–1847.

Boger RH, Sullivan LM, Schwedhelm E, et al. Plasma asymmetric dimethylarginine and incidence of cardiovascular disease and death in the community. *Circulation* 2009;119:1592–1600.

Bolinder G, de FU. Ambulatory 24-h blood pressure monitoring in healthy, middle-aged smokeless tobacco users, smokers, and nontobacco users. *Am J Hypertens* 1998;11:1153–1163.

Bonita JS, Mandarano M, Shuta D, et al. Coffee and cardiovascular disease: In vitro, cellular, animal, and human studies. *Pharmacol Res* 2007;55:187–198.

Borst JG, Borst-De Geus A. Hypertension explained by Starling's theory of circulatory homoeostasis. *Lancet* 1963;1: 677–682.

Bouillon R, Carmeliet G, Verlinden L, et al. Vitamin D and human health: Lessons from vitamin D receptor null mice. *Endocr Rev* 2008;29:726–776.

Bowman TS, Gaziano JM, Buring JE, et al. A prospective study of cigarette smoking and risk of incident hypertension in women. *J Am Coll Cardiol* 2007;50:2085–2092.

Brenner BM, Chertow GM. Congenital oligonephropathy and the etiology of adult hypertension and progressive renal injury. *Am J Kidney Dis* 1994;23:171–175.

Brondolo E, Libby DJ, Denton EG, et al. Racism and ambulatory blood pressure in a community sample. *Psychosom Med* 2008; 70:49–56.

Brook RD. Cardiovascular effects of air pollution. *Clin Sci (Lond)* 2008;115:175–187.

Browning JD, Szczepaniak LS, Dobbins R, et al. Prevalence of hepatic steatosis in an urban population in the United States: Impact of ethnicity. *Hepatology* 2004;40:1387–1395.

Brunner HR, Laragh JH, Baer L, et al. Essential hypertension: Renin and aldosterone, heart attack and stroke. *N Engl J Med* 1972;286:441–449.

Burns J, Sivananthan MU, Ball SG, et al. Relationship between central sympathetic drive and magnetic resonance imaging-determined left ventricular mass in essential hypertension. *Circulation* 2007;115:1999–2005.

Burt VL, Whelton P, Roccella EJ, et al. Prevalence of hypertension in the US adult population. Results from the Third National Health and Nutrition Examination Survey, 1988–1991. *Hypertension* 1995;25:305–313.

Calhoun DA, Nishizaka MK, Zaman MA, et al. Aldosterone excretion among subjects with resistant hypertension and symptoms of sleep apnea. *Chest* 2004;125:112–117.

Campbell NR, Spence JD. Stroke prevention and sodium restriction. *Can J Neurol Sci* 2008;35:278–279.

Canham RM, Das SR, Leonard D, et al. Alpha2cDel322-325 and beta1Arg389 adrenergic polymorphisms are not associated with reduced left ventricular ejection fraction or increased left ventricular volume. *J Am Coll Cardiol* 2007;49: 274–276.

Canzanello VJ, Baranco-Pryor E, Rahbari-Oskoui F, et al. Predictors of blood pressure response to the angiotensin receptor blocker candesartan in essential hypertension. *Am J Hypertens* 2008;21:61–66.

Carey RM, Padia SH. Angiotensin AT$_2$ receptors: Control of renal sodium excretion and blood pressure. *Trends Endocrinol Metab* 2008;19:84–87.

Carroll D, Smith GD, Shipley MJ, et al. Blood pressure reactions to acute psychological stress and future blood pressure status: A 10-year follow-up of men in the Whitehall II study. *Psychosom Med* 2001;63:737–743.

Carvajal CA, Romero DG, Mosso LM, et al. Biochemical and genetic characterization of 11 beta-hydroxysteroid dehydrogenase type 2 in low-renin essential hypertensives. *J Hypertens* 2005;23:71–77.

Champagne CM. Magnesium in hypertension, cardiovascular disease, metabolic syndrome, and other conditions: A review. *Nutr Clin Pract* 2008;23:142–151.

Charkoudian N, Joyner MJ, Johnston CP, et al. Balance between cardiac output and sympathetic nerve activity in resting humans: Role in arterial pressure regulation. *J Physiol* 2005;568: 315–321.

Chen J, Gu D, Jaquish CE, et al. Association between blood pressure responses to the cold pressor test and dietary sodium intervention in a Chinese population. *Arch Intern Med* 2008a; 168:1740–1746.

Chen L, Davey SG, Harbord RM, et al. Alcohol intake and blood pressure: A systematic review implementing a Mendelian randomization approach. *PLoS Med* 2008b;5:e52.

Chen MJ, Yang WS, Yang JH, Chen CL, et al. Relationship between androgen levels and blood pressure in young women with polycystic ovary syndrome. *Hypertension* 2007;49:1442–1447.

Chien KL, Hsu HC, Chen PC, et al. Urinary sodium and potassium excretion and risk of hypertension in Chinese: Report from a community-based cohort study in Taiwan. *J Hypertens* 2008;26:1750–1756.

Chun TY, Bankir L, Eckert GJ, et al. Ethnic differences in renal responses to furosemide. *Hypertension* 2008;52:241–248.

Colman RJ, Anderson RM, Johnson SC, et al. Caloric restriction delays disease onset and mortality in rhesus monkeys. *Science* 2009;325:201–204.

Cooper R, Rotimi C, Ataman S, et al. The prevalence of hypertension in seven populations of west African origin. *Am J Public Health* 1997;87:160–168.

Cooper RS, Wolf-Maier K, Luke A, et al. An international comparative study of blood pressure in populations of European vs. African descent. *BMC Med* 2005;3:2.

Cornelis MC, El-Sohemy A, Kabagambe EK, et al. Coffee, CYP1A2 genotype, and risk of myocardial infarction. *JAMA* 2006;295: 1135–1141.

Correia ML, Haynes WG. Obesity-related hypertension: Is there a role for selective leptin resistance? *Curr Hypertens Rep* 2004;6: 230–235.

Cowley AW. Renal medullary oxidative stress, pressure-natriuresis, and hypertension. *Hypertension* 2008;52:777–786.

Crowley SD, Coffman TM. In hypertension, the kidney breaks your heart. *Curr Cardiol Rep* 2008;10:470–476.

Cumming RG, Mitchell P, Smith W. Dietary sodium intake and cataract: The Blue Mountains Eye Study. *Am J Epidemiol* 2000; 151:624–626.

Curtis JJ, Luke RG, Dustan HP, et al. Remission of essential hypertension after renal transplantation. *N Engl J Med* 1983;309: 1009–1015.

da Silva AA, do Carmo JM, Kanyicska B, et al. Endogenous melanocortin system activity contributes to the elevated arterial pressure in spontaneously hypertensive rats. *Hypertension* 2008; 51:884–890.

Dahl LK, Heine M. Primary role of renal homografts in setting chronic blood pressure levels in rats. *Circ Res* 1975;36:692–696.

Dall'Asta C, Vedani P, Manunta P, et al. Effect of weight loss through laparoscopic gastric banding on blood pressure, plasma renin activity and aldosterone levels in morbid obesity. *Nutr Metab Cardiovasc Dis* 2009;19:110–114.

Danser AH. Prorenin: Back into the arena. *Hypertension* 2006;47: 824–826.

de Boer MP, Ijzerman RG, de Jongh RT, et al. Birth weight relates to salt sensitivity of blood pressure in healthy adults. *Hypertension* 2008;51:928–932.

de la Sierra A, Giner V, Bragulat E, et al. Lack of correlation between two methods for the assessment of salt sensitivity in essential hypertension. *J Hum Hypertens* 2002;16:255–260.

de Wardener HE, He FJ, MacGregor GA. Plasma sodium and hypertension. *Kidney Int* 2004;66:2454–2466.

Dechering DG, van der Steen MS, Adiyaman A, et al. Reproducibility of the ambulatory arterial stiffness index in hypertensive patients. *J Hypertens* 2008;26:1993–2000.

Denton D, Weisinger R, Mundy NI, et al. The effect of increased salt intake on blood pressure of chimpanzees. *Nat Med* 1995;1: 1009–1016.

Devereux RB, Case DB, Alderman MH, et al. Possible role of increased blood viscosity in the hemodynamics of systemic hypertension. *Am J Cardiol* 2000;85:1265–1268.

Dhingra R, Sullivan L, Jacques PF, et al. Soft drink consumption and risk of developing cardiometabolic risk factors and the metabolic syndrome in middle-aged adults in the community. *Circulation* 2007;116:480–488.

DiBona GF. Physiology in perspective: The Wisdom of the Body. Neural control of the kidney. *Am J Physiol Regul Integr Comp Physiol* 2005;289:R633–R641.

Dickhout JG, Mori T, Cowley AW Jr. Tubulovascular nitric oxide crosstalk: Buffering of angiotensin II-induced medullary vasoconstriction. *Circ Res* 2002;91:487–493.

Donato AJ, Eskurza I, Silver AE, et al. Direct evidence of endothelial oxidative stress with aging in humans: Relation to impaired endothelium-dependent dilation and upregulation of nuclear factor-kappaB. *Circ Res* 2007;100:1659–1666.

Doughan AK, Harrison DG, Dikalov SI. Molecular mechanisms of angiotensin II–mediated mitochondrial dysfunction: Linking mitochondrial oxidative damage and vascular endothelial dysfunction. *Circ Res* 2008;102:488–496.

Dries DL, Victor RG, Rame JE, et al. Corin gene minor allele defined by 2 missense mutations is common in blacks and associated with high blood pressure and hypertension. *Circulation* 2005;112:2403–2410.

du Cailar G, Mimran A, Fesler P, et al. Dietary sodium and pulse pressure in normotensive and essential hypertensive subjects. *J Hypertens* 2004;22:697–703.

Duprez DA. Role of the renin-angiotensin-aldosterone system in vascular remodeling and inflammation: A clinical review. *J Hypertens* 2006;24:983–991.

Eaton SB, Eaton SB, III, Konner MJ, et al. An evolutionary perspective enhances understanding of human nutritional requirements. *J Nutr* 1996;126:1732–1740.

Ehret GB, Morrison AC, O'Connor AA, et al. Replication of the Wellcome Trust genome-wide association study of essential hypertension: The Family Blood Pressure Program. *Eur J Hum Genet* 2008;4:1–5.

Elliott P, Kesteloot H, Appel LJ, et al. Dietary phosphorus and blood pressure: International study of macro- and micronutrients and blood pressure. *Hypertension* 2008;51:669–675.

Elliott P, Stamler J, Nichols R, et al. Intersalt revisited: Further analyses of 24 hour sodium excretion and blood pressure within and across populations. Intersalt Cooperative Research Group. *Br Med J* 1996;312:1249–1253.

Engeli S, Bohnke J, Gorzelniak K, et al. Weight loss and the renin-angiotensin-aldosterone system. *Hypertension* 2005;45:356–362.

Ericsson F. Potassium in skeletal muscle in untreated primary hypertension and in chronic renal failure, studied by X-ray fluorescence technique. *Acta Med Scand* 1984;215:225–230.

Esler M, Eikelis N, Lambert E, et al. Neural mechanisms and management of obesity-related hypertension. *Curr Cardiol Rep* 2008b;10:456–463.

Esler M, Eikelis N, Schlaich M, et al. Human sympathetic nerve biology: Parallel influences of and epigenetics in essential hypertension and panic disorder. *Ann N Y Acad Sci* 2008;1148:338–348.

Esler M, Eikelis N, Schlaich M, et al. Chronic mental stress is a cause of essential hypertension: Presence of biological markers of stress. *Clin Exp Pharmacol Physiol* 2008a;35:498–502.

Esler M, Julius S, Zweifler A, et al. Mild high-renin essential hypertension. Neurogenic human hypertension? *N Engl J Med* 1977;296:405–411.

Esler M, Straznicky N, Eikelis N, et al. Mechanisms of sympathetic activation in obesity-related hypertension. *Hypertension* 2006; 48:787–796.

Falkner B, Hulman S, Kushner H. Birth weight versus childhood growth as determinants of adult blood pressure. *Hypertension* 1998;31:145–150.

Fang J, Alderman MH. Serum uric acid and cardiovascular mortality the NHANES I epidemiologic follow-up study, 1971-1992. National Health and Nutrition Examination Survey. *JAMA* 2000;283:2404–2410.

Feig DI, Kang DH, Johnson RJ. Uric acid and cardiovascular risk. *N Engl J Med* 2008a;359:1811–1821.

Feig DI, Soletsky B, Johnson RJ. Effect of allopurinol on blood pressure of adolescents with newly diagnosed essential hypertension: A randomized trial. *JAMA* 2008b;300:924–932.

Feldt S, Batenburg WW, Mazak I, et al. Prorenin and renin-induced extracellular signal-regulated kinase 1/2 activation in monocytes is not blocked by aliskiren or the handle-region peptide. *Hypertension* 2008;51:682–688.

Ferguson RK, Turek DM, Rovner DR. Spironolactone and hydrochlorothiazide in normal-renin and low-renin essential hypertension. *Clin Pharmacol Ther* 1977;21:62–69.

Fisher ND, Hurwitz S, Ferri C, et al. Altered adrenal sensitivity to angiotensin II in low-renin essential hypertension. *Hypertension* 1999;34:388–394.

Flaa A, Eide IK, Kjeldsen SE, et al. Sympathoadrenal stress reactivity is a predictor of future blood pressure: An 18-year follow-up study. *Hypertension* 2008;52:336–341.

Floras JS, Aylward PE, Victor RG, et al. Epinephrine facilitates neurogenic vasoconstriction in humans. *J Clin Invest* 1988;81: 1265–1274.

Folkow B. Pathogenesis of structural vascular changes in hypertension. *J Hypertens* 2004;22:1231–1233.

Forman JP, Curhan GC, Taylor EN. Plasma 25-hydroxyvitamin D levels and risk of incident hypertension among young women. *Hypertension* 2008;52:828–832.

Forman JP, Giovannucci E, Holmes MD, et al. Plasma 25-hydroxyvitamin D levels and risk of incident hypertension. *Hypertension* 2007;49:1063–1069.

Forte JG, Miguel JM, Miguel MJ, et al. Salt and blood pressure: A community trial. *J Hum Hypertens* 1989;3:179–184.

Frank H, Heusser K, Geiger H, et al. Temporary reduction of blood pressure and sympathetic nerve activity in hypertensive patients after microvascular decompression. *Stroke* 2009;40:47–51.

Franklin SS. Arterial stiffness and hypertension: A two-way street? *Hypertension* 2005;45:349–351.

Franklin SS. Hypertension in older people: Part 1. *J Clin Hypertens (Greenwich)* 2006;8:444–449.

Franklin SS, Barboza MG, Pio JR, et al. Blood pressure categories, hypertensive subtypes, and the metabolic syndrome. *J Hypertens* 2006;24:2009–2016.

Franklin SS, Pio JR, Wong ND, et al. Predictors of new-onset diastolic and systolic hypertension: The Framingham Heart Study. *Circulation* 2005;111:1121–1127.

Frohlich ED. The role of salt in hypertension: The complexity seems to become clearer. *Nat Clin Pract Cardiovasc Med* 2008; 5:2–3.

Fukuda M, Goto N, Kimura G. Hypothesis on renal mechanism of non-dipper pattern of circadian blood pressure rhythm. *Med Hypotheses* 2006;67:802–806.

Fung MM, Nguyen C, Mehtani P, et al. Genetic variation within adrenergic pathways determines in vivo effects of presynaptic stimulation in humans. *Circulation* 2008;117:517–525.

Ganguli MC, Grimm RH Jr, Svendsen KH, et al. Higher education and income are related to a better Na: K ratio in blacks: baseline results of the Treatment of Mild Hypertension Study (TOMHS) data. *Am J Hypertens* 1997;10:979–984.

Gariepy CE, Ohuchi T, Williams SC, et al. Salt-sensitive hypertension in endothelin-B receptor-deficient rats. *J Clin Invest* 2000; 105:925–933.

Geleijnse JM, Witteman JC, Stijnen T, et al. Sodium and potassium intake and risk of cardiovascular events and all-cause mortality: The Rotterdam Study. *Eur J Epidemiol* 2007;22: 763–770.

Gerber Y, Jacobsen SJ, Killian JM, et al. Seasonality and daily weather conditions in relation to myocardial infarction and sudden cardiac death in Olmsted County, Minnesota, 1979 to 2002. *J Am Coll Cardiol* 2006;48:287–292.

Giles TD, Berk BC, Black HR, et al. Expanding the definition and classification of hypertension. *J Clin Hypertens (Greenwich)* 2005;7:505–512.

Giovannucci E, Liu Y, Hollis BW, et al. 25-hydroxyvitamin D and risk of myocardial infarction in men: A prospective study. *Arch Intern Med* 2008;168:1174–1180.

Gosse P, Papaioanou G, Coulon P, et al. Can ambulatory blood-pressure monitoring provide reliable indices of arterial stiffness? *Am J Hypertens* 2007;20:831–838.

Grassi G, Quarti-Trevano F, Dell'Oro R, et al. Essential hypertension and the sympathetic nervous system. *Neurol Sci* 2008a; 29(Suppl. 1):S33–S36.

Grassi G, Quarti-Trevano F, Seravalle G, et al. Blood pressure lowering effects of rimonabant in obesity-related hypertension. *J Neuroendocrinol* 2008b;20(Suppl. 1):63–68.

Grassi G, Seravalle G, Calhoun DA, et al. Mechanisms responsible for sympathetic activation by cigarette smoking in humans. *Circulation* 1994;90:248–253.

Grassi G, Seravalle G, Trevano FQ, et al. Neurogenic abnormalities in masked hypertension. *Hypertension* 2007;50:537–542.

Greenfield JR, Miller JW, Keogh JM, et al. Modulation of blood pressure by central melanocortinergic pathways. *N Engl J Med* 2009;360:44–52.

Grundy SM. Metabolic syndrome: A multiplex cardiovascular risk factor. *J Clin Endocrinol Metab* 2007;92:399–404.

Grundy SM. Metabolic syndrome pandemic. *Arterioscler Thromb Vasc Biol* 2008;28:629–636.

Gu JW, Anand V, Shek EW, et al. Sodium induces hypertrophy of cultured myocardial myoblasts and vascular smooth muscle cells. *Hypertension* 1998;31:1083–1087.

Guidi E, Menghetti D, Milani S, et al. Hypertension may be transplanted with the kidney in humans: A long-term historical prospective follow-up of recipients grafted with kidneys coming from donors with or without hypertension in their families. *J Am Soc Nephrol* 1996;7:1131–1138.

Guo GB, Thames MD, Abboud FM. Arterial baroreflexes in renal hypertensive rabbits. Selectivity and redundancy of baroreceptor influence on heart rate, vascular resistance, and lumbar sympathetic nerve activity. *Circ Res* 1983;53:223–234.

Guyenet PG. The sympathetic control of blood pressure. *Nat Rev Neurosci* 2006;7:335–346.

Guyton AC. Physiologic regulation of arterial pressure. *Am J Cardiol* 1961;8:401–407.

Guyton AC. Blood pressure control—special role of the kidneys and body fluids. *Science* 1991;252:1813–1816.

Guyton AC. Kidneys and fluids in pressure regulation. Small volume but large pressure changes. *Hypertension* 1992;19:I2–I8.

Guyton AC, Coleman TG. Quantitative analysis of the pathophysiology of hypertension. *Circ Res* 1969;24:1–19.

Guzik TJ, Hoch NE, Brown KA, et al. Role of the T cell in the genesis of angiotensin II induced hypertension and vascular dysfunction. *J Exp Med* 2007;204:2449–2460.

Haddy FJ, Overbeck HW. The role of humoral agents in volume expanded hypertension. *Life Sci* 1976;19:935–947.

Haentjens P, Van MA, Moscariello A, et al. The impact of continuous positive airway pressure on blood pressure in patients with obstructive sleep apnea syndrome: Evidence from a meta-analysis of placebo-controlled randomized trials. *Arch Intern Med* 2007;167:757–764.

Hainsworth R, Drinkhill MJ, Rivera-Chira M. The autonomic nervous system at high altitude. *Clin Auton Res* 2007;17:13–19.

Hales CN, Barker DJ. The thrifty phenotype hypothesis. *Br Med Bull* 2001;60:5–20.

Hall JE, Brands MW, Shek EW. Central role of the kidney and abnormal fluid volume control in hypertension. *J Hum Hypertens* 1996a;10:633–639.

Hall JE, Guyton AC, Brands MW. Pressure-volume regulation in hypertension. *Kidney Int Suppl* 1996b;55:S35–S41.

Halperin RO, Gaziano JM, Sesso HD. Smoking and the risk of incident hypertension in middle-aged and older men. *Am J Hypertens* 2008;21:148–152.

Hansen J, Sander M. Sympathetic neural overactivity in healthy humans after prolonged exposure to hypobaric hypoxia. *J Physiol* 2003;546:921–929.

Harrison DG. Vascular mediators of hypertension. ASH Clinical Hypertension Review Course Syllabus. American Society of Hypertension, 2007, pp.107–125.

Harrison DG, Guzik TJ, Goronzy J, et al. Is hypertension an immunologic disease? *Curr Cardiol Rep* 2008;10:464–469.

Harsha DW, Bray GA. Weight loss and blood pressure control (Pro). *Hypertension* 2008;51:1420–1425.

Hart EC, Charkoudian N, Wallin BG, et al. Sex differences in sympathetic neural-hemodynamic balance: Implications for human blood pressure regulation. *Hypertension* 2009;53:571–576.

Hatsukami D, Mooney M, Murphy S, et al. Effects of high dose transdermal nicotine replacement in cigarette smokers. *Pharmacol Biochem Behav* 2007;86:132–139.

He FJ, MacGregor GA. Importance of salt in determining blood pressure in children: Meta-analysis of controlled trials. *Hypertension* 2006;48:861–869.

He FJ, MacGregor GA. Salt, blood pressure and cardiovascular disease. *Curr Opin Cardiol* 2007;22:298–305.

He J, Klag MJ, Whelton PK, et al. Migration, blood pressure pattern, and hypertension: The Yi Migrant Study. *Am J Epidemiol* 1991;134:1085–1101.

Helmer OM. Renin activity in blood from patients with hypertension. *CMAJ* 1964;90:221–225.

Hemachandra AH, Howards PP, Furth SL, et al. Birth weight, postnatal growth, and risk for high blood pressure at 7 years of age: Results from the Collaborative Perinatal Project. *Pediatrics* 2007;119:e1264–e1270.

Herrera J, Ferrebuz A, MacGregor EG, et al. Mycophenolate mofetil treatment improves hypertension in patients with psoriasis and rheumatoid arthritis. *J Am Soc Nephrol* 2006;17:S218–S225.

Hertz RP, Unger AN, Ferrario CM. Diabetes, hypertension, and dyslipidemia in Mexican Americans and non-Hispanic whites. *Am J Prev Med* 2006;30:103–110.

Heusser K, Tank J, Luft FC, et al. Baroreflex failure. *Hypertension* 2005;45:834–839.

Hinchliffe SA, Lynch MR, Sargent PH, et al. The effect of intrauterine growth retardation on the development of renal nephrons. *Br J Obstet Gynaecol* 1992;99:296–301.

Holland OB, Gomez-Sanchez C, Fairchild C, et al. Role of renin classification for diuretic treatment of black hypertensive patients. *Arch Intern Med* 1979;139:1365–1370.

Hovi P, Andersson S, Eriksson JG, et al. Glucose regulation in young adults with very low birth weight. *N Engl J Med* 2007;356:2053–2063.

Huang Y, Wongamorntham S, Kasting J, et al. Renin increases mesangial cell transforming growth factor-beta1 and matrix proteins through receptor-mediated, angiotensin II-independent mechanisms. *Kidney Int* 2006;69:105–113.

Hughson MD, Gobe GC, Hoy WE, et al. Associations of glomerular number and birth weight with clinicopathological features of African Americans and whites. *Am J Kidney Dis* 2008;52:18–28.

Hulsen HT, Nijdam ME, Bos WJ, et al. Spurious systolic hypertension in young adults; prevalence of high brachial systolic blood pressure and low central pressure and its determinants. *J Hypertens* 2006;24:1027–1032.

Hunyor SN, Zweifler AJ, Hansson L, et al. Effect of high dose spironolactone and chlorthalidone in essential hypertension: Relation to plasma renin activity and plasma volume. *Aust N Z J Med* 1975;5:17–24.

Huxley R, Neil A, Collins R. Unravelling the fetal origins hypothesis: Is there really an inverse association between birthweight and subsequent blood pressure? *Lancet* 2002;360:659–665.

Intersalt Cooperative Research Group. Intersalt: An international study of electrolyte excretion and blood pressure. Results for 24 hour urinary sodium and potassium excretion. *Br Med J* 1988;297:319–328.

Iwamoto T. Na^+/Ca^{2+} exchange as a drug target—insights from molecular pharmacology and genetic engineering. *Ann N Y Acad Sci* 2007;1099:516–528.

Ji W, Foo JN, O'Roak BJ, et al. Rare independent mutations in renal salt handling genes contribute to blood pressure variation. *Nat Genet* 2008;40:592–599.

Johnson RJ, Feig DI, Nakagawa T, et al. Pathogenesis of essential hypertension: Historical paradigms and modern insights. *J Hypertens* 2008;26:381–391.

Jood K, Jern C, Wilhelmsen L, et al. Body mass index in mid-life is associated with a first stroke in men: A prospective population study over 28 years. *Stroke* 2004;35:2764–2769.

Joossens JV, Hill MJ, Elliott P, et al. Dietary salt, nitrate and stomach cancer mortality in 24 countries. European Cancer Prevention (ECP) and the INTERSALT Cooperative Research Group. *Int J Epidemiol* 1996;25:494–504.

Joyner MJ, Charkoudian N, Wallin BG. A sympathetic view of the sympathetic nervous system and human blood pressure regulation. *Exp Physiol* 2008;93:715–724.

Julius S, Krause L, Schork NJ, et al. Hyperkinetic borderline hypertension in Tecumseh, Michigan. *J Hypertens* 1991;9:77–84.

Kannel WB, Garrison RJ, Dannenberg AL. Secular blood pressure trends in normotensive persons: The Framingham Study. *Am Heart J* 1993;125:1154–1158.

Karppanen H, Mervaala E. Sodium intake and hypertension. *Prog Cardiovasc Dis* 2006;49:59–75.

Katagiri H, Yamada T, Oka Y. Adiposity and cardiovascular disorders: Disturbance of the regulatory system consisting of humoral and neuronal signals. *Circ Res* 2007;101:27–39.

Kato M, Hisatome I, Tomikura Y, et al. Status of endothelial dependent vasodilation in patients with hyperuricemia. *Am J Cardiol* 2005;96:1576–1578.

Kawasaki T, Delea CS, Bartter FC, et al. The effect of high-sodium and low-sodium intakes on blood pressure and other related variables in human subjects with idiopathic hypertension. *Am J Med* 1978;64:193–198.

Keller G, Zimmer G, Mall G, et al. Nephron number in patients with primary hypertension. *N Engl J Med* 2003;348:101–108.

Kempner W. Treatment of hypertensive vascular disease with rice diet. *Am J Med* 1948;4:545–577.

Kenchaiah S, Evans JC, Levy D, et al. Obesity and the risk of heart failure. *N Engl J Med* 2002;347:305–313.

Khalid ME, Ali ME, Ahmed EK, et al. Pattern of blood pressures among high and low altitude residents of southern Saudi Arabia. *J Hum Hypertens* 1994;8:765–769.

Khaw KT, Barrett-Connor E. Dietary potassium and stroke-associated mortality. A 12-year prospective population study. *N Engl J Med* 1987;316:235–240.

Khaw KT, Bingham S, Welch A, et al. Blood pressure and urinary sodium in men and women: The Norfolk Cohort of the European Prospective Investigation into Cancer (EPIC-Norfolk). *Am J Clin Nutr* 2004;80:1397–1403.

Khraibi AA, Smith TL, Hutchins PM, et al. Thymectomy delays the development of hypertension in Okamoto spontaneously hypertensive rats. *J Hypertens* 1987;5:537–541.

Kienitz T, Quinkler M. Testosterone and blood pressure regulation. *Kidney Blood Press Res* 2008;31:71–79.

Kloner RA, Rezkalla SH. To drink or not to drink? That is the question. *Circulation* 2007;116:1306–1317.

Knaus AE, Muthig V, Schickinger S, et al. Alpha2-adrenoceptor subtypes—unexpected functions for receptors and ligands derived from gene-targeted mouse models. *Neurochem Int* 2007;51:277–281.

Kobori H, Nangaku M, Navar LG, et al. The intrarenal renin-angiotensin system: From physiology to the pathobiology of hypertension and kidney disease. *Pharmacol Rev* 2007;59:251–287.

Koga M, Sasaguri M, Miura S, et al. Plasma renin activity could be a useful predictor of left ventricular hypertrophy in essential hypertensives. *J Hum Hypertens* 1998;12:455–461.

Kohan DE. The renal medullary endothelin system in control of sodium and water excretion and systemic blood pressure. *Curr Opin Nephrol Hypertens* 2006;15:34–40.

Konje JC, Bell SC, Morton JJ, et al. Human fetal kidney morphometry during gestation and the relationship between weight, kidney morphometry and plasma active renin concentration at birth. *Clin Sci (Lond)* 1996;91:169–175.

Krum H, Schlaich M, Whitbourn R, et al. Catheter-based renal sympathetic denervation for resistant hypertension: A multicentre safety and proof-of-principle cohort study. *Lancet* 2009;373:1275–1281.

Kupper N, Willemsen G, Riese H, et al. Heritability of daytime ambulatory blood pressure in an extended twin design. *Hypertension* 2005;45:80–85.

Lakoski SG, Cushman M, Palmas W, et al. The relationship between blood pressure and C-reactive protein in the Multi-Ethnic Study of Atherosclerosis (MESA). *J Am Coll Cardiol* 2005;46:1869–1874.

Lambert E, Straznicky N, Schlaich M, et al. Differing pattern of sympathoexcitation in normal-weight and obesity-related hypertension. *Hypertension* 2007;50:862–868.

Landin K, Tengborn L, Smith U. Elevated fibrinogen and plasminogen activator inhibitor (PAI-1) in hypertension are related to metabolic risk factors for cardiovascular disease. *J Intern Med* 1990;227:273–278.

Landmesser U, Cai H, Dikalov S, et al. Role of p47(phox) in vascular oxidative stress and hypertension caused by angiotensin II. *Hypertension* 2002;40:511–515.

Landsberg L. A teleological view of obesity, diabetes and hypertension. *Clin Exp Pharmacol Physiol* 2006;33:863–867.

Laragh JH. Vasoconstriction-volume analysis for understanding and treating hypertension: The use of renin and aldosterone profiles. *Am J Med* 1973;55:261–274.

Laragh JH. Laragh's 25 lessons in pathophysiology and 12 clinical pearls for treating hypertension. *Am J Hypertens* 2001;14:1173–1177.

Laragh JH, Sealey JE. Relevance of the plasma renin hormonal control system that regulates blood pressure and sodium balance for correctly treating hypertension and for evaluating ALLHAT. *Am J Hypertens* 2003;16:407–415.

Larsson SC, Virtanen MJ, Mars M, et al. Magnesium, calcium, potassium, and sodium intakes and risk of stroke in male smokers. *Arch Intern Med* 2008;168:459–465.

Lawes CM, Vander HS, Rodgers A. Global burden of blood-pressure-related disease, 2001. *Lancet* 2008;371:1513–1518.

Lawlor DA, Najman JM, Sterne J, et al. Associations of parental, birth, and early life characteristics with systolic blood pressure at 5 years of age: Findings from the Mater-University study of pregnancy and its outcomes. *Circulation* 2004;110:2417–2423.

Leal AK, Williams MA, Garry MG, et al. Evidence for functional alterations in the skeletal muscle mechanoreflex and metaboreflex in hypertensive rats. *Am J Physiol Heart Circ Physiol* 2008;295:H1429–H1438.

Lee AJ. Haemorheological, platelet and endothelial factors in essential hypertension. *J Hum Hypertens* 2002;16:529–531.

Leiba A, Vald A, Peleg E, et al. Does dietary recall adequately assess sodium, potassium, and calcium intake in hypertensive patients? *Nutrition* 2005;21:462–466.

Levy BI, Schiffrin EL, Mourad JJ, et al. Impaired tissue perfusion: A pathology common to hypertension, obesity, and diabetes mellitus. *Circulation* 2008;118:968–976.

Levy EI, Scarrow AM, Jannetta PJ. Microvascular decompression in the treatment of hypertension: Review and update. *Surg Neurol* 2001;55:2–10.

Lewington S, Clarke R, Qizilbash N, et al. Age-specific relevance of usual blood pressure to vascular mortality: A meta-analysis of individual data for one million adults in 61 prospective studies. *Lancet* 2002;360:1903–1913.

Li JL, Canham RM, Vongpatanasin W, et al. Do allelic variants in alpha2A and alpha2C adrenergic receptors predispose to hypertension in blacks? *Hypertension* 2006;47:1140–1146.

Liew G, Wang JJ, Duncan BB, et al. Low birthweight is associated with narrower arterioles in adults. *Hypertension* 2008;51:933–938.

Lifton RP, Gharavi AG, Geller DS. Molecular mechanisms of human hypertension. *Cell* 2001;104:545–556.

Lohmeier TE, Dwyer TM, Irwin ED, et al. Prolonged activation of the baroreflex abolishes obesity-induced hypertension. *Hypertension* 2007;49:1307–1314.

Loscalzo J. Association studies in an era of too much information: Clinical analysis of new biomarker and genetic data. *Circulation* 2007;116:1866–1870.

Lucas A, Morley R. Does early nutrition in infants born before term programme later blood pressure? *Br Med J* 1994;309:304–308.

Luft FC. A brief history of renin. *J Mol Med* 2008;86:611–613.

Luft FC, Weinberger MH. Heterogeneous responses to changes in dietary salt intake: The salt-sensitivity paradigm. *Am J Clin Nutr* 1997;65:612S–617S.

Mackenzie HS, Brenner BM. Fewer nephrons at birth: A missing link in the etiology of essential hypertension? *Am J Kidney Dis* 1995;26:91–98.

Majid DS, Kopkan L. Nitric oxide and superoxide interactions in the kidney and their implication in the development of salt-sensitive hypertension. *Clin Exp Pharmacol Physiol* 2007;34:946–952.

Manalich R, Reyes L, Herrera M, et al. Relationship between weight at birth and the number and size of renal glomeruli in humans: A histomorphometric study. *Kidney Int* 2000;58:770–773.

Mancia G, Bousquet P, Elghozi JL, et al. The sympathetic nervous system and the metabolic syndrome. *J Hypertens* 2007;25:909–920.

Marchesi C, Paradis P, Schiffrin EL. Role of the renin-angiotensin system in vascular inflammation. *Trends Pharmacol Sci* 2008;29:367–374.

Margolis KL, Ray RM, Van HL, et al. Effect of calcium and vitamin D supplementation on blood pressure: The Women's Health Initiative Randomized Trial. *Hypertension* 2008;52:847–855.

Mark AL. Dietary therapy for obesity: An emperor with no clothes. *Hypertension* 2008;51:1426–1434.

Mark AL, Correia ML, Rahmouni K, et al. Loss of leptin actions in obesity: Two concepts with cardiovascular implications. *Clin Exp Hypertens* 2004;26:629–636.

Martin D, Glass TA, Bandeen-Roche K, et al. Association of blood lead and tibia lead with blood pressure and hypertension in a community sample of older adults. *Am J Epidemiol* 2006;163:467–478.

Martin RM, Ness AR, Gunnell D, et al. Does breast-feeding in infancy lower blood pressure in childhood? The Avon Longitudinal Study of Parents and Children (ALSPAC). *Circulation* 2004;109:1259–1266.

Matthews KA, Katholi CR, McCreath H, et al. Blood pressure reactivity to psychological stress predicts hypertension in the CARDIA study. *Circulation* 2004;110:74–78.

Mayer G. An update on the relationship between the kidney, salt and hypertension. *Wien Med Wochenschr* 2008;158:365–369.

McEniery CM, Yasmin, Wallace S, et al. Increased stroke volume and aortic stiffness contribute to isolated systolic hypertension in young adults. *Hypertension* 2005;46:221–226.

McKeigue PM, Reynard JM. Relation of nocturnal polyuria of the elderly to essential hypertension. *Lancet* 2000;355:486–488.

Meade TW, Cooper JA, Peart WS. Plasma renin activity and ischemic heart disease. *N Engl J Med* 1993;329:616–619.

Meisinger C, Koenig W, Baumert J, et al. Uric acid levels are associated with all-cause and cardiovascular disease mortality independent of systemic inflammation in men from the general population: The MONICA/KORA cohort study. *Arterioscler Thromb Vasc Biol* 2008;28:1186–1192.

Melamed ML, Michos ED, Post W, et al. 25-hydroxyvitamin D levels and the risk of mortality in the general population. *Arch Intern Med* 2008;168:1629–1637.

Melikian N, Wheatcroft SB, Ogah OS, et al. Asymmetric dimethylarginine and reduced nitric oxide bioavailability in young Black African men. *Hypertension* 2007;49:873–877.

Mene P, Punzo G. Uric acid: Bystander or culprit in hypertension and progressive renal disease? *J Hypertens* 2008;26:2085–2092.

Menke A, Muntner P, Batuman V, et al. Blood lead below 0.48 micromol/L (10 microg/dL) and mortality among US adults. *Circulation* 2006;114:1388–1394.

Mercuro G, Vitale C, Cerquetani E, et al. Effect of hyperuricemia upon endothelial function in patients at increased cardiovascular risk. *Am J Cardiol* 2004;94:932–935.

Miller KA, Siscovick DS, Sheppard L, et al. Long-term exposure to air pollution and incidence of cardiovascular events in women. *N Engl J Med* 2007;356:447–458.

Mitchell GF, Conlin PR, Dunlap ME, et al. Aortic diameter, wall stiffness, and wave reflection in systolic hypertension. *Hypertension* 2008a;51:105–111.

Mitchell GF, Guo CY, Benjamin EJ, et al. Cross-sectional correlates of increased aortic stiffness in the community: The Framingham Heart Study. *Circulation* 2007;115:2628–2636.

Mitchell P, Liew G, Rochtchina E, et al. Evidence of arteriolar narrowing in low-birth-weight children. *Circulation* 2008b;118:518–524.

Modesti PA, Morabito M, Bertolozzi I, et al. Weather-related changes in 24-hour blood pressure profile: Effects of age and implications for hypertension management. *Hypertension* 2006;47:155–161.

Mohaupt MG, Schmidli J, Luft FC. Management of uncontrollable hypertension with a carotid sinus stimulation device. *Hypertension* 2007;50:825–828.

Mort JR, Kruse HR. Timing of blood pressure measurement related to caffeine consumption. *Ann Pharmacother* 2008;42:105–110.

Mueller A, Kiesewetter F, Binder H, et al. Long-term administration of testosterone undecanoate every 3 months for testosterone supplementation in female-to-male transsexuals. *J Clin Endocrinol Metab* 2007;92:3470–3475.

Mueller CF, Laude K, McNally JS, et al. ATVB in focus: Redox mechanisms in blood vessels. *Arterioscler Thromb Vasc Biol* 2005;25:274–278.

Munzel T, Sinning C, Post F, et al. Pathophysiology, diagnosis and prognostic implications of endothelial dysfunction. *Ann Med* 2008;40:180–196.

Myers MG. Effect of caffeine on blood pressure beyond the laboratory. *Hypertension* 2004;43:724–725.

Narayan KM, Boyle JP, Thompson TJ, et al. Lifetime risk for diabetes mellitus in the United States. *JAMA* 2003;290:1884–1890.

Narkiewicz K, Wolf J, Lopez-Jimenez F, et al. Obstructive sleep apnea and hypertension. *Curr Cardiol Rep* 2005;7:435–440.

Navas-Acien A, Guallar E, Silbergeld EK, et al. Lead exposure and cardiovascular disease—a systematic review. *Environ Health Perspect* 2007;115:472–482.

Neimann AL, Shin DB, Wang X, et al. Prevalence of cardiovascular risk factors in patients with psoriasis. *J Am Acad Dermatol* 2006;55:829–835.

Nesbitt SD, Julius S, Leonard D, et al. Is low-risk hypertension fact or fiction? cardiovascular risk profile in the TROPHY study. *Am J Hypertens* 2005;18:980–985.

Niskanen L, Laaksonen DE, Nyyssonen K, et al. Inflammation, abdominal obesity, and smoking as predictors of hypertension. *Hypertension* 2004;44:859–865.

Norman M. Low birth weight and the developing vascular tree: A systematic review. *Acta Paediatr* 2008;97:1165–1172.

Norris SL, Kansagara D, Bougatsos C, et al. Screening adults for type 2 diabetes: A review of the evidence for the U.S. Preventive Services Task Force. *Ann Intern Med* 2008;148:855–868.

O'Connor DT, Zhu G, Rao F, et al. Heritability and genome-wide linkage in US and australian twins identify novel genomic regions controlling chromogranin a: Implications for secretion and blood pressure. *Circulation* 2008;118:247–257.

O'Keefe JH, Bybee KA, Lavie CJ. Alcohol and cardiovascular health: The razor-sharp double-edged sword. *J Am Coll Cardiol* 2007;50:1009–1014.

O'Rourke MF, Hashimoto J. Mechanical factors in arterial aging: A clinical perspective. *J Am Coll Cardiol* 2007;50:1–13.

Oliver PM, John SW, Purdy KE, et al. Natriuretic peptide receptor 1 expression influences blood pressures of mice in a dose-dependent manner. *Proc Natl Acad Sci U S A* 1998;95: 2547–2551.

Oliver WJ, Cohen EL, Neel JV. Blood pressure, sodium intake, and sodium related hormones in the Yanomamo Indians, a "no-salt" culture. *Circulation* 1975;52:146–151.

Ong KL, Cheung BM, Man YB, et al. Prevalence, awareness, treatment, and control of hypertension among United States adults 1999–2004. *Hypertension* 2007;49:69–75.

Oparil S. Women and hypertension: What did we learn from the Women's Health Initiative? *Cardiol Rev* 2006;14:267–275.

Orlov SN, Mongin AA. Salt-sensing mechanisms in blood pressure regulation and hypertension. *Am J Physiol Heart Circ Physiol* 2007;293:H2039–H2053.

Ottaviani C, Shapiro D, Goldstein IB, et al. Hemodynamic profile, compensation deficit, and ambulatory blood pressure. *Psychophysiology* 2006;43:46–56.

Ottaviani C, Shapiro D, Goldstein IB, et al. Vascular profile, delayed recovery, inflammatory process, and ambulatory blood pressure: Laboratory-to-life generalizability. *Int J Psychophysiol* 2007;66:56–65.

Page LB, Vandevert DE, Nader K, et al. Blood pressure of Qash'qai pastoral nomads in Iran in relation to culture, diet, and body form. *Am J Clin Nutr* 1981;34:527–538.

Pak CY. Medical stone management: 35 years of advances. *J Urol* 2008;180:813–819.

Panoulas VF, Douglas KM, Milionis HJ, et al. Prevalence and associations of hypertension and its control in patients with rheumatoid arthritis. *Rheumatology (Oxford)* 2007;46:1477–1482.

Panoulas VF, Metsios GS, Pace AV, et al. Hypertension in rheumatoid arthritis. *Rheumatology (Oxford)* 2008;47:1286–1298.

Paravicini TM, Touyz RM. Redox signaling in hypertension. *Cardiovasc Res* 2006;71:247–258.

Paravicini TM, Touyz RM. NADPH oxidases, reactive oxygen species, and hypertension: Clinical implications and therapeutic possibilities. *Diabetes Care* 2008;31(Suppl. 2):S170–S180.

Pechman KR, Basile DP, Lund H, et al. Immune suppression blocks sodium-sensitive hypertension following recovery from ischemic acute renal failure. *Am J Physiol Regul Integr Comp Physiol* 2008;294:R1234–R1239.

Perlstein T, Weuve J, Schwartz J, et al. Cumulative community-level lead exposure and pulse pressure: The normative aging study. *Environ Health Perspect* 2007;115:1696–1700.

Perry IJ, Beevers DG. Salt intake and stroke: A possible direct effect. *J Hum Hypertens* 1992;6:23–25.

Peters A, Barendregt JJ, Willekens F, et al. Obesity in adulthood and its consequences for life expectancy: A life-table analysis. *Ann Intern Med* 2003;138:24–32.

Pham PC, Pham PM, Pham SV, et al. Hypomagnesemia in patients with type 2 diabetes. *Clin J Am Soc Nephrol* 2007;2:366–373.

Phillips CL, Yang Q, Williams A, et al. The effect of short-term withdrawal from continuous positive airway pressure therapy on sympathetic activity and markers of vascular inflammation in subjects with obstructive sleep apnoea. *J Sleep Res* 2007; 16:217–225.

Pickering G. Systemic arterial hypertension. In: Fisherman A, Richards C, eds. *Circulation of the Blood: Men and Ideas.* Bethesda, MD: American Physiological Society; 1964:487–544.

Pickering TG. Could hypertension be a consequence of the 24/7 society? The effects of sleep deprivation and shift work. *J Clin Hypertens (Greenwich)* 2006;8:819–822.

Pickering TG, Eguchi K, Kario K. Masked hypertension: A review. *Hypertens Res* 2007;30:479–488.

Pilz B, Brasen JH, Schneider W, et al. Obesity and hypertension-induced restrictive cardiomyopathy: A harbinger of things to come. *Hypertension* 2004;43:911–917.

Pimenta E, Calhoun DA. Aldosterone, dietary salt, and renal disease. *Hypertension* 2006;48:209–210.

Pimenta E, Calhoun DA. Resistant hypertension and aldosteronism. *Curr Hypertens Rep* 2007;9:353–359.

Poli KA, Tofler GH, Larson MG, et al. Association of blood pressure with fibrinolytic potential in the Framingham offspring population. *Circulation* 2000;101:264–269.

Porkert M, Sher S, Reddy U, et al. Tetrahydrobiopterin: A novel antihypertensive therapy. *J Hum Hypertens* 2008;22:401–407.

Poulter NR, Khaw KT, Hopwood BE, et al. The Kenyan Luo migration study: Observations on the initiation of a rise in blood pressure. *Br Med J* 1990;300:967–972.

Pratt JH, Rebhun JF, Zhou L, et al. Levels of mineralocorticoids in whites and blacks. *Hypertension* 1999;34:315–319.

Pratt-Ubunama MN, Nishizaka MK, Boedefeld RL, et al. Plasma aldosterone is related to severity of obstructive sleep apnea in subjects with resistant hypertension. *Chest* 2007;131:453–459.

Preston RA, Materson BJ, Reda DJ, et al. Age-race subgroup compared with renin profile as predictors of blood pressure response to antihypertensive therapy. Department of Veterans Affairs Cooperative Study Group on Antihypertensive Agents. *JAMA* 1998b;280:1168–1172.

Qiao X, McConnell KR, Khalil RA. Sex steroids and vascular responses in hypertension and aging. *Gend Med* 2008;5(Suppl. A):S46–S64.

Randin D, Vollenweider P, Tappy L, et al. Suppression of alcohol-induced hypertension by dexamethasone. *N Engl J Med* 1995; 332:1733–1737.

Rao F, Wen G, Gayen JR, et al. Catecholamine release-inhibitory peptide catestatin (chromogranin A(352–372)): Naturally occurring amino acid variant Gly364Ser causes profound changes in human autonomic activity and alters risk for hypertension. *Circulation* 2007a;115:2271–2281.

Rao F, Zhang L, Wessel J, et al. Tyrosine hydroxylase, the rate-limiting enzyme in catecholamine biosynthesis: Discovery of common human genetic variants governing transcription, autonomic activity, and blood pressure in vivo. *Circulation* 2007b;116:993–1006.

Richart T, Li Y, Staessen JA. Renal versus extrarenal activation of vitamin D in relation to atherosclerosis, arterial stiffening, and hypertension. *Am J Hypertens* 2007;20:1007–1015.

Ridker PM, Danielson E, Fonseca FA, et al. Rosuvastatin to prevent vascular events in men and women with elevated C-reactive protein. *N Engl J Med* 2008;359:2195–2207.

Rodriguez-Iturbe B, Romero F, Johnson RJ. Pathophysiological mechanisms of salt-dependent hypertension. *Am J Kidney Dis* 2007a;50:655–672.

Rodriguez-Iturbe B, Sepassi L, Quiroz Y, et al. Association of mitochondrial SOD deficiency with salt-sensitive hypertension and accelerated renal senescence. *J Appl Physiol* 2007b;102:255–260.

Romeo S, Kozlitina J, Xing C, et al. Genetic variation in PNPLA3 confers susceptibility to nonalcoholic fatty liver disease. *Nat Genet* 2008;40:1461–1465.

Romundstad PR, Davey SG, Nilsen TI, et al. Associations of prepregnancy cardiovascular risk factors with the offspring's birth weight. *Am J Epidemiol* 2007;166:1359–1364.

Rossi A, Baldo-Enzi G, Calabro A, et al. The renin-angiotensin-aldosterone system and carotid artery disease in mild-to-moderate primary hypertension. *J Hypertens* 2000;18:1401–1409.

Rossi E, Regolisti G, Perazzoli F, et al. –344C/T polymorphism of CYP11B2 gene in Italian patients with idiopathic low renin hypertension. *Am J Hypertens* 2001;14:934–941.

Rostand SG. Ultraviolet light may contribute to geographic and racial blood pressure differences. *Hypertension* 1997;30;150–156.

Rumantir MS, Jennings GL, Lambert GW, et al. The "adrenaline hypothesis" of hypertension revisited: Evidence for adrenaline release from the heart of patients with essential hypertension. *J Hypertens* 2000;18:717–723.

Saad MF, Lillioja S, Nyomba BL, et al. Racial differences in the relation between blood pressure and insulin resistance. *N Engl J Med* 1991;324:733–739.

Sagnella GA. Why is plasma renin activity lower in populations of African origin? *J Hum Hypertens* 2001;15:17–25.

Sander M, Chavoshan B, Victor RG. A large blood pressure-raising effect of nitric oxide synthase inhibition in humans. *Hypertension* 1999;33:937–942.

Sander M, Hansen J, Victor RG. The sympathetic nervous system is involved in the maintenance but not initiation of the hypertension induced by N (omega)-nitro-L-arginine methyl ester. *Hypertension* 1997;30:64–70.

Savoia C, Schiffrin EL. Inflammation in hypertension. *Curr Opin Nephrol Hypertens* 2006;15:152–158.

Savoia C, Touyz RM, Volpe M, et al. Angiotensin type 2 receptor in resistance arteries of type 2 diabetic hypertensive patients. *Hypertension* 2007;49:341–346.

Schefe JH, Neumann C, Goebel M, et al. Prorenin engages the (pro)renin receptor like renin and both ligand activities are unopposed by aliskiren. *J Hypertens* 2008;26:1787–1794.

Schiffrin EL. Effects of aldosterone on the vasculature. *Hypertension* 2006;47:312–318.

Schillaci G, Parati G. Ambulatory arterial stiffness index: Merits and limitations of a simple surrogate measure of arterial compliance. *J Hypertens* 2008;26:182–185.

Schlaich MP, Kaye DM, Lambert E, et al. Relation between cardiac sympathetic activity and hypertensive left ventricular hypertrophy. *Circulation* 2003;108:560–565.

Schlaich MP, Lambert E, Kaye DM, et al. Sympathetic augmentation in hypertension: Role of nerve firing, norepinephrine reuptake, and Angiotensin neuromodulation. *Hypertension* 2004;43:169–175.

Schneider MP, Ge Y, Pollock DM, et al. Collecting duct-derived endothelin regulates arterial pressure and Na excretion via nitric oxide. *Hypertension* 2008;51:1605–1610.

Schreuder MF, Langemeijer ME, Bokenkamp A, et al. Hypertension and microalbuminuria in children with congenital solitary kidneys. *J Paediatr Child Health* 2008;44:363–368.

Scragg R, Sowers M, Bell C. Serum 25-hydroxyvitamin D, ethnicity, and blood pressure in the Third National Health and Nutrition Examination Survey. *Am J Hypertens* 2007;20:713–719.

Seaberg EC, Munoz A, Lu M, et al. Association between highly active antiretroviral therapy and hypertension in a large cohort of men followed from 1984 to 2003. *AIDS* 2005;19:953–960.

Sealy JE. and Laragh JH. "Prorenin" in human plasma? *Circ Res* 1975;36(Suppl 1):10–16.

Sealey JE, Blumenfeld JD, Bell GM, et al. On the renal basis for essential hypertension: Nephron heterogeneity with discordant renin secretion and sodium excretion causing a hypertensive vasoconstriction-volume relationship. *J Hypertens* 1988;6:763–777.

Sealey JE, Gordon RD, Mantero F. Plasma renin and aldosterone measurements in low renin hypertensive states. *Trends Endocrinol Metab* 2005;16:86–91.

Selkurt EE. Effect of pulse pressure and mean arterial pressure modification on renal hemodynamics and electrolyte and water excretion. *Circulation* 1951;4:541–551.

Sesso HD, Buring JE, Rifai N, et al. C-reactive protein and the risk of developing hypertension. *JAMA* 2003;290:2945–2951.

Shankar A, Marshall S, Li J. The association between plasma adiponectin level and hypertension. *Acta Cardiol* 2008;63:160–165.

Shibao C, Gamboa A, Diedrich A, et al. Autonomic contribution to blood pressure and metabolism in obesity. *Hypertension* 2007;49:27–33.

Shih PA, O'Connor DT. Hereditary determinants of human hypertension: Strategies in the setting of genetic complexity. *Hypertension* 2008;51:1456–1464.

Shinozaki N, Yuasa T, Takata S. Cigarette smoking augments sympathetic nerve activity in patients with coronary heart disease. *Int Heart J* 2008;49:261–272.

Simonetti GD, Raio L, Surbek D, et al. Salt sensitivity of children with low birth weight. *Hypertension* 2008;52:625–630.

Singhal A, Cole TJ, Fewtrell M, et al. Breastmilk feeding and lipoprotein profile in adolescents born preterm: Follow-up of a prospective randomised study. *Lancet* 2004;363:1571–1578.

Singhal A, Lucas A. Early origins of cardiovascular disease: Is there a unifying hypothesis? *Lancet* 2004;363:1642–1645.

Sjostrom CD, Peltonen M, Wedel H, et al. Differentiated long-term effects of intentional weight loss on diabetes and hypertension. *Hypertension* 2000;36:20–25.

Sjostrom L, Lindroos AK, Peltonen M, et al. Lifestyle, diabetes, and cardiovascular risk factors 10 years after bariatric surgery. *N Engl J Med* 2004;351:2683–2693.

Smallegange C, Hale TM, Bushfield TL, et al. Persistent lowering of pressure by transplanting kidneys from adult spontaneously hypertensive rats treated with brief antihypertensive therapy. *Hypertension* 2004;44.89–94.

Smith S, Julius S, Jamerson K, et al. Hematocrit levels and physiologic factors in relationship to cardiovascular risk in Tecumseh, Michigan. *J Hypertens* 1994;12:455–462.

Smith WC, Crombie IK, Tavendale RT, et al. Urinary electrolyte excretion, alcohol consumption, and blood pressure in the Scottish heart health study. *Br Med J* 1988;297:329–330.

Sontia B, Touyz RM. Magnesium transport in hypertension. *Pathophysiology* 2007;14:205–211.

Soro A, Ingram MC, Tonolo G, et al. Evidence of coexisting changes in 11 beta-hydroxysteroid dehydrogenase and 5 beta-reductase activity in subjects with untreated essential hypertension. *Hypertension* 1995;25:67–70.

Spraul M, Ravussin E, Fontvieille AM, et al. Reduced sympathetic nervous activity. A potential mechanism predisposing to body weight gain. *J Clin Invest* 1993;92:1730–1735.

Staessen JA, Wang J, Bianchi G, et al. Essential hypertension. *Lancet* 2003;361:1629–1641.

Stamler J, Elliott P, Appel L, et al. Higher blood pressure in middle-aged American adults with less education-role of multiple dietary factors: The INTERMAP study. *J Hum Hypertens* 2003;17:655–775.

Stamler J, Rose G, Stamler R, et al. INTERSALT study findings. Public health and medical care implications. *Hypertension* 1989;14:570–577.

Steptoe A, Marmot M. Impaired cardiovascular recovery following stress predicts 3-year increases in blood pressure. *J Hypertens* 2005;23:529–536.

Stewart D, Johnson W, Saunders E. Hypertension in black Americans as a special population: Why so special? *Curr Cardiol Rep* 2006;8:405–410.

Sun Q, Wang A, Jin X, et al. Long-term air pollution exposure and acceleration of atherosclerosis and vascular inflammation in an animal model. *JAMA* 2005;294:3003–3010.

Sundstrom J, Sullivan L, D'Agostino RB, et al. Relations of serum uric acid to longitudinal blood pressure tracking and hypertension incidence. *Hypertension* 2005;45:28–33.

Suonsyrja T, Hannila-Handelberg T, Paavonen KJ, et al. Laboratory tests as predictors of the antihypertensive effects of amlodipine, bisoprolol, hydrochlorothiazide and losartan in men: Results from the randomized, double-blind, crossover GENRES Study. *J Hypertens* 2008;26:1250–1256.

Takahashi Y, Sasaki S, Okubo S, et al. Blood pressure change in a free-living population-based dietary modification study in Japan. *J Hypertens* 2006;24:451–458.

Tan EK, Chan LL. Neurovascular compression syndromes and hypertension: Clinical relevance. *Nat Clin Pract Neurol* 2007;3: 416–417.

Taylor EN, Mount DB, Forman JP, et al. Association of prevalent hypertension with 24-hour urinary excretion of calcium, citrate, and other factors. *Am J Kidney Dis* 2006;47:780–789.

Taylor JA, Studinger P. Counterpoint: Cardiovascular variability is not an index of autonomic control of the circulation. *J Appl Physiol* 2006;101:678–681.

Thomas GD, Zhang W, Victor RG. Nitric oxide deficiency as a cause of clinical hypertension: Promising new drug targets for refractory hypertension. *JAMA* 2001;285:2055–2057.

Tian N, Gu JW, Jordan S, et al. Immune suppression prevents renal damage and dysfunction and reduces arterial pressure in salt-sensitive hypertension. *Am J Physiol Heart Circ Physiol* 2007;292:H1018–H1025.

Timio M, Saronio P, Venanzi S, et al. Blood pressure in nuns in a secluded order: A 30-year follow-up. *Miner Electrolyte Metab* 1999;25:73–79.

Timmers HJ, Wieling W, Karemaker JM, et al. Cardiovascular responses to stress after carotid baroreceptor denervation in humans. *Ann N Y Acad Sci* 2004;1018:515–519.

Tobian L, Lange J, Ulm K, et al. Potassium reduces cerebral hemorrhage and death rate in hypertensive rats, even when blood pressure is not lowered. *Hypertension* 1985;7:I110–I114.

Tobin MD, Tomaszewski M, Braund PS, et al. Common variants in genes underlying monogenic hypertension and hypotension and blood pressure in the general population. *Hypertension* 2008;51:1658–1664.

Touyz RM, Schiffrin EL. Reactive oxygen species and hypertension: A complex association. *Antioxid Redox Signal* 2008;10: 1041–1044.

Trachtman H. Treatment of hyperuricemia in essential hypertension. *Hypertension* 2007;49:e45.

Turban S, Miller ER III, Ange B, et al. Racial differences in urinary potassium excretion. *J Am Soc Nephrol* 2008;19:1396–1402.

Turner ST, Schwartz GL, Chapman AB, et al. C825T polymorphism of the G protein beta(3)-subunit and antihypertensive response to a thiazide diuretic. *Hypertension* 2001;37:739–743.

Umemura S, Nyui N, Tamura K, et al. Plasma angiotensinogen concentrations in obese patients. *Am J Hypertens* 1997;10: 629–633.

Uno H, Kario K. Focus on masked workplace hypertension: The next step for perfect 24-hour blood pressure control. *Hypertens Res* 2006;29:937–940.

Urch B, Silverman F, Corey P, et al. Acute blood pressure responses in healthy adults during controlled air pollution exposures. *Environ Health Perspect* 2005;113:1052–1055.

Usui K, Bradley TD, Spaak J, et al. Inhibition of awake sympathetic nerve activity of heart failure patients with obstructive sleep apnea by nocturnal continuous positive airway pressure. *J Am Coll Cardiol* 2005;45:2008–2011.

Vague J. The degree of musculine differentiation of obesities: A factor determining predisposition to diabetes, atherosclerosis, gout and uric calculous disease. *Am J Clin Nutr* 1956;4: 20–34.

Vallance P, Leone A, Calver A, et al. Accumulation of an endogenous inhibitor of nitric oxide synthesis in chronic renal failure. *Lancet* 1992;339:572–575.

Vasan RS, Evans JC, Larson MG, et al. Serum aldosterone and the incidence of hypertension in nonhypertensive persons. *N Engl J Med* 2004;351:33–41.

Vaughan ED Jr, Laragh JH, Gavras I, et al. Volume factor in low and normal renin essential hypertension. Treatment with either spironolactone or chlorthalidone. *Am J Cardiol* 1973;32:523–532.

Vaziri ND. Mechanisms of lead-induced hypertension and cardiovascular disease. *Am J Physiol Heart Circ Physiol* 2008;295: H454–H465.

Verberk WJ, Kessels AG, de Leeuw PW. Prevalence, causes, and consequences of masked hypertension: A meta-analysis. *Am J Hypertens* 2008;21:969–975.

Verdecchia P, Schillaci G, Borgioni C, et al. Cigarette smoking, ambulatory blood pressure and cardiac hypertrophy in essential hypertension. *J Hypertens* 1995;13:1209–1215.

Victor RG. Pathophysiology of target-organ disease: Does angiotensin II remain the key? *J Clin Hypertens (Greenwich)* 2007;9: 4–10.

Victor RG, Haley RW, Willett DL, et al. The Dallas Heart Study: A population-based probability sample for the multidisciplinary study of ethnic differences in cardiovascular health. *Am J Cardiol* 2004;93:1473–1480.

Victor RG, Leimbach WN Jr, Seals DR, et al. Effects of the cold pressor test on muscle sympathetic nerve activity in humans. *Hypertension* 1987;9:429–436.

Victor RG, Shafiq MM. Sympathetic neural mechanisms in human hypertension. *Curr Hypertens Rep* 2008;10:241–247.

Vinson JA. Caffeine and incident hypertension in women. *JAMA* 2006;295:2135.

Vitart V, Rudan I, Hayward C, et al. SLC2A9 is a newly identified urate transporter influencing serum urate concentration, urate excretion and gout. *Nat Genet* 2008;40:437–442.

Vloet LC, Pel-Little RE, Jansen PA, et al. High prevalence of postprandial and orthostatic hypotension among geriatric patients admitted to Dutch hospitals. *J Gerontol A Biol Sci Med Sci* 2005;60:1271–1277.

Vongpatanasin W, Thomas GD, Schwartz R, et al. C-reactive protein causes downregulation of vascular angiotensin subtype 2 receptors and systolic hypertension in mice. *Circulation* 2007; 115:1020–1028.

Wallin BG, Charkoudian N. Sympathetic neural control of integrated cardiovascular function: Insights from measurement of human sympathetic nerve activity. *Muscle Nerve* 2007;36: 595–614.

Wang L, Manson JE, Buring JE, et al. Dietary intake of dairy products, calcium, and vitamin D and the risk of hypertension in middle-aged and older women. *Hypertension* 2008a;51:1073–1079.

Wang NY, Young JH, Meoni LA, et al. Blood pressure change and risk of hypertension associated with parental hypertension: The Johns Hopkins Precursors Study. *Arch Intern Med* 2008b; 168:643–648.

Wang TJ, Gona P, Larson MG, et al. Multiple biomarkers for the prediction of first major cardiovascular events and death. *N Engl J Med* 2006;355:2631–2639.

Wang TJ, Pencina MJ, Booth SL, et al. Vitamin D deficiency and risk of cardiovascular disease. *Circulation* 2008c;117:503–511.

Wang W, Liao X, Fukuda K, et al. Corin variant associated with hypertension and cardiac hypertrophy exhibits impaired zymogen activation and natriuretic peptide processing activity. *Circ Res* 2008d;103:502–508.

Wang X, Villar VA, Armando I, et al. Dopamine, kidney, and hypertension: Studies in dopamine receptor knockout mice. *Pediatr Nephrol* 2008e;23:2131–2146.

Weinberger MH, Miller JZ, Luft FC, et al. Definitions and characteristics of sodium sensitivity and blood pressure resistance. *Hypertension* 1986;8:II127–II134.

Weiner DE, Tighiouart H, Elsayed EF, et al. Uric acid and incident kidney disease in the community. *J Am Soc Nephrol* 2008;19: 1204–1211.

Weir MR, Saunders E. Renin status does not predict the anti-hypertensive response to angiotensin-converting enzyme inhibition in African-Americans. Trandolapril Multicenter Study Group. *J Hum Hypertens* 1998;12:189–194.

Wellcome Trust Case Control Consortium. Genome-wide association study of 14,000 cases of seven common disease and 3,000 shared controls. *Nature* 2007;447:661–678.

Whelton PK, Appel LJ, Espeland MA, et al. Sodium reduction and weight loss in the treatment of hypertension in older persons: A randomized controlled trial of nonpharmacologic interventions in the elderly (TONE). TONE Collaborative Research Group. *JAMA* 1998;279:839–846.

Widlansky ME, Sesso HD, Rexrode KM, et al. Body mass index and total and cardiovascular mortality in men with a history of cardiovascular disease. *Arch Intern Med* 2004;164:2326–2332.

Wild S, Roglic G, Green A, et al. Global prevalence of diabetes: Estimates for the year 2000 and projections for 2030. *Diabetes Care* 2004;27:1047–1053.

Williams JS, Williams GH, Jeunemaitre X, et al. Influence of dietary sodium on the renin-angiotensin-aldosterone system and prevalence of left ventricular hypertrophy by EKG criteria. *J Hum Hypertens* 2005a;19:133–138.

Williams GH, Dluhy RG, Lifton RP, et al. Non-modulation as an intermediate phenotype in essential hypertension. *Hypertension* 1992;20:788–796.

Williams TA, Mulatero P, Filigheddu F, et al. Role of HSD11B2 polymorphisms in essential hypertension and the diuretic response to thiazides. *Kidney Int* 2005b;67:631–637.

Wilson DM, Luetscher JA. Plasma prorenin activity and complications in children with insulin-dependent diabetes mellitus. *N Engl J Med* 1990;323:1101–1106.

Winkelmayer WC, Stampfer MJ, Willett WC, et al. Habitual caffeine intake and the risk of hypertension in women. *JAMA* 2005;294:2330–2335.

Wolfel EE, Selland MA, Mazzeo RS, et al. Systemic hypertension at 4,300 m is related to sympathoadrenal activity. *J Appl Physiol* 1994;76:1643–1650.

Woods LL, Weeks DA, Rasch R. Programming of adult blood pressure by maternal protein restriction: Role of nephrogenesis. *Kidney Int* 2004;65:1339–1348.

Wu H, Ghosh S, Perrard XD, et al. T-cell accumulation and regulated on activation, normal T cell expressed and secreted upregulation in adipose tissue in obesity. *Circulation* 2007; 115:1029–1038.

Wu JN, Berecek KH. Prevention of genetic hypertension by early treatment of spontaneously hypertensive rats with the angiotensin converting enzyme inhibitor captopril. *Hypertension* 1993;22:139–146.

Wu Y, Huxley R, Li L, et al. Prevalence, awareness, treatment, and control of hypertension in China: Data from the China National Nutrition and Health Survey 2002. *Circulation* 2008; 118:2679–2686.

Yang R, Barouch LA. Leptin signaling and obesity: Cardiovascular consequences. *Circ Res* 2007;101:545–559.

Zacchigna L, Vecchione C, Notte A, et al. Emilin1 links TGF-beta maturation to blood pressure homeostasis. *Cell* 2006;124: 929–942.

Zethelius B, Berglund L, Sundstrom J, et al. Use of multiple biomarkers to improve the prediction of death from cardiovascular causes. *N Engl J Med* 2008;358:2107–2116.

Zhang L, Rao F, Zhang K, et al. Discovery of common human genetic variants of GTP cyclohydrolase 1 (GCH1) governing nitric oxide, autonomic activity, and cardiovascular risk. *J Clin Invest* 2007;117:2658–2671.

Zhang WZ, Venardos K, Chin-Dusting J, et al. Adverse effects of cigarette smoke on NO bioavailability: Role of arginine metabolism and oxidative stress. *Hypertension* 2006;48.278–285.

Zhao L, Stamler J, Yan LL, et al. Blood pressure differences between northern and southern Chinese: Role of dietary factors. The International Study on Macronutrients and Blood Pressure. *Hypertension* 2004;43:1332–1337.

Zhou BF, Stamler J, Dennis B, et al. Nutrient intakes of middle-aged men and women in China, Japan, United Kingdom, and United States in the late 1990s: The INTERMAP study. *J Hum Hypertens* 2003;17:623–630.

Zimmerman MC, Lazartigues E, Lang JA, et al. Superoxide mediates the actions of angiotensin II in the central nervous system. *Circ Res* 2002;91:1038–1045.

Zinner SH, McGarvey ST, Lipsitt LP, et al. Neonatal blood pressure and salt taste responsiveness. *Hypertension* 2002;40: 280–285.

Primary Hypertension: Natural History and Evaluation

Now that the probable causes of primary hypertension have been considered, we turn to its clinical course and complications. We will first view the natural history of the disease if left untreated, examining the specific manner by which hypertension leads to premature cardiovascular damage and how such damage is clinically expressed. Additional coverage is provided for special populations—the elderly, women, blacks and other ethnic groups, diabetics, the obese—who may follow somewhat different courses. Based on this background, guidelines for evaluating the newly diagnosed hypertensive patient are presented.

As noted in previous chapters, hypertension seems logically divided into three main categories: isolated diastolic hypertension in the young; diastolic with systolic hypertension, and isolated systolic hypertension in the elderly (see Fig. 1-6 in Chapter 1). Table 4-1 delineates some of the main differences between the 2 types seen in those over age 30. They may overlap. For example, about one third of ISH patients started with combined systolic and diastolic hypertension (Franklin et al., 2005). Most of the following relates to both forms but the majority of studies on the natural history of hypertension involved younger patients with combined disease. Only recently has ISH received its deserved recognition (Franklin et al., 2001; McEniery et al., 2005; Wallace et al., 2007).

NATURAL HISTORY OF PRIMARY HYPERTENSION

The natural history of hypertension, simplistically depicted in Figure 4-1, starts when some combination of hereditary and environmental factors sets into motion transient but repetitive perturbations of cardiovascular homeostasis (*prehypertension*), not enough to raise the blood pressure (BP) to levels defined as abnormal but enough to begin the cascade that, over many years, leads to BPs that usually are elevated (*early hypertension*). Some people, abetted by lifestyle changes, may abort the process and return to normotension. The majority, however, progress into *established hypertension*, which, as it persists, may induce a variety of complications identifiable as target organ damage and disease.

As was noted in Chapter 1, the higher the BP and the longer it remains elevated, the greater the morbidity and mortality. Although some patients with markedly elevated, untreated BP never have trouble, we have no way of accurately identifying in advance those who will have an uncomplicated course, the few who will enter a rapidly progressing, accelerated-malignant phase, and the many who will more slowly but progressively develop cardiovascular complications. Even without such foreknowledge, as BP and other risk factors are increasingly being treated, rates of morbidity and mortality related to hypertension have fallen (Menotti et al., 2009). Evidence for these changes is provided in Chapter 5 and the methods to achieve them in Chapters 6 and 7.

It should be noted that the role of hypertension probably is underestimated from morbidity and mortality statistics, which are largely based on death certificates. When a patient dies from a stroke, a heart attack, or renal failure—all directly attributable to uncontrolled hypertension—the stroke, the heart attack, or the renal failure, but *not* the hypertension, usually is listed as the cause of death.

TABLE 4.1	Differences Between Combined Systolic and Diastolic Versus ISH	
	Combined	**ISH**
Age of Onset	30–50	>55
Mechanisms	Multiple	Atherosclerotic stiffness
Progression	Slow, variable	More rapid, continuous
Consequences	Coronary artery disease, nephrosclerosis	Stroke, CHF
Response to therapy	Renin-angiotensin blockers	Diuretics, calcium channel blockers

PREHYPERTENSION

Very few people are born with hypertension, although babies with intrauterine birth retardation who are therefore small for gestational age have a higher propensity to develop hypertension in adult life (Davies et al., 2006). The natural history of hypertension starts with normal BP, i.e., below 120/80 mm Hg, that typically slowly rises until middle age when hypertension, i.e., 140/90 mm Hg or higher, appears. In many people, only the systolic rises with further aging, inducing ISH, which is the most common form of hypertension in people over age 60.

As perhaps best seen in data from the Framingham cohort shown in Figure 4-2, the BP tends to track over many years, remaining in the same relative position over time (Franklin et al., 1997). Subjects in each BP segment tend to remain in that segment, with a slow, gradual rise over the 30 years of follow-up. In a later survey of the Framingham population, hypertension developed over a 4-year interval in only 5% of men and women with BP less than 120/80 mm Hg, in 18% with a BP less than 130/85 mm Hg, and in 37% with a BP 130 to 139/85 to 89 mm Hg (Vasan et al., 2001).

Naturally, the progressive rise in pressure proceeds from 120/80 to 140/90 mm Hg through levels that were traditionally labeled "high-normal." However, more and more evidence showed the appearance of cardiovascular risk factors and even target organ damage among these people (Carrington, 2009; Kshirsagar et al., 2006; Toprak et al., 2009; Vasan et al., 2001). Therefore, the 2003 Joint National Committee (JNC-7) report introduced the term "prehypertension" to cover those with sustained BP levels from 120/80 to 139/89 mm Hg (Chobanian et al., 2003). Although "prehypertension" was not accepted in the 2007 European guidelines (Task Force, 2007) and has been accused of simply being a gift to marketers of antihypertensive drugs (Marshall, 2009), the term has gained increasing acceptance (Delles, 2008). It should be recognized for the rationale stated in JNC-7:

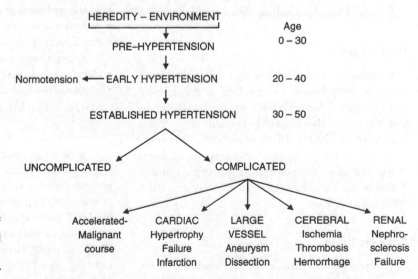

FIGURE 4-1 Representation of the natural history of untreated essential hypertension.

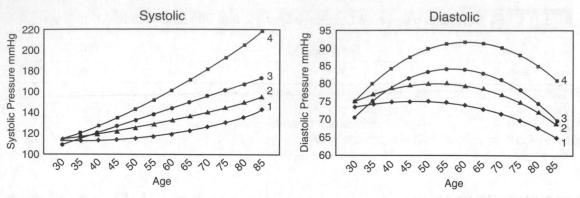

FIGURE 4-2   Tracking systolic and diastolic blood pressures by age for up to 30 years in the Framingham Heart Study. Subjects who were stratified by their systolic BP in middle age: less than 120, 120 to 139, 140 to 159, and ≤160 mm Hg. The curves are derived from averaged individual regression analysis. (Modified from Franklin SS, Gustin W IV, Wong ND, et al. Hemodynamic patterns of age-related changes in blood pressure: The Framingham Heart Study. *Circulation* 1997;96:308–315.)

Prehypertension is not a disease category. Rather it is a designation chosen to identify individuals at high risk of developing hypertension, so that both patients and clinicians are alerted to this risk and encouraged to intervene and prevent or delay the disease from developing. The goal for individuals with prehypertension and no compelling indications is to lower BP to normal with lifestyle changes and prevent the progressive rise in BP using the recommended lifestyle modifications.

Prevalence

As many or more people are prehypertensive as are hypertensive, with an average number in surveys of the U.S. population of 60 million (Elliott & Black, 2007).

Predictors

Since prehypertension is one step toward hypertension, the same factors are involved in the development of both. Obesity is foremost, with male gender and black race also involved (Franklin et al., 2005; Toprak et al., 2009). In addition, these factors are associated with more prehypertension: diabetes, impaired glucose tolerance, the metabolic syndrome, dyslipidemia and smoking (Elliott & Black, 2007; Parikh et al., 2008).

Associations

As best portrayed in the Prospective Studies Collaboration (2002), an increase in BP from 115/75 to 135/85 mm Hg doubles the mortality rate for both ischemic heart disease and stroke (see Fig. 1-1 in Chapter 1). The evidences for target organ damage in prehypertension include these:

- Left ventricular hypertrophy (LVH) (Kokkinos et al., 2007)
- Coronary calcification (Pletcher et al., 2008)
- Reduced coronary flow reserve (Erdogan et al., 2007)
- Progression of coronary atherosclerosis (Sipahi et al., 2006)
- Increases in ischemic coronary disease and stroke (Kshirsagar et al., 2006)
- Poor cognitive function (Knecht et al., 2008)
- Retinal vascular changes (Nguyen et al., 2007)
- Proteinuria (Kim et al., 2007)
- Renal arteriosclerosis (Ninomiya et al., 2007)
- Elevated serum uric acid (Syamala et al., 2007)
- Increased levels of various markers of cardiovascular risk, including C-reactive protein (CRP) (Bo et al., 2009)

With all of these indices of impending or existing target organ damage, attempts have been made to prevent prehypertension or at least to slow its progression into hypertension. As will be described more fully in Chapters 6 and 7, these have focused on lifestyle changes (Bavikati et al., 2008) but the difficulties in achieving lasting effects from lifestyle changes have led to trials of antihypertensive drugs (Julius et al., 2006; Luders et al., 2008; Skov et al., 2007).

EARLY HYPERTENSION: COURSE OF THE BLOOD PRESSURE

In most people who become hypertensive, the hypertension persists, but in some the BP returns to normal, presumably not to rise again. As emphasized in Chapter 2, hypertension should be confirmed by multiple readings before the diagnosis is made and therapy is begun. Initial readings may be higher than subsequent readings because of a greater alerting reaction and, as with all biologic variables, a tendency for initially higher readings to come down from regression toward the mean. If subsequent readings are considerably lower and the patient is free of obvious vascular complications, the patient should be advised to adhere to a healthy lifestyle and either to return every few months for repeat BP measurement or to self-monitor the BP at home.

The wisdom of this course is shown by data from the Australian therapeutic trial (Management Committee, 1982); 12.8% of the patients whose diastolic BPs averaged more than 95 mm Hg on two sets of initial readings obtained 2 weeks apart had a subsequent fall to less than 95 mm Hg that persisted over the next year, such that the patients could not be entered into the trial. An even larger portion (47.5%) of those who entered the trial with a diastolic BP above 95 mm Hg and who received only placebo tablets for the next 3 years maintained their average diastolic BP at less than 95 mm Hg. A significant portion remained below 90 mm Hg while on placebo, including 11% of those whose initial diastolic BP was as high as 105 to 109 mm Hg. On the other hand, 12.2% of the placebo-treated patients experienced a progressive rise in diastolic BP to more than 110 mm Hg.

From these data and others that will be described, a number of implications can be made:

- Multiple BP readings over at least 6 weeks may be needed to establish the diagnosis of hypertension.
- Many patients who are not given antihypertensive drugs will have a significant decline in their BP, often to levels considered safe and not requiring therapy.
- Patients who are at low overall cardiovascular risk and free of target organ damage and whose diastolic BPs are lower than 90 mm Hg can safely be left off active drug therapy for at least a few years.
- If not treated, patients must be kept under close observation since a significant number will have a rise in pressure to levels requiring active therapy.

These conclusions form part of the basis of the approach toward initial management of patients with relatively mild hypertension that is presented in Chapter 5.

ESTABLISHED HYPERTENSION

As delineated in Chapter 1 and shown in Figure 1-1, the long-term effects of progressively higher levels of BP on the incidence of stroke and coronary heart disease (CHD) are clear: In 61 prospective observational studies involving almost 1 million people with BP starting as low as 115/75 mm Hg who were followed for up to 25 years, the associations were "positive, continuous and apparently independent" (Prospective Studies Collaboration, 2002).

Uncontrolled Long-term Observations

In addition to these major studies, smaller groups of patients with fairly severe hypertension were followed up by investigators before effective therapies became available (Bechgaard, 1976). Perera (1955) followed 500 patients with an office diastolic BP of 90 mm Hg or higher—150 patients from before disease onset and 350 from an uncomplicated phase—until their death. The mean age of onset was 32 years, and the mean survival time was 20 years. Perera (1955) summarized his survey of the natural history of hypertension as follows:

> ...a chronic illness, more common in women, beginning as a rule in early adult life, related little if at all to pregnancy, and persisting for an average period of two decades before its secondary complicating pathologic features cause death at an average age fifteen to twenty years less than the normal life expectancy. Hypertensive vascular disease may progress at a highly variable rate, but on the whole the patient with this disorder spends most of his hypertensive life with insignificant symptoms and without complications.

Age of Onset

One additional point about Perera's data is worth emphasizing: Few of his patients experienced the onset of hypertension after age 45. A similar finding was observed in the Cooperative Study of Renovascular Hypertension, wherein the diagnosis of primary hypertension was made with even greater certainty in 1,128 patients (Maxwell, 1975). Of these, the onset of an elevated BP was documented to have occurred at an age younger than 20 years in 12% and older than 50 years in only 7%.

On the other hand, in a more recent prospective study of a large, more representative population than the one followed up by Perera or seen in the Cooperative Study, 20% of people aged 40 to 69 years who developed a diastolic BP of 90 mm Hg or higher over a 5-year period were 60 years of age or older (Buck et al., 1987). Moreover, the rate of developing a significant cardiovascular event among the newly discovered hypertensives was almost as high among those in their forties as among those aged 60 to 65 years. The middle-aged hypertensives were much more likely to develop an event than were normotensives of the same age but, as Buck et al. (1987) stated, "age overtakes hypertension as a cause of cardiovascular disease," so that among those aged 60 to 65, there was little difference in the rate.

Untreated Patients in Clinical Trials

To those patients left untreated during the 1940s and 1950s when no effective therapy was readily available, we can add those patients who served as the control populations in the trials of the therapy of hypertension up to the mid-1990s, at which time placebo-controlled trials were no longer considered ethical, with the exception of one in the very elderly wherein no data were available. Although these trials were not designed to observe the natural history of hypertension, their data can help to define further the course of untreated disease (Table 4-2). The trials involving elderly patients will be considered separately.

The types of patients included in these randomized, controlled trials (RCTs) and the manner in which they were followed up differ considerably, so comparisons between them are largely inappropriate. Moreover, the patients enrolled in these RCTs were, in general, much healthier than the general population. In most, they had to be free of major debilities and, often, any coexisting diseases, such as diabetes. For example, only 1.1% of those screened were eligible for enrollment in the Systolic Hypertension in the Elderly Program (SHEP) trial (SHEP Cooperative Research Group, 1991). Therefore, the rate of complications seen during the few years of follow-up on no therapy can be considered the minimum. In the overall population, much higher rates of cardiovascular

TABLE 4.2   Complications Among Control Groups in Trials of Nonelderly Hypertensives

Factor	Veterans Administration Cooperative[a] 1967	1970	USPHS[b]	Australia[c]	Oslo[d]	Medical Research Council[e]
Mean age (year)	51	52	44	50	45	52
Range of diastolic BP (mm Hg)	115–129	90–114	90–115	95–109	90–110	95–109
Number of subjects on placebo	70	194	196	1,617	379	8,654
Average follow-up (year)	1.3	3.3	7.0	3.0	5.5	5.5
Coronary disease[f]						
Fatal	1.0	6.0	2.0	0.4	0.5	1.1
Nonfatal	3.0	1.0	26.0	4.9	2.9	1.6
Congestive heart failure[f]	3.0	6.0	1.0	0.1	0.2	—
Cerebrovascular disease[f]	16.0	11.0	3.0	1.5	1.8	1.3
Renal insufficiency[f]	4.0	2.0	1.0	0.1	—	—
Progression of hypertension[f]	4.0	10.0	12.0	12.1	17.2	11.7
Total mortality[f]	6.0	10.0	2.0	1.2	2.4	2.9

USPHS, U.S. Public Health Service.
[a]Data from Veterans Administration Cooperative Study Group on Antihypertensive Agents. Effects of treatment on morbidity in hypertension. *JAMA* 1967;202:116–122;1970;213:1143–1152.
[b]Data from Smith WM. Treatment of mild hypertension. *Circ Res* 1977;40(Suppl. 1):98–115.
[c]Data from Management Committee. The Australian therapeutic trial in mild hypertension. *Lancet* 1980;1:1261–1267.
[d]Data from Helgeland A. Treatment of mild hypertension. *Am J Med* 1980;69:725–732.
[e]Data from Medical Research Council Working Party. Medical Research Council trial of treatment of mild hypertension. *Br Med J* 1985;291:97–104.
[f]Data reported as rate per 100 patients for the entire trial.

TABLE 4.3 Complications Among Control Groups in Trials of Elderly Hypertensives

Complication	Australian[a]	EWPHE[b]	Coope and Warrender[c]	SHEP[d]	STOP-HT[e]	MRC-2[f]	Syst-Eur[g]	HYVET[h]
Mean age (year)	64	72	69	72	76	70	70	84
BP at entry (mm Hg)								
Systolic	<200	160–239	190–230	160–219	<180–230	160–209	160–219	160–199
Diastolic	95–109	90–119	105–120	<90	90–120	<115	<95	<110
Mean	165/101	182/101	197/110	170/77	195/102	185/91	174/85	173/91
Number of subjects on placebo	289	424	435	2,371	815	2,113	2,297	1,912
Average follow-up (year)	3.0	4.6	4.4	4.5	2.1	5.7	2.0	1.8
Coronary disease[i]								
Fatal	1.3	11.8	6.0	3.4	2.5	5.2	1.8	
Nonfatal	8.3	2.8	2.2	3.4	2.7	2.3	1.4	
Congestive heart failure[i]	—	5.4	1.7	4.5	4.8	—	2.1	-6.4-
Cerebrovascular disease[i]	4.2	13.7	9.4	6.8	6.6	6.4	3.4	-8.0-
Progression of hypertension[i]	—	6.8	—	15.0	9.3	8.3	5.5	
Total mortality[i]	3.1	35.1	14.8	10.2	7.9	15.0	6.0	-22.0-

EWPHE, European Working Party on Hypertension in the Elderly; MRC, Medical Research Council; SHEP, Systolic Hypertension in the Elderly Program; STOP-HT, Swedish Trial in Old Patients with Hypertension; Syst-Eur, Systolic Hypertension in Europe Trial.

[a]Data from Management Committee. Treatment of mild hypertension in the elderly. Med J Aust 1981;2:398–402.

[b]Data from Amery A, Birkenäger W, Brixko P, et al. Mortality and morbidity results from the European Working Party on High Blood Pressure in the Elderly Trial. Lancet 1985;1:1349–1354.

[c]Data from Coope J, Warrender TS. Randomized trial of treatment of hypertension in elderly patients in primary care. Br Med J 1986;293:1145–1151.

[d]Data from SHEP Cooperative Research Group. Prevention of stroke by antihypertensive drug treatment in older persons with isolated systolic hypertension. JAMA 1991;266:3255–3264.

[e]Data from Dahlöf B, Lindholm LH, Hansson L, et al. Morbidity and mortality in the Swedish Trial in Older Patients with Hypertension. Lancet 1991;338:1281–1285.

[f]Data from Medical Research Council Working Party. Medical Research Council trial of treatment of older adults. Br Med J 1992;304:405–412.

[g]Data from Staessen JA, Fagard R, Thijs L, et al. Randomized double-blind comparison of placebo and active treatment for older patients with isolated systolic hypertension. Lancet 1997;350:757–764.

[h]Data from Beckett NS, Peters R, Fletcher AE, et al. Treatment of hypertension in patients 80 years of age or older. N Engl J Med 2008;358:1887–1898.

[i]Data reported as rate per 100 patients for the entire trial.

[j]Data in HYVET are rates per 100 patient years.

diseases (CVDs) would be expected, and the dangers of untreated hypertension would obviously expand over a longer time. More about these trials is covered in Chapter 5.

Untreated Elderly Patients in Trials

Table 4-3 summarizes data from seven RCTs of elderly hypertensives, two of them (SHEP Cooperative Research Group [1991] and the Systolic Hypertension in Europe Trial [Staessen et al., 1997]) including only patients with ISH, the others including a portion with ISH. The control patients in these trials had much higher rates of the various end points than were seen in the trials of younger hypertensives listed in Table 4-2.

Systolic Versus Diastolic Pressure

A meta-analysis of all published trials of elderly patients until 2000 (Staessen et al., 2000) reconfirmed what has been repeatedly shown in multiple observational studies: Rises in systolic levels and falls in diastolic levels, with the resultant widening of pulse pressure, are typical changes that occur with aging and all predict risk. As shown in Figure 4-3, risk

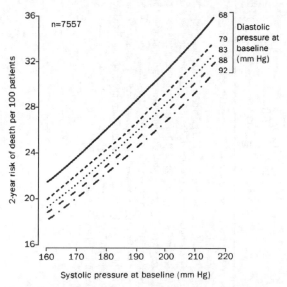

FIGURE 4-3   The 2-year probability of death associated with systolic BP at different levels of diastolic pressure at baseline in untreated elderly women with ISH but no prior cardiovascular complications enrolled in eight RCTs. (Modified from Staessen JA, Gasowski J, Wang JG, et al. Risks of untreated and treated isolated systolic hypertension in the elderly. *Lancet* 2000;355:865–872.)

of death rises steeply for every increment of systolic BP but, at every level of systolic BP, the risk increases further the lower the diastolic BP. As noted in Chapter 1, the widened pulse pressure is not as predictive of risk as is the higher systolic level.

From these multiple sources, the picture of the natural history of hypertension shown in Figure 4-1 is derived. We now will examine the various complications shown at the bottom of that figure.

COMPLICATIONS OF HYPERTENSION

The end of the natural history of untreated hypertension is an increased likelihood of premature disability or death from CVD. Before considering the specific types of organ damage and the causes of death related to hypertension, the underlying basis for the arterial pathology caused by hypertension and the manner in which this pathology is expressed clinically will be examined.

As described in Chapter 3, the pathogenesis of combined systolic and diastolic hypertension involves structural changes in the resistance arterioles subsumed under the terms *remodeling* and *hypertrophy*. These same changes almost certainly are also involved in the development of the small-vessel arteriosclerosis that is responsible for much of the target organ damage seen in long-standing hypertension. As people age, large-artery atherosclerosis becomes an increasing factor, aggravated by the high shear stress of hypertension (Lakatta & Levy, 2003) but involving "several highly interrelated processes, including lipid disturbances, platelet activation, thrombosis, endothelial dysfunction, inflammation, oxidative stress, vascular smooth cell activation, altered matrix metabolism, remodeling, and genetic factors" (Faxon et al., 2004). Small-vessel arterial and arteriolar sclerosis may be considered secondary consequences of typical combined systolic-diastolic hypertension, whereas large-vessel atherosclerosis is primarily responsible for the predominantly systolic hypertension so common among the elderly.

Types of Arterial Lesions

The more common vascular lesions found in hypertension are

• Fibrinoid necrosis, seen with acute and severe rises in BP.
• Hyperplastic or proliferative arteriolar sclerosis.

- Hyaline arteriolar sclerosis, with thickening and hyalinization of the intima and media.
- Miliary aneurysms in small cerebral penetration arterioles, usually at their first branching, which represent poststenotic dilations beyond areas of intimal thickening and which, when they rupture, cause the cerebral hemorrhages so typical of hypertension.
- Atherosclerotic plaques where thrombi form and which likely are responsible for the ischemia and infarction of heart, brain, kidney, and other organs that occur more frequently among hypertensives.
- Medial damage in the wall of the aorta may lead to the formation of large plaques with eventual aneurysmal dilation and rupture, as well as aortic dissections.

Most of the premature morbidity and mortality associated with hypertension is related to atherosclerosis. Although usually only one of the multiple risk factors involved, hypertension has an independent role (Agmon et al., 2000) that can be related to subclinical atherosclerosis even in children and adolescents (Berenson et al., 1998; Vos et al., 2003). There are variable rates of atherosclerotic stiffness between genders (Waddell et al., 2001) and ethnic groups (Chaturvedi et al., 2004), which may explain the variability in vascular damage between them. Noninvasive measures of arterial compliance are being used to identify such early atherosclerosis (Herrington et al., 2004).

Causes of Death

Death may result when these arterial lesions either rupture or become occluded enough to cause ischemia or infarction of the tissues they supply. The overall increase in mortality associated with hypertension was examined in Chapter 1; The causes of death in hypertensives, mostly from series published before the availability of effective therapy, can be summarized thusly:

- CVDs are responsible for a higher proportion of deaths as the severity of the hypertension worsens.
- Heart disease remains the leading cause of death overall but strokes become increasingly more common in populations over age 65 (Kjeldsen et al., 2001).
- Heart failure becomes increasingly common in the elderly (Tocci et al., 2008).

TARGET ORGAN INVOLVEMENT

We will now examine in more detail the pathophysiology and consequences of these various complications. Thereafter, the clinical and laboratory manifestations of the target organ damage will be incorporated into guidelines for evaluating the hypertensive patient.

Hypertensive Heart Disease

Hypertension more than doubles the risk for symptomatic coronary disease, including acute myocardial infarction (MI) and sudden death, and more than triples the risk for congestive heart failure (CHF) (Kannel, 1996). As shown in Figure 4-4, hypertension, usually in concert with a number of other risk factors, often leads to LVH and/or myocardial ischemia and/or infarction. These processes, in turn, precipitate systolic and diastolic dysfunction which often progresses to overt CHF (Krum & Alexandar, 2009) (Figure 4-5).

FIGURE 4-4 Risk of cardiovascular events by hypertensive status in subjects aged 35 to 64 years from the Framingham study at 36-year follow-up. Coronary disease includes clinical manifestations such as MI, angina pectoris, sudden death, other coronary deaths, and coronary insufficiency syndrome; peripheral artery disease is manifested as intermittent claudication. Left bars in each set of columns represent normotensives; right bars represent hypertensives. (Modified from Kannel WB. Blood pressure as a cardiovascular risk factor. *JAMA* 1996;275:1571–1576.)

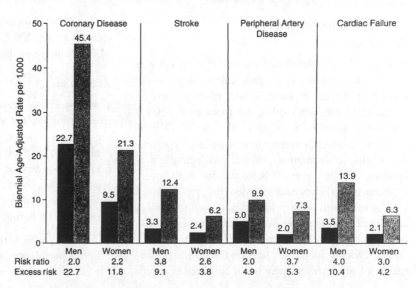

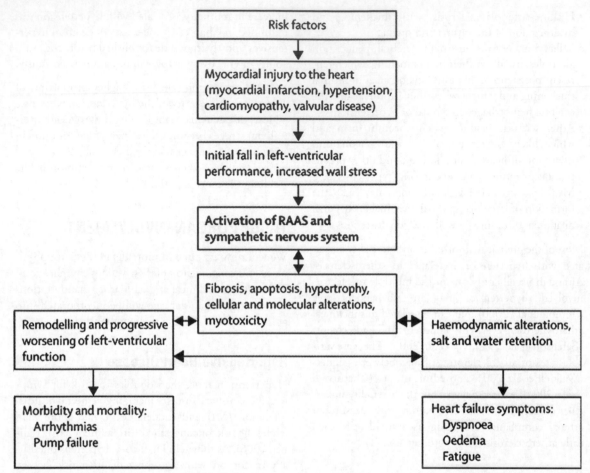

FIGURE 4-5   A simplified view of the pathophysiology of heart failure (From Krum H and Abraham WT. Heart failure. *Lancet* 2009;373:941–955.

Left Ventricular Hypertrophy

Prevalence

Whereas LVH is identified by electrocardiography in only 5% to 18% of hypertensives, dependent on the criteria used (Ang & Lang, 2008), when present by ECG, LVH predicts strokes (Ishikawa et al., 2009) and renal damage (Sciaretta et al., 2009). LVH is found by echocardiography in many more hypertensive adults, in as many as 30% of unselected hypertensives, and in up to 90% of persons with severe hypertension (Schmieder & Messerli, 2000). More LVH is seen with obesity, high dietary sodium intake, anemia of end-stage renal disease, alcohol abuse, diabetes, and hypercholesterolemia (de Simone et al., 2001). Despite its greater sensitivity, routine performance of echocardiography is not indicated (Cuspidi

et al., 2008). Nonetheless, hand-carried ultrasound (Martin et al., 2009) and contrast-enhanced cardiac MRI (Rudolph et al., 2009) are being advocated.

Associations

The association between LVH and hypertension is stronger for systolic levels, which contribute most of the relation between pulse pressure and LVH (Mulè et al., 2003). Increased pulse pressure is related to LV mass independent of other pressure components (de Simone et al., 2005). In addition to the stress and strain invoked by increased BP per se, other factors contribute, including:

• Genotype which is a likely mechanism for the higher prevalence of LVH in black than in white hypertensives (Kizer et al., 2004).

- A polymorphism of the angiotensin type-2 receptor gene (-1332G/A) (Alfakih et al., 2004).
- An important role of the renin-angiotensin system is supported by the impressive effect of ACEIs and ARBs in causing regression of LVH and preventing remodeling after an MI (Kenchaiah et al., 2004).
- In women, but not in men, an association between serum aldosterone and cardiac remodeling (Vasan et al., 2004) which could reflect increased renin-angiotensin activity.
- In view of the profibrotic effects of aldosterone described in Chapter 3, this may be involved in the increased collagen type and carbdiac remoneling 1 synthesis noted in patients with hypertensive heart failure (Querejeta et al., 2004).
- Increased cardiac sympathetic nervous activity (Schlaich et al., 2003).

Patterns

The patterns of LVH differ by the type of hemodynamic load: Volume overload leads to eccentric hypertrophy, whereas pure BP overload leads to an increase in LV wall thickness without concomitant increase in cavity volume, i.e., concentric hypertrophy. The pattern of LVH can also be modified by increased arterial stiffness, increased pulse-wave velocity, and blood viscosity.

In Wachtell et al.'s (2001) series of 913 patients with varying stages of hypertension, these percentages of various patterns were found by echocardiography: 19%, normal geometry; 11%, concentric remodeling; 47%, eccentric hypertrophy; and 23%, concentric hypertrophy.

Most find that concentric hypertrophy is most ominous (Akinboboye et al., 2004), but some find that LVH is a determinant of LV dysfunction independent of chamber geometry (Schillaci et al., 2002).

Consequences

Even without LVH, early hypertensives may have a significantly reduced coronary flow reserve from an impaired capacity for coronary vasodilation (Kawecka-Jaszcz et al., 2008). The conversion of echocardiographic concentric remodeling to LVH is associated with increased mortality (Milani et al., 2006). The presence of LVH is consistently and strongly related to subsequent cardiovascular morbidity (mean risk ratio, 2.3) and mortality (mean risk ratio, 2.5) (Vakili et al., 2001). The increased risk for sudden death in hypertensives is likely connected to alterations in ventricular conduction and repolarization associated with LVH (Oikarinen et al., 2004).

Regression

Regression of LVH was noted in 52% of the 937 hypertensives treated for 4.8. years in the LIFE study (Gerdts et al., 2008). Regression reduces the risk of stroke (Verdecchia et al., 2006). The effects of various antihypertensive agents are covered in Chapter 7.

Systolic and Diastolic Dysfunction

de Simone et al. (2004) use the term "inappropriate" left ventricular mass (LVM) when the LVM exceeds the theoretical value predicted by gender, body size, and stroke work. Such excessive LVM translates into concentric LV geometry and both systolic and diastolic dysfunction that, in turn, are the predecessors for systolic and diastolic heart failure. Patients with asymptomatic LV systolic dysfunction are at increased risk of heart failure and death, even with only mildly reduced ejection fractions (Verdecchia et al., 2005). Similarly, diastolic dysfunction, defined as an echocardiographic normal ejection fraction but abnormal LV filling in an asymptomatic hypertensive with LVH, is a precursor to diastolic heart failure (Aurigemma & Gaasch, 2004).

Congestive Heart Failure

Hypertension is present in over two thirds of patients who develop CHF (Yancy et al., 2006). Hypertension remains the major preventable factor in the disease that is now the leading cause of hospitalization in the United States for adults over age 65 (Curtis et al., 2008). It is likely that antihypertensive drugs used in treatment do not completely prevent CHF but postpone its development by several decades and are responsible for the improved survival in CHF (Roger et al., 2004).

Most episodes of CHF in hypertensive patients are associated with diastolic dysfunction, as reflected in a preserved ejection fraction (Bursi et al., 2006) (Table 4-4). Vasan and Benjamin (2001) explain the susceptibility of hypertensives, particularly those with LVH, to diastolic heart failure in this manner:

> When hemodynamically challenged by stress (such as exercise, tachycardia, increased afterload, or excessive preload), persons with hypertension are unable to increase their end-diastolic volume (i.e., they have limited preload reserve), because of decreased LV relaxation and compliance. Consequently, a cascade begins, in which the LV end-diastolic BP rises, left atrial pressure increases, and pulmonary edema develops.

TABLE 4.4   **Characteristics of Patients with Systolic or Diastolic Heart Failure**

Characteristics	Systolic Heart Failure	Diastolic Heart Failure
Age	All ages, typically 50–70 years	Frequently elderly
Sex	More often male	Frequently female
Left ventricular ejection fraction	Depressed, approximately 40% or lower	Preserved or normal, 40% or higher
Left ventricular cavity size	Usually dilated	Usually normal, often with concentric LVH
LVH on electrocardiography	Sometimes present	Usually present
Chest radiography	Congestion and cardiomegaly	Congestion with or without cardiomegaly
Gallop rhythm present	Third heart sound	Fourth heart sound

Management of CHF in hypertensive patients is covered in Chapter 7.

Coronary Heart Disease

As described in Chapter 1, hypertension is quantitatively the largest risk factor for CHD. The development of myocardial ischemia reflects an imbalance between myocardial oxygen supply and demand. Hypertension, by reducing the supply and increasing the demand, can easily tip the balance.

Clinical Manifestations

Hypertension may play an even greater role in the pathogenesis of CHD than is commonly realized for two reasons. First, hypertensives suffer more silent ischemia (Boon et al., 2003) and painless MI (Kannel et al., 1985) than do normotensives. Second, preexisting hypertension may go unrecognized in patients first seen after an MI. Although acute rises in BP may follow the onset of ischemic pain, the BP often falls immediately after the infarct if pump function is impaired.

Once an MI occurs, the prognosis is worsened in the presence of both preexisting and subsequent hypertension (Thune et al., 2008). On the other hand, an increase in post-MI mortality has been noted among those with systolic pressure below 120 mm Hg on admission (Gheorghiade et al., 2006) or 6 months later (Thune et al., 2008).

A particular concern when thrombolytic therapy is given for acute MI is the threat for stroke that is imposed by the presence of hypertension. In the Global Utilization of Streptokinase and Tissue Plasminogen Activator for Occluded Coronary Arteries-I (GUSTO-I) trial, the incidence of stroke went from 1.2% for normotensives to 3.4% in those with systolic BP greater than 175 mm Hg (Aylward et al., 1996).

Atrial Fibrillation

In a 16-year follow-up of 2,482 previously untreated hypertensives, 61 developed atrial fibrillation, a rate of 0.46 per 100 person years (Verdecchia et al., 2003). The likelihood increased with increasing age, levels of BP, LVM, and left atrial diameter. The risk of atrial fibrillation was reduced by over 60% in hypertensives treated down to a level below 120/80 mm Hg (Young-Xe & Ravid, 2004).

Aortic Stenosis

Among 193 patients with symptomatic aortic stenosis, hypertension was present in 32% and the additional workload was likely responsible for symptoms developing at larger value areas and lower stroke work loss (Antonini-Canterin et al., 2003). On the other hand, the severity of aortic stenosis may be masked by the presence of coexisting hypertension (Kaden & Haghi, 2008).

Large-vessel Disease

Abdominal Aortic Aneurysm

The incidence of abdominal aortic aneurysms is increasing, likely as a consequence of the increasing number of elderly people who carry cardiovascular risks from middle age (Rodin et al., 2003). Although hypertension is one of these risk factors, ultrasonography uncovered such an aneurysm in only 3% of mild hypertensives aged 60 to 75 years but in 11% of those with systolic BP above 195 mm Hg and either cerebral or peripheral vascular disease (PVD) (Simon et al., 1996). Onetime ultrasonographic screening is recommended for men over age 65 who have ever smoked (Earnshaw et al., 2004). Aneurysms over 5 cm in diameter are now best repaired endovascularly (Prinssen et al., 2004).

Aortic Dissection

As many as 80% of patients with aortic dissection have hypertension (Golledge & Eagle, 2008). The mechanism of dissection likely involves the combination of high pulsatile wave stress and accelerated atherosclerosis, because the higher the pressure, the greater the likelihood of dissection.

Aortic dissection may occur either in the ascending aorta (proximal, or type A), which requires surgery, or in the descending aorta (distal, or type B), which usually can be treated medically (Golledge & Eagle, 2008). Hypertension is more frequently a factor with distal dissections, whereas Marfan syndrome, Ehlers-Danlos syndrome, and cystic medial necrosis are seen more frequently with the proximal lesion (Patel & Deeb, 2008).

Peripheral Vascular Disease

The presence of symptomatic PVD, usually manifested by intermittent claudication, poses a high risk of subsequent cardiovascular mortality (Arain & Cooper, 2008). By measurement of the ankle-brachial BP index (ABI) with a Doppler device, PVD was identified in 4.3% of U.S. adults over age 40, more frequently in those who were older, black, diabetic, smoker, or hypertensive (Selvin & Erlinger, 2004). A low ABI, below 0.9, improves the accuracy of the Framingham Risk Score (Ankle Brachial Index Collaboration, 2008).

Takayasu Arteritis

Hypertension is present in nearly half of patients with Takayasu disease, an idiopathic, chronic inflammatory disease of large arteries that is reported most frequently in Japan and India (Weaver et al., 2004).

Carotid Artery Disease

The presence of a bruit over the carotid artery is indicative of twice the risk of MI and cardiovascular mortality compared with people who do not have a bruit (Pickett et al., 2008).

Increased carotid intima-media thickness is commonly used as a surrogate for hypertensive vascular disease and predicts the occurrence of ischemic strokes (Prati et al., 2008).

Cerebrovascular Disease

Stroke is the second leading cause of death worldwide, the leading cause of permanent neurological disability in adults, and the most common indication for use of hospital and chronic care home beds (Donnan et al., 2008). The stroke death rate is even higher (by 50%) among blacks who live in the southeastern United States (Obisesan et al., 2000), a rate similar to that noted in numerous other groups with inadequate health care worldwide (Donnan et al., 2008). Mortality rates from stroke have fallen markedly from the 1950s to the present in most industrialized countries, attributable to improved control of risk factors including hypertension. The incidence of stroke is increasing largely related to the increasing number of elderly people (Bejot et al., 2008).

Role of Hypertension

Even more than with heart disease, hypertension is the major cause of stroke. About 50% of strokes are attributable to hypertension, the risk rising in tandem with increasing BP (Gorelick, 2002). Hypertensives are at three to four times greater risk for stroke and those with BP above 130/85 at 1.5 times greater risk than normotensives.

In hypertensives, nearly 80% of strokes are ischemic, caused by either arterial thrombosis or embolism, 15% are caused by intraparenchymal hemorrhage, another 5% by subarachnoid hemorrhage (Donnan et al., 2008). Transient ischemic attacks—acute episodes of focal loss of cerebral or visual function lasting less than 24 hours and attributed to inadequate blood supply—may arise from emboli from atherosclerotic plaques in the carotids or thrombi in the heart (Flemming et al., 2004) and are followed by a high risk of stroke (Daffertshofer et al., 2004).

ISH in the elderly is associated with a 2.7 times greater incidence of strokes than is seen in normotensive people of the same age (Qureshi et al., 2002). Elderly hypertensives more often have silent cerebrovascular disease (Vermeer et al., 2002) and cerebral white matter lesions on MRI (van Dijk et al., 2004) which eventually may lead to brain atrophy and vascular dementia.

Brain microbleeds have been found in 15% of hypertensive patients, particularly in those with nocturnal hypertension detected by ambulatory monitors (Henskens et al., 2008). A widening pulse pressure during sleep is associated with a significantly increased risk of stroke (Kario et al., 2004), presumably reflecting the role of arterial stiffness (Laurent et al., 2003).

Whether hypertensive or normotensive before their stroke, the majority of stroke patients at the time they are first seen will have a transient elevation of BP that spontaneously falls within a few days

(Vemmos et al., 2004). Therefore, caution is advised in lowering the BP in the immediate poststroke period, as noted further in Chapter 7. On the other hand, as will be noted, long-term reduction of BP is the most effective protection against both initial and recurrent strokes (Donnan et al., 2008).

Cognitive Impairment and Dementia

Both high and low BPs are associated with impaired cognition even in the absence of clinically evident cerebrovascular disease (Birns & Kalra, 2009). A similar nonlinear relation has been noted with pulse pressure: both excessively wide pulse pressure (reflecting arterial stiffness) and narrow pulse pressure (reflecting reduced cerebral perfusion) are associated with increased risk for Alzheimer disease and dementia (Qiu et al., 2003). BP typically begins to decline 3 years before dementia becomes overt and continues to decline thereafter (Qiu et al., 2004).

Renal Disease

Hypertension plays an important role in renal damage, whether manifested as proteinuria, reduced glomerular filtration rate (GFR), or progression to end-stage renal disease (ESRD). However, the manner by which hypertension injures the kidneys and the frequency of renal damage arising from hypertension are not settled.

Assessment

Microalbuminuria is widely recognized to be an early manifestation of renal damage from any cause (Cirillo et al., 2008). Even albumin levels below 30 mg/L or an albumin-to-creatinine ratio below 20 mg/g have been found to accompany and predict hypertension and CVDs (Danziger, 2008). Therefore, lower levels of albuminuria, as low as 5 to 7 mg/L, are being recommended as the threshold for the presence of microalbuminuria (Zamora & Cubeddu, 2009). The incidence of hypertension is clearly predicted by the presence of microalbuminuria in levels well below 30 mg/L (Brantsma et al., 2006; Forman et al., 2008; Wang et al., 2005).

The presence of microalbuminuria likely reflects the presence of hypertension since it has been noted even in prehypertensives without diabetes or atherosclerotic vascular disease (Hsu et al., 2009).

Estimated glomerular filtration rate (eGFR) based on formulas including serum creatinine are increasingly being used as an indicator of renal damage,

independent of microalbuminuria but additive to its presence as predictors of cardiovascular risk (Hallan et al., 2007).

Serum cystatin C levels, both in absolute terms and as a replacement for serum creatinine to estimate GFR (Stevens et al., 2006), are being increasingly used to assess renal function. Cystatin C is a protein that is freely filtered by the glomerulus but largely reabsorbed or catabolized by the tubular epithelial cells. Since its level is not dependent on muscle mass, it may be a better maker of renal function than serum creatinine (Stevens et al., 2008). Increased serum levels are found in individuals who develop hypertension without clinical kidney or CVD (Kestenbaum et al., 2008).

Consequences

As more extensively described in Chapter 9, conventional beliefs have linked hypertension and chronic kidney disease (CKD) as a two-way street: hypertension causes CKD and CKD causes hypertension. A commonly accepted sequence for hypertension causing CKD is a loss of renal autoregulation which normally attenuates the transmission of increased systemic pressure to the glomeruli (Bidani & Griffin, 2004). As a consequence, patients with renal damage have an increased risk of both progressive renal dysfunction and CVDs (Färbom et al., 2008). Moreover, reduction of BP can slow if not stop the progression of renal diseases and accompanying cardiovascular events (Ibsen et al., 2005). The progress of hypertension into CKD has been termed "hypertensive nephrosclerosis" and this diagnosis is considered the second most common cause of CKD, below diabetic nephropathy.

However, Freedman and Sedor (2008) have questioned the hypertension causing CKD concept. First, they point out that "Hypertensive nephrosclerosis is a vaguely defined clinical entity, most commonly applied to African Americans with hypertension and advanced CKD in the absence of other causes for renal failure." While agreeing that hypertension accelerates the progress of CKD that can lead to ESRD, they then note:

> ...the epidemiologic evidence supporting mild to moderate essential hypertension as an initiator of kidney damage has always been weak. Recent molecular genetic breakthroughs now demonstrate that genetic variants within a molecular motor protein, nonmuscle myosin IIA, are associated with nondiabetic kidney disease in African Americans, suggesting it may often be kidney injury that generates the high BP and not the other way around.

The molecular genetic breakthroughs they refer to are from Kopp et al. (2008) and Kao et al. (2008). Kopp et al. reported an association in African Americans with focal and segmental glomerulosclerosis (FSGS) and a genetic marker on chromosome 22q that centers on single nucleotide polymorphisms in intron 23 of the nonmuscle myosin IIA heavy chain gene MYH9. The attributable risk for carriage of this haplotype was 72% in African Americans and 4% in European-Americans with idiopathic FSGS. Kao et al. (2008) found a close association of the MYH9 gene in patients with nondiabetic ESRD but not in patients with diabetic ESRD.

These findings may have important clinical applications. In the African American Study of Kidney Disease and Hypertension (AASK), intensive lowering of BP with ACEI did not slow the progression of renal damage (Appel et al., 2008). As stated by Freedman and Sedor (2008): "Hopefully studies of the mechanisms by which MYH9 gene variants cause CKD will result in new diagnostic tests to allow presymptomatic detection of high-risk individuals and will allow for new strategies to preserve renal function."

NATURAL HISTORY OF SPECIAL POPULATIONS

Before turning to evaluation, we will describe groups of people whose hypertension, for various reasons, may follow a different course from that seen in the predominantly male, white, middle-aged populations observed in most clinical trials and long-term observational studies. These special groups include a major part of the hypertensive population: the elderly, women, blacks and other ethnic groups, diabetics, and the obese.

Elderly

Two patterns of hypertension are seen in the elderly: combined systolic and diastolic—the carryover of primary (essential) hypertension common to middle age and ISH—the more frequent form in those over age 60. However, because the major consequences and, as is noted in Chapter 7, the therapy for both are quite similar, most of this discussion will not make a distinction between the two.

Prevalence of Hypertension

As noted in Chapter 1, whereas diastolic BPs tend to plateau before age 60 and drop thereafter, systolic BPs

rise progressively. Therefore, the incidence of ISH—defined as systolic pressure of 140 mm Hg or more and diastolic pressure of 90 mm Hg or less—progressively rises with age. In the National Health and Nutrition Examination Survey III, the proportion of various types of hypertension seen with advancing age progressively shifted from diastolic and combined hypertension to ISH (Franklin et al., 2001). In those older than 60 years, ISH was the pattern of hypertension in 87% of those who were untreated. In Framingham, nearly half of those who developed ISH did not have antecedent diastolic hypertension and only 29% had a prior diastolic level of 95 mm Hg or higher (Franklin et al., 2005). Systolic levels usually continue to rise after age 70 in those who remain healthy but tend to fall if chronic debilitating diseases occur (Starr et al., 1998). Almost 90% of Framingham subjects who were normotensive at age 55 or 65 developed hypertension 20 years later (Vasan et al., 2002).

As described in Chapter 2, two cautions are needed in evaluating BP levels in the elderly. First, the white-coat effect is more common and significant in the elderly than in younger people (Fotherby & Potter, 1993) so out-of-office readings should be obtained if possible. Second, the elderly may have artificially elevated BPs by usual indirect cuff measurements (i.e., pseudohypertension) because of increased stiffness of the large arteries, which may preclude compression and collapse of the brachial artery by the cuff (Spence, 1997).

Risks of Hypertension

As seen in Table 4-3 in the data from the placebo-treated half of the elderly patients enrolled in seven RCTs over the last 20 years, mortality in elderly hypertensives is significant, particularly from strokes, even in the brief 2- to 5-year interval of these trials. As noted, the patients enrolled tend to be healthier than the general population, so the risks of both combined systolic-diastolic and ISH are even greater than shown in Table 4-3.

A different pattern appears in the very elderly who have more chronic debility. In the subjects aged 75 to 94 years followed up in the Framingham study, risks for all-cause and cardiovascular mortality increased at the lower levels of systolic BP (<120 mm Hg). Most of this increase occurred in those with existing CVD. As Kannel et al. (1997) note:

There appears to be a different morbidity and mortality rate curve in the elderly that appears to be quadratic

(U-shaped) in those who have already had a cardiovascular event and linear in those free of cardiovascular disease. The excess mortality rate at low BP levels could be a reflection of poor ejection fractions rather than the impact of low BP…. It is thus likely that BP elevation remains a detrimental risk factor even in the very old.

The validity of this conclusion was shown in a subsequent analysis showing increased cardiovascular risk related to hypertension in those over age 80 compared to those who were younger (Lloyd-Jones et al., 2005).

In addition to increased mortality seen with either low systolic BP (<120 to 130 mm Hg) or high systolic BP (>180 mm Hg) in the very elderly, both are associated with the development of cognitive impairment (Waldstein et al., 2005).

Pathophysiology of Isolated Systolic Hypertension

The basic mechanism for the usual progressive rise in systolic BP with age is the loss of distensibility and elasticity in the large capacitance arteries, a process that was nicely demonstrated more than 50 years ago (Hallock & Benson, 1937) (Fig. 4-6). Increasing volumes of saline were infused into the tied-off aortas

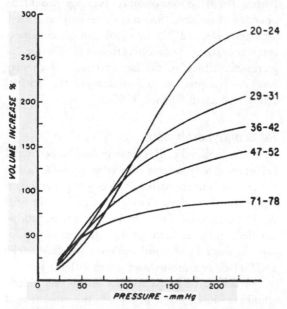

FIGURE 4-6 Curves showing the relation of the percentage of increase in pressure to the increase in volume infused into aortas excised at autopsy from people in five different age groups. The curves were constructed from the mean values obtained from a number of aortas. (Reprinted from Hallock P, Benson IC. Studies of the elastic properties of human isolated aorta. *J Clin Invest* 1937;16:595–602, with permission.)

taken from patients at death whose ages ranged from the 20s to the 70s. The pressure within the aortas from the elderly subjects rose much higher with small increases in volume as compared to that in aortas from the younger subjects, reflecting the rigidity of the vessels.

Subsequently, the progressive rise in systolic pressure with age has been found to reflect a reduced cross-sectional area of the peripheral vascular bed and stiffer aorta and large arteries, producing an increased pulse-wave velocity and an early return of pulse-wave reflection in systole (Safar & Benetos, 2003). The early return of the reflected pressure wave augments aortic pressure throughout systole, increasing both systolic and pulse pressures, further increasing the work of the left ventricle while decreasing the diastolic aortic pressure that supports coronary blood flow (Pierini et al., 2000).

Postural Hypotension

As is covered in Chapter 7, therapy of hypertension in the elderly is vital but oftentimes must be tempered by the need first to overcome coexisting postural hypotension.

Definition and Incidence

A fall in systolic pressure of 20 mm Hg or more after 1 minute of quiet standing is defined as postural hypotension. Postural hypotension was found in 68% of 489 patients with a mean age of 81.6 years in a geriatric ward (Weiss et al., 2002). In the generally healthy population of elderly men and women enrolled in the SHEP, postural hypotension was found in 10.4% at 1 minute after rising from a seated position and in 12.0% at 3 minutes, with 17.3% having hypotension at one or both intervals (Applegate et al., 1991). The prevalence would likely have been higher if the patients had been correctly tested after rising from a supine position. Although there are multiple, mainly neurological, causes for postural hypotension (Ejaz et al., 2004), the only predisposing factor for postural hypotension found in an unselected elderly population was hypertension (Räihä et al., 1995). As seen in Figure 4-7, the higher the basal supine systolic BP, the greater was the tendency for a postural fall (Lipsitz et al., 1985).

Mechanism

Normal aging is associated with various changes that may lead to postural hypotension. The two most common changes in patients with supine or seated hypertension are venous pooling in the legs and reduced baroreceptor sensitivity (Jones et al., 2003).

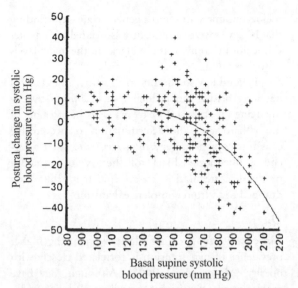

FIGURE 4-7   Relationship between basal supine systolic BP and postural change in systolic BP for aggregate data from older subjects. (Modified from Lipsitz LA, Storch HA, Minaker KL, et al. Intra-individual variability in postural BP in the elderly. *Clin Sci* 1985;69:337–341.)

Even though elderly hypertensives have intact baroreceptor modulation of sympathetic nerve traffic, they have marked impairment of baroreceptor control of heart rate and of cardiopulmonary reflex control of the peripheral circulation (Grassi et al., 2000). In addition, splanchnic pooling of blood after eating may lead to profound postprandial hypotension (Puisieux et al., 2000).

Women

Before age 50, women have a lower prevalence of hypertension than men but, after age 55, women have a greater age-related increase in proximal aortic stiffness which leads to a higher incidence of systolic hypertension in older women (Pemu & Ofili, 2008). In addition, women have two other features which tend to lower diastolic BP and widen pulse pressure: first, shorter stature which causes a more rapid return of the pulse wave to augment the peak systolic pressure; second, a faster heart rate which induces a shorter diastolic period (Safar & Smulyan, 2004).

Consequences
Women at all ages have a lower incidence of heart attacks and strokes than men but they maintain a

strong, continuous, and linear association between systolic BP and cardiovascular events (Mason et al., 2004). An increased risk of CVD, including higher BP levels, has been noted in women who have significant menopausal symptoms (Gast et al., 2008) or migraine with aura (Kurth et al., 2008).

The usual increase in intravascular volume during the luteal phase of the menstrual cycle may be related to the higher levels of plasma aldosterone, rising from an average of 11.2 μg/dL in the follicular phase to 17.8 μg/dL in the luteal phase (Fommei et al., 2009). This normal rise in plasma aldosterone may give rise to falsely positive aldosterone to renin ratios used for screening for primary aldosteronism.

Blacks

Death from hypertension is the single most common reason for the higher mortality rate for blacks than for nonblacks in the United States (Minor et al., 2008). Blacks have more hypertension and suffer more from it, at least in part because of their lower socioeconomic status and resultant reduced access to necessary health care (Jha et al., 2003). Their higher prevalence of hypertension likely reflects both genetic and environmental factors. If appropriate therapy is provided, most of their excessive morbidity and mortality related to hypertension can be relieved.

Prevalence of Hypertension
Blacks in the United States
The higher BP levels in U.S. blacks begin during childhood and adolescence and are established by early adulthood. Most of the higher BPs in young blacks are attributed to a larger body weight and size (Toprak et al., 2009). In middle age, blacks and whites have similar incidences of hypertension given the same baseline BP and BMI (He et al., 1998). However, hypertension in blacks is a greater risk factor for coronary disease, strokes, and in particular, ESRD than in whites (Minor et al., 2008). In most studies, blacks usually have higher sleeping BPs, as recorded by ambulatory monitoring (Harshfield et al., 2002a) but no greater early morning surge in BP (Haas et al., 2005).

Blacks Outside the United States
In their survey of blacks in seven populations of African origin, Cooper et al. (1999) found the rates of hypertension to be 7% in rural Nigeria, 26% in Jamaica, and 33% in the United States. These higher rates were associated with increased BMI and sodium intake.

Pathophysiology of Hypertension

Table 4-5 lists some of the numerous genotypic and phenotypic features found in black hypertensives that may explain their higher prevalence and greater degree of target organ damage. Whatever else is responsible, poverty, racial discrimination, and barriers to health care obviously are involved in the higher hypertension-related morbidity and mortality seen in U.S. blacks (Jha et al., 2003).

Stress

As described in Chapter 3, a large body of literature attests to an association between the stresses of low socioeconomic status and hypertension. A good example of the likely interaction between low

socioeconomic status and a genetic trait is the finding that BP levels were significantly associated with darker skin color but only in those blacks in the lower levels of socioeconomic status (Klag et al., 1991).

Beyond low socioeconomic status, James (1994) has long held to an influence of a coping strategy involving an active effort to manage the stressors of life by hard work and determination to succeed. He calls this coping strategy *John Henryism*, after a legendary uneducated black folk hero who defeated a mechanical steam drill in an epic battle but then dropped dead from complete exhaustion.

Diet

Particularly among older black women, the higher prevalence of hypertension is correlated closely with obesity (Minor et al., 2008). Although they have greater pressor sensitivity to sodium (Palacios et al., 2004), blacks do not appear to ingest more sodium than do non-blacks (Ganguli et al., 1999). However, their intake of both potassium and calcium is lower (Langford & Watson, 1990), they have more unprovoked hypokalemia (Andrew et al., 2002), and lower urinary potassium excretion apparently more than attributable to their lower intake of potassium (Turban et al., 2008).

Responsiveness to Growth Factors

Dustan (1995) attempted to explain the increased prevalence of severe hypertension in blacks by hypothesizing an increased responsiveness to vascular growth factors comparable to that noted in fibroblasts that form keloids, which are more common in blacks.

Complications of Hypertension

Hypertension is not only more common in blacks, but is also more severe, less well managed and, therefore, more deadly. As best as can be ascertained, blacks at any given level of BP do not suffer more vascular damage than do nonblacks; rather, they display a shift to the right of the BP distribution, yielding a higher overall prevalence and a higher proportion of severe disease (Cooper & Liao, 1996). The only apparent exception is the much higher rate of ESRD in blacks as described under "Renal Disease" earlier in this chapter.

Other Ethnic Groups

Much less is known about the special characteristics of other ethnic groups as compared to blacks in the United States, so only a few generalizations will be made about them.

TABLE 4.5	Features of Hypertension in Blacks

Genotype

Angiotensinogen (Cooper et al., 1999)
Epithelial sodium channel (Pratt et al., 2002)
G protein β_3-subunit (Dong et al., 1999)
Transforming growth factor-β_1 (Suthanthiran et al., 2000)

Intermediate Phenotype

Activation of intrarenal-renin system (Price et al., 2002)
Decreased kallikrein excretion (Song et al., 2000)
Decreased nitric oxide–dependent and nitric oxide–independent vasodilation (Campia et al., 2004)
Decreased potassium intake (Morris et al., 1999)
Diabetes mellitus (Brancati et al., 2000)
Glomerular hyperfiltration (Aviv et al., 2004a)
Increased adrenergic vasoconstriction (Abate et al., 2001)
Increased circulating endothelin-1 (Campia et al., 2004)
Decreased stress-induced pressure natriuresis (Harshfield et al., 2002b)
Increased sodium sensitivity (Aviv et al., 2004b)
Increased retention of sodium load (Palacios et al., 2004)
Obesity (Jones, 1999)
Sodium-induced renal vasoconstriction (Schmidlin et al., 1999)
Lesser fall in nocturnal BP (Hinderliter et al., 2004)

Phenotype

Aortic stiffness (Chaturvedi et al., 2004)
CHF (Dries et al., 1999)
LVH (Kizer et al., 2004)
Left ventricular systolic dysfunction (Devereux et al., 2001)
Microalbuminuria (Aviv et al., 2004a)
Nephrosclerosis (Toto, 2003)
Stroke (Gillum, 1996)

Primitive Versus Industrialized Environment

People of any race living a rural, more primitive lifestyle tend to ingest less sodium, remain less obese, and have less hypertension. When they migrate into urban areas and adapt more modern lifestyles, they ingest more sodium, gain weight, and develop more hypertension (Cooper et al., 1999). Rather dramatic changes in the prevalence of hypertension and the nature of cardiovascular complications have been seen when formerly isolated ethnic groups move to an industrialized environment, as seen among South Asians who move to England (Khattar et al., 2000).

Persistence of Ethnic Differences

Although environmental changes often alter BP and other cardiovascular traits, some ethnic groups preserve characteristics that presumably reflect stronger genetic influences. Examples include Bedouins in Israel (Paran et al., 1992) and Native Americans in the United States (Howard, 1996). In the United States, Hispanics, particularly Mexican-Americans, have a lesser prevalence of hypertension, despite their high prevalence of obesity, diabetes, and insulin resistance (Aranda et al., 2008). These factors contribute to the proportionately higher rate of CVDs in Mexican Americans, particularly strokes (Lisabeth et al., 2008).

Diabetes and Hypertension

The combination of diabetes and hypertension poses a major public health challenge, leading to the recommendation that all adults with BP greater than 135/80 mm Hg be screened for diabetes (U.S. Preventive Services Task Force, 2008).

- The incidence of type 2 diabetes is rapidly increasing with a lifetime risk in the United States now estimated to be 33% for men and 39% for women (Narayan et al., 2003).
- 71% of U.S. adult diabetics have hypertension (Geiss et al., 2002) and a significant number of hypertensives have unrecognized diabetes (Salmasi et al., 2004).
- Coexisting diabetes and hypertension are associated with greater degrees of arterial stiffness (Tedesco et al., 2004) leading to earlier rises in systolic and pulse pressures (Ronnback et al., 2004), the pattern of accelerated arterial aging.
- The presence of diabetes, either type 1 (Knerr et al., 2008) or type 2 (Mazzone et al., 2008), increases the rate of atherosclerotic CVDs, including stroke (Air & Kissela, 2007).
- Even with effective antihypertensive therapy, resistance arteries from diabetic hypertensives have persistently marked remodeling (Endermann et al., 2004).
- The microvascular complications of diabetes are also accelerated by hypertension, retinopathy in particular (Gallego et al., 2008).

As will be noted in Chapters 5 and 7, these high risks mandate earlier and more intensive therapy in hypertensives with diabetes.

Obesity and Hypertension

Even in the absence of type 2 diabetes, obesity is one of the most common factors responsible for hypertension (Schlaich et al., 2009). In the National Health and Nutrition Examination Survey III, a progressive increase in the prevalence of hypertension was seen

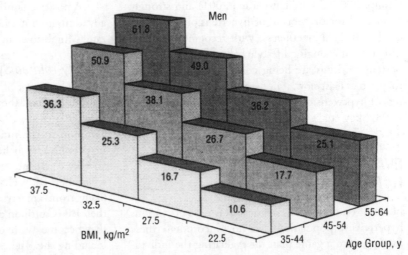

FIGURE 4-8 Estimated risk (%) of hypertension by age group and body mass index (BMI) among men in the National Health and Nutrition Examination Survey III. (Modified from Thompson D, Edelsberg J, Colditz GA, et al. Lifetime health and economic consequences of obesity. *Arch Intern Med* 1999;159: 2177–2183.)

with increasing BMI at all ages (Thompson et al., 1999) (Fig. 4-8). The prevalence is increased further when obesity is predominantly abdominal (Allemann et al., 2001). The presence of sleep apnea further increases the risk for stroke (Valham et al., 2008). In the elderly with CKD, the cardiovascular risks of obesity diminish, but abdominal obesity remains a risk factor for cardiovascular events (Elsayed et al., 2008).

ALTERING THE NATURAL HISTORY

Now that the possible mechanisms, natural history, major consequences, and special populations of untreated primary hypertension have been covered, an additional word about prevention is in order.

Most efforts to alter the natural history of hypertension involve both nondrug and drug therapies of existing disease. However, attempts to *prevent* hypertension must also be more widely promoted and followed. Without knowledge of the specific causes of this disease, no single preventive measure can be promoted with the assurance that it will work. However, to insist that specific causes be known before prevention is attempted is akin to saying that John Snow should not have closed the pump because he had no proof that *Vibrio cholera* organisms were the cause of death in those who drank the polluted water. The preventive measures likely to help—moderation in sodium intake, reduction of obesity, maintenance of physical conditioning, avoidance of stress, and greater attention to the other coexisting risk factors for premature CVD—will do no harm and may do a great deal of good.

Their value has been proved for prevention of diabetes (Diabetes Prevention Program Research Group, 2002; Tuomilehto et al., 2001) and strongly supported for prevention of hypertension (Whelton et al., 2002). Nonetheless, with recognition of the difficulty of changing lifestyle habits, trials of antihypertensive drugs are being conducted to prove that they can at least slow, if not stop, the inexorable progress of hypertension (Julius et al., 2006; Luders et al., 2008; Skov et al., 2007).

EVALUATION OF THE HYPERTENSIVE PATIENT

Having examined the natural history of various hypertensive populations, we now incorporate these findings into a game plan for evaluating the individual hypertensive patient.

There are three main reasons to evaluate patients with hypertension: (a) to determine the type of hypertension, specifically looking for identifiable causes; (b) to assess the impact of the hypertension on target organs; and (c) to estimate a patient's overall risk profile for the development of premature CVD. Such evaluation can be accomplished with relative ease and should be part of the initial examination of every newly discovered hypertensive. The younger the patient and the higher the BP, the more intensive the search for identifiable causes should be. Among middle-aged and older persons, greater attention should be directed to the overall cardiovascular risk profile, as these populations are more susceptible than others to immediate catastrophe unless preventive measures are taken.

History

The patient history should focus on the duration of the elevated BP and any prior treatment, the current use of various drugs that may cause it to rise, and symptoms of target organ dysfunction (Table 4-6). Attention should also be directed toward the patient's psychosocial status, looking for such information as the degree of knowledge about hypertension, the willingness to make necessary changes in lifestyle and to take medication, and the ability to obtain sometimes expensive therapies. An area of great importance is sexual dysfunction, often neglected until it arises after antihypertensive therapy is given. Erectile dysfunction, often attributed to antihypertensive drugs, may be present in as many as one third of untreated hypertensive men and is most likely related to their underlying vascular disease (see Chapter 7).

A positive family history of hypertension is usually accurate but a negative report is only 33% accurate (Murabito et al., 2003).

Anxiety-related Symptoms

Although many, if not most, hypertensives have symptoms that they ascribe to their elevated BP (Kjellgren et al., 1998), most of these symptoms are common to the functional somatic syndromes seen in people who believe they have a serious disease (Barsky & Borus, 1999). Many believe they can tell when their BP is elevated but, if so, the perception is likely from anxiety which, in turn, may be raising their BP (Cantillon et al., 1997). If questioned before they become aware of being hypertensive, symptoms including headaches, epistaxis, tinnitus, dizziness, and fainting were no more common among those

TABLE 4.6	**Important Aspects of the Patient's History**

Duration of the hypertension	Presence of other risk factors
Last known normal BP	Smoking
Course of the BP	Diabetes
Prior treatment of the hypertension	Dyslipidemia
Drugs: types, doses, side effects	Physical inactivity
Intake of agents that may interfere	Concomitant diseases
Nonsteroidal anti-inflammatory drugs	Dietary history
Oral contraceptives	Weight change
Sympathomimetics	Fresh vs. processed foods
Adrenal steroids	Sodium
Excessive sodium intake	Saturated fats
Alcohol (>2 drinks/day)	Sexual function
Herbal remedies	Features of sleep apnea
Family history	Early morning headaches
Hypertension	Daytime somnolence
Premature CVD or death	Loud snoring
Familial diseases: pheochromocytoma,	Erratic sleep
renal disease, diabetes, gout	
Symptoms of secondary causes	Ability to modify lifestyle and maintain therapy
Muscle weakness	Understanding the nature of hypertension and
Spells of tachycardia, sweating, tremor	the need for regimen
Thinning of the skin	Ability to perform physical activity
Flank pain	Source of food preparation
Symptoms of target organ damage	Financial constraints
Headaches	Ability to read instructions
Transient weakness or blindness	Need for care providers
Loss of visual acuity	
Chest pain	
Dyspnea	
Edema	
Claudication	

with hypertension than among those with normal BP (Weiss, 1972).

Many of the symptoms described by hypertensives are secondary to anxiety over having "the silent killer" (as hypertension frequently is described), anxiety that often is expressed as recurrent acute hyperventilation or panic attacks (Davies et al., 1999; Smoller et al., 2003). Many of the symptoms described by hypertensives, such as bandlike headaches, dizziness and light-headedness, fatigue, palpitations, and chest discomfort, reflect recurrent hyperventilation, a common problem among all patients (DeGuire et al., 1992) but likely even more common among hypertensives who are anxious over their diagnosis and its implications (Kaplan, 1997). Anxiety and panic attacks are even more common among patients who had nonspecific intolerance to multiple antihypertensive drugs (Davies et al., 2003).

The situation is similar for symptoms of depression. Symptoms of depression (and anxiety) were not found to be more common prior to the onset of hypertension (Shinn et al., 2001) but were more common after the diagnosis was made (Scherrer et al., 2003).

Headache

In cross-sectional surveys, headache is among the most common of the symptoms that are reported (Middeke et al., 2008). These headaches had usually been attributed to the psychological stress of having the "silent killer" (Friedman, 2002). However, data from prospective randomized placebo-controlled trials (RCTs) show that the prevalence of headache is often reduced when BP is lowered, irrespective of the drugs used to lower the BP (Law et al., 2005). In this meta-analysis of 94 RCTs involving over 24,000 patients, among those treated to an average 10/5 mm Hg lower BP, headaches were complained about in 8.0% versus 12.4% of those left on placebo. These data strongly implicate hypertension as a reversible cause of headache. It should be noted that sleep apnea is common among even minimally obese hypertensives, as described in Chapter 14, so early morning headaches may reflect not hypertension but nocturnal hypoxia.

Nocturia

Nocturia is more common in hypertensives, often the consequence of coexisting benign prostatic hypertrophy (Blanker et al., 2000) or simply a decreased bladder capacity (Weiss & Blaivas, 2000). At least theoretically, the altered pressure-natriuresis relationship described in Chapter 3 could delay urinary excretion, and a loss of concentrating ability may be an early sign of renal impairment.

Physical Examination

The physical examination should include a careful search for damage to target organs and for features of various identifiable causes (Table 4-7). Waist circumference should be measured, because values exceeding 88 cm (35 in.) in women and 102 cm (40 in.) in men are indicative of abdominal obesity and the metabolic syndrome (Wilson & Grundy, 2003) and serve as a cardiovascular risk factor independent of weight (Malik et al., 2004).

TABLE 4.7	Important Aspects of the Physical Examination

Accurate measurement of BP
General appearance: distribution of body fat, skin lesions, muscle strength, alertness
Funduscopy
Neck: palpation and auscultation of carotids, thyroid
Heart: size, rhythm, sounds
Lungs: rhonchi, rales
Abdomen: renal masses, bruits over aorta or renal arteries, femoral pulses, waist circumference
Extremities: peripheral pulses, edema
Neurologic assessment, including cognitive function

Funduscopic Examination

Only in the optic fundi can small blood vessels be seen with ease, but this requires dilation of the pupil, a procedure that should be more commonly practiced using a short-acting mydriatic such as 1% tropicamide. Such routine funduscopy can portray the major changes of hypertensive retinopathy (Fig. 4-9) (Pache et al., 2002; Wong & Mitchell, 2007). However, accurate recognition of the more subtle early changes that may appear even before hypertension is manifest requires digitized retinal photography (Maestri et al., 2007), now available only in ophthalmology offices but hopefully to become more accessible to all who see hypertensives.

The retinal changes have been most logically classified by Wong and Mitchell (2004) (Table 4-8). The changes progress from the initial arterial narrowing to

TABLE 4.8	Classification of Hypertensive Retinopathy	
Grade of Retinopathy	**Retinal Signs**	**Systemic Associations**
None	No detectable signs	None
Mild	Generalized arteriolar narrowing, focal arteriolar narrowing, arteriovenous nicking, opacity ("copper wiring") of arteriolar wall, or a combination of these signs	Modest association with risk of stroke, CHD, and death
Moderate	Hemorrhage (blot, dot, or flame-shaped), microaneurysm, cotton-wool spot, hard exudate, or a combination of these signs	Strong association with risk of stroke, cognitive decline, and death from cardiovascular causes
Malignant	Signs of moderate retinopathy plus bilateral swelling of the optic disk	Strong association with death

Modified from Wong TY, Mitchell P. Hypertensive retinopathy. *N Engl J Med* 2004;351:2310–2317.

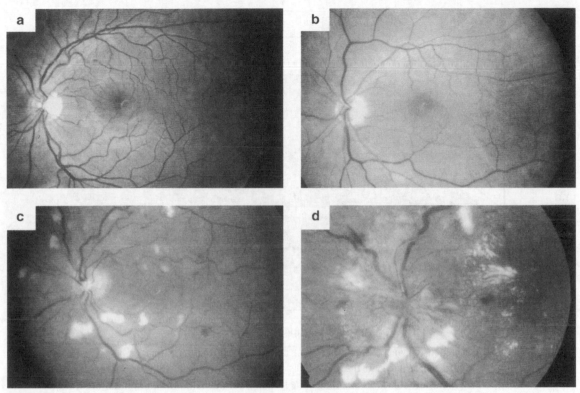

FIGURE 4-9   Retinal photographs of progressively more severe hypertensive retinopathy. *a* and *b* are grade A (nonmalignant), *c* and *d* are Grade B (malignant). (From Pache M, Kube T, Wolf S, et al. Do angiographic data support a detailed classification of hypertensive fundus changes? *J Hum Hypertens* 2002;16:405–410.)

sclerosis and then to exudation, reflected in the features shown in Figure 4-9. As Wong and Mitchell (2007) document, the "mild" changes have been seen even before hypertension is manifest. The striking association of retinal signs with the risk of stroke and the lesser but still significant association with the risk of CHD (Wang et al., 2008) make a careful retinal exam an essential part of the initial evaluation of every hypertensive with follow-up exams as indicated. Unfortunately, along with other parts of the physical exam, many practitioners do not learn or perform funduscopy very adequately.

Laboratory Tests

Routine Laboratory Testing

For most patients, a hematocrit, urine analysis, automated blood chemistry (glucose, creatinine, electrolytes, and calcium), lipid profile (LDL and HDL cholesterol, triglycerides), and a 12-lead electrocardiography are all the routine procedures needed (Task Force, 2007). The blood should be obtained after an overnight fast to improve the diagnostic accuracy of the glucose and triglyceride levels. None of these usually yields abnormal results in the early, uncomplicated phases of primary hypertension, but they should always be obtained for a baseline. The serum creatinine should be used, along with the patient's age, gender, and weight to estimate the GFR using the MDRD formula (Stevens & Levey, 2004).

As will be noted, assessment without blood or urine testing may be all that is practical in low income populations (Montalvo et al., 2008).

Dyslipidemia

Hypertriglyceridemia and, even more threatening, hypercholesterolemia are found more frequently in untreated hypertensives than in normotensives (Ruixing et al., 2009). As shown in Figure 4-10, the prevalence of hypercholesterolemia increases with the BP level and contributes to a marked increase in the incidence of fatal coronary disease (Neaton et al., 1992). Assessment and treatment of dyslipidemia is universally recommended (Cooper & O'Flynn, 2008).

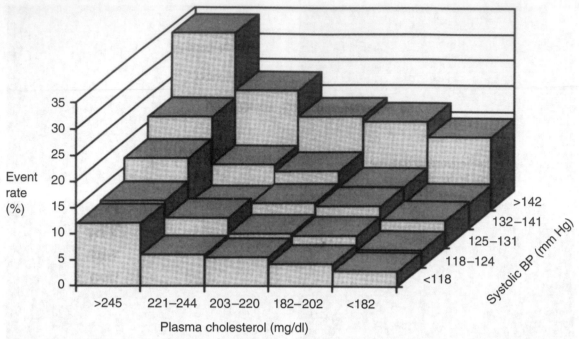

FIGURE 4-10   The associations between systolic BP, plasma cholesterol, and mortality from CHD over an average 12-year follow-up among the 316,099 men screened for the Multiple Risk Factor Intervention Trial (MRFIT). (Data adapted from Neaton JD, Wentworth D. Serum cholesterol, blood pressure, cigarette smoking, and death from coronary heart disease: Overall findings and differences by age for 316,099 white men. *Arch Intern Med* 1992;152:56–64.)

Cost Effectiveness

The performance of these few tests seems to be easily justified. A number of additional tests have been recommended in the 2007 European guidelines (Task Force, 2007). Of these, the quantitative urine albumin test is recommended as a routine test for all hypertensives. However, a cost-effectiveness analysis concluded that it should be restricted to those hypertensives who are also diabetic (Postma et al., 2008).

Similar analyses of other commonly performed laboratory tests show surprisingly high costs for one Quality Adjusted Life Year (QALY) (Boulware et al., 2003). Though these cost-effectiveness analyses are increasingly being performed in an attempt to rationalize and justify testing (as well as the use of drugs, surgical procedures, etc.), the results are often contradictory to common practice and, many would say, common sense. Nonetheless, as health care costs skyrocket, clinicians must be aware of the true costs of what they often do to individual patients at a relatively small cost when these costs are applied to large populations.

Perhaps an even better reason why testing should be limited is the likelihood of false positive results, particularly in a patient with a low likelihood of having the condition being tested for. In such patients, a positive test result would more likely be a false positive rather than a true positive. Therefore, repeat and additional, evermore expensive procedures would need to be done to rule out the diagnosis.

The bottom line is that individual practitioners dealing with individual patients must use testing selectively, recognizing both their hidden costs and their potential for false positive results mandating additional tests. Therefore, the tests that will now be described should be used only if they are known to be cost-effective, providing information needed for improved care of patients. Obviously, some tests such as blood glucose and lipids may be justified because they are needed for overall risk assessment; others for uncovering target organ damage, such as an ECG or an analysis for microalbuminuria. But tests should be reserved for recognition of conditions that can be helped by available therapies.

Nonroutine Laboratory Testing
Microalbuminuria

A measure of urinary albumin excretion is considered an "optional" test in JNC-7, but a routine test in the

2007 European guidelines (Task Force, 2007). As noted earlier in this chapter, microalbuminuria is a clear prognostic indicator for renal and cardiovascular risk and could influence the choice of antihypertensive therapy.

Serum Uric Acid

For many years, elevated uric acid levels have been known to be present in many hypertensives, considered to reflect preexisting renal disease or increased renal urate reabsorption by diuretic therapy. However, largely under the impetus of Richard Johnson, Daniel Feig, and colleagues (Feig et al., 2008a), the presence of hyperuricemia is now considered to be a precursor and possible pathogenetic factor for hypertension. Hyperuricemia has been repeatedly shown to predict the incidence of hypertension (Forman et al., 2009).

Nonetheless, proof of the ability to ameliorate hypertensive by lowering uric acid levels is only now being tested. A glimmer of evidence is now available: the lowering of uric acid by allopurinol was associated with lowering of the BP of 30 adolescent hypertensives (Feig et al., 2008b).

Inflammatory Markers

Assessed mainly by measurement of CRP, inflammation is emerging as a precursor and predictor of CVD, particularly in association with the metabolic syndrome and insulin resistance (Rutter et al., 2004). As with homocysteine, which appears to be a marker of inflammation, measures of CRP do not seem to add to the evaluation or management of hypertensives but they may be helpful in establishing overall cardiovascular risk (Ridker et al., 2005).

Plasma Insulin

There may be value in the addition of a fasting insulin measurement as an indirect way to assess insulin resistance. Higher plasma insulin levels were associated with an increased incidence of hypertension in middle-aged women (Forman et al., 2009). However, for routine clinical practice, the identification of insulin resistance is not necessary.

Plasma Renin Activity

For many years, Laragh (2001) has emphasized the value of ascertaining the plasma renin level coupled with the level of 24-hour urinary sodium excretion, the renin-sodium profile. In various guidelines by expert committees, including JNC-7 (Chobanian et al., 2003) and the European guidelines (Task Force, 2007), this profile is not recommended as part of the routine evaluation of all hypertensives but rather as a diagnostic tool if other features of low-renin states (e.g., primary aldosteronism) or high-renin states (e.g., renovascular disease) are present.

Additional Tests

Additional tests are recommended for selective use in the 2007 European guidelines (Task Force, 2007) including these:

- Echocardiogram
- Carotid ultrasound
- ABI
- Home and 24-hour ambulatory BP monitoring
- Pulse wave velocity

The value of these various tests has been described earlier in this chapter. Of them, only home and ambulatory BP monitoring seems to be needed for most hypertensives, as described in Chapter 2. These and others may be useful to uncover subclinical CVD.

Search for Identifiable Causes

The frequencies of various identifiable causes of hypertension listed in Table 1-5 are quite low in the overall population with mild, asymptomatic hypertension. Nonetheless, clues to the presence of an identifiable cause should be sought in the routine evaluation of every new hypertensive. If suggestive clues are found or if the patient has features of "inappropriate" hypertension (Table 4-9), additional workup for an identifiable cause should be performed.

TABLE 4.9   Features of "Inappropriate" Hypertension

Age of onset: <20 or >50 year
Level of BP: >180/110 mm Hg
Organ damage
    Funduscopy grade II or beyond
    Serum creatinine >1.5 mg/dL
    Cardiomegaly or LVH as determined by electrocardiography
Presence of features indicative of secondary causes
    Unprovoked hypokalemia
    Abdominal bruit
    Variable pressures with tachycardia, sweating, tremor
    Family history of renal disease
Poor response to generally effective therapy

TABLE 4.10	Overall Guide to Workup for Identifiable Causes of Hypertension	
	Diagnostic Procedure	
Diagnosis	*Initial*	*Additional*
Chronic renal disease	Urinalysis; serum creatinine; renal sonography	Isotopic renogram; renal biopsy
Renovascular disease	Captopril-enhanced isotopic renogram; duplex sonography	Magnetic resonance or CT angiogram; aortogram
Coarctation	BP in legs	Echocardiogram; aortogram
Primary aldosteronism	Plasma and urinary potassium; plasma renin and aldosterone	Plasma or urinary aldosterone after saline load; adrenal venous sampling
Cushing syndrome	Morning plasma cortisol after 1 mg dexamethasone at bedtime	Urinary cortisol after variable doses of dexamethasone; adrenal CT scans and scintiscans
Pheochromocytoma	Plasma metanephrine; urine metanephrine	Urinary catechols; plasma catechols (basal and after 0.3 mg clonidine); adrenal CT scans and scintiscans

CT, computed tomography.

The studies listed in Table 4-10 as initial usually will serve as adequate screening procedures and are readily available to every practitioner. If they are abnormal, the listed additional procedures should be performed, perhaps after referral to a hypertension specialist, along with whatever other tests are needed to confirm the diagnosis. More detail about these procedures is provided in their respective chapters.

Assessment of Overall Cardiovascular Risk

Once the cause and consequences of the hypertension have been evaluated, it is necessary to assess the patient's overall cardiovascular risk status. The proper management of hypertension should involve attention to all of the risk factors that can be altered. Patients at high risk should be counseled and helped to reduce all of their risk factors. For many patients, the BP may be the easiest of the risks to control, so this may be the first priority. As described more fully in the next chapter, the overall risk profile provides a more rational basis than an arbitrary BP level for determining whether and when to start treatment and the goal of therapy. For now, the need for a complete assessment of cardiovascular risk—a simple and inexpensive undertaking—should be obvious for the proper management of all hypertensives. However, no randomized evidence has documented changes in

care or improvement in outcomes using these risk predictions (Scott, 2009).

The Framingham Formula

Most assessments are based on data from the Framingham Heart Study, the longest and most complete follow-up of a carefully studied, large population (D'Agostino et al., 2008). The latest profiles have incorporated risks for CHD, cerebrovascular disease, PVD and heart failure. From a longer list of known risk factors, the Framingham data have used those shown in Table 4-11, which converts gradations in the various risk factors into points for women. Separate tables are provided for men. These points then are used to establish the absolute 10-year risk (Table 4-12). Although age overwhelms all else in increasing risk, the other factors are modifiable and therefore demand attention.

In view of the known difficulty of obtaining blood for analyses of lipids (Montalvo et al., 2008), the 2008 model includes risk assessments based on only age, BMI, log of systolic BP treated or not treated, smoking, and history of diabetes (D'Agostino et al., 2008).

Other Formulas

Although the Framingham data have been widely used, the British have found them to underestimate risk in women of South Asian origin (Hippisley-Cox

| TABLE 4.11 | CVD Points for Women | | | | | | |

Points	Age, year	HDL	Total Cholesterol	SBP Not Treated	SBP Treated	Smoker	Diabetic
–3		60+		>120	<120		
–2		50–59					
–1							
0	30–34	45–49	<160	120–129	120–129	No	No
1	35–39	35–44	160–199	130–139			
2		<35		140–149			
3	40–44		200–239	150–159	130–139	Yes	Yes
4	45–49		240–279	160+	140–149		
5			280+				
6	50–54				150–159		
7	55–59				160+		
8							
9	60–64						
10	65–69						
11	70–74						
12	75+						
Points alloted							

SBP, systolic blood pressure.
Reprinted from D'Agostino RB Sr, Vasan RS, Pencina MJ, et al. General cardiovascular risk profile for use in primary care:
The Framingham Heart Study. *Circulation* 2008;117:743–753, with permission.

et al., 2008), Therefore, they have proposed another risk algorithm based on data from two million patients, which includes these additional variables: ethnicity, family history of coronary disease in first degree relative under 60 years of age, a deprivation score, rheumatoid arthritis, CKD, and atrial fibrillation. The name given to this algorithm is QRISK2.

One problem with both the Framingham and U.K. formulas is the importance given to age. As stated by Christiaens (2008):

> Age is such an important risk factor for developing cardiovascular problems within the next 10 years that all risk tables are misleading. Becoming older is by far the strongest predictor for morbidity and mortality—this is a biological fact. By looking at the risk tables, anyone can see what happens: by age 65, a large group has reached the 20% risk threshold, and lipid lowering drugs are prescribed for the rest of their lives.

> A better way of using risk tables would be to compare the risk of an individual with the minimal risk of people of the same sex and age. Treatment should be considered when he or she has, for example, three times that minimal risk for his or her age and sex. This will prevent overtreatment of elderly people whose high risk is related to age and undertreatment of younger people who are at high risk.

Other Risk Factors

As counted by Scott (2009), at least 28 other disease markers have been suggested for inclusion in risk assessments. Folsom et al. (2006) assessed the association of 19 of these new risk markers with the incidence of CHD in 15,792 adults followed for 24 years and found none of them to be useful for risk assessment.

However, others have found one or more of these new markers to be useful for assessment of cardiovascular risk. These include

- Increased pulse pressure (Thomas et al., 2008)
- Hemoglobin A1C (Simmons et al., 2008)
- Homocysteine (de Ruijter et al., 2009)
- The combination of troponin 1, N-terminal pro-brain natriuretic peptide, cystatin C, and CRP (Zethelius et al., 2008)

The greater accuracy of the Zethelius et al. (2008) data may reflect their restriction of their study to lean white men of the same age at study entry. As de Lemos and Lloyd-Jones (2008) note: "This restriction mitigates the powerful influence of age in the established risk factor model."

For now, the revised Framingham formula seems most appropriate for use in the United States and will

TABLE 4.12	CVD Risk for Women
Points	**Risk**
≤−2	<1
−1	1.0
0	1.2
1	1.5
2	1.7
3	2.0
4	2.4
5	2.8
6	3.3
7	3.9
8	4.5
9	5.3
10	6.3
11	7.3
12	8.6
13	10.0
14	11.7
15	13.7
16	15.9
17	18.5
18	21.5
19	24.8
20	28.5
21+	>30

be the basis for the decision to start drug therapy in the next chapter. Patients need to be advised in a clear, understandable manner about their own risk status, both to motivate them to take necessary lifestyle changes and medications and to bring them into the decision-making process, providing them with greater autonomy. As Christiaens (2008) notes: "Estimating risk is not the problem; using it to tailor treatment to individuals is."

With the natural history in mind, we now turn to issues as to why, when, and how much therapies are needed for the appropriate management of hypertension.

REFERENCES

Abate NI, Mansour YH, Tuncel M, et al. Overweight and sympathetic overactivity in Black Americans. *Hypertension* 2001;37:379–383.

Agmon Y, Khandheria BK, Meissner I, et al. Independent association of high blood pressure and aortic atherosclerosis. *Circulation* 2000;102:2087–2093.

Air EL, Kissela BM. Diabetes, the metabolic syndrome, and ischemic stroke: Epidemiology and possible mechanisms. *Diabetes Care* 2007;30:3131–3140.

Akinboboye OO, Chou R-L, Bergmann SR. Myocardial blood flow and efficiency in concentric and eccentric left ventricular hypertrophy. *Am J Hypertens* 2004;17:433–438.

Alfakih K, Maqbool A, Sivananthan M, et al. Left ventricle mass index and the common, functional, X-linked angiotensin II type-2 receptor gene polymorphism (-1332 G/A) in patients with systemic hypertension. *Hypertension* 2004;43:1189–1194.

Allemann Y, Hutter D, Aeschbacher BC, et al. Increased central body fat deposition precedes a significant rise in resting blood pressure in male offspring of essential hypertensive patients: A 5 year follow-up study. *J Hypertens* 2001;19:2143–2148.

Andrew ME, Jones DW, Wofford MR, et al. Ethnicity and unprovoked hypokalemia in the Atherosclerosis Risk in Communities Study. *Am J Hypertens* 2002;15:594–599.

Ang D, Lang C. The prognostic value of the ECG in hypertension: Where are we now? *J Hum Hypertens* 2008;22:460–467.

Ankle Brachial Index Collaboration. Ankle brachial index combined with Framingham Risk Score to predict cardiovascular events and mortality: A meta-analysis. *JAMA* 2008;300:197–208.

Antonini-Canterin F, Huang G, Cervesato E, et al. Symptomatic aortic stenosis: Does systemic hypertension play an additional role? *Hypertension* 2003;41:1268–1272.

Appel LJ, Wright JT Jr, Greene T, et al. Long-term effects of renin-angiotensin system-blocking therapy and a low blood pressure goal on progression of hypertensive chronic kidney disease in African Americans. *Arch Intern Med* 2008;168:832–839.

Applegate WB, Davis BR, Black RH, et al. Prevalence of postural hypotension at baseline in the Systolic Hypertension in the Elderly Program (SHEP) cohort. *J Am Geriatr Soc* 1991;39:1057–1065.

Arain FA, Cooper LT Jr. Peripheral arterial disease: Diagnosis and management. *Mayo Clin Proc* 2008;83:944–949.

Aranda JM Jr, Calderon R, Aranda JM Sr. Clinical characteristics and outcomes in hypertensive patients of Hispanic descent. *Prev Cardiol* 2008;11:116–120.

Aurigemma GP, Gaasch WH. Diastolic heart failure. *N Engl J Med* 2004;351:1097–1105.

Aviv A, Hollenberg NK, Weder AB. Sodium glomerulopathy: Tubuloglomerular feedback and renal injury in African Americans. *Kidney Int* 2004a;65:361–368.

Aviv A, Hollenberg N, Weder A. Urinary potassium excretion and sodium sensitivity in blacks. *Hypertension* 2004b;43:707–713.

Aylward PE, Wilcox RG, Horgan JH, et al. Relation of increased arterial blood pressure to mortality and stroke in the context of contemporary thrombolytic therapy for acute myocardial infarction. *Ann Intern Med* 1996;125:891–900.

Barsky AJ, Borus JF. Functional somatic syndromes. *Ann Intern Med* 1999;130:910–921.

Bavikati VV, Sperling LS, Salmon RD, et al. Effect of comprehensive therapeutic lifestyle changes on prehypertension. *Am J Cardiol* 2008;102:1677–1680.

Bechgaard P. A 40 years' follow-up study of 1000 untreated hypertensive patients. *Clin Sci Mol Med Suppl* 1976;3:673S–675S.

Bejot Y, Catteau A, Caillier M, et al. Trends in incidence, risk factors, and survival in symptomatic lacunar stroke in Dijon, France, from 1989 to 2006: A population-based study. *Stroke* 2008;39:1945–1951.

Berenson GS, Srinivasan SR, Bao W, et al. Association between multiple cardiovascular risk factors and atherosclerosis in children and young adults. *N Engl J Med* 1998;338:1650–1656.

Bidani AK, Griffin KA. Pathophysiology of hypertensive renal damage: Implications for therapy. *Hypertension* 2004;44:595–601.

Birns J, Kalra L. Cognitive function and hypertension. *J Hum Hypertens* 2009;23:86–96.

Blanker MH, Bohnen AM, Groeneveld FPMJ, et al. Normal voiding patterns and determinants of increased diurnal and nocturnal voiding frequency in elderly men. *J Urol* 2000;164:1201–1205.

Bo E, Gambino P, Gentile L, et al. High-normal blood pressure is associated with a cluster of cardiovascular and metabolic risk factors: A population-based study. *J Hypertens* 2009;27:102–108.

Boon D, van Goudoever J, Piek JJ, et al. ST segment depression criteria and the prevalence of silent cardiac ischemia in hypertensives. *Hypertension* 2003;41:476–481.

Boulware LE, Jaar BG, Tarver-Carr ME, et al. Screening for proteinuria in US adults: A cost-effectiveness analysis. *JAMA* 2003;290:3101–3114.

Brancati FL, Kao WHL, Folson AR, et al. Incident type 2 diabetes mellitus in African American and white adults. *JAMA* 2000;283:2253–2259.

Brantsma AH, Bakker SJ, de ZD, et al. Urinary albumin excretion as a predictor of the development of hypertension in the general population. *J Am Soc Nephrol* 2006;17:331–335.

Buck C, Baker P, Bass M, et al. The prognosis of hypertension according to age at onset. *Hypertension* 1987;9:204–208.

Bursi F, Weston SA, Redfield MM, et al. Systolic and diastolic heart failure in the community. *JAMA* 2006;296:2209–2216.

Campia U, Cardillo C, Panza JA. Ethnic differences in the vasoconstrictor activity of endogenous endothelin-1 in hypertensive patients. *Circulation* 2004;109:3191–3195.

Cantillon P, Morgan M, Dundas R, et al. Patients' perceptions of changes in their blood pressure. *J Hum Hypertens* 1997;11:221–225.

Carrington M. Prehypertension causes a mounting problem of harmful cardiovascular disease risk in young adults. *J Hypertens* 2009;27:214–215.

Chaturvedi N, Bulpitt CJ, Leggetter S, et al. Ethnic differences in vascular stiffness and relations to hypertensive target organ damage. *J Hypertens* 2004;22:1731–1737.

Chobanian AV, Bakris GL, Black HR, et al. Seventh report of the Joint National Committee on Prevention, Detection, Evaluation, and Treatment of High Blood Pressure. *Hypertension* 2003;42:1206–1252.

Christiaens T. Cardiovascular risk tables. *Br Med J* 2008;336:1445–1446.

Cirillo M, Lanti MP, Menotti A, et al. Definition of kidney dysfunction as a cardiovascular risk factor: Use of urinary albumin excretion and estimated glomerular filtration rate. *Arch Intern Med* 2008;168:617–624.

Cooper A, O'Flynn N. Risk assessment and lipid modification for primary and secondary prevention of cardiovascular disease: Summary of NICE guidance. *Br Med J* 2008;336:1246–1248.

Cooper RS, Liao Y, Rotimi C. Is hypertension more severe among U.S. blacks, or is severe hypertension more common? *Ann Epidemiol* 1996;6:173–180.

Cooper RS, Rotimmi CN, Ward R. The puzzle of hypertension in African-Americans. *Sci Am* 1999;Feb:56–63.

Curtis LH, Greiner MA, Hammill BG, et al. Early and long-term outcomes of heart failure in elderly persons, 2001–2005. *Arch Intern Med* 2008;168:2481–2488.

Cuspidi C, Valerio C, Sala C, et al. The Hyper-Pract Study: A multicentre survey on the accuracy of the echocardiographic assessment of hypertensive left ventricular hypertrophy in clinical practice. *Blood Press* 2008;17:124–128.

D'Agostino RB Sr, Vasan RS, Pencina MJ, et al. General cardiovascular risk profile for use in primary care: The Framingham Heart Study. *Circulation* 2008;117:743–753.

Daffertshofer M, Mielke O, Pullwitt A, et al. Transient ischemic attacks are more than "ministrokes." *Stroke* 2004;35:2453–2458.

Danziger J. Importance of low-grade albuminuria. *Mayo Clin Proc* 2008;83:806–812.

Davies AA, Smith GD, May MT, et al. Association between birth weight and blood pressure is robust, amplifies with age, and may be underestimated. *Hypertension* 2006;48:431–436.

Davies SJC, Ghahramani P, Jackson PR, et al. Association of panic disorder and panic attacks with hypertension. *Am J Med* 1999;107:310–316.

Davies SJC, Jackson PR, Ramsay LE, et al. Drug intolerance due to nonspecific adverse effects related to psychiatric morbidity in hypertensive patients. *Arch Intern Med* 2003;163:592–600.

de Lemos JA, Lloyd-Jones DM. Multiple biomarker panels for cardiovascular risk assessment. *N Engl J Med* 2008;358:2172–2174.

de Ruijter W, Westendorp RG, Assendelft WJ, et al. Use of Framingham risk score and new biomarkers to predict cardiovascular mortality in older people: Population based observational cohort study. *Br Med J* 2009;338:a3083.

de Simone G, Kitzman DW, Palmieri V, et al. Association of inappropriate left ventricular mass with systolic and diastolic dysfunction. *Am J Hypertens* 2004;17:828–833.

de Simone G, Pasanisi F, Contraldo F. Link of nonhemodynamic factors to hemodynamic determinants of left ventricular hypertrophy. *Hypertension* 2001;38:13–18.

de Simone G, Roman MJ, Alderman MH, et al. Is high pulse pressure a marker of preclinical cardiovascular disease? *Hypertension* 2005;45:575–579.

DeGuire S, Gevirty R, Kawahara Y, et al. Hyperventilation syndrome and the assessment of treatment for functional cardiac symptoms. *Am J Cardiol* 1992;70:673–677.

Delles C. Risk factors and target organ damage: Is there a special case for prehypertension? *J Hypertens* 2008;26:2268–2270.

Devereux RB, Bella JN, Palmieri V, et al. Left ventricular systolic dysfunction in a biracial sample of hypertensive adults. *Hypertension* 2001;38:417–423.

Diabetes Prevention Program Research Group. Reduction in the incidence of type 2 diabetes with lifestyle intervention or metformin. *N Engl J Med* 2002;346:393–403.

Dong Y, Zhu H, Sagnella GA, et al. Association between the C825T polymorphism of the G protein β3-subunit gene and hypertension in blacks. *Hypertension* 1999;34:1193–1196.

Donnan GA, Fisher M, Macleod M, et al. Stroke. *Lancet* 2008;371:1612–1623.

Dries DL, Exner DV, Gersh BJ, et al. Racial differences in the outcome of left ventricular dysfunction. *N Engl J Med* 1999;340:609–616.

Dustan HP. Does keloid pathogenesis hold the key to understanding black/white differences in hypertension severity? *Hypertension* 1995;26:858–862.

Earnshaw JJ, Shaw E, Whyman WR, et al. Screening for abdominal aortic aneurysms in men. *Br Med J* 2004;328:1122–1124.

Ejaz AA, Haley WE, Wasiluk A, et al. Characteristics of 100 consecutive patients presenting with orthostatic hypotension. *Mayo Clin Proc* 2004;79:890–894.

Elliott WJ, Black HR. Prehypertension. *Nat Clin Pract Cardiovasc Med* 2007;4:538–548.

Elsayed EF, Tighiouart H, Weiner DE, et al. Waist-to-hip ratio and body mass index as risk factors for cardiovascular events in CKD. *Am J Kidney Dis* 2008;52:49–57.

Endermann DH, Pu Q, De Ciuceis C, et al. Persistent remodeling of resistance arteries in type 2 diabetic patients on antihypertensive treatment. *Hypertension* 2004;43(Part 2):399–404.

Erdogan D, Yildirim I, Ciftci O, et al. Effects of normal blood pressure, prehypertension, and hypertension on coronary microvascular function. *Circulation* 2007;115:593–599.

Farbom P, Wahlstrand B, Almgren P, et al. Interaction between renal function and microalbuminuria for cardiovascular risk in hypertension: The nordic diltiazem study. *Hypertension* 2008;52:115–122.

Faxon DP, Creager MA, Smith SC Jr, et al. Atherosclerotic Vascular Disease Conference: Executive summary. *Circulation* 2004;109: 2595–2604.

Feig DI, Kang DH, Johnson RJ. Uric acid and cardiovascular risk. *N Engl J Med* 2008a; 359:1811–1821.

Feig DI, Soletsky B, Johnson RJ. Effect of allopurinol on blood pressure of adolescents with newly diagnosed essential hypertension: A randomized trial. *JAMA* 2008b;300:924–932.

Flemming KD, Brown RD Jr, Petty GW, et al. Evaluation and management of transient ischemic attack and minor cerebral infarction. *Mayo Clin Proc* 2004;79:1071–1086.

Folsom AR, Chambless LE, Ballantyne CM, et al. An assessment of incremental coronary risk prediction using C-reactive protein and other novel risk markers: The atherosclerosis risk in communities study. *Arch Intern Med* 2006;166:1368–1373.

Fommei E, Ghione S, Ripoli A, et al. The ovarian cycle as a factor of variability in the laboratory screening for primary aldosteronism in women. *J Hum Hypertens* 2009;23:130–135.

Forman JP, Choi H, Curhan GC. Uric acid and insulin sensitivity and risk of incident hypertension. *Arch Intern Med* 2009;169: 155–162.

Forman JP, Fisher ND, Schopick EL, et al. Higher levels of albuminuria within the normal range predict incident hypertension. *J Am Soc Nephrol* 2008;19:1983–1988.

Fotherby MD, Potter JF. Reproducibility of ambulatory and clinic blood pressure measurements in elderly hypertensive subjects. *J Hypertens* 1993;11:573–579.

Franklin SS, Gustin W IV, Wong ND, et al. Hemodynamic patterns of age-related changes in blood pressure: The Framingham Heart Study. *Circulation* 1997;96:308–315.

Franklin SS, Jacobs MJ, Wong ND, et al. Predominance of isolated systolic hypertension among middle-aged and elderly US hypertensives. *Hypertension* 2001;37:869–874.

Franklin SS, Pio JR, Wong ND, et al. Predictors of new-onset diastolic and systolic hypertension: The Framingham Heart Study. *Circulation* 2005;111:1121–1127.

Freedman BI, Sedor JR. Hypertension-associated kidney disease: Perhaps no more. *J Am Soc Nephrol* 2008;19:2047–2051.

Friedman D. Headache and hypertension: Refuting the myth. *J Neurol Neurosurg Psychiatry* 2002;72:431.

Gallego PH, Craig ME, Hing S, et al. Role of blood pressure in development of early retinopathy in adolescents with type 1 diabetes: Prospective cohort study. *Br Med J* 2008;337:a918.

Ganguli MC, Grimm RH Jr, Svendsen KH, et al. Urinary sodium and potassium profile of blacks and whites in relation to education in two different geographic urban areas. *Am J Hypertens* 1999;12:69–72.

Gast GC, Grobbee DE, Pop VJ, et al. Menopausal complaints are associated with cardiovascular risk factors. *Hypertension* 2008; 51:1492–1498.

Geiss LS, Rolka DB, Engelgau MM. Elevated blood pressure among U.S. adults with diabetes, 1988–1994. *Am J Prev Med* 2002; 22:42–48.

Gerdts E, Cramariuc D, de SG, et al. Impact of left ventricular geometry on prognosis in hypertensive patients with left ventricular hypertrophy (the LIFE study). *Eur J Echocardiogr* 2008;9:809–815.

Gheorghiade M, Abraham WT, Albert NM, et al. Systolic blood pressure at admission, clinical characteristics, and outcomes in patients hospitalized with acute heart failure. *JAMA* 2006;296: 2217–2226.

Gillum RF. The epidemiology of cardiovascular disease in black Americans. *N Engl J Med* 1996;335:1597–1599.

Golledge J, Eagle KA. Acute aortic dissection. *Lancet* 2008;372: 55–66.

Gorelick PB. Stroke prevention therapy beyond antithrombotics: Unifying mechanisms in ischemic stroke pathogenesis and implications for therapy: An invited review. *Stroke* 2002; 33:862–875.

Grassi G, Seravalle G, Bertinieri G, et al. Sympathetic and reflex alterations in systo-diastolic and systolic hypertension in the elderly. *J Hypertens* 2000;18:587–593.

Haas DC, Gerber LM, Schwartz JE D, et al. A comparison of morning blood pressure surge in African-Americans and whites. *J Clin Hypertens* 2005;7:205–209.

Hallan S, Astor B, Romundstad S, et al. Association of kidney function and albuminuria with cardiovascular mortality in older vs younger individuals: The HUNT II Study. *Arch Intern Med* 2007;167:2490–2496.

Hallock P, Benson IC. Studies of the elastic properties of human isolated aorta. *J Clin Invest* 1937;16:595–602.

Harshfield GA, Treiber FA, Wilson ME, et al. A longitudinal study of ethnic differences in ambulatory blood pressure patterns in youth. *Am J Hypertens* 2002a;15:525–530.

Harshfield GA, Wilson ME, Hanevold C, et al. Impaired stress-induced pressure natriuresis increases cardiovascular load in African American youths. *Am J Hypertens* 2002b;15:903–906.

He J, Klag MJ, Appel LJ, et al. Seven-year incidence of hypertension in a cohort of middle-aged African Americans and whites. *Hypertension* 1998;31:1130–1135.

Henskens LH, van Oostenbrugge RJ, Kroon AA, et al. Brain microbleeds are associated with ambulatory blood pressure levels in a hypertensive population. *Hypertension* 2008;51:62–68.

Herrington DM, Brown V, Mosca L, et al. Relationship between arterial stiffness and subclinical aortic atherosclerosis. *Circulation* 2004;110:432–437.

Hinderliter AL, Blumenthal JA, Waugh R, et al. Ethnic differences in left ventricular structure: Relations to hemodynamics and diurnal blood pressure variation. *Am J Hypertens* 2004;17: 43-49.

Hippisley-Cox J, Coupland C, Vinogradova Y, et al. Predicting cardiovascular risk in England and Wales: Prospective derivation and validation of QRISK2. *Br Med J* 2008;336:1475–1482.

Howard BV. Blood pressure in 13 American Indian communities. *Public Health Rep* 1996;111:47–48.

Hsu CC, Brancati FL, Astor BC, et al. Blood pressure, atherosclerosis, and albuminuria in 10,113 participants in the atherosclerosis risk in communities study. *J Hypertens* 2009;27:397–409.

Ibsen H, Olsen MH, Wachtell K, et al. Reduction in albuminuria translates to reduction in cardiovascular events in hypertensive patients: Losartan Intervention for Endpoint Reduction in Hypertension study. *Hypertension* 2005;45:198–202.

Ishikawa J, Ishikawa K, Kabutoya T, et al. Cornell product left ventricular hypertrophy in electrocardiogram and the risk of stroke in a general population. *Hypertens* 2009;53:28–34.

James SA. John Henryism and the health of African-Americans. *Cult Med Psychiatry* 1994;18:163–182.

Jha AK, Varosy PD, Kanaya AM, et al. Differences in medical care and disease outcomes among black and white women with heart disease. *Circulation* 2003;108:1089–1094.

Jones DW. What is the role of obesity in hypertension and target organ injury in African Americans? *Am J Med Sci* 1999;317:147–151.

Jones PP, Christou DD, Jordan J, et al. Baroreflex buffering is reduced with age in healthy men. *Circulation* 2003;107:1770–1774.

Hinderliter AL, Blumenthal JA, Waugh R, et al. Ethnic differences in left ventricular structure: Relations to hemodynamics and diurnal blood pressure variation. Am J Hypertens 2004;17:43-49.

Julius S, Nesbitt SD, Egan BM, et al. Feasibility of treating prehypertension with an angiotensin-receptor blocker. *N Engl J Med* 2006;354:1685–1697.

Kaden JJ, Haghi D. Hypertension in aortic valve stenosis—a Trojan horse. *Eur Heart J* 2008;29:1934–1935.

Kannel WB. Blood pressure as a cardiovascular risk factor. *JAMA* 1996;275:1571–1576.

Kannel WB, D'Agostino RB, Silbershatz H. Blood pressure and cardiovascular morbidity and mortality rates in the elderly. *Am Heart J* 1997;134:758–763.

Kannel WB, Dannenberg AL, Abbott RD. Unrecognized myocardial infarction and hypertension. *Am Heart J* 1985;109: 581–585.

Kao WH, Klag MJ, Meoni LA, et al. MYH9 is associated with nondiabetic end-stage renal disease in African Americans. *Nat Genet* 2008;40:1185–1192.

Kaplan NM. Anxiety-induced hyperventilation. *Arch Intern Med* 1997;157:945–948.

Kario K, Ishikawa J, Eguchi K, et al. Sleep pulse pressure and awake mean pressure as independent predictors for stroke in older hypertensive patients. *Am J Hypertens* 2004;17:439–445.

Kawecka-Jaszcz K, Czarnecka D, Olszanecka A, et al. Myocardial perfusion in hypertensive patients with normal coronary angiograms. *J Hypertens* 2008;26:1686–1694.

Kenchaiah S, David BR, Braunwald E, et al. Antecedent hypertension and the effect of captopril on the risk of adverse cardiovascular outcomes after acute myocardial infarction with left ventricular systolic dysfunction: Insights from the Survival and Ventricular Enlargement trial. *Am Heart J* 2004;148:356–364.

Kestenbaum B, Rudser KD, de Boer IH, et al. Differences in kidney function and incident hypertension: The multi-ethnic study of atherosclerosis. *Ann Intern Med* 2008;148:501–508.

Khattar RS, Swales JD, Senior R, et al. Racial variation in cardiovascular morbidity and mortality in essential hypertension. *Heart* 2000;83:267–271.

Kim BJ, Lee HJ, Sung KC, et al. Comparison of microalbuminuria in 2 blood pressure categories of prehypertensive subjects. *Circ J* 2007;71:1283–1287.

Kizer JR, Arnett DK, Bella JN, et al. Differences in left ventricular structure between black and white hypertensive adults: The Hypertension Genetic Epidemiology Network Study. *Hypertension* 2004;43:1182–1188.

Kjeldsen SE, Julius S, Hedner T, et al. Stroke is more common than myocardial infarction in hypertension: Analysis based on 11 major randomized intervention trials. *Blood Press* 2001;10: 190–192.

Kjellgren KI, Ahlner J, Dahlöf B, et al. Perceived symptoms amongst hypertensive patients in routine clinical practice. *J Intern Med* 1998;244:325–332.

Klag MJ, Whelton PK, Coresh J, et al. The association of skin color with blood pressure in US blacks with low socioeconomic status. *JAMA* 1991;265:599–602.

Knecht S, Wersching H, Lohmann H, et al. High-normal blood pressure is associated with poor cognitive performance. *Hypertension* 2008;51:663–668.

Knerr I, Dost A, Lepler R, et al. Tracking and prediction of arterial blood pressure from childhood to young adulthood in 868 patients with type 1 diabetes: A multicenter longitudinal survey in Germany and Austria. *Diabetes Care* 2008;31:726–727.

Kokkinos P, Pittaras A, Narayan P, et al. Exercise capacity and blood pressure associations with left ventricular mass in prehypertensive individuals. *Hypertension* 2007;49:55–61.

Kopp JB, Smith MW, Nelson GW, et al. MYH9 is a major-effect risk gene for focal segmental glomerulosclerosis. *Nat Genet* 2008;40:1175–1184.

Krum H, Abraham WT. Heart Failure. *Lancet* 2009;373:941–955.

Kshirsagar AV, Carpenter M, Bang H, et al. Blood pressure usually considered normal is associated with an elevated risk of cardiovascular disease. *Am J Med* 2006;119:133–141.

Kurth T, Schurks M, Logroscino G, et al. Migraine, vascular risk, and cardiovascular events in women: Prospective cohort study. *Br Med J* 2008;337:a636.

Lakatta EG, Levy D. Arterial and cardiac aging: Major shareholders in cardiovascular disease enterprises. *Circulation* 2003;107: 139–146.

Langford HG, Watson RL. Potassium and calcium intake, excretion, and homeostasis in blacks, and their relation to blood pressure. *Cardiovasc Drug Ther* 1990;4:403–406.

Laragh J. Laragh's lessons in pathophysiology and clinical pearls for treating hypertension. *Am J Hypertens* 2001;14:186–194.

Laurent S, Katsahian S, Fassot C, et al. Aortic stiffness is an independent predictor of fatal stroke in essential hypertension. *Stroke* 2003;34:1203–1206.

Law M, Morris J, Jordan R, Wald N. High blood pressure and headaches; Results from a meta-analysis of 94 randomised placebo controlled trials with 24000 participants. *Circulation* 2005; 2301–2306.

Lipsitz LA, Storch HA, Minaker KL, et al. Intra-individual variability in postural BP in the elderly. *Clin Sci* 1985;69:337–341.

Lisabeth LD, Smith MA, Sanchez BN, et al. Ethnic disparities in stroke and hypertension among women: The BASIC project. *Am J Hypertens* 2008;21:778–783.

Lloyd-Jones DM, Evans JC, Levy D. Hypertension in adults across the age spectrum: Current outcomes and control in the community. *JAMA* 2005;294:466–472.

Luders S, Schrader J, Berger J, et al. The PHARAO study: Prevention of hypertension with the angiotensin-converting enzyme inhibitor ramipril in patients with high-normal blood pressure: A prospective, randomized, controlled prevention trial of the German Hypertension League. *J Hypertens* 2008;26:1487–1496.

Maestri MM, Fuchs SC, Ferlin E, et al. Detection of arteriolar narrowing in fundoscopic examination: Evidence of a low performance of direct ophthalmoscopy in comparison with a microdensitometric method. *Am J Hypertens* 2007;20:501–505.

Malik S, Wong ND, Franklin SS, et al. Impact of the metabolic syndrome on mortality from coronary heart disease, cardiovascular disease, and all causes in United States adults. *Circulation* 2004;110:1245–1250.

Management Committee. Untreated mild hypertension. *Lancet* 1982;1:185–191.

Marshall T. The rise of the term "prehypertension." *Ann Intern Med* 2009;150:145.

Martin LD, Howell EE, Ziegelstein RC, et al. Hand-carried ultrasound performed by hospitalists: Does it improve the cardiac physical examination? *Am J Med* 2009;122:35–41.

Mason PJ, Manson JE, Sesso HD, et al. Blood pressure and risk of secondary cardiovascular events in women: The Women's Antioxidant Cardiovascular Study (WACS). *Circulation* 2004;109: 1623–1629.

Maxwell MH. Cooperative study of renovascular hypertension: Current status. *Kidney Int Suppl* 1975;8:153–160.

Mazzone T, Chait A, Plutzky J. Cardiovascular disease risk in type 2 diabetes mellitus: Insights from mechanistic studies. *Lancet* 2008;371:1800–1809.

McEniery CM, Yasmin Wallace S, et al. Increased stroke volume and aortic stiffness contribute to isolated systolic hypertension in young adults. *Hypertension* 2005; 46:221–226.

Menotti A, Lanti M, Angeletti M, et al. Twenty-year cardiovascular and all-cause mortality trends and changes in cardiovascular risk factors in Gubbio, Italy: The role of blood pressure changes. *J Hypertens* 2009;27:266–274.

Middeke M, Lemmer B, Schaaf B, et al. Prevalence of hypertension-attributed symptoms in routine clinical practice: A general practitioners-based study. *J Hum Hypertens* 2008;22:252–258.

Milani RV, Lavie CJ, Mehra MR, et al. Left ventricular geometry and survival in patients with normal left ventricular ejection fraction. *Am J Cardiol* 2006;97:959–963.

Minor DS, Wofford MR, Jones DW. Racial and ethnic differences in hypertension. *Curr Atheroscler Rep* 2008;10:121–127.

Montalvo G, Avanzini F, Anselmi M, et al. Diagnostic evaluation of people with hypertension in low income country: Cohort study of "essential" method of risk stratification. *Br Med J* 2008;337:a1387.

Morris RC Jr, Sebastian A, Forman A, et al. Normotensive salt sensitivity. *Hypertension* 1999;33:18–23.

Mulè G, Nardi E, Andronico G, et al. Pulsatile and steady 24-h blood pressure components as determinants of left ventricular mass in young and middle-aged essential hypertensives. *J Human Hypertens* 2003;17:231–238.

Murabito JM, Evans JC, Lawson MG, et al. The ankle-brachial index in the elderly and risk of stroke, coronary disease, and death: The Framingham Study. *Arch Intern Med* 2003;163 :1939–1942.

Narayan KMV, Boyle JP, Thompson TJ, et al. Lifetime risk for diabetes mellitus in the United States. *JAMA* 2003;290:1884–1890.

Neaton JD, Wentworth D. Serum cholesterol, blood pressure, cigarette smoking, and death from coronary heart disease: Overall findings and differences by age for 316,099 white men. *Arch Intern Med* 1992;152:56–64.

Nguyen TT, Wang JJ, Wong TY. Retinal vascular changes in pre-diabetes and prehypertension: New findings and their research and clinical implications. *Diabetes Care* 2007;30:2708–2715.

Ninomiya T, Kubo M, Doi Y, et al. Prehypertension increases the risk for renal arteriosclerosis in autopsies: The Hisayama Study. *J Am Soc Nephrol* 2007;18:2135–2142.

Obisesan TO, Vargas CM, Gillum RF. Geographic variation in stroke risk in the United States. *Stroke* 2000;31:19–25.

Oikarinen L, Nieminen MS, Viitasalo M, et al. QRS duration and QT interval predict mortality in hypertensive patients with left ventricular hypertrophy: The Losartan Intervention for End-point Reduction in Hypertension Study. *Hypertension* 2004; 43:1029–1034.

Pache M, Kube T, Wolf S, et al. Do angiographic data support a detailed classification of hypertensive fundus changes? *J Hum Hypertens* 2002;16:405–410.

Palacios C, Wigertz K, Maritn BR, et al. Sodium retention in black and white female adolescents in response to salt intake. *J Clin Endocrin Metab* 2004;89:1858–1863.

Paran E, Galily Y, Abu-Rabia Y, et al. Environmental and genetic factors of hypertension in a biracial Beduin population. *J Hum Hypertens* 1992;6:107–112.

Parikh NI, Pencina MJ, Wang TJ, et al. A risk score for predicting near-term incidence of hypertension: The Framingham Heart Study. *Ann Intern Med* 2008;148:102–110.

Patel HJ, Deeb GM. Ascending and arch aorta: Pathology, natural history, and treatment. *Circulation* 2008;118:188–195.

Pemu PI, Ofili E. Hypertension in women: Part I. *J Clin Hypertens* 2008;40:406–410.

Perera GA. Hypertensive vascular disease. *J Chron Dis* 1955;1: 33–42.

Pickett CA, Jackson JL, Hemann BA, et al. Carotid bruits as a prognostic indicator of cardiovascular death and myocardial infarction: A meta-analysis. *Lancet* 2008;371:1587–1594.

Pierini A, Bertinieri G, Pagnozzi G, et al. Effects of systemic hypertension on arterial dynamics and left ventricular compliance in patients 70 years of age. *Am J Cardiol* 2000;86:882–886.

Pletcher MJ, Bibbins-Domingo K, Lewis CE, et al. Prehypertension during young adulthood and coronary calcium later in life. *Ann Intern Med* 2008;149:91–99.

Postma MJ, Boersma C, Gansevoort RT. Pharmacoeconomics in nephrology: Considerations on cost-effectiveness of screening for albuminuria. *Nephrol Dial Transplant* 2008;23:1103–1106.

Prati P, Tosetto A, Vanuzzo D, et al. Carotid intima media thickness and plaques can predict the occurrence of ischemic cerebrovascular events. *Stroke* 2008;39:2470–2476.

Pratt JH, Ambrosius WT, Agarwal R, et al. Racial differences in the activity of amiloride-sensitive epithelial sodium channel. *Hypertension* 2002;40:903–908.

Price DA, Fisher NDL, Lansang MC, et al. Renal perfusion in blacks: Alterations caused by insuppressibility of intrarenal renin with salt. *Hypertension* 2002;40:186–189.

Prinssen M, Verhoeven ELG, Buth J, et al. A randomized trial comparing conventional and endovascular repair of abdominal aortic aneurysms. *N Engl J Med* 2004;351:1607–1618.

Prospective Studies Collaboration. Age-specific relevance of usual blood pressure to vascular mortality: A meta-analysis of individual data for one million adults in 61 prospective studies. *Lancet* 2002;360:1903–1913.

Puisieux F, Bulckaen H, Fauchais AL, et al. Ambulatory blood pressure monitoring and postprandial hypotension in elderly persons with falls or syncopes. *J Gerontol* 2000;55A:M535–M540.

Qiu C, von Strauss E, Winblad B, et al. Decline in blood pressure over time and risk of dementia: A longitudinal study from the Kungsholmen project. *Stroke* 2004;35:1810–1815.

Qiu C, Winblad B, Viitanen M, et al. Pulse pressure and risk of Alzheimer disease in persons aged 75 years or older: A community-based, longitudinal study. *Stroke* 2003;34:594–599.

Querejeta R, Lopez B, Gonzalez A, et al. Increased collagen type I synthesis in patients with heart failure of hypertensive origin: Relation to myocardial fibrosis. *Circulation* 2004;110: 1263–1268.

Qureshi AI, Suri FK, Mohammad Y, et al. Isolated and borderline isolated systolic hypertension relative to long-term risk and type of stroke: A 20-year follow-up of the National Health and Nutrition Survey. *Stroke* 2002;33:2781–2788.

Räihä I, Luutonen S, Piha J, et al. Prevalence, predisposing factors, and prognostic importance of postural hypotension. *Arch Intern Med* 1995;155:930–935.

Ridker PM, Cannon CP, Morrow D, et al. C-reactive protein levels and outcomes after statin therapy. *N Engl J Med* 2005;352:20–28.

Rodin MB, Daviglus ML, Wong GC, et al. Middle age cardiovascular risk factors and abdominal aortic aneurysm in older age. *Hypertension* 2003;42:61–68.

Roger VL, Weston SA, Redfield MM, et al. Trends in heart failure incidence and survival in a community-based population. *JAMA* 2004;292:344–350.

Ronnback M, Fagerudd J, Forsblom C, et al. Altered age-related blood pressure pattern in type 1 diabetes. *Circulation* 2004;110: 1076–1082.

Rudolph A, Abdel-Aty H, Bohl S, et al. Noninvasive detection of fibrosis applying contrast-enhanced cardiac magnetic resonance in different forms of left ventricular hypertrophy relation to remodeling. *J Am Coll Cardiol* 2009;53:284–291.

Ruixing Y, Jinzhen W, Weixiong L, et al. The environmental and genetic evidence for the association of hyperlipidemia and hypertension. *J Hypertens* 2009;27:251–258.

Rutter MK, Meigs JB, Sullivan LM, et al. C-reactive protein, the metabolic syndrome, and prediction of cardiovascular events in the Framingham Offspring Study. *Circulation* 2004;110:380–385.

Safar ME, Benetos A. Factors influencing arterial stiffness in systolic hypertension in the elderly: Role of sodium and the renin-angiotensin system. *Am J Hypertens* 2003;16:249–258.

Safar ME, Smulyan H. Hypertension in women. *Am J Hypertens* 2004;17:82–87.

Salmasi A-M, Alimo A, Dancy M. Prevalence of unrecognized abnormal glucose tolerance in patients attending a hospital hypertension clinic. *Am J Hypertens* 2004;17:483–488.

Scherrer JF, Xian H, Bucholz KK, et al. A twin study of depression symptoms, hypertension, and heart disease in middle-aged men. *Psychosom Med* 2003;65:548–557.

Schillaci G, Vaudo G, Pasqualini L, et al. Left ventricular mass and systolic dysfunction in essential hypertension. *J Hum Hypertens* 2002;16:117–122.

Schlaich MP, Grassi G, Lambert GW, et al. European Society of Hypertension Working Group on Obesity Obesity-induced hypertension and target organ damage: Current knowledge and future directions. *J Hypert* 2009;27:207–211.

Schlaich MP, Kaye DM, Lambert E, et al, Relation between cardiac sympathetic activity and hypertensive left ventricular hypertrophy. *Circulation* 2003;108:560–565.

Schmidlin O, Forman A, Tanaka M, et al. NaCl-induced renal vasoconstriction in salt-sensitive African Americans: antipressor and hemodynamic effects of potassium bicarbonate. *Hypertension* 1999;33(2):633–639.

Schmieder RE, Messerli FH. Hypertension and the heart. *J Hum Hypertens* 2000;14:597–604.

Sciarretta S, Pontremoli R, Rosei EA, et al. Independent association of ECG abnormalities with microalbuminuria and renal damage in hypertensive patients without overt cardiovascular disease: Data from Italy-Developing Education and awareness on MicroAlbuminuria in patients with hypertensive Disease study. *J Hypertens* 2009;27:410–417.

Scott IA. Evaluating cardiovascular risk assessment for asymptomatic people. *Br Med J* 2009;338:a2844.

Selvin E, Erlinger TP. Prevalence of and risk factors for peripheral arterial disease in the United States: Results from the National Health and Nutrition Examination Survey, 1999–2000. *Circulation* 2004;110:738–743.

SHEP Cooperative Research Group. Prevention of stroke by antihypertensive drug treatment in older persons with isolated systolic hypertension. *JAMA* 1991;265:3255–3264.

Shinn EH, Poston WSC, Kimball KT, et al. Blood pressure and symptoms of depression and anxiety: A prospective study. *Am J Hypertens* 2001;14:660–664.

Simmons RK, Sharp S, Boekholdt SM, et al. Evaluation of the Framingham risk score in the European Prospective Investigation of Cancer-Norfolk cohort: Does adding glycated hemoglobin improve the prediction of coronary heart disease events? *Arch Intern Med* 2008;168:1209–1216.

Simon G, Nordgren D, Connelly S, et al. Screening for abdominal aortic aneurysms in a hypertensive patient population. *Arch Intern Med* 1996;156:2081–2084.

Sipahi I, Tuzcu EM, Schoenhagen P, et al. Effects of normal, prehypertensive, and hypertensive blood pressure levels on progression of coronary atherosclerosis. *J Am Coll Cardiol* 2006;48:833–838.

Skov K, Eiskjaer H, Hansen HE, et al. Treatment of young subjects at high familial risk of future hypertension with an angiotensin-receptor blocker. *Hypertension* 2007;50:89–95.

Smoller JW, Pollack MH, Wassertheil-Smoller S, et al. Prevalence and correlates of panic attacks in postmenopausal women: Results from an ancillary study to the Women's Health Initiative. *Arch Intern Med* 2003;163:2041–2050.

Song CK, Martinez JA, Kailasam MT, et al. Renal kallikrein excretion: Role of ethnicity, gender, environment, and genetic risk of hypertension. *J Hum Hypertens* 2000;14:461–468.

Spence JD. Pseudo-hypertension in the elderly. *J Hum Hypertens* 1997;11:621–623.

Staessen JA, Fagard R, Thijs L, et al. Randomized double-blind comparison of placebo and active treatment for older patients with isolated systolic hypertension. *Lancet* 1997;350:757–764.

Staessen JA, Gasowski J, Wang JG, et al. Risks of untreated and treated isolated systolic hypertension in the elderly. *Lancet* 2000;355:865–872.

Starr JM, Inch S, Cross S, et al. Blood pressure and ageing. *Br Med J* 1998;317:513–514.

Stevens LA, Coresh J, Greene T, et al. Assessing kidney function—measured and estimated glomerular filtration rate. *N Engl J Med* 2006;354:2473–2483.

Stevens LA, Coresh J, Schmid CH, et al. Estimating GFR using serum cystatin C alone and in combination with serum creatinine: A pooled analysis of 3,418 individuals with CKD. *Am J Kidney Dis* 2008;51:395–406.

Stevens LA, Levey AS. Clinical implications of estimating equations for glomerular filtration rate. *Ann Intern Med* 2004, 141:959–961.

Suthanthiran M, Li B, Song JO, et al. Transforming growth factor-β_1 hyperexpression in African-American hypertensives. *Proc Natl Acad Sci USA* 2000;97:3479–3484.

Syamala S, Li J, Shankar A. Association between serum uric acid and prehypertension among US adults. *J Hypertens* 2007; 25:1583–1589.

Task Force for the Management of Arterial Hypertension of the European Society of Hypertension (ESH) and of the European Society of Cardiology (ESC). 2007 Guidelines for the Management of Arterial Hypertension. *J Hypertens* 2007;25:1105–1187.

Tedesco MA, Natale F, Di Salvo G, et al. Effects of coexisting hypertension and type II diabetes mellitus on arterial stiffness. *J Human Hypertens* 2004;18:469–473.

Thomas F, Blacher J, Benetos A, et al. Cardiovascular risk as defined in the 2003 European blood pressure classification: The assessment of an additional predictive value of pulse pressure on mortality. *J Hypertens* 2008;26:1072–1077.

Thompson D, Edelsberg J, Colditz GA, et al. Lifetime health and economic consequences of obesity. *Arch Intern Med* 1999;159: 2177–2183.

Thune JJ, Signorovitch J, Kober L, et al. Effect of antecedent hypertension and follow-up blood pressure on outcomes after high-risk myocardial infarction. *Hypertension* 2008;51:48–54.

Tocci G, Sciarretta S, Volpe M. Development of heart failure in recent hypertension trials. *J Hypertens* 2008;26:1477–1486.

Toprak A, Wang H, Chen W, et al. Prehypertension and black-white contrasts in cardiovascular risk in young adults: Bogalusa Heart Study. *J Hypertens* 2009;27:243–250.

Toto RB. Hypertensive nephrosclerosis in African Americans. *Kidney Int* 2003;64.2331–2341.

Tuomilehto J, Linström J, Eriksson JG, et al. Prevention of type 2 diabetes mellitus by changes in lifestyle among subjects with impaired glucose tolerance. *N Engl J Med* 2001;344:1343–1350.

Turban S, Miller ER III, Ange B, et al. Racial differences in urinary potassium excretion. *J Am Soc Nephrol* 2008;19:1396–1402.

U.S. Preventive Services Task Force. Screening for type 2 diabetes mellitus in adults: U.S. Preventive Services Task Force recommendation statement. *Ann Intern Med* 2008;148:846–854.

Vakili BA, Okin PM, Devereux RB. Prognostic implications of left ventricular hypertrophy. *Am Heart J* 2001;141:334–341.

Valham F, Mooe T, Rabben T, et al. Increased risk of stroke in patients with coronary artery disease and sleep apnea: A 10-year follow-up. *Circulation* 2008;118:955–960.

van Dijk EJ, Breteler MMB, Schmidt R, et al. The association between blood pressure, hypertension, and cerebral white matter lesions: Cardiovascular Determinants of Dementia study. *Hypertension* 2004;44:625–630.

Vasan RS, Beiser A, Seshadri S, et al. Residual lifetime risk for developing hypertension in middle-aged women and men: The Framingham Heart Study. *JAMA* 2002;287:1003–1010.

Vasan RS, Benjamin EJ. Diastolic heart failure. *N Engl J Med* 2001;344:56–59.

Vasan RS, Evans JC, Benjamin EJ, et al. Relations of serum aldosterone to cardiac structure: Gender-related differences in the Framingham Heart Study. *Hypertension* 2004;43:957–962.

Vasan RS, Larson MG, Leip EP, et al. Impact of high-normal blood pressure on the risk of cardiovascular disease. *N Engl J Med* 2001;345:1291–1297.

Vemmos KN, Spengos K, Tsivgoulis G, et al. Factors influencing acute blood pressure values in stroke subtypes. *J Hum Hypertens* 2004;18:253–259.

Verdecchia P, Angeli F, Gattobigio R, et al. Asymptomatic left ventricular systolic dysfunction in essential hypertension: Prevalence, determinants and prognostic value. *Hypertension* 2005; 45:412–418.

Verdecchia P, Angeli F, Gattobigio R, et al. Regression of left ventricular hypertrophy and prevention of stroke in hypertensive subjects. *Am J Hypertens* 2006;19:493–499.

Verdecchia P, Reboldi GP, Gattobigio R, et al. Atrial fibrillation in hypertension: Predictors and outcome. *Hypertension* 2003; 41:218–223.

Vermeer SE, Koudstaal PJ, Oudkerk M, et al. Prevalence and risk factors of silent brain infarcts in the population-based Rotterdam Scan Study. *Stroke* 2002;33:21–25.

Vos LE, Oren A, Uiterwaal C, et al. Adolescent blood pressure and blood pressure tracking into young adulthood are related to subclinical atherosclerosis: The Atherosclerosis Risk in Young Adults (ARYA) study. *Am J Hypertens* 2003;16:549–555.

Wachtell K, Rokkedal J, Bella JN, et al. Effect of electrocardiographic left ventricular hypertrophy on left ventricular systolic function in systemic hypertension. *Am J Cardiol* 2001;87:54–60.

Waddell TK, Dart AM, Gatzka CD, et al. Women exhibit a greater age-related increase in proximal aortic stiffness than men. *J Hypertens* 2001;19:2205–2212.

Waldstein SR, Giggey PP, Thayer JF, et al. Nonlinear relations of blood pressure to cognitive function: The Baltimore Longitudinal Study of Aging. *Hypertension* 2005;45:374–379.

Wallace SM, Yasmin, McEniery C, et al. Isolated systolic hypertension is characterized by increased aortic stiffness and endothelial dysfunction. *Hypertension* 2007;51:119–126.

Wang L, Wong TY, Sharrett AR, et al. Relationship between retinal arteriolar narrowing and myocardial perfusion: Multi-ethnic study of atherosclerosis. *Hypertension* 2008;51:119–126.

Wang TJ, Evans JC, Meigs JB, et al. Low-grade albuminuria and the risks of hypertension and blood pressure progression. *Circulation* 2005;111:1370–1376.

Weaver FA, Kumar SR, Yellin AE, et al. Renal revascularization in Takayasu arteritis-induced renal artery stenosis. *J Vasc Surg* 2004;39:749–757.

Weiss A, Grossman E, Beloosesky Y, et al. Orthostatic hypotension in acute geriatric ward: Is it a consistent finding? *Arch Intern Med* 2002;162:2369–2374.

Weiss JP, Blaivas JG. Nocturia. *J Urol* 2000;163:5–12.

Weiss NS. Relation of high blood pressure to headache, epistaxis, and selected other symptoms. *N Engl J Med* 1972;287:631–633.

Whelton PK, He J, Appel LJ, et al. Primary prevention of hypertension: Clinical and public health advisory from the National High Blood Pressure Education Program. *JAMA* 2002;288: 1882–1888.

Wilson PWF, Grundy SM. The metabolic syndrome: Practical guide to origins and treatment: Part I. *Circulation* 2003;108: 1422–1425.

Wong TY, Mitchell P. Hypertensive retinopathy. *N Engl J Med* 2004;351:2310–2317.

Wong TY, Mitchell P. The eye in hypertension. *Lancet* 2007;369: 425–435.

Yancy CW, Lopatin M, Stevenson LW, et al. Clinical presentation, management, and in-hospital outcomes of patients admitted with acute decompensated heart failure with preserved systolic function: A report from the Acute Decompensated Heart Failure National Registry (ADHERE) Database. *J Am Coll Cardiol* 2006;47:76–84.

Young-Xu Y, Ravid S. Optimal blood pressure control for the prevention of atrial fibrillation [Abstract]. *Circulation* 2004;110 (Suppl. 3):III-768.

Zamora CR, Cubeddu LX. Microalbuminuria: Do we need a new threshold? *J Hum Hypertens* 2009;23:146–149.

Zethelius B, Berglund L, Sundstrom J, et al. Use of multiple biomarkers to improve the prediction of death from cardiovascular causes. *N Engl J Med* 2008;358:2107–2116.

CHAPTER 5

Treatment of Hypertension: Why, When, How Far

In the preceding four chapters, the epidemiology, natural history, and pathophysiology of primary (essential) hypertension were reviewed. We will now turn to its treatment, examining the benefits and costs of therapy in this chapter and the use of nondrug and drug treatments in the two chapters that follow.

In this chapter, three main questions are addressed:

• First, what is the evidence that treatment is beneficial?
• Second, at what level of blood pressure (BP) should active drug therapy be started? Lifestyle modifications, which will be examined in the next chapter, can be justified for everyone, hypertensive or not.
• Third, what is the goal of therapy and, further, are there different goals for different patients?

To answer these questions, in this chapter, only data comparing active drug therapy against untreated or placebo-treated patients will be considered. In Chapter 7, data comparing one or another form of therapy will be examined.

EVIDENCE FOR BENEFITS OF THERAPY

The evidence for benefits of therapy comes in part from epidemiologic and experimental evidence but mainly from the results of large-scale therapeutic trials.

Epidemiologic Evidence

Epidemiologic evidence, covered in Chapter 1, provides a clear conclusion: The risks of cardiovascular morbidity and mortality rise progressively with increasing BP

levels (Prospective Studies Collaboration, 2002). As an aside, it seems intuitive that reducing BP would decrease these risks to a similar degree. However, mortality rates remain higher in hypertensives treated to a lower BP than in subjects with the same BP without antecedent hypertension (Asayama et al., 2009). Reasons for this residual risk will be examined when evidence from trials of treatments is reviewed.

Despite this residual risk, community-wide surveys document that improved BP control has been accompanied by reductions in BP-related mortality (Ingelsson et al., 2008).

Interrupting the Progress of Hypertension

The 15- to 17-year longitudinal study of Welshmen by Miall and Chinn (1973) and the 24-year follow-up of American aviators by Oberman et al. (1967) showed that hypertension begets further hypertension. In both studies, the higher the BP, the greater was the rate of change of pressure, pointing to an obvious conclusion: Progressive rises in BP can be prevented by keeping the pressure down. This conclusion is further supported by the results of the major placebo-controlled trials of antihypertensive therapy: Whereas 10% to 17% of those on placebo progressed beyond the threshold of diastolic pressure above 110 mm Hg, only a small handful of those on drug treatment did so (see Chapter 4, Tables 4-2 and 4-3).

Evidence from Natural Experiments in Humans

Vascular damage and the level of BP have been closely correlated in three situations: unilateral renal vascular disease, coarctation, and pulmonary hypertension. These three experiments of nature provide evidence that what is important is the level of the BP flowing through a vascular bed and not some other deleterious effect associated with systemic hypertension. Tissues with lower BP are protected; those with higher pressure are damaged.

- The kidney with renal artery stenosis is exposed to a lower pressure than is the contralateral kidney without stenosis. Arteriolar nephrosclerosis develops in the high-pressure nonstenotic kidney, occasionally to such a degree that hypertension can be relieved only by removal of the nonstenotic kidney, along with repair of the stenosis (Thal et al., 1963).
- The vessels exposed to the high pressure above the coarctation develop atherosclerosis to a much greater degree than do the vessels below the coarctation, where the pressure is low (Hollander et al., 1976).
- The low pressure within the pulmonary artery ordinarily protects these vessels from damage. When patients develop pulmonary hypertension secondary to mitral stenosis or certain types of congenital heart disease, both arteriosclerosis and arteriolar necrosis often develop within the pulmonary vessels (Heath & Edwards, 1958).

Evidence from Animal Experiments

Just as hypertension accelerates and worsens atherosclerosis in humans, animals that are made hypertensive develop more atherosclerosis than do normotensive animals fed the same high-cholesterol diet (Chobanian, 1990). In animals, the lesions caused by hypertension, including accelerated atherosclerosis, can be prevented by lowering the pressure with antihypertensive agents (Chobanian et al., 1992).

Evidence from Clinical Trials of Antihypertensive Therapy

The last piece of evidence—that there is benefit from lowering an elevated BP—is the most important. Over the last five decades, since oral antihypertensive therapy has become available, protection with antihypertensive therapy has been demonstrated at progressively lower levels of pressure and, more recently, in the elderly (Beckett et al., 2008). The benefits of individual drugs against placebo are so compelling as to preclude the performance of such trials, so attention has turned to trials

contrasting a set of one or two drugs against another set of one or two. The data in multiple meta-analyses (Blood Pressure Lowering Treatment Trialists' Collaboration, 2008; Staessen et al., 2003; Wang et al., 2007) validate the conclusion of the European societies' guidelines that "the main benefits of antihypertensive therapy are due to lowering of BP per se" (Task Force, 2007).

As will be noted, this wide umbrella covers disparate groups of patients who may differ in their responses to different drugs (Wang et al., 2007; Zanchetti et al., 2009). However, the overall message is clear: the lower the BP, the greater the protection.

Problems in Applying Trial Results to Clinical Practice

Before examining the results of the multiple randomized clinical trials (RCTs) and their meta-analyses, that are used to inform guidelines for clinical practice, a few cautionary comments are in order. Practitioners must be aware of the features, both good and bad, of both the performance and the presentation of clinical trials since they are the foundation of *evidence-based medicine*, i.e., the decision to use a therapy based on systematic analyses of unbiased scientific evidence.

Problems with Trials

As noted, RCTs are required to assess reliably the modest effects of antihypertensive treatment on the major outcomes expected in typical hypertensive patients over a relatively short time, 3 to 5 years, wherein close observation remains possible (Mancia, 2006). RCTs are needed because, as concluded by Vandenbroucke (2004), "observational studies about therapy will be credible only in exceptional circumstances."

As essential as they are, RCTs may be misleading, partly by their nature and partly because of human foibles (Mancia, 2006). In particular, the increasing financial sponsorship of clinical trials by drug marketers, although often essential for their performance, has been associated with selection of an inappropriate comparator and poorer quality of methods (Lexchin et al., 2003), selective reporting of outcomes (Chan et al., 2004), and more positive conclusions than seen in trials funded by nonprofit sources (Yank et al., 2007).

Beyond these often subtle and unrecognized biases toward the financial sponsor, a number of other factors may either, on the one hand, exaggerate or, on the other, diminish the apparent benefits of therapy.

Possible Underestimations of Benefit

Results of trials may underestimate the true benefits of antihypertensive therapy for a number of reasons, including the following:

Mislabeling of Patients: The ascertainment of hypertension for enrollment into trials is usually based on two or three sets of office-based BP measurements over 1 to 2 months. As amply noted in Chapter 2, such limited measurements are likely to capture a large number of transient or isolated clinic (white-coat) hypertensives, thereby diminishing the efficacy of therapy, as all antihypertensive drugs lower BP more in relation to a higher starting BP, and most drugs lower BP very little in the absence of persistent hypertension.

Intervention Too Late: Hypertension may produce damages well before patients have sufficiently high BP to be eligible for enrollment. Even if effectively treated, these damages may be irreversible, particularly if other risk factors are also not corrected.

Too Short Duration of Treatment: The duration of the trials is usually less than 5 years. However, the benefit of drugs may take much longer to become fully manifest, thereby minimizing the drugs' apparent efficacy.

Inadequate Therapy: The approximately 12/6 mm Hg overall decreases in BP, accomplished in most clinical trials, are likely too little to reduce the damages of hypertension maximally. The degree of damage clearly relates to the level of BP achieved during therapy and not to the pretreatment level (Adler et al., 2000). Because as many as 40% of patients in some trials did not reach the goal BP (Mancia, 2006), the benefits may then be less than what could have been obtained by more intensive therapy.

Patients Lost to Follow-Up: In some trials, as many as 25% of patients have been lost to follow-up before completion. In general, more high-risk patients are lost, weakening the evidence for benefit (Mancia, 2006).

Switching of Patients: In all trials, a sizable number of patients initially randomized to placebo were switched to active therapy because their BP rose beyond the predetermined ceiling of presumed safety. As noted by Ramsay et al. (1996), "treatment of these high-risk patients in the control groups will inevitably have reduced the cardiovascular disease event rates and led to underestimates of the absolute benefit."

Harm from Drugs: The drugs available and chosen for almost all the earlier trials in subjects younger than 60 years old were high doses of diuretics and adrenergic inhibitors, mostly nonselective β-blockers. As is noted in Chapter 7, multiple metabolic abnormalities, which particularly aggravate lipid and glucose-insulin levels, have been amply documented with these therapies. These drug-induced abnormalities may have blunted or reversed the improvement in coronary risk provided by reduction of the BP.

Noncompliance with Therapy: Patients assigned to active drug therapy may not have taken all of their medication and thereby have had less benefit. Although pill counts are usually performed, no truly accurate assessment of compliance is available.

Possible Overestimates of Benefit

On the other hand, antihypertensive therapy may be less effective than is seen in controlled trials, because of poor external validity for application of the results to routine clinical practice and individual patients (Kent & Hayward, 2007). Data from clinical trials may overestimate the benefits of therapy as they are applied to the universe of hypertensives for the following reasons.

Inclusion of Inappropriate End Points: To maximize the impact of therapy, multiple end points may be combined, some of questionable significance such as hospitalizations which occur at the subjective discretion of the investigator (Lim et al., 2008). Lauer and Topol (2003) argue that only all-cause mortality should be the primary end point since it is objective, unbiased, and clinically relevant. As they note, "any end point that requires a measurement involving human judgment is inherently subject to bias."

Exclusion of High-Risk Patients: In many early RCTs, patients with various symptomatic cardiovascular diseases, target organ damage, or major risk factors were excluded, leaving a fairly healthy population who may respond better than the usual mix of patients (Uijen et al., 2007).

Better Compliance with Therapy: Patients enrolled in trials in which medications and all health care are free and follow-up is carefully monitored are likely to be more compliant with therapy than patients in clinical practice. Therefore, they may achieve greater benefit.

Overemphasis on Initial Reports: The first report of a trial of a new drug is often more positive than are subsequent reports, but the first one is more likely to be cited and publicized (Ioannidis, 2005).

Relative versus Absolute Changes: In most reports of RCTs, the reductions in coronary heart disease (CHD)

TABLE 5.1	Calculations of Relative and Absolute Risk Reduction and Numbers Needed to Be Treated for Patients with Hypertension				
	Stroke in 5 Years		Relative Risk Reduction, $(P_c - P_a)/P_c$	Absolute Risk Reduction, $P_c - P_a$	Number Needed to Treat, $1/(P_c - P_a)$
Hypertension	Control Group	Active Treatment Group			
Diastolic ≤ 115 mm Hg					
Event rate (P)	0.20	0.12	0.40	0.08	13
Total number of patients	16,778	16,898			
Diastolic ≤ 110 mm Hg					
Event rate (P)	0.015	0.009	0.40	0.006	167
Total number of patients	15,165	15,238			

Modified from Cook RJ, Sackett DL. The number to treat: A clinically useful measure of treatment and effect. *Br Med J* 1995;310:452–454. Based on the results of Collins R, Peto R, MacMahon S, et al. Blood pressure, stroke and coronary heart disease. Part 2: Short-term reductions in blood pressure. *Lancet* 1990;335:827–838.

and stroke are relative—that is, they are the difference between the rates seen in treated versus untreated patients. However, as documented in Table 5-1, large relative differences may translate into small absolute differences. The 40% relative risk reduction by treatment of "mild" hypertension translates into only a 0.6% absolute risk reduction. The presentation of trial data as large relative reductions in risk is much more attractive to the public and the practitioners than the usually much smaller absolute reductions; however, the relative data may easily mislead the unwary into thinking that many more patients will be helped than is possible.

As shown in the far right column of Table 5-1, these investigators propose the use of the measure *number needed to treat* (*NNT*), calculated as the inverse of the absolute risk reduction, because it "conveys both statistical and clinical significance to the doctor" and "can be used to extrapolate published findings to a patient at an arbitrary specified baseline risk" (Cook & Sackett, 1995).

The need for using absolute risk, or the NNT, is well demonstrated in Figure 5-1 (Lever & Ramsay, 1995). Figure 5-1A shows the quite similar reductions in relative risk for stroke in six major trials in the elderly and in the earlier Medical Research Council trial of younger hypertensives. Figure 5-1B shows the same data in absolute terms, clearly portraying the progressively greater benefit of therapy with increasing pretherapy risk, as reflected in the rates in the placebo groups.

The use of NNTs based on absolute risk reduction is clearly more accurate than the portrayal of relative risks. The NNT must be related to the duration of the trial. This is best done by using the *hazard difference*, expressed as mortality per unit of patient-time (Lubsen et al., 2000). However, in most recent reports, results are presented as *survival curves*, showing differences in outcomes that change over time, using the Kaplan-Meier life table methods for estimating the proportion of patients who experience an event by time since randomization (Pocock et al., 2002). When properly constructed, i.e., showing both the number of subjects remaining in the trial over time and a display of statistical uncertainty, such survival curves portray RCT results very well.

Admixture of Drugs: To achieve the preset goal of therapy, e.g., BP below 140/90, most trials comparing a drug versus placebo (as examined in this chapter) or one drug versus another (as examined in Chapter 7) must add additional drugs to the study drug. In some trials, 80% or more of the patients end up on two or more. What is ascribed to only the study drug may represent the effect of many others (McAlister et al., 2003).

Solutions to the Problems of Trials

Obviously those who perform and report RCTs must follow established guidelines such as CONSORT (Rennie, 2001) or the GRADE system (Guyatt et al., 2008). However, clinicians themselves

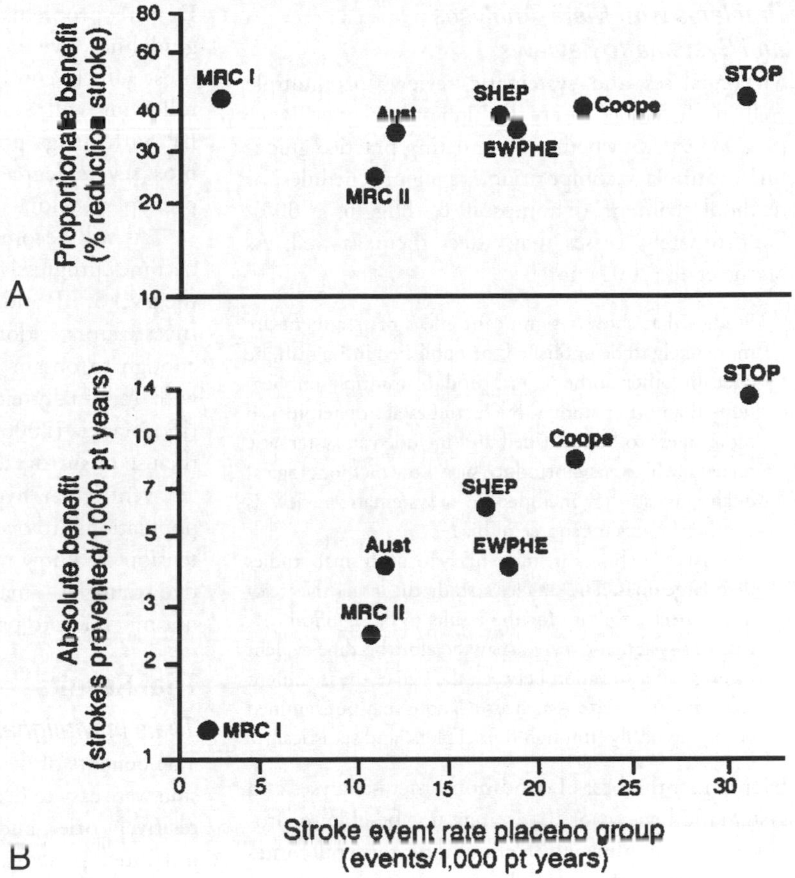

FIGURE 5-1 Comparison of (**A**) proportionate (relative) and (**B**) absolute benefit from reduction in the incidence of stroke in six trials in the elderly and in one other trial (Medical Research Council I [MRC-I]) having a similar design but in which the absolute stroke risk was much lower. Event rates are for fatal and nonfatal stroke combined. Aust, Australian study; EWPHE, European Working Party on High BP in the Elderly trial; Coope, Coope and Warrender; SHEP, Systolic Hypertension in the Elderly Program; STOP, Swedish Trial in Old Patients with Hypertension. (Modified from Lever AF, Ramsay LE. Treatment of hypertension in the elderly. *J Hypertens* 1995;13:571–579.)

must be prepared to assess the validity of trial data, since in the words of Montori et al. (2004):

> Science is often not objective. Emotional investment in particular ideas and personal interest in academic success may lead investigators to overemphasize the importance of their findings and the quality of their work. Even more serious conflicts arise when for-profit organizations, including pharmaceutical companies, provide funds for research and consulting, conduct data management and analyses, and write reports on behalf of the investigators.

Montori et al. (2004) provide this set of guides for clinicians to avoid being misled by biased presentation and interpretation of trial data:

• Read the "Methods and Results" sections. Remember that the "Discussion" section often offers inferences that differ from those a dispassionate reader would draw.
• Read abstracts and comments in objective secondary publications such as the *ACP Journal Club*, *Evidence-based Medicine, Up-To-Date, the Medical Letter*, etc.

• Beware of faulty comparators. A weak comparator is often chosen in comparative trials, perhaps the most egregious being the β-blocker atenolol (Carlberg et al., 2004).
• Beware of composite end points; as noted previously, all-cause mortality can hardly be fudged.
• Beware of small treatment effects, particularly when the data are reported as differences in relative risks. If the 95% confidence interval (CI) crosses the midline, beware.
• Beware of subgroup analyses. A number of provisos should be met to ensure that apparent differences in subgroup responses are real, particularly that only a small number of hypotheses were tested that were specified before the results became available (Rothwell, 2005).

Meanwhile, students and practitioners need to take better advantage of available sources of evidence-based clinical information (Demaerschalk, 2004). The Cochrane Library is now the most prolific provider, but more and more sources are available, many at no cost.

Problems with Meta-Analyses and Systematic Reviews

Meta-analyses and systematic reviews of multiple well-conducted RCTs are the highest level of evidence used by experts whether formulating practice guidelines, formulary composition, payment schedules, or textbook content (Thompson & Higgins, 2005). Unfortunately, biases may affect them as well. As Sterne et al. (2001) note:

> Studies that show a significant effect of treatment are more likely to be published, be published in English, be cited by other authors, and produce multiple publications than other studies. Such studies are therefore also more likely to be identified and included in systematic reviews, which may introduce bias. Low methodological quality of studies included in a systematic review is another important source of bias.
>
> All these biases are more likely to affect small studies than large ones. The smaller a study the larger the treatment effect necessary for the results to be significant.... Bias in a systematic review may therefore become evident through an association between the size of the treatment effect and study size—such associations may be examined both graphically [through funnel plots] and statistically.

Even under the best of conditions, meta-analyses and systematic reviews of RCTs may not be able to provide adequate information about long-term outcomes of such chronic diseases as hypertension, since almost all RCTs are of relatively short-term duration.

Problems with Guidelines

The most authoritative recommendations on how to best manage hypertension are the guidelines issued by national, or international, expert committees such as the U.S. Joint National Committee (Chobanian et al., 2003a,b) or the European Societies of Hypertension and Cardiology (Task Force, 2007).

However, there are problems with current guidelines, including these:

• Their recommendations may differ substantially.
• They are too long to be used when needed, although shorter "Practice Guidelines" are now being provided.
• The targets for therapy are too stringent and fail to take patients' beliefs and abilities into account (Campbell & Murchie, 2004).
• The participants in guideline committees may be too narrow in outlook, beholden to commercial interests, or not include the most critical observers (Alderman et al., 2002).

Despite problems with trials, meta-analyses, and guidelines, we must use them to determine the most effective way to manage hypertension. The following will examine the evidence that lowering BP with drugs provides benefit, starting with the most severe degree of hypertension and ending with prehypertension.

As will become obvious, the evidence of benefit becomes progressively more difficult to document as the level of BP and the overall degree of risk decrease. Investigators seldom live long enough or have funds enough to obtain "hard" outcome data on patients with minimally elevated BP or little cardiovascular risk. Mancia (2006) among others has recommended the use of surrogate end points, such as regression of left ventricular hypertrophy or proteinuria in such populations "to overcome the paradox that in hypertension we know much about cardiovascular preventive strategies—mainly in patients in whom there is not much left to prevent" (Mancia, 2006).

Trial Results

Trials in Malignant Hypertension

The benefits of drug therapy in malignant hypertension were easy to demonstrate in view of its predictable, relatively brief, and almost uniformly fatal course in untreated patients. Starting in 1958, a number of studies appeared showing a significant effect of medical therapy in reducing mortality in malignant hypertension (see Chapter 8).

Trials in Less Severe Hypertension

Demonstrating that therapy made a difference in nonmalignant, primary hypertension took a great deal longer. However, during the late 1950s and early 1960s, reports began to appear that suggested that therapy of nonmalignant hypertension was helpful (Hodge et al., 1961; Hood et al., 1963; Leishman, 1961). The first placebo-controlled, albeit small, study by Hamilton et al. (1964) showed a marked decrease in complications over a 2- to 6-year interval for 26 effectively treated patients as compared to 31 untreated patients.

Veterans Administration Cooperative Study

The first definitive proof of the protection provided by antihypertensive therapy in nonmalignant hypertension came from the Veterans Administration Cooperative Study begun in 1963. The value of therapy in the 73 men with diastolic BPs of 115 to 129 mm Hg given hydrochlorothiazide, reserpine, and hydralzine versus the 70 men given placebo became obvious after less than 1.5 years, with a reduction in deaths from four to zero and, in major complications, from twenty-three to two (Veterans Administration Cooperative Study Group [VA], 1967).

Along with the men with diastolic BPs of 115 to 129 mm Hg, another 380 with diastolic BPs between 90 and 114 mm Hg also were assigned randomly to either placebo or active therapy. It took a longer time—up to 5.5 years, with an average of 3.3 years—to demonstrate a statistically clear advantage of therapy in this group (VA, 1970). A total of 19 of the placebo group, but only eight of the treated group, died of hypertensive complications, and serious morbidity occurred more often among the placebo group. Overall, major complications occurred in 29% of the placebo group and 12% of the treated group.

The promising results of the Veterans Administration study prompted the initiation of a number of additional controlled trials of therapy of hypertension. Data from trials completed before 1995, primarily with diuretics and β-blockers, are separated from those completed since 1995, primarily with angiotensin converting enzyme inhibitors (ACEIs), calcium channel blockers (CCBs), and angiotensin II receptor blockers (ARBs).

Trials Before 1995

The 21 trials listed in Table 5-2 included a total of 56,078 patients followed up for an average of 5 years (Psaty et al., 1997; 2003). In all these trials, the primary drugs were either β-blockers or diuretics; in trials done before the mid-1980s, almost all used higher doses of diuretic. It should be noted that the entry BP criterion for all of the trials before the Systolic Hypertension in the Elderly Program-Pilot Study (SHEP-P) in 1989 was the diastolic level, reflecting

---

TABLE 5.2	**Randomized Placebo-Controlled Trials of Antihypertensive Drug Treatment Published Before 1995**

Trial (Reference)	Number of Patients	Entry BP, mm Hg	Mean Age, Years	Duration, Years	Primary Drugs
VA Coop I (1967)	143	186/121	51	1.5	D-high
VA Coop II (1970)	380	163/104	51	3.3	D-high
Carter (1970)	97	>160/110	60–79	4.0	D-high
Barraclough et al. (1973)	116	—/109	56	2.0	D-high
Hypertension-Stroke (1974)	452	167/100	59	2.3	D-high
USPHS (Smith, 1977)	389	148/99	44	7.0	D-high
VA-NHLBI (Perry et al., 1978)	1,012	—/93	38	1.5	D-high
HDFP (1979)	10,940	170/101	51	5.0	D-high
Oslo (Hegeland, 1980)	785	155/97	45	5.5	D-high
Australian (Management Comm, 1980)	3,427	165/101	50	4.0	D-high
Kuramoto et al. (1981)	91	168/86	76	4.0	D-high
MRC-I (1985)	17,354	161/98	52	5.0	β-B/D-high
EWPHE (Amery et al., 1985)	840	182/101	72	4.7	D-low
HEP (Coope & Warrender, 1986)	884	197/100	60	4.4	β-B
SHEP-P (Perry et al., 1989)	551	172/75	72	2.8	D-low
SHEP (1991)	4,736	170/77	72	4.5	D-low
STOP-H (Dahlöf et al., 1991)	1,627	195/102	76	2.0	β-B
MRC-II (1992)et al.	4,396	185/91	70	5.8	β-B/D-low
Dutch TIA (1993)	1,473	157/91	52% > 65	2.6	β-B
PATS (1995)	5,665	154/93	60	2.0	D-high
TEST (Eriksson, 1995)	720	161/89	70	2.6	β-B

β-B, beta-blocker; BP, blood pressure; D-high, diuretic dose ≥ 50 mg hydrochlorothiazide; D-low, diuretic dose < 50 mg hydrochlorothiazide; EWPHE, European Working Party on Hypertension in the Elderly; HDFP, Hypertension Detection and Follow-up Program; MRC, Medical Research Council; NHLBI, National Heart, Lung, and Blood Institute; PATS, Post-Stroke Antihypertensive Treatment; SHEP, Systolic Hypertension in the Elderly Program; SHEP-P, SHEP Pilot Study; STOP-H, Swedish Trial in Old Patients with Hypertension; TEST, Tenormin after Stroke and TIA; USPHS, U.S. Public Health Service; VA, Veterans Administration.

the greater emphasis placed, until recently, on diastolic rather than systolic BP as the major determinant of risk.

The trials published before 1985 mainly involved younger patients; those in the early 1990s enrolled elderly hypertensives with either combined hypertension or isolated systolic hypertension (ISH), who will be examined separately.

Separation of the Data by Doses

Psaty et al. (1997) separated the nine trials that involved high doses of diuretic (equivalent to 50 mg or more of hydrochlorothiazide) from the four that involved lower doses (equivalent to 12.5 to 25.0 mg hydrochlorothiazide) and the four that used a β-blocker as the primary drug (Fig. 5-2). The Hypertension Detection and Follow-up Program study was considered separately, as it was not placebo controlled: Half of the patients were more intensively treated (stepped care); the other half were less intensively treated (referred care).

The separation of the data by doses clearly reveals the lack of protection from CHD by high doses of diuretic and β-blockers, whereas all therapies had a significant impact on stroke. The later four studies with low doses of diuretic showed excellent protection against CHD.

Conclusion

Based on these trials, primarily in middle-aged patients with combined systolic and diastolic hypertension, the evidence was clear: Reductions in BP of 10 to 12 mm Hg systolic and 5 to 6 mm Hg diastolic for a few years conferred relative reductions of 38% for stroke and 16% for CHD (Collins & MacMahon, 1994).

Placebo-Controlled Trials after 1995

After 1995, a new series of trials were completed, and many more started, to determine the effects of the newer antihypertensive agents—ACEIs, CCBs, and ARBs—and to broaden the patient population to those with associated conditions including coronary disease, diabetes, and renal insufficiency (Table 5-3).

Figure 5-3 is an overview of data from 31 RCTs showing the relation between odds ratios for cardiovascular events and differences in systolic BP (Staessen et al., 2003). The Figure portrays data from 15 of the 21 placebo-controlled trials published before 1995 that are listed in Table 5-2, the others being too small or too short to be included. Most of the placebo-controlled trials published before 2003 are included. In addition, data from some of the comparative trials to be covered in Chapter 7 are included, since the purpose of the graph is to show the degree of protection with varying differences of systolic BP. In some of the comparative trials, higher systolic BP was seen with the "comparator" drug, with resultant increases in cardiovascular events.

The message of Figure 5-3 is clear: the degree of BP reduction is the primary determinant of cardiovascular

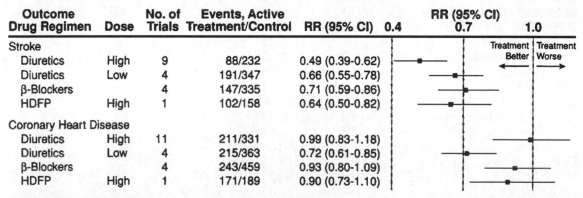

FIGURE 5-2 Meta-analysis of randomized, placebo-controlled clinical trials in hypertension according to first-line treatment strategy. For these comparisons, the numbers of participants randomized to active therapy and placebo were 7,758 and 12,075 for high-dose diuretic therapy; 4,305 and 5,116 for low-dose diuretic therapy; and 6,736 and 12,147 for β-blocker therapy. HDFP, Hypertension Detection and Follow-up Program; RR, relative risk; CI, confidence interval. (Adapted from Psaty BM, Smith NL, Siscovick DS, et al. Health outcomes associated with antihypertensive therapies used as first-line agents. *JAMA* 1997;277:739–745.)

TABLE 5.3	Randomized Placebo-Controlled Trials of Antihypertensive Drug Treatment Published After 1995				
Trial (Reference)	No. of Patients	Entry BP, mm Hg	Mean Age, Years	Duration, Years	Primary Drugs
ACEI vs. Placebo					
HOPE (Heart Outcomes, 2000)	9,297	139/79	66	5	Ramipril
PART 2 (MacMahon et al., 2000)	617	133/79	61	4	Ramipril
OUIET (Cashin-Hemphill et al., 1999)	1,750	123/74	58	2	Quinapril
SCAT (Teo et al., 2000)	460	130/78	61	5	Enalapril
PROGRESS (2001)	6,150	147/86	64	4	Perindopril, Indapamide
CCB vs. Placebo					
STONE (Gong, 1996)	1,632	169/98	67	2	Nifedipine
SYST-EUR (Staessen et al., 1997)	4,695	174/86	70	2	Nitrendipine
SYST-CHINA (Liu, 1998)	2,394	170/86	67	3	Nitrendipine
PREVENT (Pitt et al., 2000)	825	129/79	57	3	Amlodipine
IDNT (Lewis et al., 2001)	1,136	159/97	59	3	Amlodipine
ARB vs. Placebo					
IDNT (Lewis, 2001)	1,148	160/87	60	3	Irbesartan
RENAAL (Brenner et al., 2001)	1,513	152/82	60	4	Losartan
SCOPE (Lithell, 2003)	4,937	166/90	76	4	Candesartan

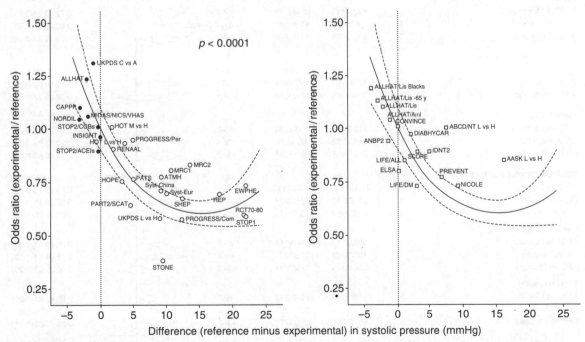

FIGURE 5-3 Relationship between odds ratio for cardiovascular events and corresponding differences in systolic BP in trials published before (left) and after (right) 2000. Odds ratios were calculated for experimental versus reference treatment. BP differences were obtained by subtracting achieved levels of experimental groups from those in reference groups. Negative values indicate tighter BP on control than on reference treatment. The regression lines were plotted with 95% CI and were weighted for the inverse of the variance of the individual odds ratios. (Modified from Staessen JA, Wang J-G, Thijs L. Cardiovascular protection and blood pressure reduction: A quantitative overview updated until 1 March 2003. *J Hypertens* 2003;21:1055–1076.)

protection, not the type of drug that provided the reduction in BP.

The only apparent exception, to be described in more detail in Chapter 7, is that β-blocker–based therapy has not been as protective against stroke as other drugs, despite equal reduction in BP (Carlberg et al., 2004).

In placebo-controlled trials of ACEIs, ARBs, and CCBs, published before 2003, the only apparent difference is lesser protection against heart failure by CCBs (Blood Pressure Lowering Treatment Trialists' Collaboration, 2003) (Fig. 5-4). Subsequent trials with the CCB amilodipine have shown better protective effects with this agent (Wang et al., 2007).

Trial Results: Special Populations

Trials in the Elderly with Isolated Systolic Hypertension

Although both the earlier and the later trials listed in Tables 5-2 and 5-3 include some elderly patients with ISH, defined in most of these trials as a systolic BP 160 mm Hg or higher with a diastolic BP below 95 mm Hg, the fact that such patients make up the largest portion of hypertensive patients now and will do so, to an even greater degree, in the future, justifies a closer, separate look at the data on their therapy. Staessen et al. (2000) have provided a meta-analysis of these trials, which are listed in Table 5-4.

	Trials	Events/Participants		Difference in BP (mean, mm Hg)	Relative Risk (95%)
		Drug	Placebo		
Stroke					
ACEI vs Placebo	5	473/9111	660/9118	-5/-2	0·72 (0·64-0·81)
CA vs Placebo	4	76/3794	119/3688	-8/-4	0·62 (0·47-0·82)
ARB vs Placebo	3	132/3461	141/2888	-3/-2	0·79 (0·63-0·99)
Coronary Heart Disease					
ACEI vs Placebo	5	667/9111	834/9118	-5/-2	0·80 (0·73-0·88)
CA vs Placebo	4	125/3794	156/3688	-8/-4	0·78 (0·62-0·99)
ARB vs Placebo	3	191/4183	177/3614	-3/-2	0·94 (0·77-1·14)
Heart Failure					
ACEI vs Placebo	5	219/8233	269/8246	-5/-2	0·82 (0·69-0·98)
CA vs Placebo	3	104/3382	88/3274	-8/-4	1·21 (0·93-1·58)
ARB vs Placebo	2	242/1655	240/1091	-3/-2	0·71 (0·60-0·83)
Major Cardiovascular Events					
ACEI vs Placebo	5	1283/9111	1648/9118	-5/-2	0·78 (0·73-0·83)
CA vs Placebo	3	280/3382	337/3274	-8/-4	0·82 (0·71-0·95)
ARB vs Placebo	3	755/3619	680/3111	-3/-2	0·96 (0·88-1·06)
Cardiovascular Death					
ACEI vs Placebo	5	488/9111	614/9118	-5/-2	0·80 (0·71-0·89)
CA vs Placebo	4	107/3382	135/3274	-8/-4	0·78 (0·61-1·00)
ARB vs Placebo	3	234/3359	198/2831	-3/-2	1·00 (0·83-1·20)
Total Mortality					
ACEI vs Placebo	5	839/9111	951/9118	-5/-2	0·88 (0·81-0·96)
CA vs Placebo	4	239/3794	263/3688	-8/-4	0·89 (0·75-1·05)
ARB vs Placebo	3	587/3787	514/3277	-3/-2	0·99 (0·89-1·11)

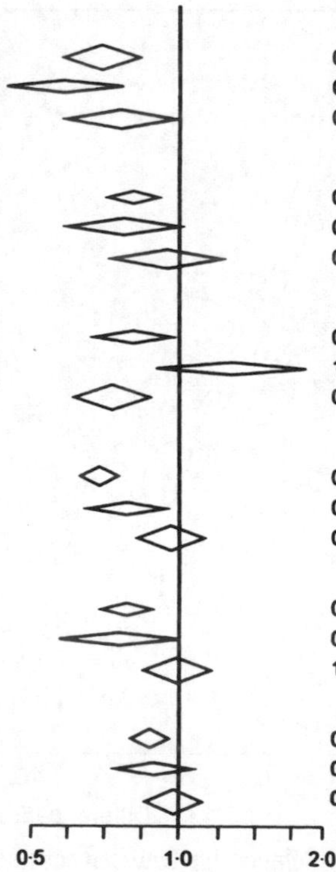

FIGURE 5-4 Comparisons of the effects of therapy based on ACEI, angiotensin converting enzyme inhibitor; CA, calcium antagonist; ARB, angiotensin II receptor blocker; and all versus placebo on cardiovascular events and mortality. (Modified from Blood Pressure Lowering Treatment Trialists' Collaboration. Effects of different blood-pressure-lowering regimens on major cardiovascular events: Results of prospectively-designed overviews of randomised trials. *Lancet* 2003;362: 1527–1535.)

TABLE 5.4	Randomized Placebo-Controlled Trials of Antihypertensive Drug Treatment in Elderly Patients with Isolated Systolic Hypertension above 160 mm Hg[a]				
Trial (Reference)	Number of Patients	Entry BP, mm Hg	Mean Age, years	Duration, years	Primary Drugs
EWPHE (Amery et al., 1985)	172	178/92	73	4.3	Diuretic
MRC-I (1985)	428	174/92	62	5.2	β-B/Diuretic
HEP (Coope & Warrender, 1985)	349	191/85	70	3.6	β-B
SHEP (1991)	4,736	170/77	72	4.4	Diuretic
STOP-H (Dahlöf et al., 1991)	268	194/91	76	1.9	β-B/Diuretic
MRC-II (1992)	2,651	182/83	70	6.1	β-B/Diuretic
Syst-Eur (Staessen et al., 1997)	4,695	174/85	70	2.0	CCB
Syst-China (Liu et al., 1998)	2,394	170/86	67	3.0	CCB

[a]Diagnosis of systolic hypertension based on systolic BP above 160, diastolic blood pressure below 95 mm Hg in all trials except SHEP, which required a diastolic blood pressure of ≤90 mm Hg.

β-B, beta-blocker; CCB, calcium channel blocker; EWPHE, European Working Party on Hypertension in the Elderly; MRC, Medical Research Council; SHEP, Systolic Hypertension in the Elderly Program; STOP-H, Swedish Trial in Old Patients with Hypertension; Syst-China, Systolic Hypertension in China trial; Syst-Eur, Systolic Hypertension in Europe trial.

Figure 5-5 summarizes the data from these eight trials of 15,693 elderly patients with ISH. The average BP at entry was 174/83 mm Hg and the mean fall in BP over the median 3.8-year follow-up was 10.4/4.1 mm Hg. Therapy significantly reduced all-cause and cardiovascular mortality by 13% and 18%, respectively, but had an even greater impact on morbidity: Coronary events were reduced by 23% and strokes by 30%.

In these trials, the absolute benefits of active therapy were greater in men, older patients, and those with prior cardiovascular complications, reflecting the higher initial risk status of such patients. To prevent one major cardiovascular event, the numbers of patients that needed to be treated for 5 years were 18 men versus 38 women, 19 patients who were 79 years or older versus 39 patients who were 60 to 69 years old, and 16 of those with prior cardiovascular complications versus 37 of those without (Staessen et al., 2000). Moreover, in a 15-year follow-up of a portion of the participants in the SHEP trial, a persistent reduction in fatal plus nonfatal cardiovascular events was found among the original drug-treated group compared to the placebo group, 58% versus 79%, despite the eventual use of antihypertensive therapy in 65% of the placebo group, compared to 72% of the active group (Sutton-Tyrrell et al., 2003).

As impressive as these data are, they must be recognized as covering only the higher range (Stage 2) of ISH, i.e., systolics of 160 mm Hg or higher, which has uniformly been the criterion for entry into the trials shown in Table 5-4 and Figure 5-5. Most ISH is between 140 and 159 mm Hg, and most premature cardiovascular events occur in patients in that range

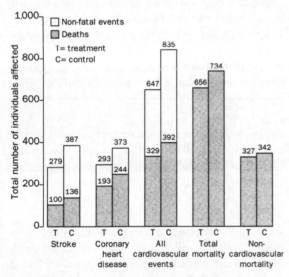

FIGURE 5-5 Summarized results in 15,693 older patients with isolated systolic hypertension above 160 mm Hg enrolled in eight trials of antihypertensive drug treatment. BP at entry averaged 174/83 mm Hg. During follow-up (median, 3.8 years), the mean difference in BP between the treated and control patients was 10.4 mm Hg systolic and 4.1 mm Hg diastolic. (Modified from Staessen JA, Gasowski J, Wang JG, et al. Risks of untreated and treated isolated systolic hypertension in the elderly. *Lancet* 2000;355:865–872.)

rather than in those with higher systolic BP (Chaudhry et al., 2004). As of now, there are no RCTs documenting the benefit for those with Stage 1 ISH.

Trials in Those over Age 80

Data are now available on the effect of therapy for patients over the age of 80 years, percentage-wise the fastest growing demographic group (Beckett et al., 2008). The Hypertension in the Very Elderly Trial (HYVET) included 3,845 hypertensives over age 80 with a sustained systolic BP of 160 mm Hg or higher. Their mean seated BP was 173/91 mm Hg. Half were assigned to placebo; the other half to active therapy, starting with the diuretic indapamide and adding the ACEI perindopril, if needed, to achieve the goal of 150 mm Hg. With the average additional decrease in BP of 15/6 mm Hg over placebo, the actively treated half achieved significantly greater protection against stroke, heart failure, and all-cause mortality after a median follow-up of only 1.8 years.

These impressive results are in keeping with the observation that older patients derive greater *absolute* benefit from any reduction in BP than do younger patients. As shown by Wang et al. (2005), the relative slopes of decreasing events with therapy are similar in the younger, older, and very old but since the older start at higher degrees of risk, they achieve a greater absolute benefit (Fig. 5-6). Wang et al. (2005) further show that the lowering of systolic pressure is the critical element of therapy, regardless of the magnitude of the fall in diastolic pressure.

The results of all published antihypertensive RCTs on major cardiovascular events in patients under age 65, and those 65 years and older (not including HYVET), show similar risk reductions (Table 5-5) (Blood Pressure Lowering Treatment Trialists' Collaboration, 2008). Thus, age per se is not a defining issue: Patients at any age with a reasonable life expectancy deserve antihypertensive therapy if their systolic BP is above 160 mm Hg.

The data in Table 5-5 cover RCTs with either an ACEI or CCB versus placebo. The trials with an ARB were not placebo controlled.

Trials in Women

In the various previously described trials, women achieve slightly less benefit from antihypertensive therapy than do men with similar levels of BP (Gueyffier et al., 1997). This reflects the lesser risk status for women than men, so they achieve less absolute benefit. However, when women with equal

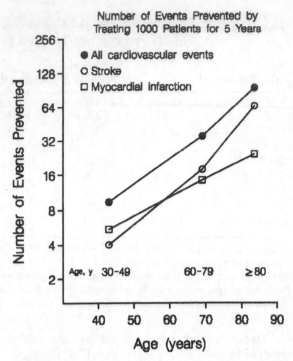

FIGURE 5-6 Absolute benefits in the prevention of fatal and nonfatal cardiovascular events, stroke, and myocardial infarction in three age-groups. Symbols represent the number of events that can be prevented by treating 1,000 patients for 5 years. (Modified from Wang J-G, Staessen JA, Franklin SS, et al. Systolic and diastolic blood pressure lowering as determinants of cardiovascular outcome on antihypertensive drug treatment. *Hypertension* 2005;45:907–913.)

degrees of risk as men are treated, they achieve virtually identical relative reductions in coronary disease and slightly greater protection against strokes (Gueyffier et al., 1997).

Trials in Blacks

BP in blacks responds less to renin-inhibiting drugs than it does in whites, and, in the ALLHAT trial, blacks on the ACEI lisinopril had more heart failure and strokes than those on the diuretic chlorthalidone (Wright et al., 2008).

Trials in Diabetic Patients

Ten RCTs have compared the effect of ACEIs (in four trials), ARBs (in two trials), or CCBs (in four trials) against placebo in hypertensives with, or without, diabetes (Table 5-6) (Blood Pressure Lowering Treatment Trialists' Collaboration, 2005). The greater falls in BP with active therapy were accompanied, in general,

| TABLE 5.5 | Mean Differences in Blood Pressure Between Randomized Groups in Younger and Older Adults |

Treatment comparison	Age <65 (n=96 466)		Age ≥ 65 (n=94 140)	
	Age (years)	Difference in SBP/DBP (mm Hg)	Age (years)	Difference in SBP/DBP (mm Hg)
ACE-I v placebo	57	−4.6/−2.1	70	−4.2/−2.0
CA v placebo	58	−7.2/−2.9	72	−9.3/−3.8
More v less*	57	−4.3/−3.5	70	−3.5/−3.4
ARB v other	56	−1.7/−0.3	75	−2.0/−1.2
ACE-I v D/BB	55	1.3/0.2	73	2.0/0.5
CA v D/BB	58	1.1/−0.2	72	0.5/−0.4
ACE-I v CA	59	0.9/0.6	73	1.0/1.0

SBP/DBP – systolic/diastolic blood pressure; ACE-I = angiotensin converting enzyme inhibitor; CA = calcium antagonist; ARB = angiotensin receptor blocker; D/BB = diuretic or β blocker.
*More v less intensive blood pressure lowering regimen.
(From Blood Pressure Lowering Treatment Trialists' collaboration. *BMJ* 2008;336:1121.)

| TABLE 5.6 | RCTs of Treatment of Hypertension with Diabetes |

Trials (number)	Difference in SBP/DBP, mm Hg	Relative Risk (95% CI)
Stroke		
ACEI vs. Placebo		
Diabetes (4)	−3.6/−1.9	0.69 (0.55–0.86)
No diabetes (4)	−5.8/−2.7	0.73 (0.62–0.85)
CCB vs. Placebo		
Diabetes (4)	−6.3/−3.0	0.47 (0.28–0.78)
No diabetes (3)	−6.2/−3.7	0.70 (0.49–0.99)
CHD		
ACEI vs. Placebo		
Diabetes (4)	−3.6/−1.9	0.91 (0.62–1.34)
No diabetes (4)	−5.8/−2.7	0.78 (0.69–0.88)
CCB vs. Placebo		
Diabetes (4)	−6.3/−3.0	1.00 (0.89–1.13)
No diabetes (3)	−9.2/−3.7	1.01 (0.93–1.10)
Heart Failure		
ACEI vs. Placebo		
Diabetes (4)	−3.6/−1.9	0.88 (0.67–1.16)
No diabetes (4)	−5.8/−2.7	0.78 (0.62–0.98)
CCB vs. Placebo		
Diabetes (3)	−5.9/−3.1	1.29 (0.97–1.72)
No diabetes (2)	−9.3/−3.9	1.07 (0.43–2.62)

Composed from Blood Pressure Lowering Treatment Trialists' Collaboration. Effects of different blood pressure-lowering regimens on major cardiovascular events in individuals with and without diabetes mellitus: Results of prospectively designed overviews of randomized trials. *Arch Intern Med* 2005;165:1410–1419.

with equal protection in the two groups against stroke, coronary disease, and, to a lesser degree, heart failure. In the two trials of diabetes with nephropathy, those treated with an ARB had slowing progression of renal damage (Berl et al., 2003; Brenner et al., 2001).

Trials in Cardiac Patients

In addition to the documentation that CHD morbidity and mortality have been significantly prevented by low-dose diuretics, CCBs, ACEIs, and ARBs reviewed earlier in this chapter (Figs. 5-2, 5-4), additional RCTs have examined the effect of antihypertensive agents in patients with preexisting coronary disease.

Angina and Coronary Disease

Nitrates, β-blockers, and CCBs had been used for many years on the basis of efficacy in reducing symptoms with little or no hard outcome data. More recently, trials of longer duration, and with adequate power, to provide hard outcome data have shown that the ACEIs ramipril (Heart Outcomes, 2000) and perindopril (European Trial on Reduction, 2003) reduce major cardiovascular events, whereas the CCB nifedipine GITS had no effect on survival (Poole-Wilson et al., 2004). However, the CAMELOT trial (Nissen et al., 2004) showed that a CCB, but not an ACEI, further protected patients with coronary artery disease (CAD) even when they were normotensive. Data are not available on the ability of antihypertensive therapy to protect patients who remain hypertensive after a myocardial infarction (Thune et al., 2008).

Congestive Heart Failure

Multiple trials, a few placebo-controlled and mostly of short duration, have shown reduction in hospitalizations and mortality in patients with chronic heart failure with diuretics, β-blockers, ACEIs, ARBs, aldosterone antagonists (Klein et al., 2003; Lee et al., 2004), and, in blacks, a combination of hydralazine and nitrate (Taylor et al., 2004).

Trials in Patients with Brain Disease
Stroke

A reduction in stroke events and mortality by treatment of hypertension has been clearly documented in patients initially free of cerebrovascular disease as well as in those with preexisting disease (Zhang et al., 2006). ARBs have been found to preserve cerebral blood flow in poststroke patients which could add to their safety (Moriwaki et al., 2004). In the PROGRESS trial, an ACEI alone did not reduce the stroke recurrence, but the addition of a diuretic did (PROGRESS, 2001). CCBs and low doses of diuretics may be most efficacious, but all classes, except β-blockers, protect against stroke equally (Papadopoulos & Papademetriou, 2008).

Along with antihypertensive therapy, reduction of blood cholesterol with statins has provided another 21% reduction in stroke incidence in high-risk patients (Heart Protection Study, 2004) and a 27% reduction in hypertensives (Sever et al., 2003), an effect which may be greater than expected from the fall in BP usually seen with statin therapy (Ferrier et al., 2002).

Cognitive Function

In observational studies, antihypertensive therapy preserves cognitive function (Staessen et al., 2007). The only specific drug that has been shown in a RCT to prevent dementia is the CCB nitrendipine in the Syst-Eur trial (McGuinness et al., 2008).

An Overview of the Benefits of Therapy

Despite all of the preceding evidence that treatment of hypertension reduces cardiovascular disease, the overall role of antihypertensive therapy in the impressive falls in coronary and stroke mortality seen in most developed societies over the past 40 years turns out to be rather small. Recall from Chapter 1 that the best available evidence gives the treatment of hypertension only 3% and population-wide lowering of BP 9.5% of the credit for the 62% decline in men and the 45% decline in women in coronary mortality in England and Wales between 1981 and 2000 (Unal et al., 2004).

The reasons for this limited role are multiple, including:

- Poor rates of adequate control of hypertension, in turn related to the basic nature of the condition and the inadequacies of current management.
- Inadequate attention to concomitant risk factors, leaving a large residual of risk even among those treated (Blacher et al., 2004).
- Too high levels of BP, both for initiation of therapy and for the goals of therapy, according to the recognition that risk increases above 115/75 mm Hg.
- Inability to provide effective preventive therapy, before the inexorable progress of hypertension-related complications.

These issues and others are addressed in the remainder of this chapter and in Chapter 7, but first we will examine one of the more attractive aspects of treating hypertension, namely its cost-effectiveness.

Cost-Effectiveness of Treating Hypertension

The treatment of hypertension is among the most cost-effective measures now available for preventing avoidable death. Using various mathematical modeling techniques and Markov decision analyses, most recent estimates find that treatment of hypertension provides additional quality-adjusted life-years (QALYs) for a far lower cost than treatment of dyslipidemia or diabetes. Perhaps the best analysis of the cost-effectiveness of various therapies has been provided by the CDC Diabetes Cost-Effectiveness Group (2002) who estimate these costs of one QALY in type 2 diabetic patients: $41,384 for intensive glycemic control; $51,889 for reduction in serum cholesterol; and a positive + $1,959 for intensive control of hypertension. The reduction in cost reflects the decrease in money spent for care of the various complications provided by intensive control for hypertension.

These cost-effectiveness estimates often assume the use of the least expensive forms of therapy. With the current JNC-7 recommendations to start most patients with a low-dose diuretic and to use other medications as needed for various compelling indications, Fischer and Avorn (2004) project a savings of about $1.2 billion in the United States alone.

Such less expensive choices could obviously save the health care system money but the seemingly insatiable desire of both practitioners and patients to mainly use those brand name products that are so heavily advertised on TV and in print will continue to inflate U.S. drug costs.

Although the concept of a polypill containing a statin, three antihypertensives, aspirin, and folic acid to be given to everyone over age 55 and everyone with existing cardiovascular disease (Wald & Law, 2003) may seem far-fetched, but the increasing need for inexpensive but effective preventive therapies may bring such a strategy to fruition (Law et al., 2009).

Potential Constraints on Treatment of Hypertension

Such issues of cost-effectiveness may seem remote and almost irrelevant to those who care for hypertensive patients. However, there are three reasons for everyone to pay attention to such issues. First, there are unintended risks of continued growth of medical care

under the assumption that more is better, particularly in an increasingly fatter and older population (Fisher & Welch, 1999). Second, financial constraints are being imposed everywhere on health care, so the decision to treat hypertension may need to be based on cost-effectiveness. Third, worldwide inequalities in health care are widening and availability of less costly but effective care is essential to overcome these inequalities (Gwatkin et al., 2004).

On the surface, the United States seems to be the exception, as health care spending will soon reach $2.2 trillion and, if current trends continue, will consume 25% of the gross national product by the year 2030 (Blumenthal, 2001). Even in the United States, however, the need to constrain the growth of the major federally financed programs Medicare and Medicaid is being recognized, particularly with the rapid growth in the number of people older than 65 years of age (American College of Physicians, 2008). And, although the political will to provide universal health care coverage has only recently come forth, attention paid to the 45 million people in the United States who have no health insurance will increase the overall cost of health care, at least in the beginning of coverage.

As these constraints increase, a collision may occur between the inherent desire to expand the number of hypertensive people under treatment and the societal need to limit health care expenditures. The late Swales (2000), who served in the United Kingdom government for 3 years, wrote of this issue:

> The success of science has created painful dilemmas for health care across the world, whether funded through taxation or private insurance. A gap is opening up between aspiration and affordability. The treatment of hypertension provides an illuminating example of the problems this creates for clinical practice. These lead inevitably to social and political issues.
>
> The continuous gradient of risk associated with blood pressure implies that the benefits of reversing that risk will also be continuous. The lower the blood pressure level at which treatment is recommended, the smaller the probability of the individual benefiting and the greater the number of patients eligible for treatment. There is a continuous, inverse relationship between individual benefit and the total cost of health care. At some point a decision has to be made that the cost of treating a low level of risk is not justified.... The final decision concerning treatment clearly cannot be independent of the resources made available for treatment either by governments or private healthcare funders.

Treatment of a hypertensive patient has to take place in the real world of constrained healthcare systems.... Excluding the social dimension can lead to serious errors and can weaken the case for more resources to be put into treating disorders such as hypertension. The cost of treating a large proportion of the population may be high, but the cost of not treating hypertension in terms of both hospital and social care is also high. The combined hospital and social care costs of treating stroke in England is 4 times the cost of managing hypertension, and there is actually a net return to society as a result of treating elderly hypertensives in terms of reduced indirect healthcare costs.

Constraints on the treatment of hypertension should be fairly easily resisted, because such a treatment has been shown to be beneficial at costs that are low in comparison to most other therapies. As the demand for evidence-based medicine has grown, the treatment of hypertension stands as one of the prime examples wherein conclusive evidence is available for cost-effectiveness. At the same time, the critical decision as to when to institute therapy has been more rationally defined.

WHEN SHOULD DRUG THERAPY BE STARTED?

Before addressing the question, "When should drug therapy be started?" one caveat must always be recalled: An initially elevated BP, above 140 mm Hg systolic or 90 mm Hg diastolic, must always be remeasured at least three times over at least 4 weeks to ensure that hypertension is present. Only if the level is very high (>180/110 mm Hg) or if symptomatic target organ damage is present should therapy be begun before the diagnosis is carefully established.

On the other hand, in view of the risks of even "high-normal" BP (Vasan et al., 2001), therapy in the future may be indicated for many more patients even without hypertension as currently defined.

Problems with Past Guidelines

In the past, guidelines for the institution of therapy have been based solely on the level of BP, giving rise to major irrationalities and inconsistencies. As noted by Jackson et al. (1993):

This has led to the situation in which a 60-year-old woman with a diastolic BP of 100 mm Hg but no other risk factors (her absolute risk of cardiovascular disease is

about 10% in 10 years) may meet the criteria for treatment, whereas a 70-year-old man with multiple risk factors but a diastolic BP of 95 mm Hg (his absolute risk is about 50% in 10 years) may not. The treatment of these two patients would be expected to reduce the absolute risk in the 60-year-old woman by nearly 3% in 10 years (30% of 10%) but in the 70-year-old man by approximately 17% (30% of 50%).

Guidelines Using Overall Risk

The situation has recently changed dramatically for the better with widespread acceptance of targeting treatment rationally on absolute cardiovascular risk rather than arbitrarily on certain levels of BP (Jackson et al., 2005). The change has been spurred on by numerous factors, including these:

• The repeated presentation of cardiovascular risk profiles covering the entire adult population from the phenomenally productive Framingham Heart Study (Kannel & Wolf, 2008). The Framingham bar graph surely is recognized everywhere (Fig. 5-7).
• The presentation of relatively simple, easily used nomograms that translate the concept of risk assessment into a practical method (Jackson et al., 2005; Mendis et al., 2007) (Fig. 5-8). Increasingly, computers are being used to make the individual patient's overall risk assessment and provide guidance on therapeutic choices (Roberts et al., 2008).
• The recognition that simpler measures of risk, not requiring laboratory testing, are as accurate as those that do (Gaziano et al., 2008; Montalvo et al., 2008).
• The awareness that 90% or more of patients with coronary disease have multiple risk factors with hypertension being first or second in prevalence in various populations (Greenland et al., 2003; Khot et al., 2003).

Problems with Current Assessments

As will be seen, different expert committees that have recently issued national and international guidelines differ in their modes of assessing risk and the level of risk they use as criteria for treatment, in part because the Framingham-based profiles have been found to overestimate the risk in populations outside the United States (Brindle et al., 2003).

Efforts to improve the accuracy of risk assessments have been advanced. These include the addition of testing for microalbuminuria, carotid intima-media thickness by ultrasound, and left ventricular mass index by echocardiography (Task Force, 2007).

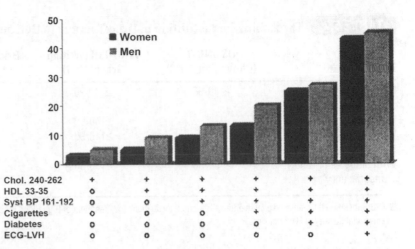

FIGURE 5-7 Risk of CHD in subjects with serum cholesterol level of 240 to 262 mg/dL by level of other risk factors. Subjects were 42 to 43 years old in the Framingham Study. (Modified from Kannel, et al. *Am Heart J* 2004;148:17.)

Only microalbuminuria has been added to recent guidelines, the others are considered to be too expensive for routine use and provide no additional accuracy (Wang et al., 2006).

Current Guidelines

The guidelines from four expert committees published since 2003 have based the decision to start active drug therapy in those with BP of less than 140/90 mm Hg on the degree of overall cardiovascular risk (Table 5-7). The British guidelines (Williams et al., 2004a,b) continue to be more conservative, recommending drug treatment in those with BP between 140–159/90–99 only if there is a target organ damage, cardiovascular complications, diabetes, or 10-year risk of cardiovascular disease greater than 20%.

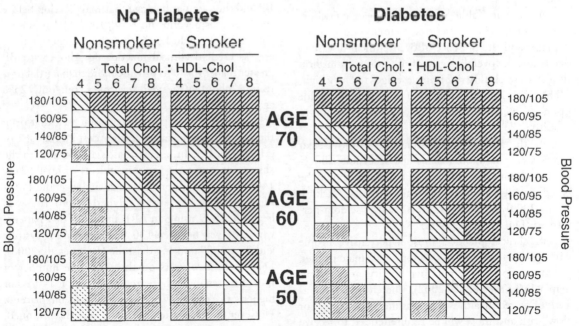

FIGURE 5-8 Risk levels for men at varying ages and levels of BP according to the presence or absence of diabetes, smoking, and various levels of the ratio between total and high-density lipoprotein (HDL) cholesterol (chol). Risk of cardiovascular event in 5 years shown by *stippled squares*, 2.5% to 5.0%; *closely hatched squares*, 5% to 10%; *open squares*, 10% to 15%; *widely hatched squares*, 15% to 20%; and *medium-hatched squares*, greater than 20%. (Modified from Core Service Committee. *Guidelines for the Management of Mildly Raised Blood Pressure in New Zealand.* Wellington, New Zealand: National Health Committee, 1995.)

TABLE 5.7	**Thresholds for Institution of Drug Therapy in Current Guidelines**			
Level of Risk	**US JNC-7 (Chobanian, 2003)**	**WHO-ISH (Writing Group, 2003)**	**British (Williams et al., 2004a,b)**	**European (Task Force, 2007)**
No target organ damage or risk factors	≥140/90	≥140/90	≥160/100	≥140/90
With risk factors		≥140/90	≥140/90	≥140/90
With target organ damage		≥140/90	≥140/90	≥140/90
With diabetes or renal insufficiency	≥130/80	≥130/80	≥140/90	≥130/85

JNC, Joint National Committee on Prevention, Detection, Evaluation, and Treatment of High Blood Pressure; WHO-ISH, World Health Organization-International Society of Hypertension.

Remarkably, all four guidelines now agree that drug therapy should be started at 140/90 if risk factors or target organ damage is present, and all but the British recommend therapy for patients with diabetes or renal insufficiency at 130/80 (US, WHO-ISH) or 130/85 (Task Force, 2007).

All but the U.S. JNC-7 continue to use overall risk assessment in determining the threshold to start therapy. The failure of JNC-7 to utilize even a crude profile will almost certainly be corrected in the new JNC-8 Report.

As seen in Table 5-8, the European guidelines (Task Force, 2007) use risk factors, target organ damage, and the presence of overt clinical disease to determine the overall degree of risk, using a stratification chart to classify risk from "average" to "very high" (Table 5-9). In turn, the level of risk is used to decide upon the need to begin therapy or to continue to monitor.

As the ability to determine the cardiovascular risk has become more reliable and accessible, all recommendations for initiation of therapy should be based on a quantitative assessment of risk (Jackson et al., 2009), although in practice, it is seldom performed (Ducher et al., 2008).

In clinical practice, most hypertensive people will have at least two risk factors, e.g., male gender, age above 55 years, abdominal obesity, and dyslipidemia (Muntner et al., 2002). Therefore, few paragons of perfect health will be classified at "average" or "low" risk and most will be recommended to receive therapy at or above 140/90.

Should the Threshold Be Lower?

As seen in Table 5-7, all current guidelines recommend antihypertensive drug therapy for patients with BP below the traditional definition of hypertension of 140/90 if they have a high overall risk status, particularly in patients with diabetes or renal insufficiency. Arguments have been made for a conservative approach to the use of active drug therapy for "mild," low-risk hypertensives (Rose, 1981).

However, as easier to take and more effective drugs have become available, some have argued that they be given to people who are not yet hypertensive in an attempt to prevent both the onset of elevated BP and the vascular damage that may develop before the level goes beyond the 140/90 mm Hg threshold. The rationale includes the inability of current therapy, as used in clinical practice, for those with BP greater than 140/90 to provide more than partial protection, about 40% against strokes, but only 25% against heart disease.

Stevo Julius, in particular, has argued that drug therapy should be started earlier despite the lack of evidence of benefit, a lack that is attributable to the absence of long-term trials in subjects with BP below 140/90 mm Hg. To provide such evidence, the TROPHY (Trial of Preventing Hypertension) trial was begun in 1999 using an ARB in half of 809 patients whose BP was between 130 and 139 mm Hg systolic and 85 and 89 mm Hg diastolic (Julius et al., 2006). During the two years on the ARB, the number of those progressing to hypertension, i.e., BP 140/90 or higher, was 66% lower than in those on placebo. However, 2 years after the ARB was discontinued, there was only a 16% lesser onset of hypertension in the previously tested group compared to the placebo group.

The average age of the TROPHY participants was 48 years. If the spontaneously hypertensive rat (SHR) can be considered a model of human

TABLE 5.8	**Factors Influencing Prognosis**
Risk Factors	**Target Organ Damage (TOD)**
• Systolic and diastolic BP levels	• Electrocardiographic LVH
• Levels of pulse pressure (in the elderly)	• Echocardiographic LVH
• Age	• Carotid wall thickening (IMT > 0.9 mm) or plaque
• Smoking	• Carotid-femoral pulse wave velocity > 12 m/s
• Dyslipidemia	• Ankle/brachial BP index < 0.9
• TC > 5.0 mmol/L (190 mg/dl) or	• Sight increase in plasma creatinine:
• LDL-C > 3.0 mmol/L (115 mg/dL) or	M: 115–133 µmol/L (1.3–1.5 mg/dL);
• HDL C: M < 1.0 mmol/L (40 mg/dL), W < 1.2 mmol/L (46 mg/dL) or	W: 107–124 µmol/L (1.2–1.4 mg/dL)
• TG > 1.7 mmol/L (150 mg/dL)	• Low estimated glomerular filtration rate (<60 mL/min/1.73 m²)
• Fasting plasma glucose 5.6–6.9 mmol/L (102–125 mg/dL)	• Microalbuminuria 30–300 mg/24 h
• Abnormal glucose tolerance test	***ESTABLISHED CARDIOVASCULAR OR RENAL DISEASE***
• Diabetes Mellitus	
• Abdominal obesity [Waist circumference > 102 cm (M), >88 cm (W)]	• Cerebrovascular disease: ischemic stroke; cerebral hemorrhage; transient ischemic attack
• Family history of premature CV disease	• Heart disease: myocardial infarction; angina; coronary revascularization; heart failure
• Family history of premature CV disease (M at age < 55 years; W at age < 65 years)	• Renal disease: renal impairment (serum creatinine M > 133, W > 124 mmol/L); proteinuria (>300 mg, 24 h)
	• Peripheral artery disease
	• Advance retinopathy: hemorrhages or exudates, papilledema

M, men; W, women; CV, cardiovascular disease; IMT, intima-media thickness; BP, blood pressure; TG, triglycerides; C, cholesterol; LVH, left ventricular hypertrophy.

hypertension, antihypertensive therapy must be given early in adolescence to prevent the future development of hypertension when they mature (Harrap et al., 1990). Therefore, to prevent the future development of hypertension, the antihypertensive drug would need to be given at a much earlier age, likely making such a study impractical, if not unethical.

Thresholds for Higher Risk Patients

As seen in Table 5-7, all current guidelines, save the British, recommend lower thresholds for initiation of drug therapy in patients with diabetes or chronic kidney disease (CKD). The increased risk of hypertensive

cardiovascular and renal damage in both diabetic and CKD patients is certain, based on large amounts of observational data (Jafar et al., 2003; Vijan & Hayward, 2003) and experimental evidence (Bidani & Griffin, 2004). But the database for recommending considerably lower BP levels for the institution of drug therapy is sparse and unconvincing (Zanchetti et al., 2009). Most of the repeatedly quoted data supporting the lower threshold do not, in fact, show what is claimed. In particular:

• For diabetes, the evidence comes from the UKPDS trial (1998) wherein better protection was seen at an achieved BP of 144/82 compared to 154/87 and from the HOT trial (Hansson et al., 1998) wherein

TABLE 5.9	Stratification of Risk to Quantify Prognosis				

	Blood Pressure, mm Hg				
Other Risk Factors and Disease History	Normal SBP 120–129 or DBP 80–84	Highnormal SBP 130–139 or DBP 85–89	Grade 1 SBP 140–159 or DBP 90–99	Grade 2 SBP 160–179 or DBP 100–109	Grade 3 SBP ≥ 180 or DBP ≥ 110
No other risk factors	Average risk	Average risk	Low added risk	Moderate added risk	High added risk
One to two risk factors	Low added risk	Low added risk	Moderate added risk	Moderate added risk	Very high added risk
Three or more risk factors or TOD or diabetes	Moderate added risk	High added risk	High added risk	High added risk	Very high added risk
ACC	High added risk	Very high added risk	Very high added risk	Very high added risk	Very high added risk

ACC, associated clinical conditions; TOD, target organ damage; SBP, systolic blood pressure; DBP, diastolic blood pressure. (Modified from Guidelines Committee, 2003. European society of Hypertension-European society of Cardiology guidelines for the management of arterrial hypertension. *J Hypertens* 2003;21:1011–1053)

better protection was seen at an achieved BP of 140/81 compared to 144/85 mm Hg.

• For chronic renal disease, the evidence comes largely from the MDRD trial, wherein better protection was seen *only in those CKD patients with proteinuria* greater than 1.0 g per day but not in those with less proteinuria at an achieved BP of about 125/75 compared to 135/82 (Peterson et al., 1995). Additional studies, though not designed to address the issue of the threshold for therapy but which provide data on the risk for progression of CKD by levels of achieved BP, found protection below 130 mm Hg only in those with proteinuria greater than 1.0 g per day and no added protection from systolics as high as 160 down to less than 110 for those with less proteinuria (Jafar et al., 2003) (Fig. 5-9). Furthermore, in the African American Study of Kidney (AASK) Disease and Hypertension, no additional benefit for the slowing of progression of hypertensive nephrosclerosis was seen with an achieved BP of 128/78 than with an achieved BP of 141/85 (Wright et al., 2002).

The preceding is not intended to deny the value of starting higher risk patients such as those with CKD or diabetes at lower levels of BP and pushing them to below that level with drug therapy. However, more widespread institution of therapy costs money and can induce side effects. We obviously need more data as noted in JNC-7 which observed that "available data are somewhat sparse to justify the lower target level of 130/80 mm Hg" (Chobanian et al., 2003b).

Patients with Coronary Artery Disease

On the other hand, the use of a lower threshold even below those now recommended for patients with target organ damage (Table 5-7) has been supported in an RCT, the CAMELOT study, of over 2,000 patients with preexisting CAD (Nissen et al., 2004). These patients were normotensive, average BP = 129/78. Most were receiving aspirin, β-blockers, and a statin and, for those 60% with prior hypertension, one or more antihypertensive drugs. They were randomly assigned to placebo, amlodipine, or enalapril. After a mean follow-up of 2.2 years, both drugs lowered BP by an average of 4.8/2.5 mm Hg. The number of cardiovascular events was significantly reduced (by 31%) but only in those who received the CCB.

Largely based on the CAMELOT data plus some experimental evidence, the 2007 Scientific Statement from the American Heart Association (Rosendorff et al., 2007) recommends a target below 130/80 for patients at high CHD risk, including those with stable angina. The statement further recommends consideration of a goal below 120/80 for patients with left ventricular dysfunction.

Overall Management

The bottom line is this: Most hypertensives have fairly mild, asymptomatic hypertension and the benefits of treatment—measured as the reduction of hard end points—progressively decline the milder the degree of hypertension. Many patients receive relatively little benefit yet are exposed both

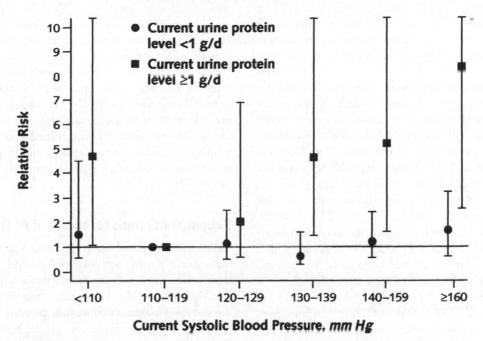

FIGURE 5-9   The relative risk for CKD progression in patients with a current urine protein excretion of 1.0 g per day or greater represents 9,336 patients (223 events), and the relative risk for patients with a current urine excretion less than 1.0 g per day represents 13,274 patients (88 events). The reference group for each is defined at a systolic BP of 110 to 119 mm Hg. CIs are truncated, as shown. (Modified from Jafar TH, Stark PC, Schmid CH, et al. Progression of chronic kidney disease: The role of blood pressure control, proteinuria, and angiotensin-converting enzyme inhibition: A patient-level meta-analysis. *Ann Intern Med* 2003;139:244–252.).

to the adverse side effects and to the fairly large financial costs of therapy. Therefore, for maximal patient benefit, a management strategy based on overall risk is rational and appropriate. On the other hand, those at higher degrees of risk likely achieve better protection when treated at lower levels of BP. The situation would obviously change if and when the earlier use of antihypertensive drug therapy is shown to prevent the progression of BP and cardiovascular damage in those with BPs lower than the currently accepted lower threshold for institution of therapy.

Now that the rationale for the institution of therapy has been described, let us turn to the issue of how far to lower the pressure.

GOAL OF THERAPY

Logically, the goal of therapy should be to lower BP below the threshold for starting therapy. Until recently, the general attitude was "the lower, the better." However, a number of factors have led to a more cautious approach, including the following:

• The progressively lower threshold for instituting therapy, previously as high as 160/110 mm Hg, now as low as 130/80 mm Hg for some patients.
• The inclusion of elderly patients with ISH and, by definition, low diastolic BP and the recognition that very low diastolic BP may be associated with increased risk whether occurring naturally or induced by therapy (Messerli et al., 2006).
• Perhaps most important, concerns over the possible existence of a J-curve for both systolic and diastolic BP, i.e., a reduction in risk as BP is lowered down to some critical level that is inadequate to maintain perfusion of vital organs, resulting in an increased risk as the pressure is lowered further (Sleight et al., 2009).

Evidence for a J-Curve

An association between reduction of BP and ischemic injury was first suggested by Stewart (1979), who reported a fivefold increase in myocardial infarction among patients whose diastolic BP was reduced to less than 90 mm Hg (Korotkoff, phase 4). Stewart's report was largely neglected until Cruickshank et al. (1987) reported the same phenomenon.

A number of long-term studies in patients with diastolic hypertension have evaluated the incidence of cardiovascular complications according to the mean in-study diastolic BP. Rather than demonstrating a progressive benefit at lower pressures, many of these trials have shown a J-curve in which the risk of cardiac events declines as the diastolic pressure falls from more than 100 to 85 mm Hg but then the risk rises back up at diastolic pressures below 70 to 75 mg Hg (Fagard et al., 2007; Messerli et al., 2006; Protogerou et al., 2007). In all three of these series, the increase in cardiovascular events occurred only in patients with preexisting CAD who logically would be most vulnerable to a further reduction in perfusion. In patients with isolated systolic hypertension who start with a diastolic below 90, an increase in stroke has been retrospectively recognized in those whose diastolic pressures were reduced by therapy to below 65 mm Hg (Somes et al., 1999; Vokó et al., 1999). Weiner et al. (2007) found an increase in strokes when systolic pressure was lowered below 120 mm Hg in patients with CKD and Sleight et al. (2009) an increase in CV mortality with further lowering of systolic BP in those with baseline systolic BP below 130 mm Hg.

In addition, apparent J-curves have been reported in the smokers enrolled in the HOT trial (Zanchetti et al., 2003), patients in the IDNT trial of diabetic nephropathy (Pohl et al., 2005), and in elderly subjects followed for the development of dementia (van Dijk et al., 2004).

Evidence Against a J-Curve

Cruickshank's concept has not gone unchallenged. In particular, questions have been raised as to the exactness of the critical level at which the break in the curve appears and the relatively few events that make up the curves (Hansson, 2000). Moreover, a decrease in coronary events has been seen in patients with left ventricular dysfunction whose initially low diastolic pressures were reduced even further by ACEI therapy, well below the break of 85 to 90 mm Hg in the J-curve (Yusuf et al., 1992), as well as in the patients with CAD starting at a BP of 129/78 (Nissen et al., 2004) who were given a CCB. Patients with preexisting cerebrovascular disease had the greatest protection against recurrence if the systolic BP was reduced below 120 mm Hg (Arima et al., 2006). As suggested in data on post-MI patients, the J-curve was assumed to reflect a decreased left ventricular function (Thune et al., 2008).

The validity of this interpretation has been supported by the meta-analysis of individual patient data from 40,233 subjects in seven RCTs (Boutitie et al., 2002). Their meticulous analysis is concluded thusly: "The increased risk for events observed in patients with low blood pressure was not related to antihypertensive treatment and was not specific to blood pressure-related events. Poor health conditions leading to low blood pressure and an increased risk for death probably explain the J-curve".

Recommendations for the Goal of Therapy

The optimal goal of antihypertensive therapy in most patients with combined systolic and diastolic hypertension who were not at high risk is a BP of less than 140/90 mm Hg. The greatest benefit is likely derived from lowering the diastolic pressure to 80 to 85 mm Hg. Not only is there no proved benefit with more intensive control, but also there is an added cost and probable increased side effects associated with more intensive antihypertensive therapy.

In elderly patients with ISH, the goal should be a systolic BP of 140 to 150 mm Hg, the level reached in the RCTs wherein benefit was shown (Becket et al., 2008). Caution is advised if, inadvertently, diastolic pressures fall below 65 mm Hg. In such an event, less-than-ideal reductions in systolic levels need to be balanced against the potential of harm if diastolic levels fall below that level.

More intensive therapy to attain a systolic pressure below 140 and/or a diastolic pressure below 90 may be desirable in some groups, including the following:

- Black patients, who are at greater risk for hypertensive complications and who may continue to have progressive renal damage despite a diastolic pressure of 85 to 90 mm Hg.
- Patients with diabetes mellitus, in whom a BP of less than 140/80 mm Hg reduces the incidence of cardiovascular events (Hansson et al., 1998).
- Patients with slowly progressive chronic renal disease excreting more than 1 g of protein per day, in whom reducing the BP to 125/75 mm Hg may slow the rate of loss of renal function (Lazarus et al., 1997).
- Patients with coronary disease, if more evidence supports their additional benefit with a BP of 125/75 (Nissen et al., 2004).

The Overriding Need: Adequate Therapy

Despite the concerns over a J-curve, we should not lose sight of the fact that the reason for the lesser protection found among most treated hypertensives reflects undertreatment, not overtreatment. Clearly, it is essential that all patients have their systolic BP brought down to 140 mm Hg and their diastolic BP to the 80- to 85-mm Hg range to provide the demonstrated benefits of therapy.

Importance of Population Strategies

Most of our current efforts are directed at the individual patient with existing hypertension. Clearly, we also need to advise the larger population to do those things that may protect against the development of hypertension, an approach directed toward the "sick populations" rather than only the sick individuals. At this time, such population strategies should not involve medications but rather should be based on lifestyle modifications. The next chapter describes these modifications.

REFERENCES

Adler AI, Stratton IM, Neil HAW, et al. Association of systolic blood pressure with macrovascular and microvascular complications of type 2 diabetes (UKPDS 36). *Br Med J* 2000;321: 412–419.

Alderman MH, Furberg CD, Kostis JB et al. Hypertension guidelines: criteria that might make them more clinically useful. *Am J Hypertens* 2002;15:917–923.

American College of Physicians. Information on cost-effectiveness: An essential product of a national comparative effectiveness program. *Ann Intern Med* 2008;148:956–961.

Amery A, Birkenhäger W, Brixko P, et al. Mortality and morbidity from the European Working Party on high blood pressure in the elderly trial. *Lancet* 1985;1:1350–1354.

Arima H, Chalmers J, Woodward M, et al. Lower target blood pressures are safe and effective for the prevention of recurrent stroke: The PROGRESS trial. *J Hypertens* 2006;24:1201–1208.

Asayama K, Ohkubo T, Yoshida S et al. Stroke risk and antihypertensive drug treatment in the general population: the Japan arteriosclerosis longitudinal study. *J Hypertens* 2009;27:357–364.

Barraclough M, Joy MD, MacGregor GA, et al. Control of moderately raised blood pressure. *BMJ* 1973;3:434–436.

Beckett NS, Peters R, Fletcher AE, et al. Treatment of hypertension in patients 80 years of age or older. *N Engl J Med* 2008;358: 1887–1898.

Berl T, Hunsicker LG, Lewis JB, et al. Cardiovascular outcomes in the Irbesartan Diabetic Nephropathy Trial of patients with type 2 diabetes and overt nephropathy. *Ann Intern Med* 2003; 138:542–549.

Bidani AK, Griffin KA. Pathophysiology of hypertensive renal damage: Implications for therapy. *Hypertension* 2004;44:595–601.

Blacher J, Evans A, Arveiler D, et al. Residual coronary risk in men aged 50-59 years treated for hypertension and hyperlipidemia in the population: The PRIME study. *J Hypertens* 2004;22: 415–423.

Blood Pressure Lowering Treatment Trialists' Collaboration. Effects of different blood-pressure-lowering regimens on major cardiovascular events: Results of prospectively-designed overviews of randomised trials. *Lancet* 2003;362:1527–1535.

Blood Pressure Lowering Treatment Trialists' Collaboration. Effects of different blood pressure-lowering regimens on major cardiovascular events in individuals with and without diabetes mellitus: Results of prospectively designed overviews of randomized trials. *Arch Intern Med* 2005;165:1410–1419.

Blood Pressure Lowering Treatment Trialist Collaboration. Effects of different regimens to lower blood pressure on major cardiovascular events in older and younger adults: Meta-analysis of randomised trials. *Br Med J* 2008;336:1121–1123.

Blumenthal D. Controlling health care expenditures. *N Engl J Med* 2001;344:766–769.

Boutitie F, Gueyffier F, Pocock S, et al. J-shaped relationship between blood pressure and mortality in hypertensive patients: New insights from a meta-analysis of individual-patient data. *Ann Intern Med* 2002;136:438–448.

Brenner BM, Cooper ME, de Zeeuw D, et al. Effects of losartan on renal and cardiovascular outcomes in patients with type 2 diabetes and nephropathy. *N Engl J Med* 2001;345:861–869.

Brindle P, Emberson J, Lampe F, et al. Predictive accuracy of the Framingham coronary risk score on British men: Prospective cohort study. *Br Med J* 2003;327:1238–1239.

Campbell NC, Murchie P. Treating hypertension with guidelines in general practice: Patients decide how low they can go, not targets. *Br Med J* 2004;329:523–524.

Carlberg B, Samuelsson O, Lindholm LH. Atenolol in hypertension: Is it a wise choice? *Lancet* 2004;364:1684–1689.

Carter AB. Hypotensive therapy in stroke survivors. *Lancet* 1970; 1:485–489.

Cashin-Hemphill L, Holmvang G, Chan R, et al. Angiotensin converting enzyme inhibition as antiatherosclerotic therapy. *Am J Cardiol* 1999;83:43–47.

Chan A-W, Hróbjartsson A, Haahr MT, et al. Empirical evidence for selective reporting of outcomes in randomized trials: Comparison of protocols to published articles. *JAMA* 2004;291: 2457–2465.

Chaudhry SI, Krumholz HM, Foody JM. Systolic hypertension in older persons. *JAMA* 2004;292:1074–1080.

Chobanian AV. Adaptive and maladaptive responses of the arterial wall to hypertension. *Hypertension* 1990;15:666–674.

Chobanian AV, Haudenschild CC, Nickerson C, et al. Trandolapril inhibits atherosclerosis in the Watanabe heritable hyperlipidemic rabbit. *Hypertension* 1992;20:473–477.

Chobanian AV, Bakris GL, Black HR, et al. The seventh report of the Joint National Committee on Prevention, Detection, Evaluation, and Treatment of High Blood Pressure: The JNC-7 report. *JAMA* 2003a;289:2560–2572.

Chobanian AV, Bakris GL, Black HR, et al. Seventh report of the Joint National Committee on Prevension, Detection, Evaluation, and Treatment of High Blood Pressure. *Hypertension* 2003b;42:1206–1252.

Collins R, MacMahon S. Blood pressure, antihypertensive drug treatment and the risks of stroke and coronary heart disease. *Br Med Bull* 1994;50:272–298.

Cook RJ, Sackett DL. The number needed to treat: A clinically useful measure of treatment effect. *Br Med J* 1995;310: 452–454.

Coope J, Warrender TS. Randomised trial of treatment of hypertension in elderly patients in primary care. *BMJ (Clin Res Ed)* 1987;294(6565):179.

Cruickshank JM, Thorp JM, Zacharias FJ. Benefits and potential harm of lowering high blood pressure. *Lancet* 1987;1: 581–584.

Dahlöf B, Lindholm LH, Hansson L, et al. Morbidity and mortality in the Swedish Trial in Old Patients with Hypertension (STOP-Hypertension). *Lancet* 1991;338:1281–1285.

Demaerschalk BM. Literature-searching strategies to improve the application of evidence-based clinical practice principles to stroke care. *Mayo Clin Proc* 2004;79:1321–1329.

Ducher M, Juillard C, Leutenegger E, et al. Major cardiovascular risk factors are not taken into account by physicians when targeting blood pressure values for uncontrolled hypertensive patients. *Am J Hypertens* 2008;21:1264–1268.

Eriksson S, Olofsson BO, Webster PO, for the TEST Study Group. Atenolol in secondary prevention after stroke. *Cerebrovasc Dis* 1995;5:21–25.

European Trial on Reduction of Cardiac Events with Perindopril in Stable Coronary Artery Disease Investigators. Efficacy of perindopril in reduction of cardiovascular events among patients with stable coronary artery disease: Randomized, double-blind, placebo-controlled, multicentre trial (The EUROPA study). *Lancet* 2003;362:782–788.

Fagard RH, Staessen JA, Thijs L, et al. On-treatment diastolic blood pressure and prognosis in systolic hypertension. *Arch Intern Med* 2007;167:1884–1891.

Ferrier KE, Muhlmann MH, Baguet J-P, et al. Intensive cholesterol reduction lowers blood pressure and large artery stiffness in isolated systolic hypertension. *J Am Coll Cardiol* 2002;39:1020–1025.

Fischer MA, Avorn J. Economic implications of evidence-based prescribing for hypertension: Can better care cost less? *JAMA* 2004;291:1850–1856.

Fisher ES, Welch HG. Avoiding the unintended consequences of growth in medical care. *JAMA* 1999;281:446–453.

Gaziano TA, Young CR, Fitzmaurice G, et al. Laboratory-based versus non-laboratory-based method for assessment of cardiovascular disease risk: the NHANES I Follow-up Study cohort. *Lancet* 2008;371:923–931.

Gong L, Zhang W, Zhu Y, et al. Shanghai trial of nifedipine in the early (STONE). *J Hypertens* 1996;14:1237–1245.

Greenland P, Knoll MD, Stamler J, et al. Major risk factors as antecedents of fatal and non-fatal coronary heart disease events. *JAMA* 2003;290:891–897.

Gueyffier F, Boutitie F, Boissel J-P, et al. Effect of antihypertensive drug treatment on cardiovascular outcomes in women and men. *Ann Intern Med* 1997;126:761–767.

Gueyffier F, Bulpitt C, Boissel J-P, et al. Antihypertensive drugs in very old people. *Lancet* 1999;353:793–796.

Guyatt GH, Oxman AD, Vist GE, et al. GRADE: An emerging consensus on rating quality of evidence and strength of recommendations. *Br Med J* 2008;336:924–926.

Gwatkin DR, Bhuiya A, Victora CG. Making health systems more equitable. *Lancet* 2004;364:1273–1280.

Hamilton M, Thompson EN, Wisniewski TKM. The role of blood-pressure control in preventing complications of hypertension. *Lancet* 1964;1:235–238.

Hansson L. Antihypertensive treatment: Does the J-curve exist? *Cardiovasc Drugs Ther* 2000;14:367–372.

Hansson L, Zanchetti A, Carruthers SG, et al. Effects of intensive blood-pressure lowering and low-dose aspirin in patients with hypertension. *Lancet* 1998;351:1755–1762.

Harrap SB, Van der Merwe WM, Griffin SA, et al. Brief angiotensin converting enzyme inhibitor treatment in young spontaneously hypertensive rats reduces blood pressure long term. *Hypertension* 1990;16:603–614.

Heart Outcomes Prevention Evaluation Study Investigators. Effects of an angiotensin-converting-enzyme inhibitor, ramipril, on cardiovascular events in high-risk patients. *N Engl J Med* 2000;342:145–153.

Heart Protection Study Collaborative Group. Effects of cholesterol-lowering with simvastatin on stroke and other major vascular events in 20,536 people with cerebrovascular disease or other high-risk conditions. *Lancet* 2004;363:757–767.

Heath D, Edwards JE. The pathology of hypertensive pulmonary vascular disease. *Circulation* 1958;18:533–547.

Hegeland A. Treatment of mild hypertension. *Am J Med* 1980; 69:725–732.

Hodge JV, McQueen EG, Smirk H. Results of hypotensive therapy in arterial hypertension. *Br Med J* 1961;1:1–7.

Hollander W, Madoff I, Paddock J, et al. Aggravation of atherosclerosis by hypertension in a subhuman primate model with coarctation of the aorta. *Circ Res* 1976;38(Suppl 2):631–672.

Hood D, Bjork S, Sannerstedt R, et al. Analysis of mortality and survival in actively treated hypertensive disease. *Acta Med Scand* 1963;174:393–402.

Ingelsson E, Gona P, Larson MG, et al. Altered blood pressure progression in the community and its relation to clinical events. *Arch Intern Med* 2008;168:1450–1457.

Ioannidis JP. Contradicted and initially stronger effects in highly cited clinical research. *JAMA* 2005;294:218–228.

Jackson R. Attributing risk to hypertension: what does it mean? *Am J Hypertens* 2009; 22(3):237–238.

Jackson R, Barham P, Biels J, et al. Management of raised blood pressure in New Zealand. *BMJ* 1993;307:107–110.

Jackson R, Lawes CMM, Bennett DA, et al. Treatment with drugs to lower blood pressure and blood cholesterol based on an individual's absolute cardiovascular risk. *Lancet* 2005;365:434–441.

Jafar TH, Stark PC, Schmid CH, et al. Progression of chronic kidney disease: The role of blood pressure control, proteinuria, and angiotensin-converting enzyme inhibition: A patient-level meta-analysis. *Ann Intern Med* 2003;139:244–252.

Julius S. Trials of antihypertensive treatment. *Am J Hypertens* 2000; 13:11S–17S.

Julius S, Nesbitt SD, Egan BM, et al. Feasibility of treating prehypertension with an angiotensin-receptor blocker. *N Engl J Med* 2006;354:1685–1697.

Kannel WB, Wolf PA. Framingham Study insights on the hazards of elevated blood pressure. *JAMA* 2008;300:2545–2547.

Kent DM, Hayward RA. Limitations of applying summary results of clinical trials to individual patients: The need for risk stratification. *JAMA* 2007;298:1209–1212.

Khot UN, Khot MB, Bajzer CT, et al. Prevalence of conventional risk factors in patients with coronary heart disease. *JAMA* 2003;290:898–904.

Klein L, O'Connor CM, Gattis WA, et al. Pharmacologic therapy for patients with chronic heart failure and reduced systolic function: Review of trials and practical considerations. *Am J Cardiol* 2003;91(Suppl):18F–40F.

Kuramoto K, Matsushita S, Kuwajima I, Murakami M. Prospective study on the treatment of mild hypertension in the aged. *Jpn Heart J* 1981;22:75–85.

Lauer MS, Topol EJ. Clinical trials: Multiple treatments, multiple end points, and multiple lessons. *JAMA* 2003;289:2575–2577.

Law MR, Morris JK, Wald NJ. Use of blood pressure lowering drugs in the prevention of cardiovascular disease: meta-analysis of 147 randomised trials in the context of expectations from prospective epidemiological studies. *BMJ* 2009;338:b1665.

Lazarus JM, Bourgoignie JJ, Buckalew VM, et al. Achievement and safety of a low blood pressure goal in chronic renal disease. *Hypertension* 1997;29:641–650.

Lee VC, Rhew DC, Dylan M, et al. Meta-analysis: Angiotensin-receptor blockers in chronic heart failure and high-risk acute myocardial infarction. *Ann Intern Med* 2004;141:693–704.

Leishman AWD. Hypertension—treated and untreated—A study of 400 cases. *Br Med J* 1961;1:1–5.

Lever AF, Ramsay LE. Treatment of hypertension in the elderly. *J Hypertens* 1995;13:571–579.

Lewis EJ, Hunsicker LG, Clarke WR, et al. Renoprotective effect of the angiotensin-receptor antagonist irbesartan in patients with nephropathy due to type 2 diabetes. *N Engl J Med* 2001;345:851–860.

Lexchin J, Bero LA, Djulbegovic B, et al. Pharmaceutical industry sponsorship and research outcome and quality: Systematic review. *Br Med J* 2003;326:1167–1176.

Lim E, Brown A, Helmy A, et al. Composite outcomes in cardiovascular research: A survey of randomized trials. *Ann Intern Med* 2008;149:612–617.

Lithell H, Hansson L, Skoog I, et al. The Study of Cognition and Prognosis in the Elderly (SCOPE): Principal results of a randomized double-blind interventional trial. *J Hypertens* 2003;21:875–886.

Liu L, Wang JG, Gong L, et al. Comparison of active treatment and placebo in older Chinese patients with isolated systolic hypertension. *J Hypertens* 1998;16:1823–1829.

Lubsen J, Hoes A, Grobbee D. Implications of trial results: The potentially misleading notions of number needed to treat and average duration of life gained. *Lancet* 2000;346:1757–1759.

MacMahon S, Neal B, Rodgers A, et al. Commentary: The PROGRESS trial three years later: Time for more action, less distraction. *Br Med J* 2004;329:970–971.

MacMahon S, Sharpe N, Gamble G, et al. Randomised, placebo-controlled trial of the angiotensin converting enzyme inhibitor, ramipril, in patients with coronary or other occlusive vascular disease. *J Am Coll Cardiol* 2000;36:438–443.

Management Committee of the Australian National Blood Pressure Study. The Australian therapeutic trial in mild hypertension. *Lancet* 1980;1:1262–1267.

Mancia G. Role of outcome trials in providing information on antihypertensive treatment: importance and limitations. *Am J Hypertens* 2006;19:1–7.

McAlister FA, Straus SE, Sackett DL, et al. Analysis and reporting of factorial trials: A systematic review. *JAMA* 2003;289:2545–2553.

McGuinness B, Todd S, Passmore AP, et al. Systematic review: blood pressure lowering in patients without prior cerebrovascular disease for prevention of cognitive impairment and dementia. *J Neurol Neurosurg Psychiatry* 2008;79:4–5.

Medical Research Council Working Party. MRC trial of treatment of mild hypertension. *BMJ* 1985;291:97–104.

Medical Research Council Working Party. Medical Research Council trial of treatment of hypertension in older adults. *BMJ* 1992;304:405–412.

Mendis S, Lindholm LH, Mancia G, et al. World Health Organization (WHO) and International Society of Hypertension (ISH) risk prediction charts: Assessment of cardiovascular risk for prevention and control of cardiovascular disease in low and middle-income countries. *J Hypertens* 2007;25:1578–1582.

Messerli FH, Mancia G, Conti CR, et al. Dogma disputed: can aggressively lowering blood pressure in hypertensive patients with coronary artery disease be dangerous? *Ann Intern Med* 2006;144:884–893.

Miall WE, Chinn S. Blood pressure and ageing. *Clin Sci Mol Med* 1973;45(Suppl):23–33.

Montalvo G, Avanzini F, Anselmi M, et al. Diagnostic evaluation of people with hypertension in low income country: Cohort study of "essential" method of risk stratification. *Br Med J* 2008;337:a1387.

Montori VM, Jaeschke R, Schünemann HJ, et al. Users' guide to detecting misleading claims in clinical research reports. *Br Med J* 2004;329:1093–1096.

Moriwaki H, Uno H, Nagakane Y, et al. Losartan, an angiotensin II (AT_1) receptor antagonists, preserves cerebral blood flow in hypertensive patients with a history of stroke. *J Hum Hypertens* 2004;18:693–699.

Muntner P, He J, Roccella EJ, et al. The impact of JNC-VI guidelines on treatment recommendations in the US population. *Hypertension* 2002;39:897–902.

Nissen SE, Tuzcu EM, Libby P, et al. Effect of antihypertensive agents on cardiovascular events in patients with coronary disease and normal blood pressure. The CAMELOT Study: A randomized controlled trial. *JAMA* 2004;292:2217–2226.

Oberman A, Lane NE, Harlan WR, et al. Trends in systolic blood pressure in the thousand aviator cohort over a twenty-four-year period. *Circulation* 1967;36:812–822.

Papadopoulos DP, Papademetriou V. Aggressive blood pressure control and stroke prevention: Role of calcium channel blockers. *J Hypertens* 2008;26:844–852.

PATS Collaborating Group. Post-stroke antihypertensive treatment study: A preliminary result. *Chinese Med J* 1995;108:710–717.

Perry HM Jr, Goldman AI, Lavin MA, et al. Evaluation of drug treatment in mild hypertension. *Ann N Y Acad Sci* 1978;304:267–288.

Perry HM Jr, Smith WM, McDonald RH, et al. Morbidity and mortality in the Systolic Hypertension in the Elderly Program (SHEP) pilot study. *Stroke* 1989;20:4–13.

Peterson JC, Adler S, Burkart JM, et al. Blood pressure control, proteinuria, and the progression of renal disease: The Modification of Diet in Renal Disease Study. *Ann Intern Med* 1995;123:754–762.

Pitt B, Byington R, Furberg C, et al. Effect of amlodipine on the progression of atherosclerosis and the occurrence of clinical events. *Circulation* 2000;102:1503–1510.

Pocock SJ, Clayton TC, Altman DG. Survival plots of time-to-event outcomes in clinical trials: Good practice and pitfalls. *Lancet* 2002;359:1686–1689.

Pohl MA, Blumenthal S, Cordonnier DJ, et al. The independent and additive impact of blood pressure control and angiotensin II receptor blockade on renal outcomes in the Irbesartan Diabetic Nephropathy Trial (IDNT): Clinical implications and limitations. *J Am Soc Nephrol* 2005;16:3027–3037.

Poole-Wilson PA, Lubsen J, Kirwan B-A, et al. Effect of long-acting nifedipine on mortality and cardiovascular morbidity in patients with stable angina requiring treatment (ACTION trial): Randomised controlled trial. *Lancet* 2004;364:849–857.

PROGRESS Collaborative Group. Randomised trial of a perindopril-based blood-pressure-lowering regimen among 6105 individuals with previous stroke or transient ischaemic attack. *Lancet* 2001;358:1033–1041.

Prospective Studies Collaboration. Age-specific relevance of usual blood pressure to vascular mortality: A meta-analysis of individual data for one million adults in 61 prospective studies. *Lancet* 2002;360:1903–1913.

Protogerou AD, Safar ME, Iaria P, et al. Diastolic blood pressure and mortality in the elderly with cardiovascular disease. *Hypertension* 2007;50:172–180.

Psaty BM, Lumly T, Furberg CD, et al. Health outcomes associated with various antihypertensive therapies used as first-line agents: A network meta-analysis. *JAMA* 2003;289:2534–2544.

Psaty BM, Smith NL, Siscovick DS, et al. Health outcomes associated with antihypertensive therapies used as first-line agents. *JAMA* 1997;277:739–745.

Ramsay LE, Hag IU, Yeo WW, et al. Interpretation of prospective trials in hypertension. *J Hypertens* 1996;14(Suppl 5):S187–S194.

Rennie D. CONSORT revised: Improving the reporting of randomized trials. *JAMA* 2001;285:2006–2007.

Roberts EB, Ramnath R, Fallows S, et al. "First-hit" heart attack risk calculators on the world wide web: Implications for laypersons and healthcare practitioners. *Int J Med Inform* 2008; 77:405–412.

Rose G. Strategy of prevention. *Br Med J* 1981;282:1847–1851.

Rosendorff C, Black HR, Cannon CP, et al. Treatment of hypertension in the prevention and management of ischemic heart disease: A scientific statement from the American Heart Association Council for High Blood Pressure Research and the Councils on Clinical Cardiology and Epidemiology and Prevention. *Circulation* 2007;115:2761–2788.

Rothwell PM. Treating individuals 2. Subgroup analysis in randomised controlled trials: importance, indications, and interpretation. *Lancet* 2005;365:176–186.

Sever PS, Dahlöf B, Poulter NR, et al. Prevention of coronary and stroke events with atorvastatin in hypertensive patients who have average or lower-than-average cholesterol concentrations, in the Anglo-Scandinavian Cardiac Outcomes Trial—Lipid-Lowering Arm (ASCOT-LLA): A multicentre randomised controlled trial. *Lancet* 2003;361:1149–1158.

SHEP Cooperative Research Group. Prevention of stroke by antihypertensive drug treatment in older persons with isolated systolic hypertension. *JAMA* 1991;265:3255–3264.

Sleight P, Redon J, Verdecchia P et al. Prognostic value of blood pressure in patients with high vascular risk in the Ongoing Telmisartan Alone and in combination with Ramipril Global Endpoint Trial study. *J Hypertens* 2009;27:1360–1369.

Smith WM. Treatment of mild hypertension. *Hypertension* 1977; 25(Suppl 1):I98–I105.

Somes GW, Pahor M, Shorr RI, et al. The role of diastolic blood pressure when treating isolated systolic hypertension. *Arch Intern Med* 1999;159:2004–2009.

Staessen JA, Fagard R, Thijs L, et al. Randomised double- blind comparison of placebo and active treatment for older patients with isolated systolic hypertension. *Lancet* 1997;350:757–764.

Staessen JA, Gasowski J, Wang JG, et al. Risks of untreated and treated isolated systolic hypertension in the elderly. *Lancet* 2000;355:865–872.

Staessen JA, Wang J-G, Thijs L. Cardiovascular protection and blood pressure reduction: A quantitative overview updated until 1 March 2003. *J Hypertens* 2003;21:1055–1076.

Staessen JA, Richart T, Birkenhager WH. Less atherosclerosis and lower blood pressure for a meaningful life perspective with more brain. *Hypertension* 2007;49:389–400.

Sterne JAC, Egger M, Smith GD. Investigating and dealing with publication and other biases in meta-analysis. *Br Med J* 2001;323:101–105.

Stewart IMG. Relation of reduction in pressure to first myocardial infarction in patients receiving treatment for severe hypertension. *Lancet* 1979;1:861–865.

Sutton-Tyrrell K, Wildman R, Newman A, et al. Extent of cardiovascular risk reduction associated with treatment of isolated systolic hypertension. *Arch Intern Med* 2003;163:2728–2731.

Swales JD. Hypertension in the political arena. *Hypertension* 2000;35:1179–1182.

Task force for the management of arterial hypertension of the European society of hypertension (ESH) and of the European society of cardiology (ESC). 2007 Guidelines for the Management of Arterial Hypertension: The Task Force for the Management of Arterial Hypertension of the European Society of Hypertension (ESH) and of the European Society of Cardiology (ESC). *J Hypertens* 2007;25:1105–1187.

Taylor AL, Ziesche S, Yancy C, et al. Combination of isosorbide dinitrate and hydralazine in blacks with heart failure. *N Engl J Med* 2004;351:2049–2057.

Teo K, Burton J, Buller C, et al. Long-term effects of cholesterol lowering and angiotensin-converting enzyme inhibition on coronary atherosclerosis. *Circulation* 2000;102:1748–1754.

Thal AP, Grage TB, Vernier RL. Function of the contralateral kidney in renal hypertension due to renal artery stenosis. *Circulation* 1963:27:36–43.

Thompson SG, Higgins JPT. Can meta-analysis help target interventions at individuals most likely to benefit? *Lancet* 2005;365:341–346.

Thune JJ, Signorovitch J, Kober L, et al. Effect of antecedent hypertension and follow-up blood pressure on outcomes after high-risk myocardial infarction. *Hypertension* 2008;51: 48–54.

Uijen AA, Bakx JC, Mokkink HG, et al. Hypertension patients participating in trials differ in many aspects from patients treated in general practices. *J Clin Epidemiol* 2007;60:330–335.

UKPDS Group. Tight blood pressure control and risk of macrovascular and microvascular complications in type 2 diabetes: UKPDS 38. *Br Med J* 1998;317:703–713.

Unal B, Critchley JA, Capewell S. Explaining the decline in coronary heart disease mortality in England and Wales between 1981 and 2000. *Circulation* 2004;109:1101–1107.

Vandenbrouke JP. When are observational studies as credible as randomized trials? *Lancet* 2004;363:1728–1731.

van Dijk EJ, Breteler MMB, Schmidt R, et al. The association between blood pressure, hypertension, and cerebral white matter lesions: Cardiovascular Determinants of Dementia study. *Hypertension* 2004;44:625–630.

Vasan RS, Larson MG, Leip EP, et al. Impact of high-normal blood pressure on the risk of cardiovascular disease. *N Engl J Med* 2001;345:1291–1297.

Veterans Administration Cooperative Study Group on Antihypertensive Agents. Effects of treatment on morbidity in hypertension. *JAMA* 1967;202:1028–1034.

Veterans Administration Cooperative Study Group on Antihypertensive Agents. Effects of treatment on morbidity in hypertension. *JAMA* 1970;213:1143–1152.

Vijan S, Hayward RA. Treatment of hypertension in type 2 diabetes mellitus: Blood pressure goals, choice of agents, and setting priorities in diabetes care. *Ann Intern Med* 2003;138:593:602.

Voko Z, Bots ML, Hofman A, et al. J-shaped relation between blood pressure and stroke in treated hypertensives. *Hypertension* 1999;34:1181–1185.

Wald NJ, Law MR. A strategy to reduce cardiovascular disease by more than 80%. *Br Med J* 2003;326:1419–1424.

Wang J-G, Staessen JA, Franklin SS, et al. Systolic and diastolic blood pressure lowering as determinants of cardiovascular outcome on antihypertensive drug treatment. *Hypertension* 2005;45:907–913.

Wang W, Lee ET, Fabsitz RR, et al. A longitudinal study of hypertension risk factors and their relation to cardiovascular disease: the Strong Heart Study. *Hypertension* 2006;47:403–409.

Wang JG, Li Y, Franklin SS, et al. Prevention of stroke and myocardial infarction by amlodipine and Angiotensin receptor blockers: a quantitative overview. *Hypertension* 2007;50:181–188.

Weiner DE, Tighiouart H, Levey AS, et al. Lowest systolic blood pressure is associated with stroke in stages 3 to 4 chronic kidney disease. *J Am Soc Nephrol* 2007;18:960–966.

WHO/ISH Writing Group. 2003 World Health Organization (WHO)/International Society of Hypertension (ISH) statement on management of hypertension. *J Hypertens* 2003;21:1983–1992.

Williams B, Poulter NR, Brown MJ, et al. British Hypertension Society guidelines for hypertension management 2004 (BHS-IV): Summary. *Br Med J* 2004a;328:634–640.

Williams B, Poulter NR, Brown MJ, et al. Guidelines for management of hypertension: Report of the fourth working party of the British Hypertension Society, 2004—BHS IV. *J Hum Hypertens* 2004b;18:139–185.

Wright JT Jr, Bakris G, Greene T, et al. Effect on blood pressure lowering and antihypertensive drug class on progression of hypertensive kidney disease: Results from the AASK trial. *JAMA* 2002;288:2421–2431.

Wright JT Jr, Harris-Haywood S, Pressel S, et al. Clinical outcomes by race in hypertensive patients with and without the metabolic syndrome: Antihypertensive and Lipid-Lowering Treatment to Prevent Heart Attack Trial (ALLHAT). *Arch Intern Med* 2008;168:207–217.

Yank V, Rennie D, Bero LA. Financial ties and concordance between results and conclusions in meta-analyses: Retrospective cohort study. *Br Med J* 2007;335:1202–1205.

Yusuf S, Pepine CJ, Garces C, et al. Effect of enalapril on myocardial infarction and unstable angina in patients with low ejection fractions. *Lancet* 1992;340:1173–1178.

Zanchetti A, Hansson L, Clement D, et al. Benefits and risks of more intensive blood pressure lowering in hypertensive patients of the HOT study with different risk profiles: Does a J-shaped curve exist in smokers? *J Hypertens* 2003;21:797–804.

Zanchetti A, Grassi G, Mancia G. When should antihypertensive drug treatment be initiated and to what levels should systolic blood pressure be lowered? A critical reappraisal. *J Hypertens* 2009;27:923–934.

Zhang H, Thijs L, Staessen JA. Blood pressure lowering for primary and secondary prevention of stroke. *Hypertension* 2006;48: 187–195.

Treatment of Hypertension: Lifestyle Modifications

With an appreciation of the benefits and costs of antihypertensive therapy, we now will consider the practical aspects of accomplishing a reduction in blood pressure (BP). In this chapter, *lifestyle modifications*—the term used rather than *nondrug therapies*—will be examined. At the end of this chapter, a number of miscellaneous therapies that are not lifestyle modifications are also covered. The next chapter covers the use of drugs.

THE PLACE FOR LIFESTYLE MODIFICATIONS

Lifestyle modifications are recommended to help treat hypertension in all current guidelines by expert committees (Canadian Hypertension Society, 2008; Chobanian et al., 2003; Task force, 2007; Williams et al., 2004). As listed in Table 6-1, the recommendations are virtually identical except for a more liberal consumption of alcohol in the European, Canadian, and British guidelines and a more specific statement about increased fruits and vegetables and reduced fat, the dietary approaches to stop hypertension (DASH) diet (Table 6-2) in the JNC-7 report (Chobanian et al., 2003).

Potential for Prevention

Lifestyle modifications may also prevent hypertension (Whelton et al., 2002). The evidence for their preventive potential remains fragmentary, and there is no proof that, individually or together, they will reduce hypertension-induced morbidity and mortality. However, the evidence that they will lower BP and reduce other major cardiovascular risk factors is incontrovertible (Elmer et al., 2006).

The benefits of a lifestyle that follows the features shown in Table 6-1 have been amply demonstrated in large populations observed over long periods. Examples include the 25% lower mortality rate in those who closely adhere to a Mediterranean diet than in those Greek adults who do not (Trichopoulou et al., 2003) and the 50% lower mortality rate in Europeans 70- to 90-year-olds who ate the Mediterranean diet, were physically active, drank alcohol in moderation, and did not smoke (Knoops et al., 2004). Another is the 7- to 10-year longer life expectancy for Seventh-Day Adventists who closely adhere to a healthy lifestyle (Fraser & Shavlik, 2001). Yet another is the lower incidence of stroke among health professionals and nurses who did not smoke, were not obese, exercised regularly, and consumed moderate amounts of alcohol (Chiuve et al., 2008).

The evidence for prevention of diabetes by lifestyle change is even stronger (Lindstrom et al., 2006). Over a 20-year period, those Chinese with initially abnormal glucose tolerance who lost weight, ate more vegetables, drank less alcohol, and exercised more, had a 43% decrease in onset of diabetes (Li et al., 2008).

There is no doubt that the unhealthy lifestyle of people in most developed societies contribute to our high incidence of hypertension, diabetes, and cardiovascular disease (Mente et al., 2009). As noted in the JNC-7 report (Chobanian et al., 2003):

> One hundred twenty-two million Americans are overweight or obese. Mean sodium intake is approximately 4100 mg per day for men and 2,750 mg per day for women, 75% of which comes from processed foods. Fewer than 20% of Americans engage in regular physical activity, and fewer than 25% consume five or more servings of fruits and vegetables daily.

TABLE 6.1	Lifestyle Therapy to Reduce the Possibility of Becoming Hypertensive and to Reduce BP and to Reduce the Risk of BP-related CV Complications in Hypertensive Patients

Healthy diet: high in fresh fruits, vegetables, low-fat dairy products, dietary and soluble fiber, whole grains, and protein from plant sources; low in saturated fat, cholesterol, and salt

Regular physical activity: accumulation of 30–60 min of moderate-intensity dynamic exercise, 4–7 days per week

Low-risk alcohol consumption (≤2 standard drinks per day and <14 standard drinks per week for men and <9 standard drinks per week for women).

Attaining and maintaining ideal body weight (BMI 18.5–24.9 kg/m²)

A waist circumference of <102 cm (men) and 88 cm (women)

Reduction in sodium intake to <100 mmol/day

A smoke-free environment

Because the lifetime risk of developing hypertension is very high, a public health strategy that complements the hypertension treatment strategy is warranted. In order to prevent BP levels from rising, primary prevention measures should be introduced to reduce or minimize those causal factors in the population, particularly in individuals with prehypertension. A population approach that decreases the BP level in the general population by even modest amounts has the potential to substantially reduce morbidity and mortality or at least delay the onset of hypertension.

Barriers to prevention include cultural norms: insufficient attention to health education by health care practitioners; lack of reimbursement for health education services; lack of access to places to engage in physical activity; larger servings of food in restaurants; lack of availability of healthy food choices in most schools, worksites, and restaurants; lack of exercise programs in schools; large amounts of sodium added to foods by the food industry and restaurants; and the higher cost of food products that are lower in sodium and calories. Overcoming the barriers will require a multipronged approach directed not only at high-risk populations but also to communities, schools, worksites, and the food industry.

Obviously, removal of these barriers will be difficult and will require major environmental changes which demand a political advocacy and governmental financing that is sorely lacking. Meanwhile, more focused, smaller attempts have been made to document the ability of lifestyle changes to delay, if not prevent,

TABLE 6.2	DASH Diet

Food Group	Daily Serving	Examples and Notes
Grains	7–8	Whole wheat bread, oatmeal, popcorn
Vegetables	4–5	Tomatoes, potatoes, carrots, beans, peas, squash, spinach
Fruits	4–5	Apricots, bananas, grapes, oranges, grapefruit, melons
Low-fat or fat-free dairy foods	2–3	Fat-free (skim)/low-fat (1%) milk, fat-free/low-fat yogurt, fat-free/low-fat cheese
Meats, poultry, fish	≤2	Select only lean meats, trim away fats; broil, roast, or boil; no frying; and remove skin from poultry
Nuts, seeds, dry beans	4–5/week	Almonds, peanuts, walnuts, sunflower seeds, soybeans, lentils
Fats and oils	2–3	Soft margarines, low-fat mayonnaise, vegetable oil (oil, corn, canola, or safflower)
Sweets	5/week	Maple syrup, sugar, jelly, jam, hard candy, sorbet

DASH eating plan available at: http://www.nhlbi.nih.gov/health/public/heart/hpb/dash/new_dash.pdf

the development of hypertension. As summarized in Table 6-3, three long-term, well-controlled preventive trials involving subjects with high-normal BP have shown that individual and combined lifestyle modifications lower BP and reduce the incidence of overt hypertension (Hypertension Prevention Trial Research Group, 1990; Stamler et al., 1989; Trials of Hypertension Prevention Collaborative Research Group, 1992, 1997).

The effects of multiple lifestyle changes have also been examined in two groups of patients with somewhat higher BPs. The Trial of Nonpharmacologic Interventions in the Elderly (TONE) enrolled 975 men and women aged 60 to 80 years whose hypertension was controlled on one antihypertensive drug (Whelton et al., 1998). They were randomly assigned to reduced sodium intake, weight loss, both of these, or no intervention (i.e., usual care). After 3 months, their antihypertensive drug was withdrawn. Over the ensuing 30 months, the proportion of patients who remained normotensive without antihypertensive drugs was only 16% in those on usual care, more than 35%

in those on one of the two interventions, and 43.6% in those on both interventions (Fig. 6-1). These impressive effects were achieved with relatively small amounts of dietary sodium reduction (an average of 40 mmol per day) or weight reduction (an average of 4.7 kg).

Another trial involved 412 adults whose average age was 48 years and who had a BP between 120 and 159 mm Hg systolic and 80 to 95 mm Hg diastolic (Sacks et al., 2001). They were randomly given one of two already prepared diets, one typical of the U.S. diet (i.e., control), the other composed of more fruits, vegetables, and low-fat dairy foods (i.e., Dietary Approaches to Stop Hypertension [the DASH diet, portrayed in Table 6-2]). In addition, they were randomly given one of three levels of sodium intake: high (150 mmol per day), intermediate (100 mmol per day), or low (50 mmol per day).

Each diet was consumed for 30 consecutive days, while weight was kept constant. Figure 6-2 shows significant falls in systolic blood pressure (SBP) noted with the DASH diet at every level of sodium intake as

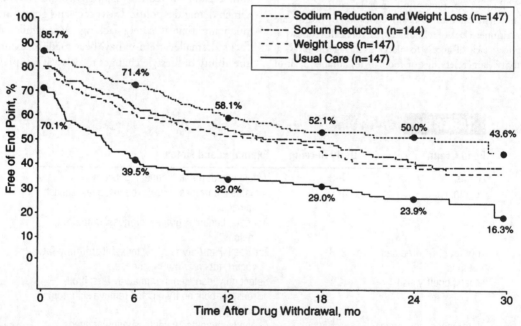

FIGURE 6-1 Percentages of the 144 participants assigned to reduced sodium intake, the 147 assigned to weight loss, the 147 assigned to reduced sodium intake and weight loss combined, and the 147 assigned to usual care (no lifestyle intervention) who remained free of cardiovascular events and high BP and in whom no antihypertensive agent was prescribed during follow-up. (Modified from Whelton PK, Appel LJ, Espeland MA, et al. Sodium reduction and weight loss in the treatment of hypertension in older persons. *JAMA* 1998;279:839–846.)

TABLE 6.3	Trials of Lifestyle Modifications on the Incidence of Hypertension			
Trial (reference)	**No. of subjects**	**Duration (year)**	**Weight loss (kg)**	**Reduction of incidence (%)**
Primary prevention trial (Stamler et al., 1989)	201	5	2.7	54
Hypertension Prevention Trial (Hypertension Prevention Trial Research Group, 1990)	252	3	1.6	23
Trials of hypertension prevention				
I (Trials of Hypertension Prevention Collaborative Research Group, 1992)	564	1.5	3.9	51
II (Trials of Hypertension Prevention Collaborative Research Group, 1997)	595	4.0	1.9	21

compared to the control diet and significant falls in SBP with progressively lower sodium intakes on either diet. The effects were seen in normotensives and hypertensives, men and women, blacks and non-blacks, and were accompanied by falls in diastolic blood pressure (DBP) as well.

As impressive as these results are, they may not be applicable to the "real" world since they were obtained in a short study that was tightly controlled. A more realistic view of what can be expected comes from the PREMIER trial wherein participants were assigned to the DASH diet but prepared their own meals (Elmer et al., 2006). Not surprisingly, at the end of 18 months, neither the extent of dietary change nor the reduction in BP was as great as seen in the original DASH trial. The additional fall in

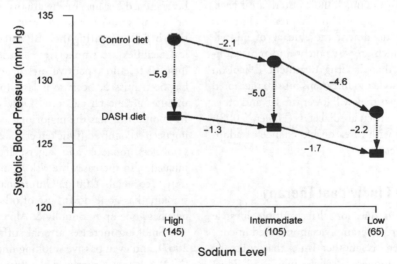

FIGURE 6-2   Reduction of SBP by dietary approaches to stop hypertension [the (DASH) diet] and reduced sodium intake. The mean SBP are shown for the high-sodium control diet. The three dietary sodium levels are expressed in terms of millimoles per day. The *solid lines* indicate changes in BP for various sodium levels, and the *dotted arrows* show the mean differences in BP between the two diets at each level of sodium intake. The order in which participants were given the sodium levels was random, with a crossover design. There was a significant difference in SBP between the high-sodium and low-sodium phases of the control diet (mean, –6.7 mm Hg) and the DASH diet (mean, –3.0 mm Hg). (Modified from Sacks FM, Svetkey LP, Vollmer WM, et al. Effects on blood pressure of reduced dietary sodium and the dietary approaches to stop hypertension (DASH) diet. *N Eng J Med* 2001;344:3–10.)

BP compared to the group only given advice was −1.1/−0.9 mm Hg.

As rational as lifestyle modifications seem to be, both for prevention and treatment of hypertension, their value must be put into perspective. As Pickering (2004) notes:

> Given that healthcare practitioners have limited resou rces to improve hypertension control, it would seem appropriate to focus on the intervention that has the greatest chance of success; there can be little doubt that drug treatment wins hands down. This conclusion is not intended to negate the importance of lifestyle changes such as the DASH diet, and patients should certainly be encouraged to adopt them, but if behavioral medicine is to progress, practitioners need to find more cost-effective methods for instituting and maintaining behavior change. In the mean time, doctors are still going to need to take out the prescription pad.

Protection Against Cardiovascular Disease

The larger issue of whether these lifestyle modifications will, in fact, reduce morbidity and mortality in hypertensive patients may never be settled. The difficulty of demonstrating such protection in the various therapeutic trials using much more potent antihypertensive drugs was described in Chapter 5. There is likely no way to document the efficacy of lifestyle modifications, which are less potent and more difficult to monitor than is drug treatment (Nicolson et al., 2004). Lifestyle modifications must be accepted on the evidence that they will lower the BP and other risk factors, in particular diabetes (Unger, 2008), without risk and with a reasonable chance of adoption by most patients.

The Problem of Individual Therapy

While there is no question that multiple lifestyle changes will lower BP as amply demonstrated in controlled trials, there is another issue that must be recognized—practitioners dealing with individual patients may find much less benefit, despite their best efforts (Christian et al., 2008; Folsom et al., 2007). Only minimal effects may be accomplished even with repeated counseling (Kastarinen et al., 2002) or other interventions (Little et al., 2004) as noted in the PREMIER trial (Elmer et al., 2006).

Clearly, lifestyle changes, for most people, can come only from societal changes. Despite proof that

tobacco kills, it took a massive financial hit from a lawsuit to slow the purveyors' promotion of their poison in the United States, resulting in an impressive reduction in smoking in the United States.

A promising beginning for governmental action to reduce sodium consumption has been made in the United Kingdom as a result of a continuous campaign led by a tenacious physician, Graham MacGregor. In the United States, the Center for Science in the Public Interest is the most forceful advocate for governmental action.

With recognition that only societal changes will lead to major changes, the effects of individual lifestyle modifications on hypertension will now be examined.

AVOIDANCE OF TOBACCO

Smoking cessation is the most effective, immediate way to reduce cardiovascular risk (Asaria et al., 2007). However, an effect on BP has not been generally thought to be involved in this risk reduction because chronic smokers as a group have a lower BP than do nonsmokers (Mikkelsen et al., 1997), likely because smokers weigh less than do nonsmokers. In fact, the role of a pressor effect of smoking has likely been missed because of the almost universal practice of having smokers abstain from smoking for some time before measuring their BP, usually because medical facilities are smoke free. Thus, the significant, immediate, and repetitive pressor effect of smoking has been missed, because it lasts for only 15 to 30 minutes after each cigarette. Only with ambulatory BP monitoring has the major pressor effect of smoking been recognized (Oncken et al., 2001). The use of smokeless tobacco and cigars, if their smoke is inhaled, also increases the risk of myocardial infarction (Teo et al., 2006). Unfortunately, as cigarette smoking has gone down, use of other tobacco products has gone up (Connolly & Alpert, 2008).

Smoking increases arterial stiffness (Jatoi et al., 2007), and even passive smoking impairs nitric oxide (NO) synthase (Argacha et al., 2008). These are likely involved in the higher incidence of hypertension in middle-aged people (Halperin et al., 2008).

Thus, hypertensives who use tobacco must be repeatedly and unambiguously told to quit and given assistance in doing so (Burke et al., 2008b). Nicotine replacement therapy may help even if they cause sympathetic stimulation (Hatsukami et al., 2008). The partial nicotine agonist, varenicline (Chantix) is superior to nicotine replacement therapy, both in relieving withdrawal symptoms and blocking the desire to continue smoking (Burke et al., 2008b). If the patient continues to smoke, any antihypertensive drugs except nonselective β blockers may attenuate the smoking-induced rise in BP (Pardell et al., 1998).

WEIGHT REDUCTION

Most Americans, as many as 80% of African American women, are overweight, defined as a BMI more than 25, and 30% are obese, defined as a BMI more than 30 (Burke et al., 2008a). The nature of modern life, with more caloric intake and less physical activity, engenders more obesity, which is now a worldwide epidemic (Romero-Corral et al., 2006), particularly in children (Ogden et al., 2008). Any degree of weight gain, even to a level that is not defined as overweight, is associated with an increasing incidence of hypertension (Redón et al., 2008) and, even more strikingly, of type 2 diabetes. A BMI more than 30 is a significant predictor of incident hypertension (Parikh et al., 2008). As more completely described in Chapter 3, the hypertensive effect of weight gain is mainly related to increased abdominal visceral fat (Orr et al., 2008), accompanied by impaired endothelial function (Pierce et al., 2008).

Despite increasing awareness of the problem, dietary habits among U.S. adult hypertensives continue to worsen (Mellen et al., 2008). Because the maintenance of significant weight loss is so difficult for most who are obese, physicians, patients, and society at large must do more to prevent weight gain, particularly among children (Ebbeling et al., 2002) in whom obesity and the metabolic syndrome are increasing so rapidly (Ogden et al., 2008). Unfortunately, even with a structured program in 7- to 11-year-old children,

weight continued to increase when the program was stopped (James et al., 2007). Here again, societal changes are needed to stop the epidemic.

Clinical Data

In their analysis of all literature available up to March 2007, Horvath et al. (2008) were able to identify only 15 studies of the effect on BP of hypertensive people caused by weight loss by diet or drug therapy that met criteria for a randomized controlled trial (RCT) where patients were followed up for at least 24 weeks (Table 6-4). These 15 studies were the distillation of 5,285 articles on weight loss that were found, an indication of how few reliable data are available. Note that, despite its rapid rise, bariatric surgery has had no valid controlled study. In a retrospective study of 180 patients who had gastric bypass, compared to 157 treated without surgery, the surgical group had a −7/−6 mm Hg greater fall in BP after a mean follow-up of 3.4 years (Batsis et al., 2008).

The data can be looked upon as positive, as do Harsha and Bray (2008), since a 6/3 mm Hg fall by diet is about half that seen with antihypertensive drugs and, if applied to the total hypertensive population, would be expected to reduce cardiovascular morbidity and mortality. However, Mark (2008) takes a negative view, arguing thusly:

> …there are questions about the pragmatism of long-term widespread lifestyle modification in the "real world." In addition, although even modest weight loss produces an early reduction in blood pressure, the long-term reductions in blood pressure are much less impressive than the short term reductions. One more nail in the coffin of the idea that weight loss is the answer to hypertension in obesity is the following: in patients undergoing bariatric surgery for morbid obesity, although blood pressure decreases initially, it returns to control levels after 6 to 8 years despite substantial and sustained

| **TABLE 6.4** | Long-term Effects of Weight-reducing Interventions in Hypertensive Patients |

	No. of RCTs	No. of Pts	Change in SBP (mm Hg)	Change in DBP (mm Hg)	Change in Body Weight (kg)
Diet	7	1632	−6.3	−3.4	−4.14
Orlistat	4	1023	−2.5	−1.7	−3.74
Sibutramine	4	360	—	+3.2	−3.72
Invasive	0	—	—	—	—

Based on data in Horvath K, Jeitler K, Siering U, et al. Long-term effects of weight reducing interventions in hypertensive patients: Systematic review and meta-analysis. *Arch Intern Med* 2008;168(6):571–580.

decreases in body weight. In summary, chronic blood pressure reduction during dieting and weight loss is not as sustained or pronounced as generally assumed.

Mark's (2008) pessimistic conclusion is tempered by the argument that, since obesity is a "genetic neurobiological" condition, it may take combinations of drugs given over a lifetime to bring it under control, analogous to type 2 diabetes mellitus. Obviously, there is no value of short-term crash-diet programs that offer instant relief but almost always result in further frustration and often are followed by weight gain beyond the prediet level.

To be sure, a few people who are overweight and hypertensive can benefit from diet plus currently available drugs. Perhaps the best example is the Trials of Hypertension Prevention II study (Stevens et al., 2001) in which 595 moderately obese subjects (10% to 65% above ideal body weight) with high-normal BP (DBPs, 83 to 89 mm Hg) were assigned to an intensive weight loss program and then compared to another 596

subjects who were simply observed. Over the 3-year follow-up, only 13% of the active participants were able to maintain a substantial weight loss of 4.5 kg or more but, as shown in Figure 6-3, those subjects experienced a significant fall in BP and a 65% lower relative risk for the onset of hypertension as compared to the control group. Even those for whom weight loss was not sustained (i.e., the relapse group) had a 25% lower risk for developing hypertension by the end of the 3 years.

Recommendations

To begin, the waist circumference should be measured along with the BMI (Nyamdorj et al., 2008). A structured, low-calorie diet, along the lines of the Weight Watchers program (Tsai & Wadden, 2005), should be advised while avoiding "crash" diets and the latest fad of the moment. Dietary counseling and behavioral therapies are of limited benefit (Svetkey et al., 2008). The ability to lose weight is greatly

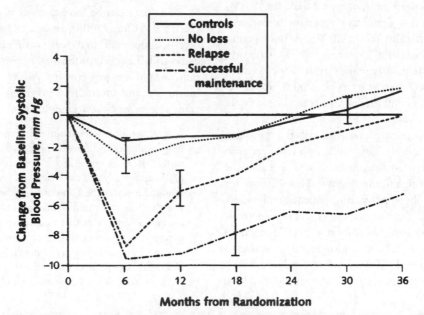

FIGURE 6-3 Long-term changes in weight and SBP. Data are adjusted for age, ethnicity, and gender, according to patterns of weight change. Usual-care controls were not assigned to intervention. Participants with successful maintenance of weight loss were defined as those who lost 4.5 kg or more at 6 months and maintained at least 4.5 kg of weight loss at 36 months. Participants with relapse were those who lost at least 4.5 kg at 6 months but whose weight loss at 36 months was less than 2.5 kg. Participants registered as having no weight loss had weight loss of 2.5 kg or less at 6 and 36 months. Error bars represent 95% confidence intervals. (Modified from Stevens VJ, Obarzanek E, Cook NR, et al. Long-term weight loss and changes in blood pressure: Results of the Trials of Hypertension Prevention, phase II. *Ann Intern Med* 2001;134:1–11.)

enhanced by an accompanying regularly performed program of physical activity (Jakicic et al., 2008). It takes fairly vigorous exercise to overcome the decline in resting metabolic rate that occurs during dieting. An average of 275 minutes per week of moderate activity is needed to prevent weight gain after successful weight loss (Jakicic et al., 2008).

As seen in Table 6-4, among currently available drug therapies, orlistat does not raise BP. Sibutramine reduces central sympathetic activity while increasing peripheral activity, so its effect on BP is related to the baseline level of peripheral nerve activity: Those with high levels, measured as muscle sympathetic nerve activity, tend to have no change or a fall in BP; those with low levels tend to have a rise in BP (Heusser et al., 2007).

In view of the extremely limited success of medical regimens in those with marked obesity, bariatric surgery is being increasingly performed with significant weight loss in more than 90% of patients (Sjöström et al., 2007). As noted in Chapter 3, unfortunately the modest initial reductions in BP are usually not sustained (Sjöström et al., 2004).

We are left with a rapidly growing epidemic that brings multiple damages, some related to hypertension, which is seemingly uncontrollable. Perhaps, as with tobacco, the cure must require legal action, as noted by Gostin (2007):

> Despite the undoubted political risks, should public health agencies push for strong measures to control obesity, perhaps even banning hazardous foods? The justification lies with the epidemic rates of overweight and obesity, the preventable morbidity and mortality, and the stark health disparities based on race and socioeconomic status. If the problem were related to pathogens, tobacco, or lead paint, most would support aggressive measures to protect innocent individuals from hazards created by others. But comfort foods also have hidden hazards—it is difficult to tell if they are laden with fat and, if so, what kind. Although the public dislikes paternalism, it is at least worth considering whether such an approach is ever justified to regulate harms that are apparently self-imposed, but also are deeply socially embedded and pervasively harmful to the public.

DIETARY SODIUM REDUCTION

Background

No food in its natural state is high in sodium. Salt was originally added to preserve foods that spoil without refrigeration. Although infants do not prefer saltier liquids, the presence of increased salt in virtually all processed food quickly leads to an acquired preference. Food processors are able to bulk up their products with water held by the salt. Soft drink and beer drinkers are enticed to consume more fluid to quench the saltiness of food and bar condiments.

Except for a few well-paid consultants to the salt industry lobby, led by M. Alderman (Alderman, 2008; Cohen et al., 2008), moderate dietary sodium reduction is advocated by individual experts, national and international guideline reports, governmental health agencies, and medical organizations, including the American Medical Association (Havas et al., 2007). Unfortunately, the one official U.S. document that prevents the occurrence of this desired societal change is the U.S. Food and Drug Administration regulations that continue to designate salt as "an ingredient recognized as safe (GRAS)," thereby allowing food processors to add as much salt as they wish and delivering 77% of individual American's sodium intake. Unlike other countries which have begun to address dietary sodium intake, the United States refuses to do so, despite the repeated presentation of solid scientific evidence for both the pathogenic role of excess sodium and the benefit of moderate sodium reduction. In their analysis, Dickinson and Havas (2007) estimate that "moderate sodium reduction could prevent at least 150,000 deaths annually in the United States."

Rigid restriction of dietary sodium intake was one of the first effective therapies for hypertension (Kempner, 1948). However, after thiazides were introduced during the late 1950s and their mode of action was shown to involve a mild state of sodium depletion, both physicians and patients eagerly adopted this form of therapy in place of dietary sodium reduction. In discarding rigid salt restriction, physicians disregarded the benefits of modest reduction both for its inherent antihypertensive effect and for its potential of reducing diuretic-induced potassium loss.

This same misguided designation allows large amounts of sodium in medications without its presence acknowledged and required on the label. One 325 mg acetaminophen tablet in the United Kingdom has almost 1,000 mg of sodium (Jarrett, 2008), but Tylenol sold in the United States has less then 1 mg per tablet.

Evidence for Antihypertensive Effect

Moderate sodium reduction to a level of 2.4 g per day (6 g NaCl per day, 100 mmol per day) has been found to have a moderate, but substantial, antihypertensive effect and a possible preventative effect. Analyses show a significant fall in BP that is greater in hypertensives than in normotensives and correlates with the degree of sodium reduction (He & MacGregor, 2003) (Fig. 6-4). This analysis was restricted to 26 trials that lasted 4 weeks or longer but very similar results were found in an analysis of 40 trials that lasted only 2 weeks or longer (Geleijnse et al., 2003) (Table 6-5). These two meta-analyses reported an average decrease in daily sodium excretion of over 75 mmol per day. However, the third meta-analysis, that of Hooper et al. (2002), was restricted to trials that lasted 6 months or longer, a few for 5 years. In these relatively few trials, the degree of sustained sodium reduction was obviously less and the degree of BP reduction considerably less. These data highlight the problem of individual action to reduce sodium intake. In discussing their results, Hooper et al. (2002) comment:

Despite a great deal of ongoing encouragement and support used in the trials included in this review, it seems that salt reduction attenuates over time. In routine primary care, the intervention is likely to be less intense and therefore of more limited impact.

Despite this sobering conclusion, the same argument can be made about attempts to get obese people to lose weight or addicted smokers to quit: Most good advice is not readily accepted but the goals seem worth pursuing.

This likely inability to maintain enough dietary sodium reduction to achieve a meaningful effect on BP over a longer period of time has led to a concerted effort to convince food processors to reduce the amount of sodium added to processed foods and drinks, the source of about three fourths of current sodium consumption (Dickinson & Havas, 2007). In the meantime, patients should be advised to read the label on processed products, avoiding those with more than 300 mg per portion. In addition, a number of books

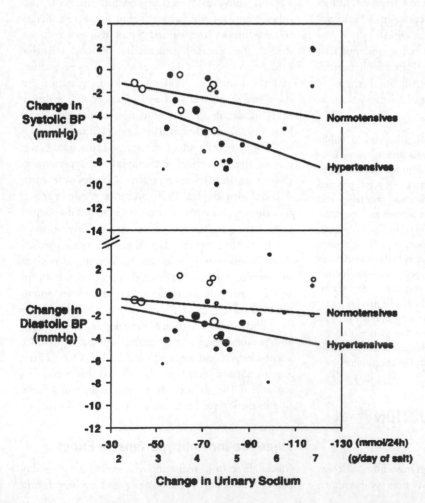

FIGURE 6-4 Relationship between the net change in 24-hour urinary sodium excretion and BP in a meta-analysis of 26 trials. *Open circles*, normotensive. *Solid circles*, hypertensives. The slope is weighted by the inverse of the variance of the net change in BP. The size of the circle is proportional to the weight of the trial. (Modified from He FJ, MacGregor GA. How far should salt intake be reduced? *Hypertension* 2003;42:1093–1099.)

TABLE 6.5	Meta-analyses of Trials of Dietary Sodium Reduction				

| | | | | Reduction in BP | |
| | | | | Normotensive syst/dias | Hypertensive syst/dias |
Reference	No. of Trials	Duration	Reduction in 24-h Sodium Excretion (mmol)		
Geleijnse et al. (2003)	40	>2 weeks	−77	−1.3/−1.1	−5.2/−3.7
He and MacGregor (2003)	26	>4 weeks	−78	−2.0/−1.0	−5.0/−2.7
Hooper et al. (2002)	7	6–12 months	−49	−2.5/−1.2	
	4	13–60 months	−35	−1.1/−0.6	

and Web sites, such as the American Heart Association, provide advice and recipes for lower sodium diets.

Mechanisms of Antihypertensive Effect

Despite considerable research, neither the mechanisms by which excessive sodium intake raises BP nor the mechanisms by which moderate sodium restriction lowers BP are well characterized. However, the structure and function of the heart and kidneys may be improved after prolonged, moderate sodium reduction: Left ventricular hypertrophy decreases (Messerli et al., 1997), and glomerular hyperfiltration and proteinuria are reduced (Weir, 2004).

The fall in BP tends to be greater in those with lower plasma renin and higher atrial natriuretic peptide levels (Melander et al., 2007). The BP sensitivity to sodium tends to be enhanced in hypertensives, in blacks and older people, all associated with lower renin, so that these patients tend to respond more to sodium reduction (Vollmer et al., 2001; Weinberger, 1996).

Sodium Sensitivity

As detailed in Chapter 3, people vary as to their BP response to either sodium loads or reduction, i.e., sodium sensitivity. This sensitivity is greater in adults who had a low birth weight (de Boer et al., 2008). Blacks, who are more likely to have been of low birth weight, tend to be more sodium sensitive (Schmidlin et al., 2007). More sodium-sensitive people developed hypertension over a 15-year follow-up (Barba et al., 2007); they have more cardiovascular disease and shorter survival (Franco & Oparil, 2006).

Despite these associations, there seems to be no need to ascertain the individual patient's degree of sodium sensitivity before recommending moderate sodium reduction, particularly as testing may not be reliable or reproducible (Gerdts et al., 1999). Those who respond more to sodium reduction likely are more sodium sensitive, but there is no harm and, as noted in Table 6-6, there are other potential benefits of moderate sodium reduction in

TABLE 6.6	Additional Benefits of Moderate Sodium Reduction

Improvement in large artery compliance (Gates et al., 2004)
Enhancement of efficacy of antihypertensive drugs (Vogt et al., 2008)
Reduction of diuretic-induced potassium loss (Crippa et al., 1996)
Regression of left ventricular hypertrophy (Messerli et al., 1997)
Reduction in proteinuria (Weir, 2004)
Reduction in urine calcium excretion (Carbone et al., 2003; Sakhaee et al., 1993)
Decrease in osteoporosis (Martini et al., 2000)
Decreased prevalence of stomach cancer (Fock et al., 2008)
Decreased prevalence of stroke (Joossens & Kesteloot, 2008)
Decreased prevalence of asthma (Peat, 1996)
Decreased prevalence of cataract (Cumming et al., 2000)
Protection against onset of hypertension (Whelton et al., 2002)

all hypertensives. All should be encouraged to reduce their levels to the 100 mmol per day goal, particularly since there is no certain way to predict who will develop hypertension.

Additional Benefits of Sodium Reduction

In addition to lowering BP, other benefits have been observed with moderate sodium reduction, as summarized in Table 6-6.

Enhancement of Efficacy of Antihypertensive Drugs

Moderate sodium reduction clearly increases the antihypertensive efficacy of all classes of antihypertensive drugs, with the possible exception of calcium channel blockers (Chrysant et al., 2000; Morgan et al., 1986). As is noted in Chapter 7, calcium channel blockers have an intrinsic natriuretic effect, which may explain the lesser potentiation with sodium reduction.

Protection from Diuretic-induced Potassium Loss

High levels of dietary sodium make patients more vulnerable to the major side effect of diuretic therapy, potassium loss. The diuretic inhibits sodium reabsorption proximal to that part of the distal convoluted tubule where secretion of potassium is coupled with sodium reabsorption under the influence of aldosterone. When a diuretic is given daily while the patient ingests large amounts of sodium, the initial diuretic-induced sodium depletion shrinks plasma volume, activating renin release and secondarily increasing aldosterone secretion. As the diuretic continues to inhibit sodium reabsorption, more sodium is delivered to this distal site. The increased amounts of aldosterone act to increase sodium reabsorption, thereby increasing potassium secretion; the potassium is swept into the urine.

With modest sodium reduction, less sodium is delivered to the distal exchange site, and therefore less potassium is swept into the urine. This modest restriction should not further activate the renin-angiotensin-aldosterone mechanism to cause more distal sodium-for-potassium exchange, because that usually occurs only with more rigid sodium restriction. This postulate was confirmed in a test of 12 hypertensive patients who were given one of three diuretics f or 4-week intervals while ingesting a diet inclusive of either 72 or 195 mmol per day of sodium (Ram et al., 1981). While on the modestly restricted diet, patients' total body potassium levels fell only half as much.

Similar results have been observed with the diuretic indapamide (Crippa et al., 1996).

A Dissenting View

There are a few dissenters to the value of such moderate sodium reduction. Their dissent is based on the possibility that such reduction may cause hazards that outweigh its benefits. These putative dangers include the following:

- *An increase in myocardial infarction* (Alderman et al., 1995). These data showed an increase in myocardial infarctions (but not strokes) in men (but not women) with the lowest urinary sodium excretion who were followed up for 3.8 years. These data have been faulted because of the small number of events (46 in 2,937 subjects), the failure to ascertain long-term sodium intake, and the likely presence of multiple confounding factors (Cook et al., 1995).
- *An increase in mortality* (Alderman et al., 1998; Cohen et al., 2006; 2008). These data, based on a single-day dietary recall, showed increased all-cause mortality with lower sodium intake in a representative sample of U.S. adults surveyed in the National Health and Nutrition Examination Surveys (NHANES) I, II, and III. These data have been questioned mainly for the inadequacy of the measure of sodium intake, a single 24-hour recall, resulting in a level so low (30 mmol per day) as to be impossible to achieve in a free-living population; the presence of known and (likely) unknown confounding factors; and the inability to ascertain long-time sodium intake (de Wardener, 1999; Poulter, 1998). Moreover, when the same data from NHANES were looked at separately for the 6,797 nonobese and the 2,688 obese subjects, highly significant direct associations between increased sodium intake and stroke, coronary heart disease, and cardiovascular and all-cause mortality were found among the obese subjects (He et al., 1999).

Methodologically stronger prospective data from Finland further document the *positive* correlation between higher sodium intake, ascertained from 24-hour urinary sodium excretion, and the risk of coronary heart disease in men, an association that was independent of other risk factors including BP and also primarily seen in those who were overweight (Tuomilehto et al., 2001).

- *Potentially harmful perturbations in various hormonal, lipid, and physiologic responses* (Graudal et al., 1998).

These perturbations have usually been noted only when sodium intake has been severely restricted to as low as 10 mmol per day over short intervals.

• *Lack of outcome data on safety.* RCT of moderate sodium intake on hard outcomes are not feasible, providing the dissenters a gratuitous objection. However, a 10- to 15-year follow-up of 2,415 people, who had maintained a lower than usual dietary sodium intake after participating in 1.5- to 4-year randomized trials of lower sodium intake, reported a 25% lower rate of cardiovascular events among those previously on reduced sodium versus those on a usual diet (Cook et al., 2007). Admittedly, these are soft data, but they are better than purely observational data.

Conclusions

High sodium intake is harmful and moderate sodium reduction is worthwhile and feasible. The reduction of BP possible with a universal reduction in sodium intake of 50 mmol per day down to the recommended level of 100 mmol per day has been estimated to translate into a 22% reduction of the incidence of stroke and a 16% reduction in the incidence of coronary disease (Law, 1997). Such estimates may be valid: Repeated surveys from 1966 to 1986 in Belgium showed a progressive decrease in average sodium intake from 203 to 144 mmol per day; these falls correlated closely with lesser rises in BP with increasing age and decreased stroke mortality in the population (Joossens & Kesteloot, 1991). Such population-wide reductions in sodium intake are likely both to improve health and reduce costs to society (Asaria et al., 2007). The real potential for benefit, with the remote possibility of harm, makes moderate sodium reduction a desirable goal both for the individual hypertensive patient and for the population at large. As noted by Havas et al. (2007):

> ...substantial cooperation among the government, the food industry, clinicians, and the public will be required to accomplish meaningful change and enable a larger proportion of the population to experience the benefits of reduced dietary sodium. With an appropriate food industry response, counseling of patients, public education, and knowledgeable use of food labels, sodium intake could be reduced without inconvenience or loss of food enjoyment.

POTASSIUM SUPPLEMENTATION

Many of the benefits of reduced sodium intake could reflect an increased potassium intake, although in the TONE study the antihypertensive effects of the two were independent of each other (Appel et al., 2001). Intracellular potassium levels are lower in hypertensives and, as the most abundant ion in the cell, it may be a fundamental factor in BP control (Delgado, 2004).

Clinical Data

He and Whelton (1999) identified 33 RCTs of the effect of oral potassium supplementation on BP, 20 in hypertensives. A pooled analysis of the 33 trials found an overall reduction of 4.4/2.5 mm Hg (Fig. 6-5). Greater effects were seen in the 28 trials wherein potassium excretion was increased by 20 mmol per day or more and in the 28 trials wherein no antihypertensive drugs were given. Overall, the response was greater in blacks, the higher the baseline BP and the greater the sodium intake. Another analysis of 27 trials found that an average 44 mmol per day increase in potassium intake provided an average 3.5/2.5 mm Hg fall in BP among hypertensive subjects (Geleijnse et al., 2003). However, with much stricter criteria applied to all published studies, only six were accepted, covering 483 patients (Dickinson et al., 2006a). The authors' conclusion was:

> This systematic review found no statistically significant effect of potassium supplementation on blood pressure. Because of the small number of participants in the two high quality trials, the short duration of follow-up, and the unexplained heterogeneity between trials, the evidence about the effect of potassium supplementation on blood pressure is not conclusive.

The potassium supplement in almost all these trials was potassium chloride (KCl), given in amounts from 48 to 120 mmol per day. Two RCTs have found a greater fall in BP after either potassium citrate (Overlack et al., 1995) or potassium bicarbonate (Morris et al., 1995) than after equal amounts of KCl. Potassium citrate also prevented the kaluresis and bone resorption caused by a high salt intake (Sellmeyer et al., 2002).

Protection Against Strokes

Increased potassium intake may protect against strokes. This was suggested by Acheson and Williams (1983) and supported by the finding that an increase in potassium intake of 10 mmol per day was associated with a 40% reduction in stroke mortality among 859 older people (Khaw & Barrett-Connor, 1987). Among men in the Framingham Heart

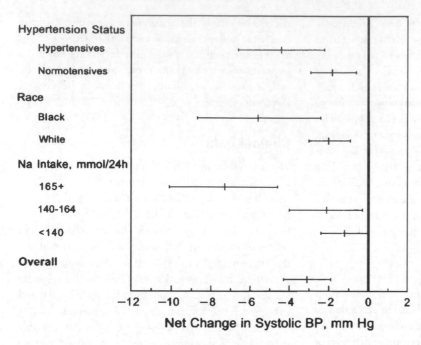

FIGURE 6-5 Pooled net change in SBP by participants' characteristics in 33 randomized, controlled trials of potassium supplementation. Na, sodium. (Modified from Jiang H, Whelton PK. What is the role of dietary sodium and potassium in hypertension and target organ injury? *Am J Med Sci* 1999;317:152–159.)

Study, an increased intake of three servings per day of potassium-rich fruits and vegetables was associated with a 22% lesser risk for stroke over a 20-year follow-up (Gillman et al., 1995). In three even larger populations, increased dietary potassium intake was associated with fewer strokes (Ascherio et al., 1998; Bazzano et al., 2001; Fang et al., 2000) and lower all-cause mortality (Tunstall-Pedoe, 1999). Although fruits and vegetables provide other protective ingredients than potassium, the significant reductions in stroke seen in eight cohort studies, an 11% reduction in those who consumed three to five portions a day, and 26% in those consuming more than five portions a day may be attributed to their higher potassium content (He et al., 2006).

Recommendations

Though potassium supplements may lower the BP, they are too costly and potentially hazardous for routine use in the treatment of hypertension in normokalemic patients. They are indicated for diuretic-induced hypokalemia and, in the form of potassium-containing salt substitutes, will add little expense (Coca et al., 2005). For the larger population, a reduction of high-sodium low-potassium processed foods with an increase of low-sodium high-potassium natural foods is all that likely is needed to achieve the potential

benefits. Fruits and beans provide the largest quantity of potassium per serving.

CALCIUM SUPPLEMENTATION

Both dietary and nondietary calcium supplements have a minimal effect on BP, an effect too small to recommend their use to treat hypertension. Moreover, the 732 healthy postmenopausal women who were randomly allocated to receive one gram of elemental calcium per day had significantly *more* cardiovascular events, including heart attacks, strokes, and sudden death, over 5 years than seem among the 739 who took a placebo (Bolland et al., 2008).

Clinical Data

A 2006 Cochrane Review found only 13 RCTs that were methodologically sound, covering 485 hypertensives (Dickinson et al., 2006b). A statistically significant decrease in SBP of –2.5 mm Hg was noted, but DBP fell by an insignificant –0.8 mm Hg. The authors' conclusion was:

> In view of the poor quality of included trials and the heterogeneity between trials, the evidence in favour of causal association between calcium supplementation and blood pressure reduction is weak and is probably due to bias. This is because poor quality studies generally tend to

over-estimate the effects of treatment. Larger, longer duration and better quality double-blind placebo controlled trials are needed to assess the effect of calcium supplementation on blood pressure and cardiovascular outcomes.

Recommendations

In the absence of data showing a significant beneficial effect of calcium supplements on BP, and in the presence of data showing a significant adverse effect on cardiovascular disease, their use is not recommended for treatment of hypertension. Moreover, calcium supplements may increase further the hypercalciuria already present in many hypertensives and thereby lead to kidney stones and urinary tract infection (Curhan et al., 1997). The best course is to ensure an adequate dietary calcium intake, but not to give calcium supplements to either prevent or treat hypertension.

MAGNESIUM SUPPLEMENTATION

The advice given for calcium supplements seems to be appropriate in regard to magnesium as well. Serum and intracellular magnesium levels are normal in most untreated hypertensives (Delva et al., 1996). However, low muscle magnesium concentration has been found in half of patients on chronic high-dose diuretic therapy (Drup et al., 1993), and magnesium deficiency may be responsible if hypokalemia is not corrected by potassium repletion (Whang et al., 1992).

In another Cochrane Review, Dickinson et al. (2006c) found 12 trials covering 545 hypertensives that met their strict criteria with magnesium supplements. SBP fell by an insignificant –1.3 mm Hg, whereas DBP fell by a significant –2.2 mm Hg. As with potassium and calcium, the conclusion was: "In view of the poor quality of included trials and the heterogeneity between trials, the evidence in favor of a causal association between magnesium supplementation and BP reduction is weak and is probably due to bias…"

Therefore, rather than giving magnesium supplements, increasing dietary consumption with fresh fruits and vegetables is preferable (Larsson et al., 2008). Magnesium supplements should only be given to patients found to be magnesium deficient (Atsmon & Dolev, 2005). For those patients, 15 mmol per day of magnesium will usually be tolerated.

INCREASED PHYSICAL ACTIVITY

The evidence for protection from both the development of hypertension and CVD and all-cause mortality by regular physical activity has become incontrovertible (Williams, 2008). Nonetheless, most people in all industrialized societies are becoming less physically active in their daily lives, spending more and more time in sedentary activities (Kimm et al., 2005; Nader et al., 2008). Not only will increased physical activity and higher levels of exercise capacity reduce the risk of coronary disease (Weinstein et al., 2008) and diabetes (Sigal et al., 2007), but they will likely prevent the development of hypertension (Leary et al., 2008). In a prospective 11-year follow-up of over 12,000 Finnish people, the incidence of hypertension was reduced by 28% in men and 35% in women who engaged in high levels of physical activity such as jogging or swimming (Barengo et al., 2005). In addition, regular physical activity during pregnancy reduced the incidence of preeclampsia (Saftlas et al., 2004).

Clinical Data

BP rises during moderate to high levels of exercise, more with resistance than with aerobic (Lydakis et al., 2008), but usually falls thereafter to below pre-exercise levels (Quinn, 2000). Persistent BP reduction may be seen after repetitive aerobic exercise, even without weight loss (Williams et al., 2007). Moreover, patients with orthostatic hypotension may have less of a postural fall after performing regular exercise (Winker et al., 2005).Because the SBP rises during exercise and because the abrupt rise in BP after arising from sleep is associated with an increased incidence of cardiovascular events, concerns about exercise in the morning have been raised. However, even in patients with known coronary disease, no increase in events was noted with exercise performed in the morning versus the afternoon (Murray et al., 1993). On the other hand, strenuous physical exertion in patients who are habitually sedentary, i.e., weekend warriors, may, on occasion, precipitate an acute myocardial infarction, whereas habitual vigorous exercise reduces the risk of sudden death during exercise (Whang et al., 2006). Therefore, sedentary patients should always be advised to increase their level of activity slowly. With slowly increasing exercise, an exaggerated rise in BP, as can be seen during stress testing, can be moderated (Ketelhut et al., 2004).

Hypertensives may start with a reduced exercise capacity (Lim et al., 1996) and may experience additional difficulty if they take β-blockers, which blunt exercise-mediated increases in heart rate and cardiac output (Vanhees et al., 2000). Other antihypertensive agents should not interfere with exercise ability (Predel et al., 1996).

Concerns may arise about another activity that involves exercise—sexual intercourse, which is accompanied by significant rises in pulse and BP that are equivalent to Stage II of the standardized Bruce treadmill test for men and Stage I for women (Palmieri et al., 2007). Although actually quite rare even among patients with coronary disease, the triggering of myocardial infarction during sexual activity likely can be prevented by regular exercise (Muller et al., 1996). Moreover, erectile dysfunction may be overcome by a program of physical activity and weight loss in obese men (Esposito et al., 2004).

Recommendations

Increased levels of physical activity, either during ordinary life or with structured exercise, may lower BP and prevent the onset of hypertension and diabetes, at least in part, through prevention of obesity (Hu et al., 2003). As little as 30 minutes of walking or its equivalent per day provides improvement in cardiorespiratory fitness (Blair & LaMonte, 2005) and slows the decline in cognitive function in the elderly (Lautenschlager et al., 2008).

Despite the obvious benefits, few physicians counsel their patients about exercise (Mellen et al., 2004), even though counseling has been shown to be effective in increasing patients' level of physical activity (Grandes et al., 2009). Perhaps of all attempts to modify lifestyle, this can have the most immediate acceptance and greatest overall benefit, other than cessation of smoking.

MODERATION OF ALCOHOL

A usual portion of alcohol-containing beverage, i.e., 12 oz of beer, 4 oz of wine, or 1.5 oz of whiskey, contains 10 to 12 mL of alcohol. Consumption of more than three usual portions per day raises BP and leads to a host of other problems. There is evidence that drinking one or two portions a day is not associated with a rise in BP (McFarlane et al.,

2007) and provides benefits on total mortality (Di Castelnuovo et al., 2006) and coronary disease (Beulens et al., 2007). However, as Jackson et al. (2005) state:

> Any coronary protection from light to moderate drinking will be very small and unlikely to outweigh the harms.... If so, the public health message is clear. Do not assume there is a window in which the health benefits of alcohol are greater than the harm—there is probably no free lunch.

The putative benefits of moderate drinking may have a biochemical rationale (Vasdev et al., 2006), but Jackson et al. (2005) attribute this "artificial association" to uncontrolled confounding. Naimi et al. (2005) found that among light to moderate drinkers, 27 of 30 cardiovascular risk factors were less prevalent than among nondrinkers. Fillmore et al. (2006) conclude from a meta-analysis of 54 published prospective studies on alcohol and mortality that a systematic misclassification error of including people who had stopped drinking because of ill health as "abstainers" led to an overestimation of cardiac protection.

Effects on Blood Pressure

Acutely drinking of 60 g of ethanol, the amount contained in five usual portions, induces an immediate fall in BP averaging 4/4 mm Hg followed, after 6 hours, by a rise averaging 7/4 mm Hg (Rosito et al., 1999). Chronically, the incidence of hypertensive is increased among women who drink more than two portions a day (Thadhani et al., 2002) and among men who drink more than three per day (Fuchs et al., 2001). The BP rises during heavy binge drinking (Seppä & Sillanaukee, 1999) and, when heavy drinkers abstain, their BP usually goes down (Xin et al., 2001). An analysis of the relation between the risk of hypertension and the pattern of drinking found a slightly lower incidence among those who drank daily with meals but a 41% increased incidence in those who drank without food (Stranges et al., 2004).

These and other studies examining the effect of alcohol on BP are likely to be both inexact, as they depend on people's estimate of their own drinking habits, and biased, as they cannot account for all possible confounders. Chen et al. (2008) have provided a way to more accurately ascertain the relation between BP and alcohol consumption.

Beneficial Effects

Nonetheless, there is impressive evidence for a protective effect of moderate, regular alcohol consumption of one half to two portions per day on a host of cardiovascular and other diseases when compared to similar outcomes in nondrinkers or heavy drinkers. Protection has been seen against total mortality (Grønbæk et al., 2000), coronary heart disease (Tolstrup et al., 2006), heart failure (Djoussé & Gaziano, 2007), the incidence of type 2 diabetes (Wei et al., 2000), osteoporosis (Berg et al., 2008), and mild cognitive impairment (Stampfer et al., 2005). Beneficial effects have been attributed to improvements in the lipid profile, in hemostatic factors, insulin sensitivity (Avogaro et al., 2002), and antioxidant activity (Vasdev et al., 2006).

However, no mortality benefit is seen in young people and an increased prevalence of breast cancer has been seen in women who drink more than one portion per day (Smith-Warner et al., 1998) and of colon cancer in those who drink more than two portions per day (Cho et al., 2004). Drinking more than two portions per day was associated with an increased risk for ischemic stroke (Mukamal et al., 2005).

Wine may be more protective than beer or whiskey (Renaud et al., 2004) but wine drinkers tend to have a healthier lifestyle (Tjønneland et al., 1999), so this apparent benefit may be exaggerated. Although there is a common perception that red wine is more protective than white wine because of its increased levels of polyphenols, there is little evidence to support that conclusion (Vogel, 2003).

Recommendations

The following guidelines seem appropriate:

- Carefully assess alcohol intake, as some people drink well beyond moderate amounts without being aware of their excessive consumption or its deleterious effects.
- If intake is more than one portion per day in women or two per day in men, advise a reduction to that level.
- Strongly advise against binge drinking.
- Drink only with food intake.
- For most people who consume moderate amounts of alcohol, no change is needed. If middle-aged (45- to 64-year-old) people start to drink, they rarely go beyond recommended amounts while properly benefiting from lower rates of cardiovascular morbidity (King et al., 2008).

OTHER DIETARY FACTORS

The impressive results of the DASH diet (Fig. 6-2) strongly support an antihypertensive effect of a diet low in saturated fat and high in fiber and minerals from fresh fruits and vegetables (Sacks et al., 2001). Moreover, among 1,710 middle-aged men followed up for 7 years, the rise in SBP was significantly less with diets higher in fruits and vegetables and lower in red meats (Miura et al., 2004).

Vegetarians have less hypertension than non-vegetarians. Compared to those eating a nonvegetarian diet, those consuming a vegetarian diet under controlled conditions had a lower BP in all nine published studies (Berkow & Barnard, 2005).

Dietary Nitrate

Certain green leafy vegetables, such as spinach, lettuce, and beetroot have high inorganic nitrate (NO_3) content. In an intriguing rediscovery of the antihypertensive effect of nitrate via its endogenous bioconversion to nitrite (NO_2), partially on the tongue, Webb et al. (2008) found a significant acute BP lowering, vasoprotective and antiplatelet effect of dietary nitrate contained in 500 mL of beetroot juice. After bioconversion from nitrate, the nitrite is reduced to NO when ischemia or injury induces a more acidic environment within tissues. The NO generated from nitrite induces vasodilation, thereby lowering BP.

Fiber

One feature of a vegetarian diet is the increased amount of fiber. The benefits found in the DASH diet could reflect the increase in fiber from 9 to 31 g per day (Appel et al., 1997). A meta-analysis of all 24 randomized, placebo-controlled clinical trials published from 1966 to 2003 of the effect on BP of supplements of dietary fiber averaging 11.5 g per day found an average fall of 1.1/1.3 mm Hg (Streppel et al., 2005). In addition, a pooled analysis of ten prospective cohort studies found a decrease in the risk of coronary heart disease with increased consumption of dietary fiber (Pereira et al., 2004).

Dietary Fat

In keeping with the potential contribution of the low saturated fat content of the DASH diet, other smaller studies have shown a lowering of BP with a low-fat diet (Straznicky et al., 1999).

The type of fat may also be important. As a component of the cardiovascularly beneficial Mediterranean diet (Papamichael et al., 2008), olive oil may lower BP because of its high content of mono-unsaturated fatty acids or antioxidant polyphenols (Psaltopoulou et al., 2004). Increased intake of linoleic acid, the main dietary polyunsaturated fatty acid, is associated with a significant fall in BP (Miura et al., 2008). Omega-3 fatty acid intake in food has been shown to have a small BP lowering effect (Ueshima et al., 2007). In a crossover trial of 13 hypertensives, 100 g per day of polyphenol-rich dark chocolate eaten for 14 days was associated with a 5.1/1.8 mm Hg average fall in BP compared to the lack of effect of polyphenol-free white chocolate (Taubert et al., 2003).

Lipid-lowering Diet and Drugs

Beyond any antihypertensive effect, low saturated-fat diets may protect against CVD (Howard et al., 2006; Mustad & Kris-Etherton, 2000). Both diet and lipid-lowering drugs, in particular statins, improve the endothelial dysfunction associated with dyslipidemia (Balk et al., 2004), thereby both lowering BP (Strazzullo et al., 2007). Protection against atherosclerotic complications, including stroke, has been seen with statins in both normotensives and hypertensives (Messerli et al., 2008).

Protein Intake

Although high protein intake has been thought to be detrimental, in large part by placing an additional load on the kidney (Friedman, 2004), both INTERSALT (Stamler et al., 1996) and INTERMAP (Elliott et al., 2006) found a lower BP in people who consume a high vegetable protein diet. However, red meat intake is associated with higher SBP (Tzoulaki et al., 2008).

Antioxidants

Although the antihypertensive effect of a diet rich in fruits and vegetables has been related to the accompanying increase in antioxidant vitamins (John et al., 2002), trials of antioxidant supplements have shown no effect on preventing cardiovascular events (Katsiki & Manes, 2008). As noted in Chapter 3, these trials have used inadequate antioxidants.

Caffeine

The effects of caffeine-containing beverages are covered in Chapter 3. In summary, there seems no reason to restrict moderate amounts of caffeine-containing beverage (Lopez-Garcia et al., 2008).

MISCELLANEOUS

A large number of complementary and alternative therapies are being used for hypertension among other indications, in part because of dissatisfaction with traditional medical practices (Adams et al., 2002). When such therapies are subjected to appropriately controlled study, they often are found to be ineffectual (Canter, 2003).

Relaxation

In view of the evidence, reviewed in Chapter 3, that stress-related anxiety and job strain may be involved in the development of hypertension (Esler & Parati, 2004), various stress-relieving techniques to lower BP have been used for many years (Jacobson, 1939). More recently, a variety of cognitive-behavioral therapies—including transcendental meditation, yoga, biofeedback, tai chi, and psychotherapy—have been shown to reduce the BP of hypertensive patients at least transiently (Anderson et al., 2008; Rainforth et al., 2007; Yeh et al., 2008). Although each therapy has its advocates, none has been shown conclusively to be either practical for the majority of hypertensives or effective in maintaining a significant long-term effect (Canter & Ernst, 2004).

If available and acceptable to the patient, one or another form of relaxation therapy may be tried, as such techniques may provide additional benefits in reducing coronary risk beyond any effect on BP. Patients should be forewarned that short-term effects may not be maintained, so continued surveillance is needed.

Slow Breathing

Slow breathing guided by a device has been shown to reduce BP in some hypertensives (Meles et al., 2004; Radaelli et al., 2004), but not in others (Logtenberg et al., 2007). Whether this provides more reduction in BP than other relaxation techniques is uncertain.

Bed Rest and Sedatives

When patients, even those whose disease is difficult to control on an outpatient basis, are hospitalized, their BP frequently comes down, mainly because the sympathetic nervous system becomes less active (Nishimura et al., 1987). This fall in BP may largely reflect the removal of the white-coat effect, as little change has been noted by repeated ambulatory monitoring in hospitalized patients (Fotherby et al., 1995).

The BP usually falls considerably during sleep. However, there is no evidence that sedatives or tranquilizers lower BP (U.S. Public Health Service Cooperative Study, 1965). Monoamine oxidase inhibitors will lower the BP, but their use is limited by the potential for bad pressor reactions with tyramine-containing foods.

Garlic and Herbal Remedies

Garlic, mainly as a deodorized powder, has been found to significantly lower BP by −8.4/−7.3 mm Hg in 4 RCTs, compared to placebo in hypertensive subjects (Ried et al., 2008).

Herbal remedies are being widely used for all sorts of unproved benefits, totally unsupervised in the United States because of congressional interference with the Food and Drug Administration's surveillance (Bent, 2008). None has been shown to lower BP (with the obvious exceptions of *Rauwolfia* and *Veratrum*) and some, in fact, will raise BP, including *Ephedra* and licorice extract (De Smet, 2004).

Other Modalities

Acupuncture, though widely used, has either no effect on BP (Macklin et al., 2006) or a transient effect that disappears when acupuncture is stopped (Flachskampf et al., 2007). *Melatonin*, 2.5 mg at bedtime for 3 weeks, was found to reduce nighttime BP by 6/4 mm Hg in a crossover trial in 16 hypertensives (Scheer et al., 2004). High intake of *folate* was associated with a reduced incidence of hypertension in the Nurses Health Study (Forman et al., 2005).

Surgical Procedures

From approximately 1935 through the 1950s, surgical sympathectomy, along with a rigid low-salt diet, was about all that was available for treating hypertension. Sympathectomy was shown to be beneficial for those with severe disease (Thorpe et al., 1950). With current medical therapy, there is no place for sympathectomy. Meanwhile, a clinical study is being performed on the use of an implanted device to activate the carotid baroreflex, thereby lowering BP in patients resistant to drug therapy (Scheffers et al., 2008).

Neurovascular decompression of the rostral ventolateral medulla may have a transient antihypertensive effect (Frank et al., 2009).

CONCLUSIONS

Appropriate lifestyle modifications should be assiduously promoted in all patients. Those with mild hypertension may thereby be able to stay off drugs; those with more severe hypertension may need less medication. Hopefully, population-wide adoption of healthier lifestyles will reduce the incidence of hypertension and its complications (Fung et al., 2008). Meanwhile, most hypertensive patients will need antihypertensive drugs as described in the next chapter.

REFERENCES

Acheson RM, Williams DRR. Does consumption of fruit and vegetables protect against stroke? *Lancet* 1983;1:1191–1193.

Adams KE, Cohen MH, Eisenberg D, et al. Ethical considerations of complementary and alternative medical therapies in conventional medical settings. *Ann Intern Med* 2002;137:660–664.

Alderman MH. Salt and blood pressure in children. *J Hum Hypertens* 2008;22:1 3.

Alderman MH, Cohen H, Madhavan S. Dietary sodium intake and mortality: The National Health and Nutrition Examination Survey (NHANES I). *Lancet* 1998;351:781–785.

Alderman MH, Madhavan S, Cohen H, et al. Low urinary sodium is associated with greater risk of myocardial infarction among treated hypertensive men. *Hypertension* 1995;25:1144–1152.

Anderson JW, Liu C, Kryscio RL. Blood pressure response to transcendental meditation: A meta-analysis. *Am J Hypertens* 2008;21(3):310–316.

Appel LJ, Espeland MA, Easter L, et al. Effects of reduced sodium intake on hypertension control in older individuals: Results from the Trial of Nonpharmacologic Interventions in the Elderly (TONE). *Arch Intern Med* 2001;161:685–693.

Appel LJ, Moore TJ, Obarzanek E, et al. A clinical trial of the effects of dietary patterns on blood pressure. *N Engl J Med* 1997;336:1117–1124.

Argacha J, Adamopoulos D, Gujic M, et al. Acute effects of passive smoking on peripheral vascular function. *Hypertension* 2008;51:1506–1511.

Asaria P, Chisholm D, Mathers C, et al. Chronic disease prevention: Health effects and financial costs of strategies to reduce salt intake and control tobacco use. *Lancet* 2007;370:2044–2053.

Ascherio A, Rimm EB, Hernán MA, et al. Intake of potassium, magnesium, calcium, and fiber and risk of stroke among US men. *Circulation* 1998;98:1198–1204.

Atsmon J, Dolev E. Drug-induced hypomagnesaemia: Scope and management. *Drug Saf* 2005;28(9):763–788.

Avogaro A, Watanabe RM, Gottardo L, et al. Glucose tolerance during moderate alcohol intake: Insights on insulin action from glucose/lactate dynamics. *J Clin Endocrinol Metab* 2002;87: 1233–1238.

Balk EM, Karas RH, Jordan HS, et al. Effects of statins on vascular structure and function: A systematic review. *Am J Med* 2004;117:775–790.

Barba G, Galletti F, Cappuccio F, et al. Incidence of hypertension in individuals with different blood pressure salt-sensitivity: Results of a 15-year follow-up study. *J Hypertens* 2007;25: 1465–1471.

Barengo NC, Hu G, Kastarinen M, et al. Low physical activity as a predictor of antihypertensive drug treatment in 25—64-year-old populations in Eastern and south-western Finland. *J Hypertens* 2005;23:293–299.

Batsis JA, Romero-Corral A, Collazo-Clavell ML, et al. Effect of bariatric surgery on the metabolic syndrome: A population-based, long-term controlled study. *Mayo Clin Proc* 2008;83(8): 897–906.

Bazzano LA, He J, Ogden LG, et al. Dietary potassium intake and risk of stroke in US men and women: National Health and Nutrition Examination Survey I epidemiologic follow-up study. *Stroke* 2001;32:1473–1480.

Bent S. Herbal Medicine in the United States: Review of efficacy, safety, and regulation. *J Gen Intern Med* 2008;23(6):854–859.

Berg KM, Kunins HV, Jackson JL, et al. Association between alcohol consumption and both osteoporotic fracture and bone density. *Am J Med* 2008;121:406–418.

Berkow SE, Barnard ND. Blood pressure regulation and vegetarian diets. *Nutr Rev* 2005;63:1–8.

Beulens JWJ, Rimm EB, Ascherio A, et al. Alcohol consumption and risk for coronary heart disease among men with hypertension. *Ann Intern Med* 2007;146:10–19.

Blair SN, LaMonte MJ. How much and what type of physical activity is enough? What physicians should tell their patients. *Arch Intern Med* 2005;165:2324–2325.

Bolland MJ, Barber PA, Doughty RN, et al. Vascular events in healthy older women receiving calcium supplementation: Randomised controlled trial. *Br Med J* 2008;336:226–227.

Burke GL, Bertoni AG, Shea S, et al. The impact of obesity on cardiovascular disease risk factors and subclinical vascular disease: The multi-ethnic study of atherosclerosis. *Arch Intern Med* 2008a;168(9):928–935.

Canadian Hypertension Society. 2008 CHEP recommendations for the management of hypertension. Available at: www. Canadian Hypertension Education Program.com.

Canter PH. The therapeutic effects of meditation. *Br Med J* 2003;326:1049–1050.

Canter PH, Ernst E. Insufficient evidence to conclude whether or not transcendental meditation decreases blood pressure: Results of a systematic review of randomized controlled trials. *J Hypertens* 2004;22:2049–2054.

Carbone LD, Bush AJ, Barrow KD, et al. The relationship of sodium intake to calcium and sodium excretion and bone mineral density of the hip in postmenopausal African-American and Caucasian women. *J Bone Miner Metab* 2003;21(6):415–420.

Chen L, Smith GD, Harbord RM, et al. Alcohol intake and blood pressure: A systematic review implementing a mendelian randomization approach. *PLoS Med* 2008;5(3):e52,461–471.

Chiuve SE, Rexrode KM, Spiegelman D, et al. Primary prevention of stroke by healthy lifestyle. *Circulation* 2008;118:947–954.

Cho E, Smith-Warner SA, Ritz J, et al. Alcohol intake and colorectal cancer: A pooled analysis of 8 cohort studies. *Ann Intern Med* 2004;140:603–613.

Chobanian AV, Bakris GL, Black HR, et al. Seventh report of the Joint National Committee on Prevention, Detection, Evaluation, and Treatment of High Blood Pressure. *Hypertension* 2003;42:1206–1252.

Christian JG, Bessesen DH, Byers TE, et al. Clinic-based support to help overweight patients with type 2 diabetes increase physical activity and lose weight. *Arch Intern Med* 2008;168(2): 141–146.

Chrysant SG, Weder AB, McCarron DA, et al. Effects of isradipine or enalapril on blood pressure in salt-sensitive hypertensives during low and high dietary salt intake. *Am J Hypertens* 2000;13: 1180–1188.

Coca SG, Perazella MA, Buller GK. The cardiovascular implications of hypokalemia. *Am J Kidney Dis* 2005;45(2):233–247.

Cohen HW, Hailpern SM, Alderman MH. Sodium intake and mortality follow-up in the Third National Health and Nutritional Examination Survey (NHANES III). *J Gen Intern Med* 2008;8:645–646.

Cohen HW, Hailpern SM, Fang J, et al. Sodium intake and mortality in the NHANES II follow-up study. *Am J Med* 2006;119: 275.e7–275.e14.

Connolly GN, Alpert HR. Trends in the use of cigarettes and other tobacco products, 2000–2007. *JAMA* 2008;299(22):2629–2630.

Cook NR, Cutler JA, Hennekens CH. An unexpected result for sodium—causal or casual? *Hypertension* 1995;25:1153–1154.

Cook NR, Cutler JA, Obarzanek E, et al. Long term effects of dietary sodium reduction on cardiovascular disease outcomes: Observational follow-up of the trials of hypertension prevention (TOHP). *Br Med J* 2007;334:885–893.

Crippa G, Nuñez-Ruiz M, Sverzellati E, et al. Dietary sodium curtailment reduces indapamide kaliuretic effect and improves blood pressure control [Abstract]. *Am Soc Hypertens* 1996;9:145A.

Cumming RG, Mitchell P, Smith W. Dietary sodium intake and cataract: The Blue Mountains eye study. *Am J Epidemiol* 2000;151:624–626.

Curhan GC, Willett WC, Speizer FE, et al. Comparison of dietary calcium with supplemental calcium and other nutrients as factors affecting the risk for kidney stones in women. *Ann Intern Med* 1997;126:497–504.

de Boer MP, Ijzerman RG, de Jongh RT, et al. Birth weight relates to salt sensitivity of blood pressure in healthy adults. *Hypertension* 2008;51:928–932.

De Smet PAGM. Health risks of herbal remedies: An update. *Clin Pharmacol Ther* 2004;76:1–17.

de Wardener HE. Salt reduction and cardiovascular risk: The anatomy of a myth. *J Hum Hypertens* 1999;13:1–4.

Delgado MC. Potassium in hypertension. *Curr Hypertens Rep* 2004;6:31–35.

Delva PT, Pastori C, Degan M, et al. Intralymphocyte free magnesium in a group of subjects with essential hypertension. *Hypertension* 1996;28:433–439.

Di Castelnuovo AD, Costanzo S, Bagnardi V, et al. Alcohol dosing and total mortality in men and women: An updated meta-analysis of 34 prospective studies. *Arch Intern Med* 2006;166: 2437–2445.

Dickinson BD, Havas S. Reducing the population burden of cardiovascular disease by reducing sodium intake: A report of the Council on Science and Public Health. *Arch Intern Med* 2007;167(14):1460–1468.

Dickinson HO, Nicolson DJ, Campbell F, et al. Potassium supplementation for the management of primary hypertension in adults. *Cochrane Database Syst Rev* 2006a;3:CD004641.

Dickinson HO, Nicolson DJ, Cook JV, et al. Calcium supplementation for the management of primary hypertension in adults. *Cochrane Database Syst Rev* 2006b;2:CD004639.

Dickinson HO, Nicolson DJ, Campbell F, et al. Magnesium supplementation for the management of essential hypertension in adults. *Cochrane Database Syst Rev* 2006c;3:CD004640.

Djoussé L, Gaziano JM. Alcohol consumption and risk of heart failure in the physicians' health study I. *Circulation* 2007;115:34–39.

Drup I, Skajaa K, Thybo NK. Oral magnesium supplementation restores the concentrations of magnesium, potassium and sodium-potassium pumps in skeletal muscle of patients receiving diuretic treatment. *J Int Med* 1993;233:117–123.

Ebbeling CB, Pawlak DB, Ludwig DS. Childhood obesity: Public-health crisis, common sense cure. *Lancet* 2002;360:473–482.

Elliott P, Stamler J, Dyer AR, et al. Association between protein intake and blood pressure: The INTERMAP study. *Arch Intern Med* 2006;166:79–87.

Elmer PJ, Obarzanek E, Vollmer WM, et al. Effects of comprehensive lifestyle modification on diet, weight, physical fitness, and blood pressure control: 18-month results of a randomized trial. *Ann Intern Med* 2006;144:485–495.

Esler M, Parati G. Is essential hypertension sometimes a psychosomatic disorder? *J Hypertens* 2004;22:873–876.

Esposito K, Giugliano F, Di Palo C, et al. Effect of lifestyle changes on erectile dysfunction in obese men: A randomized controlled trial. *JAMA* 2004;291:2978–2984.

Estabrooks PA, Glasgow RE, Dzewaltowski DA. Physical activity promotion through primary care. *JAMA* 2003;289:2913–2916.

Fang J, Madhavan S, Alderman MH. Dietary potassium intake and stroke mortality. *Stroke* 2000;31:1532–1537.

Fillmore KM, Kerr WC, Stockwell T, et al. Moderate alcohol use and reduced mortality risk: Systematic error in prospective studies. *Addict Res Theory* 2006;14(2):101–132.

Flachskampf FA, Gallasch J, Gefeller O, et al. Hypertension: Randomized trial of acupuncture to lower blood pressure. *Circulation* 2007;115:3121–3129.

Fock KM, Talley N, Moayyedi P, et al. Asia-Pacific consensus guidelines on gastric cancer prevention. *Gastroenterol Hepatol* 2008;23(3):351–365.

Folsom AR, Parker ED, Harnack LJ. Degree of concordance with DASH diet guidelines and incidence of hypertension and fatal cardiovascular disease. *Am J Hypertens* 2007;20:225–232.

Forman JP, Rimm EB, Stampfer MJ, et al. Folate intake and the risk of incident hypertension among US women. *JAMA* 2005;293:320–329.

Fotherby MD, Critchley D, Potter JF. Effect of hospitalization on conventional and 24-hour blood pressure. *Age Ageing* 1995;24:25–29.

Franco V, Oparil S. Salt sensitivity, a determinant of blood pressure, cardiovascular disease and survival. *J Am Coll Nutr* 2006;25(3):247S–255S.

Frank H, Heusser K, Geiger H, et al. Temporary reduction of blood pressure and sympathetic nerve activity in hypertensive patients after microvascular decompression. *Stroke* 2009;40(1):41–51.

Fraser GE, Shavlik DJ. Ten years of life: Is it a matter of choice? *Arch Intern Med* 2001;161:1645–1652.

Friedman AN. High-protein diets: Potential effects on the kidney in renal health and disease. *Am J Kidney Dis* 2004;44:950–962.

Fuchs FD, Chambless LE, Whelton PK, et al. Alcohol consumption and the incidence of hypertension: The Atherosclerosis Risk in Communities Study. *Hypertension* 2001;37:1242–1250.

Fung TT, Chiuve SE, McCullough ML, et al. Adherence to a DASH-style diet and risk of coronary heart disease and stroke in women. *Arch Intern Med* 2008;168:713–720.

Gates PE, Tanaka H, Hiatt WR, et al. Dietary sodium restriction rapidly improves large elastic artery compliance in older adults with systolic hypertension. *Hypertension* 2004;44:35–41.

Geleijnse JM, Kok FJ, Grobbee DE. Blood pressure response to changes in sodium and potassium intake: A metaregression analysis of randomised trials. *J Hum Hypertens* 2003;17:471–480.

Gerdts E, Lund-Johansen P, Omvik P. Reproducibility of salt sensitivity testing using a dietary approach in essential hypertension. *J Hum Hypertens* 1999;13:375–384.

Gillman MW, Cupples A, Gagnon D, et al. Protective effect of fruits and vegetables on development of stroke in men. *JAMA* 1995;273:1113–1117.

Gostin LO. Law as a tool to facilitate healthier lifestyles and prevent obesity. *JAMA* 2007;297(1):87.

Grandes G, Sanchez A, Sanchez-Pinilla RO, et al. Effectiveness of physical activity advice and prescription by physicians in routine primary care: A cluster randomized trial. *Arch Intern Med* 2009;169(7):694.

Graudal N, Galløe A, Garred P. Effects of sodium restriction on blood pressure, renin, aldosterone, catecholamines, cholesterols, and triglyceride. *JAMA* 1998;279:1383–1391.

Grønbæk M, Becker U, Johansen D, et al. Type of alcohol consumed and mortality from all causes, coronary heart disease, and cancer. *Ann Intern Med* 2000;133:411–419.

Halperin RO, Gaziano JM, Sesso HD. Smoking and the risk of incident hypertension in middle-aged and older men. *Am J Hypertens* 2008;21:148–152.

Harsha DW, Bray GA. Weight loss and blood pressure control (pro). *Hypertension* 2008;51:1420–1425.

Hatsukami DK, Stead LF, Gupta PC. Tobacco addiction. *Lancet* 2008;371:2027–2038.

Havas S, Dickinson BD, Wilson M. The urgent need to reduce sodium consumption. *JAMA* 2007;298(12):1439.

He FJ, MacGregor GA. How far should salt intake be reduced? *Hypertension* 2003;42:1093–1099.

He FJ, Nowson CA, MacGregor GA. Fruit and vegetable consumption and stroke: Meta-analysis of cohort studies. *Lancet* 2006;367:320–326.

He J, Ogden LG, Vupputuri S, et al. Dietary sodium intake and subsequent risk of cardiovascular disease in overweight adults. *JAMA* 1999;282:2027–2034.

He J, Whelton PK. What is the role of dietary sodium and potassium in hypertension and target organ injury? *Am J Med Sci* 1999;317:152–159.

Heusser K, Engeli S, Tank J, et al. Sympathetic vasomotor tone determines blood pressure response to long-term sibutramine treatment. *J Clin Endocrinol Metab* 2007;92(4):1560–1563.

Hooper L, Bartlett C, Davey Smith G, et al. Systematic review of long term effects of advice to reduce dietary salt in adults. *Br Med J* 2002;325:628–632.

Horvath K, Jeitier K, Siering U, et al. Long-term effects of weight reducing interventions in hypertensive patients: Systematic review and meta-analysis. *Arch Intern Med* 2008;168(6):571–580.

Howard BV, Van Horn L, Hsia J, et al. Low-fat dietary pattern and risk of cardiovascular disease: The women's health initiative randomized controlled dietary modification trial. *JAMA* 2006;295(6):655–666.

Hu FB, Li TY, Colditz GA, et al. Television watching and other sedentary behaviors in relation to risk of obesity and type 2 diabetes mellitus in women. *JAMA* 2003;289:1785–1791.

Hypertension Prevention Trial Research Group. The Hypertension Prevention Trial: Three-year effects of dietary changes on blood pressure. *Arch Intern Med* 1990;150:153–162.

Jackson R, Broad J, Connor J, et al. Alcohol and ischaemic heart disease: Probably no free lunch. *Lancet* 2005;366:1911–1912.

Jacobson E. Variation of blood pressure with skeletal muscle tension and relaxation. *Ann Intern Med* 1939;12:1194–1212.

Jakicic JM, Marcus BH, Lang W, et al. Effect of exercise on 24-month weight loss maintenance in overweight women. *Arch Intern Med* 2008;168(14):1550–1559.

James J, Thomas P, Kerr D. Preventing childhood obesity: two year follow-up results from the Christchurch obesity prevention programme in schools (CHOPPS). *Br Med J* 2007;335:762–765.

Jarrett DRJ. Paracetamol and hypertension: Time to label sodium in drug treatments? *Br Med J* 2008;336:1324.

Jatoi NA, Jerrard-Dunne P, Feely J, et al. Impact of smoking and smoking cessation on arterial stiffness and aortic wave reflection in hypertension. *Hypertension* 2007;49:981–985.

John JH, Ziebland S, Yudkin P, et al. Effects of fruit and vegetable consumption on plasma antioxidant concentrations and blood pressure: A randomised controlled trial. *Lancet* 2002;359:1969–1974.

Joossens JV, Kesteloot H. Dietary salt, cerebrovascular disease and stomach cancer mortalities. *Acta Cardiol* 2008;63(1):9–10.

Joossens JV, Kesteloot H. Trends in systolic blood pressure, 24-hour sodium excretion, and stroke mortality in the elderly in Belgium. *Am J Med* 1991;90(Suppl. 3A):5.

Kastarinen MJ, Puska PM, Korhonen MH, et al. Non-pharmacological treatment of hypertension in primary health care: A 2-year open randomized controlled trial of lifestyle intervention against hypertension in eastern Finland. *J Hypertens* 2002;20:2505–2512.

Katsiki N, Manes C. Clinical trials of antioxidant supplementation in the prevention of cardiovascular events. *Arch Intern Med* 2008;168(7):773–774.

Kempner W. Treatment of hypertensive vascular disease with rice diet. *Am J Med* 1948;4:545–577.

Ketelhut RG, Franz IW, Scholze J. Regular exercise as an effective approach in antihypertensive therapy. *Med Sci Sports Exerc* 2004;36:4–8.

Khaw K-T, Barrett-Connor E. Dietary potassium and stroke-associated mortality: A 12-year prospective population study. *N Engl J Med* 1987;316:235–240.

Kimm SYS, Glynn NW, Obarzanek E, et al. Relation between the changes in physical activity and body-mass index during adolescence: A multicentre longitudinal study. *Lancet* 2005;366:301–307.

King DE, Mainous AG, Geesey ME. Adopting moderate alcohol consumption in middle age: Subsequent cardiovascular events. *Am J Med* 2008;121:201–206.

Knoops KTB, de Groot LCPGM, Kromhout D, et al. Mediterranean diet, lifestyle factors, and 10-year mortality in elderly European men and women: The HALE project. *JAMA* 2004;292:1433–1439.

Larsson SC, Virtanen MJ, Mars M, et al. Magnesium, calcium, potassium, and sodium intakes and risk of stroke in male smokers. *Arch Intern Med* 2008;168(5):459–465.

Lautenschlager NT, Cox KL, Flicker L, et al. Effect of physical activity on cognitive function in older adults at risk for Alzheimer disease. *JAMA* 2008;300(9):1027–1037.

Law MR. Epidemiologic evidence of salt and blood pressure. *Am J Hypertens* 1997;10:42S–45S.

Leary SD, Ness AR, Smith GD, et al. Physical activity and blood pressure in childhood: Findings from a population-based study. *Hypertension* 2008;51:92–98.

Li G, Zhang P, Wang J, et al. The long-term effect of lifestyle interventions to prevent diabetes in the China Da Qing diabetes prevention study: A 20-year follow-up study. *Lancet* 2008;371:1783–1789.

Lim PO, MacFadyen RJ, Clarkson PBM, et al. Impaired exercise tolerance in hypertensive patients. *Ann Intern Med* 1996;124:41–55.

Lindstrom J, Ilanne-Parikka M, Peltonen M, et al. Sustained reduction in the incidence of type 2 diabetes by lifestyle intervention: Follow-up of the Finnish diabetes prevention study. *Lancet* 2006;368:1673–1679.

Little P, Kelly J, Barnett J, et al. Randomised controlled factorial trial of dietary advice for patients with a single high blood pressure reading in primary care. *Br Med J* 2004;328:1054–1058.

Logtenberg SJ, Kleefstra N, Houweling ST, et al. Effect of device-guided breathing exercises on blood pressure in hypertensive patients with type 2 diabetes mellitus: A randomized controlled trial. *J Hypertens* 2007;1:241–246.

Lopez-Garcia E, van Dam RM, Li TY, et al. The relationship of coffee consumption with mortality. *Ann Intern Med* 2008;148:904–914.

Lydakis C, Momen A, Blaha C, et al. Changes of central haemodynamic parameters during mental stress and acute bouts of static and dynamic exercise. *J Hum Hypertens* 2008;22:320–328.

Macklin EA, Wayne PM, Kalish LA, et al. Stop hypertension with the acupuncture research program (SHARP): Results of a randomized, controlled clinical trial. *Hypertension* 2006;48:838–845.

Mark AL. Dietary Therapy for obesity: An emperor with no clothes. *Hypertension* 2008;51:1426–1434.

Martini LA, Cuppari L, Colugnati FAB, et al. High sodium chloride intake is associated with low bone density in calcium stone-forming patients. *Clin Nephrol* 2000;54:85–93.

McFarlane SI, von Gizycki H, Salifu M, et al. Alcohol consumption and blood pressure in the adult US population: Assessment of gender-related effects. *J Hypertens* 2007;25:965–970.

Melander O, von Wowern F, Frandsen E, et al. Moderate salt restriction effectively lowers blood pressure and degree of salt sensitivity is related to baseline concentration of renin and N-terminal atrial natriuretic peptide in plasma. *J Hypertens* 2007;25:619–627.

Meles E, Giannattasio C, Failla M, et al. Nonpharmacologic treatment of hypertension by respiratory exercise in the home setting. *Am J Hypertens* 2004;17:370–374.

Mellen PB, Gao SK, Vitolins MZ, et al. Deteriorating dietary habits among adults with hypertension. *Arch Intern Med* 2008;168(3):308–314.

Mellen PB, Palla SL, Goff DC, et al. Prevalence of nutrition and exercise counseling for patients with hypertension: United States, 1999 to 2000. *J Gen Intern Med* 2004;19:917–924.

Mente A, de Koning L, Shannon HS, et al. A systematic review of the evidence supporting a casual link between dietary factors and coronary heart disease. *Arch Intern Med* 2009;169(7):659–669.

Messerli FH, Pinto L, Tang SSK, et al. Impact of systemic hypertension on the cardiovascular benefits of statin therapy—A meta-analysis. *Am J Cardiol* 2008;101:319–325.

Messerli FH, Schmieder RE, Weir MR. Salt: A perpetrator of hypertensive target organ disease? *Arch Intern Med* 1997;157:2449–2452.

Mikkelsen KL, Wiinberg N, Hoegholm A, et al. Smoking related to 24-hr ambulatory blood pressure and heart rate. *Am J Hypertens* 1997;10:483–491.

Miura K, Greenland P, Stamler J, et al. Relation of vegetable, fruit, and meat intake to 7-year blood pressure change in middle-aged men: The Chicago Western Electric study. *Am J Epidemiol* 2004;159:572–580.

Miura K, Stamler J, Nakagawa H, et al. Relationship of dietary linoleic acid to blood pressure: The international study of macro-micronutrients and blood pressure study. *Hypertension* 2008;52:408–414.

Morgan T, Anderson A, Wilson D, et al. Paradoxical effect of sodium restriction on blood pressure in people on slow-channel calcium blocking drugs. *Lancet* 1986;1:793.

Morris RC Jr, O'Connor M, Forman A, et al. Supplemental dietary potassium with KHCO$_3$ but not KCl attenuates essential hypertension [Abstract]. *J Am Soc Nephrol* 1995;6(3):645.

Mukamal KJ, Ascherio A, Mittleman MA, et al. Alcohol and risk for ischemic stroke in men: The role of drinking patterns and usual beverage. *Ann Intern Med* 2005;142:11–19.

Muller JE, Mittleman MA, Maclure M, et al. Triggering myocardial infarction by sexual activity. *JAMA* 1996;275:1405–1409.

Murray PM, Herrington DM, Pettus CW, et al. Should patients with heart disease exercise in the morning or afternoon? *Arch Intern Med* 1993;153:833–836.

Mustad VA, Kris-Etherton PM. Beyond cholesterol lowering: Deciphering the benefits of dietary intervention on cardiovascular diseases. *Curr Atherosclerosis Rep* 2000;2:461–466.

Nader PR, Bradley RH, Houts RM, et al. Moderate-to-vigorous physical activity from ages 9 to 15 years. *JAMA* 2008;300(3): 295–305.

Naimi TS, Brown DW, Brewer RD, et al. Cardiovascular risk factors and confounders among nondrinking and moderate-drinking U.S. adults. *Am J Prev Med* 2005;28(4):369–373.

Nicolson DJ, Dickinson HO, Campbell F, et al. Lifestyle interventions or drugs for patients with essential hypertension: A systematic review. *J Hypertens* 2004;22:2043–2048.

Nishimura H, Nishioka A, Kubo S, et al. Multifactorial evaluation of blood pressure fall upon hospitalization in essential hypertensive patients. *Clin Sci* 1987;73:135–141.

Nyamdorj R, Qiao Q, Söderberg S, et al. Comparison of body mass index with waist circumference, waist-to-hip ratio, and waist-to-stature ratio as a predictor of hypertension incidence in Mauritius. *J Hypertens* 2008;26:866–870.

Ogden CL, Carroll MD, Flegal KM. High body mass index for age among US children and adolescents, 2003–2006. *JAMA* 2008;299(20):2401–2405.

Oncken CA, White WB, Cooney JL, et al. Impact of smoking cessation on ambulatory blood pressure and heart rate in postmenopausal women. *Am J Hypertens* 2001;14:942–949.

Orr J, Gentile CL, Davy BM, et al. Large artery stiffening with weight gain in humans: Role of visceral fat accumulation. *Hypertension* 2000;51.1519–1324.

Overlack A, Maus B, Ruppert M, et al. Kaliumcitrat versus kaliumchlorid bei essentieller hypertonie. Wirkung auf hämodynamische, hormonelle und metabolische parameter. *Dtsch Med Wochenschr* 1995;120:631–635.

Palmieri ST, Kostis JB, Casazza L, et al. Heart rate and blood pressure response in adult men and women during exercise and sexual activity. *Am J Cardiol* 2007;100:1795–1801.

Papamichael CM, Karatzi KN, Papaioannou TG, et al. Acute combined effects of olive oil and wine on pressure wave reflections: Another beneficial influence of the Mediterranean diet antioxidants? *J Hypertens* 2008;26:223–229.

Pardell H, Tresserras R, Saltó E, et al. Management of the hypertensive patient who smokes. *Drugs* 1998;56:177–187.

Parikh NI, Pencina MJ, Wang TJ, et al. A risk score for predicting near-term incidence of hypertension: The Framingham heart study. *Ann Intern Med* 2008;148:102–110.

Peat JK. Prevention of asthma. *Eur Resp J* 1996;9:1545–1555.

Pereira MA, O'Reilly E, Augustsson K, et al. Dietary fiber and risk of coronary heart disease: A pooled analysis of cohort studies. *Arch Intern Med* 2004;164:370–376.

Pickering TG. Lifestyle modification: Is it achievable and durable? *J Clin Hypertens* 2004;6:581–584.

Pierce GL, Beske SD, Lawson BR, et al. Weight loss alone improves conduit and resistance artery endothelial function in young and older overweight/obese adults. *Hypertension* 2008;52: 72–79.

Poulter NR. Dietary sodium intake and mortality: NHANES [Letter to the Editor]. *Lancet* 1998;352:987–988.

Predel HG, Schramm TH, Rohden C, et al. Effects of various antihypertensive treatment regimens in physically active patients with essential hypertensive (EH) [Abstract]. *J Hypertens* 1996;14 (Suppl. 1):S230.

Psaltopoulou T, Naska A, Orfanos P, et al. Olive oil, the Mediterranean diet, and arterial blood pressure: The Greek European Prospective Investigation into Cancer and Nutrition (EPIC) study. *Am J Clin Nutr* 2004;80:1012–1018.

Quinn TJ. Twenty-four hour, ambulatory blood pressure responses following acute exercise: Impact of exercise intensity. *J Hum Hypertens* 2000;14:547–553.

Radaelli A, Raco R, Perfetti P, et al. Effects of slow, controlled breathing on baroreceptor control of heart rate and blood pressure in healthy men. *J Hypertens* 2004;22:1361–1370.

Rainforth MV, Schnieider RH, Nidich SI, et al. Stress reduction programs in patients with elevated blood pressure: A systematic review and meta-analysis. *Curr Hypertens Rep* 2007;9: 520–528.

Ram CVS, Garrett BN, Kaplan NM. Moderate sodium restriction and various diuretics in the treatment of hypertension. Effects of potassium wastage and blood pressure control. *Arch Intern Med* 1981;141:1015–1019.

Redón J, Cea-Calvo L, Moreno B, et al. Independent impact of obesity and fat distribution in hypertension prevalence and control in the elderly. *J Hypertens* 2008;26:1757–1764.

Renaud SC, Guéguen R, Conard P, et al. Moderate wine drinkers have lower hypertension-related mortality: A prospective cohort study in French men. *Am J Clin Nutr* 2004;80: 621–625.

Ried K, Frank OR, Stocks NP, et al. Effect of garlic on blood pressure: A systematic review and meta-analysis. *BMC Cardiovasc Disord* 2008;8:13.

Romero-Corral A, Montori VM, Somers VK, et al. Association of bodyweight with total mortality and with cardiovascular events in coronary artery disease: A systematic review of cohort studies. *Lancet* 2006;368:666–678.

Rosito GA, Fuchs FD, Duncan BB. Dose-dependent biphasic effect of ethanol on 24 h blood pressure in normotensive subjects. *Am J Hypertens* 1999;12:236–240.

Sacks FM, Svetkey LP, Vollmer WM, et al. Effects on blood pressure of reduced dietary sodium and the dietary approaches to stop hypertension (DASH) diet. *N Engl J Med* 2001;344: 3–10.

Saftlas AF, Logsden-Sackett N, Wang W, et al. Work, leisure-time physical activity, and risk of preeclampsia and gestational hypertension. *Am J Epidemiol* 2004;160:758–765.

Sakhaee K, Harvey JA, Padalino PK, et al. The potential role of salt abuse on the risk for kidney stone formation. *J Urol* 1993;150:310–312.

Scheer FA, Van Montfrans GA, van Someren EJ, et al. Daily nighttime melatonin reduces blood pressure in male patients with essential hypertension. *Hypertension* 2004;43:192–197.

Scheffers IJ, Kroon AA, Tordoir JH, et al. Rheos® baroreflex hypertension therapy trade mark system to treat resistant hypertension. *Expert Rev Med Devices* 2008;5(1):33–39.

Schmidlin O, Forman A, Sebastian A, et al. Sodium-selective salt sensitivity: Its occurrence in blacks. *Hypertension* 2007;50: 1085–1092.

Sellmeyer DE, Schloetter M, Sebastian A. Potassium citrate prevents increased urine calcium excretion and bone resorption induced by a high sodium chloride diet. *J Clin Endocrinol Metab* 2002;87:2008–2012.

Seppä K, Sillanaukee P. Binge drinking and ambulatory blood pressure. *Hypertension* 1999;33:79–82.

Sigal RJ, Kenny GP, Boulé NG, et al. Effects of aerobic training, resistance training, or both on glycemic control in type 2 diabetes: A randomized trial. *Ann Intern Med* 2007;147: 357–369.

Sjöström L, Lindroos A, Peltonen M, et al. Lifestyle, diabetes, and cardiovascular risk factors 10 years after bariatric surgery. *N Eng J Med* 2004;351:2683–2693.

Sjöström L, Narbro K, Sjöström CD, et al. Effects of bariatric surgery on mortality in Swedish obese subjects. *N Eng J Med* 2007;357:741–752.

Smith-Warner SA, Spiegelman D, Yaun S-S, et al. Alcohol and breast cancer in women. *JAMA* 1998;279:535–540.

Stamler J, Elliott P, Kesteloot H, et al. Inverse relation of dietary protein markers with blood pressure. Findings for 10,020 men and women in the INTERSALT study. *Circulation* 1996;94: 1629–1634.

Stamler R, Stamler J, Gosch FC, et al. Primary prevention of hypertension by nutritional-hygienic means: Final report of a randomized, controlled trial. *JAMA* 1989;262:1801–1807.

Stampfer MJ, Kang JH, Chen J, et al. Effects of moderate alcohol consumption on cognitive function in women. *N Eng J Med* 2005;352:245–253.

Stevens VJ, Obarzanek E, Cook NR, et al. Long-term weight loss and changes in blood pressure: Results of the Trials of Hypertension Prevention, Phase II. *Ann Intern Med* 2001;134:1–11.

Stranges S, Wu T, Dorn JM, et al. Relationship of alcohol drinking pattern to risk of hypertension: A population-based study. *Hypertension* 2004;44:813–819.

Straznicky NE, O'Callaghan CJ, Barrington VE, et al. Hypotensive effect of low-fat, high-carbohydrate diet can be independent of changes in plasma insulin concentrations. *Hypertension* 1999;34:580–585.

Strazzullo P, Kerry SM, Barbato A, et al. Do statins reduce blood pressure? A meta-analysis of randomized, controlled trials. *Hypertension* 2007;49:792–798.

Streppel MT, Arends LR, van't Veer P, et al. Dietary fiber and blood pressure: A meta-analysis of randomized placebo-controlled trials. *Arch Intern Med* 2005;165:150–156.

Svetkey LP, Stevens VJ, Brantley PJ, et al. Comparison of strategies for sustaining weight loss: The weight loss maintenance randomized controlled trial. *JAMA* 2008;299(10):1139–1148.

Task Force for the Management of Arterial Hypertension of the European Society of Hypertension (ESH) and of the European Society of Cardiology (ESC). 2007 Guidelines for the management of arterial hypertension. *J Hypertens* 2007;25: 1105–1187.

Taubert D, Roesen R, Schömig E. Effect of cocoa and tea intake on blood pressure: A meta-analysis. *Arch Intern Med* 2007;167: 626–634.

Teo KK, Ounpuu S, Hawken S, et al. Tobacco use and risk of myocardial infarction in 52 countries in the INTERHEART study: A case-control study. *Lancet* 2006;368:647–658.

Thadhani R, Camargo CA Jr, Stampfer MJ, et al. Prospective study of moderate alcohol consumption and risk of hypertension in young women. *Arch Intern Med* 2002;162:569–574.

Thorpe JJ, Welch WJ, Poindexter CA. Bilateral thoracolumbar sympathectomy for hypertension. *Am J Med* 1950;9:500–515.

Tjønneland A, Grønbæk M, Stripp C, et al. Wine intake and diet in a random sample of 48763 Danish men and women. *Am J Clin Nutr* 1999;69:49–54.

Tolstrup J, Jensen MK, Tjønneland A, et al. Prospective study of alcohol drinking patterns and coronary heart disease in women and men. *Br Med J* 2006;332:1244–1248.

Trials of Hypertension Prevention Collaborative Research Group. The effects of nonpharmacologic interventions on blood pressure of persons with high normal levels. Results of the Trials of Hypertension Prevention, Phase I. *JAMA* 1992;267:1213–1220.

Trials of Hypertension Prevention Collaborative Research Group. Effects of weight loss and sodium reduction intervention on blood pressure and hypertension incidence in overweight people with high-normal blood pressure. *Arch Intern Med* 1997;157: 657–667.

Trichopoulou A, Costacou T, Bamia C, et al. Adherence to a Mediterranean diet and survival in a Greek population. *N Engl J Med* 2003;348:2599–2608.

Tsai AG, Wadden TA. Systematic review: An evaluation of major commercial weight loss programs in the United States. *Ann Intern Med* 2005;142:56–66.

Tunstall-Pedoe H. Does dietary potassium lower blood pressure and protect against coronary heart disease and death? Findings from the Scottish heart health study. *Semin Nephrol* 1999;19:500–502.

Tuomilehto J, Jousilahti P, Rastenyte D, et al. Urinary sodium excretion and cardiovascular mortality in Finland. *Lancet* 2001;357:848–851.

Tzoulaki I, Brown IJ, Chan Q, et al. Relation of iron and red meat intake to blood pressure: Cross sectional epidemiological study. *Br Med J* 2008;337:a258.

U.S. Public Health Service Cooperative Study. Evaluation of antihypertensive therapy. II. Double-blind controlled evaluation of mebutamate. *JAMA* 1965;193:103–105.

Ueshima H, Stamler J, Elliott P, et al. Food omega-3 fatty acid intake of individuals (total, linolenic acid, long-chain) and their blood pressure: INTERMAP study. *Hypertension* 2007;50: 313–319.

Unger RH. Reinventing type 2 diabetes: pathogenesis, treatment, and prevention. *JAMA* 2008;299(10):1185.

Vanhees L, Defoor JGM, Schepers D, et al. Effect of bisoprolol and atenolol on endurance exercise capacity in healthy men. *J Hypertens* 2000;18:35–43.

Vasdev S, Gill V, Singal PK. Beneficial effect of low ethanol intake on the cardiovascular system: possible biochemical mechanisms. *Vasc Health Risk Manag* 2006;2(3):263–276.

Vogel RA. Vintners and vasodilators: Are French red wines more cardioprotective? *J Am Coll Cardiol* 2003;41:479–481.

Vogt L, Waanders F, Boomsma F, et al. Effects of dietary sodium and hydrochlorothiazide on the antiproteinuric efficacy of losartan. *J Am Soc Nephrol* 2008;19:999–1007.

Vollmer WM, Sacks FM, Ard J, et al. for the DASH-Sodium Trial Collaborative Research Group. Effects of diet and sodium intake on blood pressure: Subgroup analysis of the DASH-sodium trial. *Ann Intern Med* 2001;135:1019–1028.

Webb AJ, Patel N, Loukogeorgakis S, et al. Nitric oxide, oxidative stress: Acute blood pressure lowering, vasoprotective, and antiplatelet properties of dietary nitrate via bioconversion to nitrite. *Hypertension* 2008;51:784–790.

Wei M, Gibbons LW, Mitchell TL, et al. Alcohol intake and incidence of type 2 diabetes in men. *Diabetes Care* 2000;23:18–22.

Weinberger MH. Salt sensitivity of blood pressure in humans. *Hypertension* 1996;27:481–490.

Weinstein AR, Sesso HD, Rexrode KM, et al. The joint effects of physical activity and body mass index on coronary heart disease risk in women. *Arch Intern Med* 2008;168(8):884–890.

Weir MR. Dietary salt, blood pressure, and microalbuminuria. *J Clin Hypertens* 2004;6(Suppl. 3):23–26.

Whang R, Whang DD, Ryan MP. Refractory potassium repletion. A consequence of magnesium deficiency. *Arch Intern Med* 1992;152:40–45.

Whang W, Manson HE, Hu FB, et al. Physical exertion, exercise, and sudden cardiac death in women. *JAMA* 2006;295(12): 1399–1403.

Whelton PK, Appel LJ, Espeland MA, et al. Sodium reduction and weight loss in the treatment of hypertension in older persons. *JAMA* 1998;279:839–846.

Whelton PK, He J, Appel LJ, et al. Primary prevention of hypertension: Clinical and public health advisory from The National High Blood Pressure Education Program. *JAMA* 2002;288: 1882–1888.

Williams PT. A cohort study of incident hypertension in relation to changes in vigorous physical activity in men and women. *J Hypertens* 2008;26:1085–1093.

Williams B, Poulter NR, Brown MJ, et al. British Hypertension Society guidelines for hypertension management 2004 (BHS-IV): Summary. *Br Med J* 2004;328:634–640.

Williams MA, Haskell WL, Ades PA, et al. Resistance exercise in individuals with and without cardiovascular disease. 2007 update: A scientific statement from the American Heart Association Council on Clinical Cardiology and Council on Nutrition, Physical Activity, and Metabolism. *Circulation* 2007;116:572–584.

Winker R, Barth A, Bidmon D, et al. Endurance exercise training in orthostatic intolerance: A randomized, controlled trial. *Hypertension* 2005;45:391–398.

Xin X, Frontini MG, Ogden LG, et al. Effects of alcohol reduction on blood pressure: A meta-analysis of randomized controlled trials. *Hypertension* 2001;38:1112–1117

Yeh GY, Wang C, Wayne PM, et al. The effect of Tai Chi exercise on blood pressure: A systematic review. *Prev Cardiol* 2008;11: 82–89.

CHAPTER 7

Treatment of Hypertension: Drug Therapy

I n the previous two chapters, the evidence for the need for blood pressure (BP) reduction and the use of lifestyle modifications to lower the BP were reviewed. This chapter begins with ways to improve on the currently inadequate control of the disease. Then each class of drugs currently available is covered. An analysis of initial drug choice and of the subsequent order of additional therapy follows; then come considerations of the management of special populations and of hypertensives with various other conditions.

BACKGROUND

As reviewed in Chapter 1, hypertension is the most common risk factor for heart attack, stroke, and heart failure and second only to diabetes for renal failure (Rosamond et al., 2008). With a longer life span and increasing obesity, this prevalence will continue to increase, particularly in developing societies (Sun et al., 2008). Since most hypertension remains inadequately treated, the demand for more effective management continues to rise (Wu et al., 2009).

Therefore the use of drugs for the treatment of hypertension, already the most common indication for prescriptions in the United States, will continue to grow. New formulations proliferate, although most are almost copies of others already marketed. With such a massive unmet market, competition for the use of each company's products is intense—as long as the product is under patent protection. Therefore, angiotension receptor blockers, all selling for $2 to $3 per pill, are the fastest growing antihypertensive agents, while equally effective generic reserpine costing a few cents is virtually unavailable.

Despite both the obvious and the hidden attractions of pharmaceutical marketing to which both authors have been willing contributors, we have assiduously maintained an objective view, both about the use of drugs overall and about the relative value of individual agents. Specific choices are often favored, in keeping with the guidelines from multiple expert committees in the United States (Chobanian et al., 2003), in the United Kingdom (Williams et al., 2004), and Europe (Task Force, 2007).

As we shall see, currently available antihypertensive drugs, used in concert with appropriate lifestyle modifications and self-monitoring, can control the BP in most hypertensives. Yet, in every survey, in only a minority of patients, is the BP lower than 140/90 mm Hg (McWilliams et al., 2009), and those in most need of tight control, such as stroke survivors, are often even less well controlled (Amar et al., 2004). Therefore, before considering the drugs that are available and their indications, the issue of how to achieve better overall control of hypertension will be addressed.

CURRENT STATE OF CONTROL OF HYPERTENSION

Most hypertensives in the United States are aware of their diagnosis, and the majority have been prescribed antihypertensive drugs (Cutler et al., 2008). However, only one third are under adequate control, usually defined as a BP of 140/90 mm Hg or lower (Cutler et al., 2008). As bad as these data are, they are considerably better than reported from most other developed countries (Wang et al., 2007b).

Reasons for Poor Control

Although practitioners are quick to blame patients as the main cause for poor control of their hypertension, all three players—physicians, patients, and therapies—are involved (Ho et al., 2008).

Problems with Physicians

Many practitioners are either unaware of the need to more intensively treat hypertension, particularly isolated systolic hypertension in the elderly, or are unwilling to do so. Admittedly, systolic levels are more difficult to bring under control even under the best of circumstances, with fewer than half of patients enrolled in controlled trials having their systolics brought to 140 mm Hg or lower, whereas 80% of diastolics were brought to 90 mm Hg or lower (Mancia & Grassi, 2002).

However, much of the problem in clinical practice is "clinical inertia," the unwillingness to push therapy to the desired goal (Phillips & Twombly, 2008). This unwillingness may reflect inaccurate perceptions: that systolic elevations "aren't that bad"; that they can't be lowered without multiple medications and side effects; and that little benefit will accompany better control.

Moreover, many practitioners do not recognize their shortcomings. They often underestimate the level of their patient's cardiovascular risk (Kerr et al., 2008) and, even though they are unwilling to intensify therapy to the levels recommended in guidelines, they usually perceive their level of adherence to guidelines as being much better than it is (Steinman et al., 2004).

Hypertension "experts" have contributed to practitioners' problems by promoting conflicting positions, often at the same time: diuretics are bad—no, they are good; β-blockers are good—no, they are bad; calcium channel blockers (CCBs) are bad—no, they are good, and so on. On a higher level, the failure of national and international groups of experts to agree on such simple measures as the classification of hypertension and the goals of therapy adds to the confusion. And then, the often subtle machinations of pharmaceutical marketers, particular in providing experts to tout somewhat hidden messages under the guise of Continuing Medical Education, must be playing a role in keeping practitioners from having a single, clear message of how best to manage hypertension.

In a capitalistic, competitive market system, multiple options will remain available, increasingly being touted directly to the public and profitably marketed to the profession. However, better directions can be provided. Attempts are being made: the National Institute for Clinical Excellence (NICE) in the United Kingdom, the Hypertension Education Program in Canada, the National Institutes of Health (NIH) and, in particular, the National High Blood Pressure Education Program in the United States, are trying to bring the best advice to practitioners. Such advice has positive impact, but the impact is often short-lived (Ma et al., 2006).

Beyond physician inertia and confusion, problems with the health care delivery system can markedly reduce long-term adherence. Particularly in inner-city clinics which in the United States serve a large portion of the elderly and poor, records are often unavailable, little continuity of care is provided, and patients are made to wait long hours for short visits without an opportunity for meaningful interaction with their physician.

As the only developed country without universal health coverage, the United States is particularly susceptible to the faults of an erratic health care delivery system. Most of these faults revolve around the lack of insurance coverage (Lenzer, 2008), so that patients are unable to obtain continuity of care or to purchase often expensive medications.

For those with adequate insurance or under a rational delivery system, adherence has been shown to be greatly improved. In the U.S. Veterans Affairs facilities, where care and drugs are almost free, adherence to therapy for up to 18 months has reached 80% (Siegel et al., 2007). Among patients in an integrated group practice, the combination of home BP monitoring (BPM), web communication, and pharmacist involvement provided a 3.3-fold improved frequency of BP control compared to patients given usual care (Green et al., 2008).

Imaginative programs have been used to improve adherence. Telementoring of home BP (Parati et al., 2009), telephone calls from a pharmacist between office visits (Wu et al., 2006), coordination of care by a nurse (Wood et al., 2008), structured collaboration between pharmacist and physician (Carter et al., 2008a), tailored feedback to patients and their physicians (Bosworth et al., 2005), and monitoring patients at a place which they frequent, i.e., their barbershop (Victor et al., 2009), have all been shown to improve adherence.

Problems with Patients

As many as half of hypertensives prescribed an antihypertensive medication will not be taking it within a year (Vrijens et al., 2008). There are many patient-related reasons for poor adherence to antihypertensive therapy, including:

- Failure to identify and deal with patients' differing perceptions about their disease and beliefs about both the benefits and the problems of therapy (Victor et al., 2008).
- The largely asymptomatic nature of hypertension, making it difficult for patients to forego immediate pleasures (salt, calories, money, etc.) for distant, unrecognized benefits, even more so if therapy makes them feel worse.
- Competing problems such as poverty (Kripalani et al., 2008), psychological depression (Eze-Niam et al., 2008), or more immediately threatening diseases such as diabetes (Wang et al., 2005).
- Inability to access and maintain contact with a health care system that is affordable, available, and appropriate to their long-term needs, including over 45 million people in the United States without health insurance (Bautista, 2008).
- Real and imaginary concerns about the safety of lifelong medication. In the past, many people were willing to take whatever they were prescribed with full confidence in their physician, but there are fewer today. The delayed recognition that a nonsteroidal antiinflammatory drug (NSAID) prescribed by thousands of physicians to millions of patients was responsible for heart attacks surely will further damage the patient-doctor relationship.

Problems with the Therapy

As noted, hypertension has all the wrong characteristics to ensure adherence to therapy, but these are often compounded by problems of therapy, including:

- Difficulty in changing unhealthy lifestyles, in particular weight gain from too many calories and too little physical activity (see Chapter 6).
- The high cost of most new, patent-protected medications. When available, generic agents that are equally efficacious (Kesselheim et al., 2008) are more likely to be taken (Shrank et al., 2006).
- The prescription of two or more doses per day when long-acting once-a-day options are available. Even worse is one daily dose of drugs, e.g. atenolol, which lack a 24 hour effect (Protogeru et al., 2009).
- Side effects of antihypertensive drugs, some not predicted such as impotence with diuretics.

- Even less obvious but perhaps more critical, the sympathetic nervous system may be chronically activated when the BP is lowered (Fu et al., 2005).
- Interactions with other medications and substances, NSAIDs the most common, grapefruit juice likely the least recognizable (Kakar et al., 2004), herbal remedies perhaps the most dangerous (Tannergren et al., 2004).
- Difficulty in assessment of adherence (Morisky et al., 2008). Although there are multiple ways to assess the degree of patients' pill taking, few have been found to be accurate (Vrijens et al., 2008).
- Variable responses to any dose of any medication. The starting and usual doses are determined by trials in only a limited number of usually uncomplicated patients. In practice, many patients respond either more or less to any drug (Law et al., 2003).

Ways to Improve Adherence to Therapy

Many books and articles have suggested ways to keep more patients on effective therapy of hypertension but the list of those that have been shown to affect clinical outcomes is relatively short (Kripalani et al., 2007). In the future, genotyping may provide a way to maximize the response but as of now, none has been reported to provide clinically useful data (van Wieren-de Wijer et al., 2009).

The guidelines in Table 7-1 have been shown to improve adherence in most but not in all careful studies (Osterberg & Blaschke, 2005; Roumie et al., 2006).

Beyond these more immediate measures, better organized and monitored healthcare as in the U.S. Veterans Administration system improves adherence (Siegel et al., 2007). Even better would be the application of nationwide system changes with computerized, easily accessed medical records and financial incentives to reward practitioners who improve the care and outcomes of their patients (Doran et al., 2006).

Patient Involvement

Involvement of the patient is helpful, not only in making initial decisions which are therefore more likely to be followed, but also in monitoring the course of the disease. Home BP readings should always be recommended, preferably taken by the patient or sometimes by other caregivers. As noted in Chapter 2, responses to therapy are more closely related to out-of-office measurements than office readings (Parati et al., 2009).

TABLE 7.1	Guidelines to Improve Maintenance of Antihypertensive Therapy

Involve the patient in decision making to the extent desired
    Assess attitudes and beliefs
    Provide individual assessments of current risks and potential benefits of control
    Inform the patient about the condition and its treatment
    If patient agrees, involve family
Articulate the goal of therapy: to reduce BP to near normotension with few or no side effects
Be alert for signs of inadequate intake of medications, e.g., absence of BP response or expected effects, e.g., bradycardia
    with β-blocker
Recognize and manage depression
Maintain contact with the patient
    Encourage visits and calls to allied health personnel
    Give feedback to the patient via home BP readings
    Make contact with patients who do not return
Keep care inexpensive and simple
    Do the least workup needed to rule out secondary causes
    Obtain follow-up laboratory data only yearly unless indicated more often
    Encourage lifestyle changes if needed
    Use home BP readings
    Use once-daily doses of long-acting drugs
    Use generic drugs and break larger doses of scored tablets in half
    If appropriate, use combination tablets
    Use calendar blister packs
    Inspect all pill containers at each visit
    If medications must be taken separately, provide clear, easily read instructions
    Use clinical protocols monitored by nurses and assistants
Prescribe according to pharmacologic principles
    Add one drug at a time
    Start with small doses, aiming for 5- to 10-mm Hg reductions at each step, unless more rapid response is indicated
    Have medication taken immediately on awakening in the morning. If morning surge of BP (above 160/100) persists, give
    at least some drugs at 6 p.m. or at bedtime
Provide feedback and validation of success

Intensity of Therapy

The rapidity of reaching goal is now in question since too fast a course may cause intolerable symptoms, but too slow may expose high-risk patients to immediate dangers. The benefit of more rapid control was graphically shown in the Valsartan Antihypertensive Long-term Use Evaluation (VALUE) trial, wherein the quicker response over the first 3 to 6 month to the CCB amlodipine than to the angiotensin II receptor blocker (ARB) valsartan, provided greater protection against heart attacks and strokes (Julius et al., 2004b). The patients in VALUE were all at high risk for cardiovascular disease, so it still seems appropriate to "start low and go low" for most, particularly the elderly with systolic hypertension. For those with higher levels of BP but, even more so, higher overall risk, a "higher and faster" approach may be more appropriate.

Timing of Dosing

The time of day to take one-a-day antihypertensive medications needs to be more carefully considered. Early morning has usually been recommended but there are two potential problems: first, the pills may not exert a full 24-hour effect, as shown for atenolol (Neutel et al., 1990); second, an even greater effect may be needed in the early morning, before today's therapy has kicked in, to keep the pressure from surging in the immediate postarising time, thereby contributing to the "morning surge" of cardiovascular catastrophes. In a study from Spain, the majority of hypertensives with well-controlled office readings had uncontrolled early morning readings (Redón et al., 2002).

The solution for the first problem is twofold: first, ensure full 24-hour control by having the patient measure early a.m. BP at home; second, choose intrinsically long-acting medications, e.g., metoprolol XL rather than atenolol, trandolapril rather than enalapril, amlodipine rather than felodipine.

The solution for the second problem seems as obvious but has never been definitely proven, i.e., take medications later in the day or even at bedtime. In the Heart Outcomes Prevention Evaluation (HOPE) trial (Heart Outcomes, 2000), the study medication, the angiotensin-converting enzyme inhibitor (ACEI) ramipril, was taken at bedtime, purposely to prevent early morning events. The positive results were said not to reflect the 3/2 mm Hg lower average clinic BP of those who took ramipril. However, the clinic pressures were taken hours after the morning surge, so the possible benefit was undetectable. This belief is supported by a HOPE substudy wherein 38 participants had 24-hour ambulatory monitoring (Svensson et al., 2001). Among the 20 given bedtime ramipril, the midday pressures were the same as those in the 18 given placebo, but the overnight BPs were significantly lower (by 17/8 mm Hg) as were the 24-hour readings (by 10/4 mm Hg) in the ramipril group.

Therefore, the concept of "chronotherapeutics" sounds logical but there are no data to either support or refute it. As Mosenkis and Townsend (2004) note:

> For now, the schedule of antihypertensive drug administration can be determined by other factors such as convenience, concurrence with the administration of other medications to foster adherence, and timing to minimize untoward effects of these medications.... If there are no other compelling timing considerations, one may choose nocturnal dosing (i.e., at bedtime for standard daily drugs and nighttime for extended-release preparations) so that their peak activities coincide with, and perhaps helps to blunt, the early morning BP increase.

Dealing with Side Effects

Some medications are easier to take than others, but some patients cannot seem to take any. Such patients with nonspecific intolerance to multiple antihypertensive drugs almost always have underlying psychological morbidity, often manifested as recurrent hyperventilation, panic attacks, generalized anxiety, or depression (Davies et al., 2003). Many people get anxious when their "silent killer" is diagnosed and even more when it cannot be easily controlled (Mena-Martin et al., 2003). Obviously, there are all grades of drug-related side effects. Fortunately, most currently available drugs do not interfere with cognitive

performance (Sink et al., 2009) or other aspects of the quality of life (QOL). However, even such senses as smell and taste that seem unrelated to hypertension can be adversely affected by various antihypertensive drugs (Doty et al., 2003).

The astute clinician will remain open to all possibilities.

Follow-up Visits

To achieve and maintain target BP with the lowest possible dosage of medication requires ongoing patient follow-up, preferably with home BPM, and may involve multiple dosage adjustments. Most patients should be seen within 1 to 2 months after the initiation of therapy to determine the adequacy of BP control, the degree of patient cooperation in taking pills, the need for more therapy, and the presence of adverse effects. Associated medical problems—including target organ damage, other major risk factors, and laboratory test abnormalities—also play a part in determining the frequency of patient follow-up. Once the BP is stabilized, follow-up at 3- to 6-month intervals (depending on the patient's status) is generally appropriate. In most patients, particularly the elderly and patients with orthostatic symptoms, monitoring should include BP measurement in the supine position and after standing for up to 5 minutes, to recognize postural hypotension (Hiitola et al., 2009).

The marked variability of usual office BP readings make them almost worthless; more home readings are needed (Keenan et al., 2009).

SPECIFICS ABOUT ANTIHYPERTENSIVE DRUGS

The modern era of antihypertensive therapy began only about 50 years ago with the pioneering work of Ed Freis in the United States and Horace Smirk in New Zealand (Piepho & Beal, 2000). Since then, a large panoply of drugs have been developed, as listed in Table 7-2. We will consider the drugs in the order shown in Table 7-2. Some that are used extensively elsewhere, but are not now available in the United States, will also be covered, along with newer agents that are on the horizon.

In 2006 in the United States, drugs used for the treatment of hypertension were the most commonly prescribed, totaling over 200 million prescriptions (Cherry et al., 2008). When these annual surveys of

TABLE 7.2	Antihypertensive Drugs Available in the United States (as of 2009)				
Diuretics	**Adrenergic inhibitors**			**Vasodilators**	
Thiazides	*Peripheral Inhibitors*	*β-Blockers*	*Direct Vasodilators*	*ACEIs*
Chlorthalidone	Guanadrel	Acebutolol	Hydralazine	Benazepril
Indapamide	Guanethidine	Atonolol	Minoxidil	Captopril
Metolazone	Reserpine	Betaxolol	*CCBs*	Enalapril
Thiazides	*Central α₂-agonists*	Bisoprolol	Dihydropyridines	Fosinopril
Loop diuretics	Clonidine	Carteolol	Amlodipine	Lisinopril
Bumetanide	Guanabenz	Metoprolol	Felodipine	Moexipril
Ethacrynic acid	Guanfacine	Nadolol	Isradipine	Quinapril
Furosemide	Methyldopa	Penbutolol	Nicardipine	Perindopril
Torsemide	*α₁-Blockers*	Pindolol	Nifedipine	Ramipril
Aldosterone blockers	Dozazosin	Propranolol	Nisoldipine	Trandolapril
Spironolactone	Prazosin	Timolol	Diltiazem	*All receptor blockers*
Eplerenone	Terazosin	*Combined α-, β-blockers*	Verapamil	Candesartan
Potassium sparers		Carvediol	Direct rennin inhibitor	Eprosartan
Amiloride		Labetalol	Aliskerin	Irbesartan
Triamterene		*Vasodilating β-blockers*		Losartan
		Nebivolol		Telmisartan
				Valsartan

drug use are compared, diuretics have continued to be the most commonly prescribed, followed by ACEIs, β-blockers, and CCBs, with ARBs rising the fastest and α-blockers continuing to fall. The initial rapid growth in the use of ARBs is almost certainly related to their intensive marketing. However, as will be noted, ARBs may be special, so their continued growth clearly reflects more than marketing.

Law et al., (2009) suggest that 2 or 3 drugs in half usual doses be given, rather than full doses of 1 or 2, both to achieve greater efficacy and to reduce dose-dependent side effects. Initial experience is promising (Indian Polycap Study, 2009) but acceptance into general practice must overcome many barriers. The use of drugs in various secondary forms of hypertension (e.g., spironolactone in primary aldosteronism) is considered in the respective chapters on these identifiable causes.

DIURETICS

Among the first orally effective drugs to become available, diuretics are being used even more frequently because their effectiveness has been reiterated and, with lower doses, their side effects minimized.

However, concerns have been raised about potential long-term disadvantages and the current choices of diuretics.

Diuretics differ in structure and major site of action within the nephron (Fig. 7-1). The site of action determines their relative efficacy, as expressed in the maximal percentage of filtered sodium chloride excreted (Brater, 2000). Agents acting in the proximal tubule (site I) are seldom used to treat hypertension.

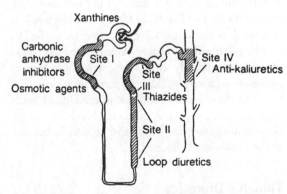

FIGURE 7-1   Diagrammatic representation of the nephron showing the four main tubular sites where diuretics interfere with sodium reabsorption.

TABLE 7.3	Diuretics and Potassium-Sparing Agents	
Drug	Daily Dosage, mg	Duration of Action, h
Thiazides		
Bendroflumethiazide	1.25–5.0	18
Benzthiazide	50–200	12–18
Chlorothiazide	250–1,000	6–12
Hydrochlorothiazide	12.5–50	12–18
Hydroflumethiazide	12.5–50	12–18
Trichlormethiazide	1.0–4.0	18–24
Related sulfonamide compounds		
Chlorthalidone	12.5–50	24–72
Indapamide	1.25–2.5	24
Metolazone	0.5–1.0	24
Mykrox	2.5–10	24
Zaroxolyn		
Loop Diuretics		
Bumetanide	0.5–5.0	4–6
Ethacrynic acid	25–100	12
Furosemide	20–480	4–6
Torsemide	5–40	12
Potassium-sparing agents		
Amiloride	5–10	24
Triamterene	50–150	12
Aldosterone blockers		
Spironolactone	25–100	8–12
Eplerenone	50–100	12

Treatment is usually initiated with a thiazide-type diuretic (acting at site III, the distal convoluted tubule). Chlorthalidone and indapamide are structurally different from, but still related to, the thiazides and will be covered with them. If renal function is significantly impaired (i.e., serum creatinine exceeding 1.5 mg/dL), a loop diuretic (acting at site II, the thick ascending limb of the loop of Henle) or metolazone likely will be needed. A potassium-sparing agent (acting at site IV) may be given with the diuretic to reduce the likelihood of hypokalemia. By themselves, potassium-sparing agents are relatively weak antihypertensives.

The diuretics now available in the United States are listed in Table 7-3. Aldosterone blockers, though potassium-sparers, are considered separately because of their additional effects.

Thiazide Diuretics

Mode of Action

The thiazide diuretics act by inhibiting sodium and chloride cotransport across the luminal membrane of the early segment of the distal convoluted tubule, where 5% to 8% of filtered sodium is normally reabsorbed (Puschett, 2000) (Fig. 7-1, site III). Plasma and extracellular fluid volume are thereby shrunken, and cardiac output falls (Wilson & Freis, 1959). Humoral and intrarenal counterregulatory mechanisms rapidly reestablish the steady state so that sodium intake and excretion are balanced within 3 to 9 days in the presence of a decreased body fluid volume (Sica, 2004a). With chronic use, plasma volume returns partially toward normal but, at the same time, peripheral resistance decreases (Conway & Lauwers, 1960; Zhu et al., 2005) (Fig. 7-2).

Determinants of Response

The degree of BP response to diuretics is predicated on their capacity to activate the counterregulatory defenses to a lower BP and a shrunken fluid volume—in particular, a reactive rise in renin and aldosterone levels. Those who start with low, suppressed plasma renin activity (PRA) and aldosterone levels and who are capable of mounting only a weak

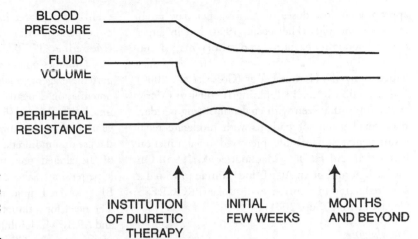

FIGURE 7-2 Scheme of the hemodynamic changes responsible for the antihypertensive effects of diuretic therapy.

rise in these levels after diuretics are initiated have been shown to be more "diuretic-responsive" (Chapman et al., 2002). This includes older, black, and hypertensive people, all of whom frequently have lower renin levels (Kaplan, 1977). Those who respond less well, with a fall in mean BP of less than 10%, were found to have a greater degree of plasma volume depletion and greater stimulation of renin and aldosterone, contributing to a persistently high peripheral resistance (van Brummelen et al., 1980). Blockade of the reactive rise in renin-angiotensin-aldosterone, as with the addition of an ACEI or ARB, will potentiate the antihypertensive action (Ram, 2004).

Pharmacogenetic studies have related the responsiveness to thiazide diuretics to various polymorphisms of genes controlling the renin-angiotensin system (Frazier et al., 2004), the 11βHSD2 enzyme (Williams et al., 2005), and sodium channels (Maitland-van der Zee et al., 2004) that vary with both gender and ethnic background. Moreover, diuretic-treated carriers of a variant of the adducin gene which is associated with increased renal sodium reabsorption have been reported to have a lower risk of heart attack and stroke than seen in diuretic-treated patients who do not carry that variant or in those who are given other antihypertensive medications (Psaty et al., 2002). These studies may foretell an application of pharmacogenetics to clinical practice.

Thiazide-like Diuretics
Chlorthalidone
Although commonly considered a thiazide, chlorthalidone is of a different chemical structure and milligram for milligram acts both stronger and longer than hydrochlorothiazide (HCTZ) (Ernst et al., 2006). Although HCTZ has become by far the most widely used diuretic to treat hypertension in the United States, chlorthalidone has been used in all trials sponsored by the NIH, with as much or more protection against heart attacks, heart failure, and strokes as seen with other agents (ALLHAT Investigators, 2002). On the other hand, there are no data showing such benefits of HCTZ in the currently recommended lower doses of 12.5 to 25 mg per day. Moreover, in a comparison of the two agents in a 8-week crossover study using both office and 24-hour ambulatory BP monitoring (ABPM), 25 mg of chlorthalidone provided a 5 mm Hg greater fall in systolic BP over the entire 24 hours and an even greater 7.1 mm Hg fall in systolic BP during the nighttime than did 50 mg of HCTZ with a similar difference in the early morning office readings (Ernst et al., 2006). A similar incidence of hypokalemia was seen with both diuretics.

As recently recalled by Ernst et al. (2009), a significantly greater reduction in mortality was seen in the patients in the Multiple Risk Factor Intervention Trial (MRFIT) (1990) who were given chlorthalidone than in those given HCTZ. And in all, chlorthalidone has been proven to be a better diuretic agent than HCTZ and hopefully more combination tablets with chlorthalidone as the diuretic will be marketed.

Indapamide
Indapamide (Lozol) is a chlorobenzene sulfonamide but has a methylindoline moiety, which may provide additional protective actions beyond its diuretic effect (Chillon & Baumbach, 2004). It is as effective in reducing the BP as are thiazides or CCBs (Emeriau et al., 2001); maintains a 24-hour effect; and, in

appropriately low doses of 1.25 mg per day, rarely raises serum lipids (Hall et al., 1994) but in larger doses, hyponatremia and hypokalemia may occur. With 1.5-mg doses, regression of left ventricular hypertrophy (LVH) was better (Gosse et al., 2000) and reduction in microalbuminuria equal to (Marre et al., 2004) that seen with enalapril, 20 mg per day. In a small group of patients with moderate renal insufficiency, indapamide preserved renal function better than did HCTZ (Madkour et al., 1995). On the background of an ACEI, indapamide provided a 43% reduction in recurrences of stroke (PROGRESS Collaborative Group, 2001).

Metolazone

Metolazone, a long-acting and more potent quinazoline thiazide derivative, maintains its effect in the presence of renal insufficiency (Paton & Kane, 1977). Small doses, 0.5 to 1.0 mg per day, of a new formulation (Mykrox) may be equal to ordinary long-acting thiazide diuretics (Miller et al., 1988); the agent is particularly useful in patients with renal insufficiency and resistant hypertension but variable absorption may interfere with its efficacy.

Antihypertensive Efficacy

When used alone, thiazide diuretics provide efficacy similar to that of other classes of drugs (Law et al., 2009). Blacks and the elderly respond better to diuretics than do nonblacks and younger patients (Brown et al., 2003) presumably because they have lower renin responsiveness. Diuretics may provide

even better protection against strokes than would be expected from their antihypertensive efficacy (Messerli et al., 2003).

Diuretics potentiate the effect of all other antihypertensive agents, including CCBs (Sica, 2004a. This potentiation depends on the contraction of fluid volume by the diuretic (Finnerty et al., 1970) and the prevention of fluid accumulation that frequently follows the use of nondiuretic antihypertensive drugs. Because of the altered pressure-natriuresis curve of primary hypertension (Saito & Kimura, 1996), whenever the BP is lowered, fluid retention is expected (Fig. 7-3). The need for a diuretic may be lessened with ACEIs and ARBs, which inhibit the renin-aldosterone mechanism, and with CCBs, which have some intrinsic natriuretic activity but potentiation persists with all classes.

Duration of Action

The durations of action listed in Table 7-3 relate to the diuretic effect; the full antihypertensive effect may not last beyond the diuretic effect. Even though HCTZ has been known to have only a 12- to 18-hour duration of diuretic action, conventional wisdom often based on BP measurements made a few hours after the daily morning dose, has been that the full antihypertensive effect would persist over 24 hours. This has been shown not to be true on the basis of 24 hour ABPM (Finkielman et al., 2005). However, not until the comparison between HCTZ and chlorthalidone using ABPM was there a clear evidence for a lessening of HCTZ antihypertensive effect during the night (Ernst et al., 2006). As Ernst et al. (2009)

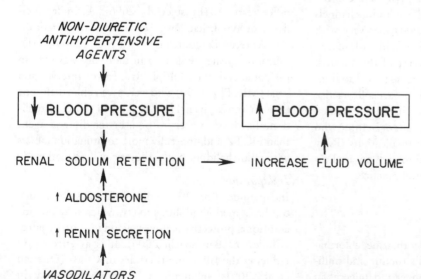

FIGURE 7-3 Manner by which nondiuretic antihypertensive agents may lose their effectiveness by reactive renal sodium retention.

argue, trials that use only 12.5 to 25 mg of HCTZ in comparison to an agent with persistent 24-hour effect (Jamerson et al., 2008) may be misleading.

Dosage
Monotherapy
The recommended daily dose of thiazide diuretics has been progressively falling from as high as 200 mg of HCTZ or equivalent doses of other thiazides in the early 1960s (Cranston et al., 1963) to as little as 12.5 mg today. In hypertensives with good renal function, most of the antihypertensive effect will be obtained from such small doses, with less hypokalemia and other side effects (Carlsen et al., 1990; Zimlichman et al., 2004). Thought most patients will have a good response to such small doses, some patients will require much more (Freis et al., 1988). However, as shown by Carlsen et al. (1990), the full antihypertensive effect of low doses of diuretic may not become apparent in 4 weeks, so patience is advised when low doses are prescribed.

Combination Therapy
Even more convincing data confirm a significant effect from small doses, even below 12.5 mg per day HCTZ, when diuretics are added to a variety of other drugs to enhance their antihypertensive efficacy. This was most clearly documented with the combination of 6.25 mg HCTZ plus the β-blocker bisoprolol (Frishman et al., 1994). Similar potentiation of ACEI efficacy with 6.25 mg HCTZ has been seen (Andrén et al., 1983).

Thiazides may also be coupled with loop diuretics in those with renal impairment, because they counter the distal nephron hypertrophy that occurs with loop diuretics alone (Brater, 2000).

The overall evidence indicates that many hypertensives will respond over time to small doses of a thiazide diuretic but that an agent with a full 24-hour duration of action, e.g., chlorthalidone, will provide greater nocturnal and early morning antihypertensive effect than the more commonly used HCTZ.

Resistance to Diuretics
Resistance to the natriuretic and antihypertensive action of diuretics may occur for numerous reasons (Ellison, 1999):

- Excessive dietary sodium intake (Winer, 1961).
- For those with renal impairment (i.e., serum creatinine >1.5 mg/dL or creatinine clearance <30 mL/

minute), thiazides likely will not work; because these drugs must be secreted into the renal tubules to work and because endogenous organic acids that build up in renal insufficiency compete with diuretics for transport into the proximal tubule, the renal response progressively falls with increasing renal damage
- Food affects the absorption and bioavailability of different diuretics to variable degrees (Neuvonen & Kivistö, 1989), so the drugs should be taken in a uniform pattern in terms of the time of day and food ingestion.
- NSAIDs may blunt the effect of most diuretics. (Cheng & Harris, 2004).

Protection Against Cardiovascular Events
Diuretics protect against cardiovascular morbidity and mortality as well as any other class of drug (Psaty et al., 2003). In the ALLHAT trial (Davis et al., 2006), chlorthalidone-based therapy lowered BP better than either ACEI or CCC-based therapy and a diuretic is recommended as the initial choice of therapy for most patients in the JNC-7 (Chobanian et al., 2003).

Side Effects
As shown in Figure 7-4, the likely pathogenesis for most of the more common complications related to diuretic use arises from the intrinsic activity of the drugs, and most complications are, therefore, related to the dose and duration of diuretic use. Logically, side effects occur with about the same frequency and severity with equipotent doses of all diuretics, and their occurrence will diminish with lower doses.

Hypokalemia
Increased urinary K^+ loss may occur for multiple reasons: (Coca et al., 2005).

The degree of hypokalemia is dose dependent. The incidence of hypokalemia (<3.5 mmol /L) is approximately 20% on higher doses (Widmer et al., 1995) and 5% to 10% on 12.5 to 25 mg per day of chlorthalidone (Franse et al., 2000). Diuretic-induced hypokalemia will be accentuated by increased amounts of sodium intake and in those with lower total body potassium stores, including many elderly patients (Flynn et al., 1989).

The major potential risks of potassium depletion are to increase the incidence of stroke (Levine & Coull, 2002) and ventricular arrhythmias causing sudden death (Grobbee & Hoes 1995). Patients on

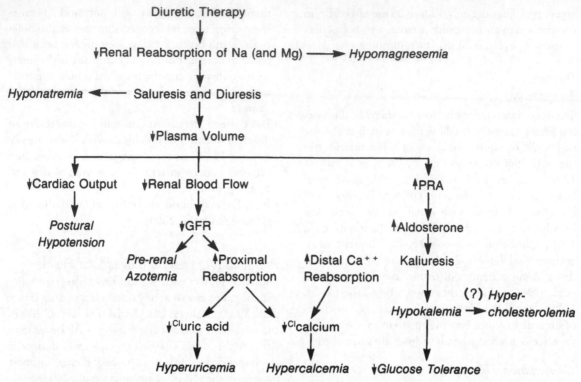

FIGURE 7-4 Mechanisms by which chronic diuretic therapy may lead to various complications. The mechanism for hypercholesterolemia remains in question, although it is shown as arising via hypokalemia. Ca, calcium; Cl, chlorine; GFR, glomerular filtration rate; Na, sodium; Mg, magnesium; PRA, plasma renin activity.

digitalis may develop toxicity, perhaps because both digitalis and hypokalemia inhibit the Na^+/K^+-adenosine triphosphatase (Na^+/K^+-ATPase) pump, the activity of which is essential to normal intracellular electrolyte balance and membrane potential (Nørgaard & Kjeldsen, 1991). Hypokalemia may raise the BP (Coca et al., 2005), and its correction may lower BP (Kaplan et al., 1985).

VENTRICULAR ARRHYTHMIAS AND SUDDEN DEATH In two case-control studies, the risk of sudden death was nearly doubled in those on large doses of naked diuretics as compared to those on thiazide plus a potassium-sparing agent (Hoes et al., 1995; Siscovick et al., 1994). In the SHEP trial, among those randomly allocated to 12.5 to 25 mg chlorthalidone, the 7.2% who developed hypokalemia had less than half the reduction in major cardiovascular events than those who remained normokalemic (Franse et al., 2000).

PREVENTION OF DIURETIC-INDUCED HYPOKALEMIA By lowering dietary sodium, increasing dietary potassium, and using the least amount of diuretic needed, potassium depletion may be avoided. A potassium-sparing agent, β-blocker, ACEI or ARB given with the diuretic will reduce the degree of potassium loss but may not prevent the development of hypokalemia (Sawyer & Gabriel, 1988). Aldosterone blockers may be even more efficient (Coca et al., 2005).

REPLETION OF DIURETIC-INDUCED HYPOKALEMIA If prevention does not work, the potassium deficiency can be replaced with supplemental K^+, preferably given as the chloride; other anions (as found in most fruits rich in potassium) will not correct the alkalosis or the intracellular K^+ deficiency as well (Kopyt et al., 1985). However, potassium citrate (Sakhaee et al., 1991) or bicarbonate (Frassetto et al., 2000) will be more effective in reducing urinary calcium loss in patients with renal stones or osteoporosis. The KCl may be given as a potassium-containing salt substitute; a number of these substitutes are available, and they are less expensive than potassium supplements.

Caution is advised in giving potassium supplements to patients receiving ACEIs, ARBs, or direct renin inhibitors (DRI) whose aldosterone levels are suppressed and who may be unable to excrete extra potassium. The problem may be compounded in diabetics who may be unable to move potassium rapidly into cells and in those with renal insufficiency who may have a limited ability to excrete potassium.

Hypomagnesemia

Some of the problems attributed to hypokalemia may be caused by hypomagnesemia instead. However, conventional doses of diuretics rarely induce magnesium deficiency (Wilcox, 1999).

Clinical features include weakness, nausea, neuromuscular irritability, and the appearance of ventricular arrhythmias, which are resistant to treatment unless both hypomagnesemia and hypokalemia are corrected (Whang et al., 1985). Since, experimentally, magnesium inhibits norepinephrine (NE) release (Shimosawa et al., 2004), hypomagenesiumia may raise BP.

Magnesium wastage is lessened by use of smaller doses of diuretics and concomitant use of a potassium-sparing agent (Schnaper et al., 1989). If repletion is needed, oral magnesium oxide, 200 to 400 mg per day (10 to 20 mmol), or potassium-magnesium citrate may be tolerated without gastrointestinal (GI) distress (Palt, 2000).

Hyponatremia

By impairing the dilution of the tubular fluid, thiazides reduce the capacity for rapid and effective elimination of free water, and slight, asymptomatic falls in serum sodium concentration are common (Wilcox, 1999). Rarely, severe, symptomatic hyponatremia develops, usually soon after diuretics are started in elderly women who appear to have an expanded fluid volume from increased water intake in the face of a decreased ability to excrete free water (Mann, 2008).

Hyperuricemia

Serum uric acid levels are high in as many as 30% of untreated hypertensives and diuretics increase renal urate reabsorption, raising uric acid levels further, rarely provoking gout. Moreover, Richard Johnson and others have provided evidence for a casual role of hyperuricemia in the pathogenesis of hypertension (Feig et al., 2008a) and renal damage (Obermayr et al., 2008).

Before the evidence presented by Johnson et al. (2005) was recognized, thiazide-induced hyperuricemia was overlooked unless a kidney stone or gout

appeared (Dykman et al., 1987). If therapy is given, the logical choice is probenecid to increase renal excretion of uric acid not allopurinol (Gutierrez-Macias et al., 2005). The ARB losartan is uricosuric and may ameliorate diuretic-induced hyperuricemia.

Calcium Metabolism Alterations

Renal calcium reabsorption also is increased with chronic thiazide therapy, and urinary calcium excretion is decreased by 40% to 50% (Friedman & Bushinsky, 1999). A slight rise in serum calcium (i.e., 0.1 to 0.2 mg/dL) is usual, and hypercalcemia is often provoked in patients with preexisting hyperparathyroidism or vitamin D-treated hypoparathyroidism. By reducing renal calcium excretion, thiazides are used to treat patients with renal stones caused by hypercalcemia from increased calcium absorption (Quereda et al., 1996). The retention of calcium in bone offers protection from osteoporosis and fractures (Schoofs et al., 2003). However, loop diuretics, which increase urinary calcium excretion, are associated with an increased rate of hip bone loss in older men (Lim et al., 2008).

Glucose Intolerance and Insulin Resistance

Insulin resistance, impairment of glucose tolerance, precipitation of overt diabetes, and worsening of diabetic control have all been observed in patients taking larger doses of thiazides (Carter et al., 2008b). In a review of data from 83 trials with thiazide, the rise in blood glucose was closely correlated with the fall in serum potassium (Zillich et al., 2006).

As with all the adverse effects of diuretics, the impairment of glucose utilization that connotes insulin resistance is seen more with high doses (Harper et al., 1995). With currently used lower doses, no increase in the incidence of diabetes was noted in a prospective cohort study of 12,500 hypertensive subjects (Gress et al., 2000). However, the incidence of new-onset diabetes among the ALLHAT trial participants who took chlorthalidone (most at a dose of 25 mg, equivalent to 40 to 50 mg of HCTZ) was 11.5% compared to 8.3% in those who started with amlodipine and 7.6% in those who started with lisinopril (Black et al., 2008). During the few years of the trial, no adverse consequences of this increase in diabetes was apparent, but the potential for future trouble should be recognized (Almgren et al., 2007). Nonetheless, those patients given chlorthalidone in the SHEP trial, despite having an increased incidence of diabetes, compared to those given a placebo, did not have an increase in cardiovascular events even after an average of 14.3-year follow-up (Kostis et al., 2005).

It is likely that part of the increases in diabetes in diuretic-treated patients comes from the concomitant use of β-blockers, the "conventional" therapy of older trials.

Effect on Lipids

With low doses, thiazides have little effect on the blood lipid profile (Weir & Moser, 2000). However, higher doses may induce significant effects on fat distribution which in turn may be associated with insulin resistance. Eriksson et al. (2008) examined the effects of a placebo, the ARB candesartan (16 to 32 mg per day) and HCTZ (50 mg per day), each given to 26 hypertensives with abdominal obesity for 12 weeks in a randomized crossover design. After the 12 weeks on the diuretic, the subjects had increases in abdominal and hepatic fat, abnormal liver function test, insulin resistance and increased C-reactive protein levels. None of these effects wwere seen after placebo or ARB.

If these adverse effects are seen with lower doses of diuretic, the advocacy of diuretics will certainly be reconsidered.

Erectile Dysfunction

Impotence may be more common with diuretics than with other drugs. In the large, randomized Medical Research Council (MRC) trial, impotence was reported by 22.6% of the men on bendrofluazide, as compared to a rate of 10.1% among those on placebo and 13.2% among those on propranolol (Medical Research Council Working Party, 1981). In the Treatment of Mild Hypertension Study (TOMHS), the men randomized to chlorthalidone had a 17.1% incidence of erection problems through 24 months, as compared to an 8.1% incidence in those on placebo (Grimm et al., 1997).

Other Side Effects

Fever and chills, blood dyscrasias, cholecystitis, pancreatitis, necrotizing vasculitis, acute interstitial nephritis, and noncardiogenic pulmonary edema have been seen rarely. Excess volume depletion may induce prerenal azotemia and favor thrombosis (Lottermoser et al., 2000). Allergic skin rashes occur in 0.28% of patients, and approximately the same percentage develops photosensitivity (Diffey & Langtry, 1989). An increased relative risk of renal

cell (and perhaps colon) cancer has been reported with diuretic therapy (Lip & Ferner, 1999), but the absolute risk is far below the proven benefits of these drugs. Weak observational data suggest an association of chronic diuretic use and end-stage renal disease (ESRD) (Hawkins, 2006) and mortality (Ahmed et al., 2006).

Conclusion

Strong controlled trial data document the benefits of diuretics in particular chlorthalidone, for the treatment of hypertension. Nonetheless, diuretics can cause multiple metabolic perturbations that could reduce their ability to protect against progressive atherosclerosis as they lower BP, including rises in uric acid, increasing insulin resistance and deranged fat distribution. These adverse effects are dose dependent and should be much less problematic with appropriately lower doses, doses that will provide most, if not all, of their antihypertensive effects.

Loop Diuretics

Loop diuretics primarily block chloride reabsorption by inhibition of the $Na^+/K^+/Cl^-$ cotransport system of the luminal membrane of the thick ascending limb of Henle's loop, the site where 35% to 45% of filtered sodium is reabsorbed (Fig. 7-1). Therefore, the loop diuretics are more potent and have a more rapid onset of action than do the thiazides. However, they are no more effective in lowering BP or less likely to cause side effects if given in equipotent amounts. Their major use is in patients with renal insufficiency, in whom large enough doses can be given to achieve an effective luminal concentration (see Chapter 9).

Furosemide

Most find that even twice-daily furosemide is less effective than twice-daily HCTZ (Anderson et al., 1971; Holland et al., 1979) or once-daily chlorthalidone (Healy et al., 1970) while producing similar hyperuricemia and hypokalemia. The maintenance of a slightly shrunken body fluid volume, which is critical for an antihypertensive action from diuretic therapy, is not met by the short duration of furosemide action (3 to 6 hours for an oral dose); during the remaining hours sodium is retained, so that net fluid balance over 24 hours is left unaltered (Wilcox et al., 1983). If furosemide is used twice daily, the first dose should be given early in the morning and the second in the midafternoon, both to provide diuretic action at the time of sodium intake and to avoid nocturia. Blacks respond more to furosemide than nonblacks, perhaps because they have a more active Na, K, 2Cl cotransporter in the thick ascending limb (Chun et al., 2008).

Loop diuretics may cause fewer metabolic problems than do longer-acting agents, because of their shorter duration of action (Reyes & Taylor, 1999). With similar durations of action, the side effects are similar.

Bumetanide

Bumetanide, although 40 times more potent and two times more bioavailable than furosemide on a weight basis, is identical in its actions when given in an equivalent dose (Brater et al., 1983).

Torsemide

Torsemide differs from the other diuretics in that it is mainly eliminated by hepatic metabolism, with only 20% being excreted unchanged in the urine (Brater, 1993). Therefore, it has a more prolonged duration of action, as long as 12 hours.

In small doses of 2.5 to 5 mg, torsemide may lower BP in uncomplicated hypertension, whereas larger doses are needed for chronic edematous states or with renal insufficiency (Dunn et al., 1995). In patients with chronic renal disease, 40 mg of torsemide once a day provided equal natriuresive and hypertensive effect as 40 mg of furosemide twice a day (Vasavada et al., 2003).

Ethacrynic Acid

Although structurally different from furosemide, ethacrynic acid also works primarily in the ascending limb of Henle's loop and has an equal potency. It is used much less than furosemide, mainly because of its greater propensity to cause permanent hearing loss. Since it does not contain a sulfonamide moiety, its main use has been in patients with sulfonamide sensitivity.

Potassium-Sparing Agents

Amiloride and triamterene act directly to inhibit sodium reabsorption by the epithelial sodium channels in the renal distal tubule, decreasing the net negative potential in the tubular lumen and thereby reducing potassium and hydrogen secretion and excretion, independent of aldosterone. Since neither are potent natriuretics, they are almost exclusively used in combination with thiazides which, by delivering more sodium to the K+-sparers' site of action,

increase their K+-sparing effect while countering the K+-wasting effect of the diuretic. Presumably, by preventing hypokalemia, the use of K+-sparing diuretics reduced the risk of death compared to the use of non–K+-sparing diuretics (Hebert et al., 2008).

Amiloride

Amiloride is usually used with a thiazide diuretic in tablets containing 50 mg of HCTZ and 5 mg of amiloride. The drug has been used as medical therapy for hyperaldosteronism in patients intolerant to aldosterone blockers and in patients with mutations of the genes regulating sodium channels that lead to the full-blown Liddle syndrome (see Chapter 11) or to a less severe prototype from the T594M polymorphism (Baker et al., 2002).

Nausea, flatulence, and skin rash have been the most frequent side effects and hyperkalemia the most serious. Moreover, a number of cases of hyponatremia in elderly patients have been reported after its use in combination with HCTZ (Mathew et al., 1990).

Triamterene

As with amiloride, triamterine (37.5 mg) is usually combined with HCTZ (25 mg). Triamterene may be excreted into the urine and may find its way into renal stones (Sörgel et al., 1985). Because triamterene is a folic acid antagonist, it should not be used during pregnancy (Hernández-Díaz et al., 2000).

Aldosterone Blockers

Greater use of these agents may be the most important recent advance in the treatment of hypertension. The first of these, spironolactone, has long been available in the United States but little used until publication of the Randomized Evaluation Study (RALES) in 1999 which showed a 30% decrease in mortality in patients with severe heart failure given 25 mg of spironolactone in addition to their other medications (Pitt et al., 1999). Since then, a large body of experimental and clinical evidence has revealed a multiorgan profibrotic effect of aldosterone so that blocking the hormone has assumed an important place in clinical medicine. At the same time, the marketing of a more specific aldosterone blocker, eplerenone, has stimulated the use of these agents.

Mode of Action

The primary mineralocorticoid aldosterone causes hypertension when present in large excess, the syndrome of primary aldosteronism covered in Chapter 11. However, even "normal" amounts of aldosterone in the presence of the relatively high sodium intake of modern societies are now known to activate mineralocorticoid receptors in multiple organs including the brain, heart, kidney, and blood vessels (Schiffrin, 2006). In turn, vasculitis and fibrosis are induced, independent of the traditional renal sodium-retaining effect of the hormone. Moreover, the incidence of hypertension over 4 years was 60% higher in those initially nonhypertensive subjects who were in the highest quartile of serum aldosterone (Vasan et al., 2004).

Eplerenone has virtual equivalence to spironolactone in blocking the mineralocorticoid receptor but a much lower blockade of androgen and progesterone receptors (Funder, 2002). In 2003, the addition of eplerenone was shown to reduce morbidity and mortality among patients with acute myocardial infarction (MI) complicated by left ventricular (LV) dysfunction in the Eplerenone Post-Acute Myocardial Infarction Heart Failure Efficacy and Survival Study (EPHESUS) (Pitt et al., 2003). Subsequently, the drug was shown to reduce mortality in these subjects whether they had been hypertensive or not (Pitt et al., 2008).

In both the RALES and EPHESUS trials, the aldosterone blocker provided additional benefit to patients receiving full doses of blockers of the renin-angiotensin system, ACEIs, or ARBs. It is now known that aldosterone synthesis is not completely suppressed with these agents, breaking through to maintain the pretreatment aldosterone levels even if angiotensin II levels remain suppressed (Sato & Saruta, 2003). Such a breakthrough was not seen in the Valsartan Heart Failure Trial (Cohn et al., 2003) but the role of breakthrough has been documented in trials of hypertension therapy wherein addition of an aldosterone blocker to ACEIs or ARBs provided additional benefit (Black, 2004).

Antihypertensive Efficacy
Spironolactone has been used alone to treat hypertension for many years, particularly in France (Jeunemaitre et al., 1988) but its major use in the United States has been as a K+-sparer in combination with a thiazide diuretic, providing an effect equivalent to 32 mmol of KCl (Toner et al., 1991) or to treat aldosteronism caused by bilateral adrenal hyperplasia. More recently, it has been found to effectively control patients with refractory hypertension (Ouzan et al., 2002;

Chapman et al., 2007). As expected, the drug lowers BP more in patients with low plasma renin and higher aldosterone levels (Weinberger, 2004). They add to the efficacy of ACEI or ARB (Black, 2004). Aldosterone blockers improve diastolic function (Grandi et al., 2002), are antiarrhythmic (Shah et al., 2007) and reduce proteinuria in patients with diabetic nephropathy (Sato et al., 2003). For these reasons, the use of aldosterone blockers will almost certainly expand to initial therapy, usually in combination with a diuretic, for more and more hypertensives.

Side Effects
The less specific spironolactone in doses of 25 to 50 mg per day induced gynecomastia in 6% of patients and biochemical abnormalities (mainly hyperkalemia) in 2% of the patients with resistant hypertension in the ASCOT Trial (Chapman et al., 2007). The more specific eplerenone induced gynecomastia in fewer than 1% of men in the EPHESUS Trial (Pitt et al., 2005). Hyperkalemia may occur with either agent but is uncommon in the absence of renal insufficiency, concomitant β-blocker, ACEI, or ARB therapy, or the use of potassium supplements (Gumieniak & Williams, 2004). However, with the much greater use of spironolactone in patients with heart failure also being treated with ACEIs after publication of the RALES trial in 1999, the rate of hospitalization for hyperkalemia in a Toronto hospital rose from 2.4 per 1,000 patients in 1994 to 11.0 per 1,000 in 2001 and mortality rose from 0.3 to 2.0 per 1,000 (Juurlink et al., 2004). Care is obviously needed in combining an aldosterone blocker with a β-blocker, ACEI, or ARB or DRI.

The possibility of upper GI bleeding has been raised in a case-control observational study wherein upper GI bleeding was 2.7-fold more likely in spironolactone users than in nonusers (Gulmez et al., 2008).

ADRENERGIC-INHIBITING DRUGS

Of the adrenergic-inhibiting agents currently used to treat hypertension, some act centrally on α_2-receptors to inhibit sympathetic nerve activity, some inhibit postganglionic sympathetic neurons, and some block the α- or β-adrenoreceptors on target organs (Fig. 7-5). Agents that act by blocking ganglia are no longer used.

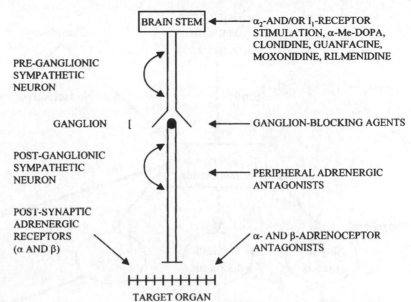

BRAIN STEM ← α₂-AND/OR I₁-RECEPTOR STIMULATION, α-Me-DOPA, CLONIDINE, GUANFACINE, MOXONIDINE, RILMENIDINE

PRE-GANGLIONIC SYMPATHETIC NEURON

GANGLION ← GANGLION-BLOCKING AGENTS

POST-GANGLIONIC SYMPATHETIC NEURON ← PERIPHERAL ADRENERGIC ANTAGONISTS

POST-SYNAPTIC ADRENERGIC RECEPTORS (α AND β) — α- AND β-ADRENOCEPTOR ANTAGONISTS

TARGET ORGAN

FIGURE 7-5 Drug targets in the sympathetic nervous system. (Modified from van Zwieten PA. Beneficial interactions between pharmacological, pathophysiological and hypertension research. *J Hypertens* 1999;17:1787–1797.)

Central α-Agonists

Central α-agents stimulates α_{2a}-adrenergic receptors that are involved in depressor sympathoinhibitory mechanisms (van Zwieten, 1999) (Fig. 7-6). Some are selective, whereas clonidine also acts on central imidazoline receptors. These drugs have well-defined effects, including:

- A marked decline in sympathetic activity reflected in lower levels of NE.
- A reduction of the ability of the baroreceptor reflex to compensate for a decrease in BP, accounting for the relative bradycardia and enhanced hypotensive action noted on standing.
- A modest decrease in both peripheral resistance and cardiac output.
- A fall in plasma renin levels.
- Fluid retention.
- Maintenance of renal blood flow despite a fall in BP.
- Common side effects reflecting their central site of action: sedation, decreased alertness, and a dry mouth.

When central α-agonists are abruptly stopped, a rapid rebound and, rarely, an overshoot of the BP may be experienced with or without accompanying features of excess sympathetic nervous activity. This discontinuation syndrome likely represents a sudden surge of catecholamine release, freed from the prior state of inhibition.

Methyldopa

From the early 1960s to the late 1970s, when β-blockers became available, methyldopa was the second most popular drug (after diuretics) used to treat hypertension.

Methyldopa is the α-methylated derivative of dopa, the natural precursor of dopamine and NE. Its mode of action involves the formation of methylnorepinephrine, which acts as a potent agonist at α-adrenergic receptors within the central nervous system (CNS) (van Zwieten, 1999).

Antihypertensive Efficacy

BP is lowered maximally approximately 4 hours after an oral dose of methyldopa, and some effect persists for up to 24 hours. For most patients, therapy should be started with 250 mg two times per day, and the daily dosage can be increased to a maximum of 3.0 g on a twice-per-day schedule. In patients with renal insufficiency, the dosage should be halved.

Side Effects

In addition to the anticipated sedative effects, postural hypotension, and fluid retention, an impairment of reticuloendothelial function (Kelton, 1985) and a variety of autoimmune side effects, including fever and liver dysfunction, can occur with methyldopa. Liver dysfunction usually disappears when the drug is stopped, but at least 83 cases

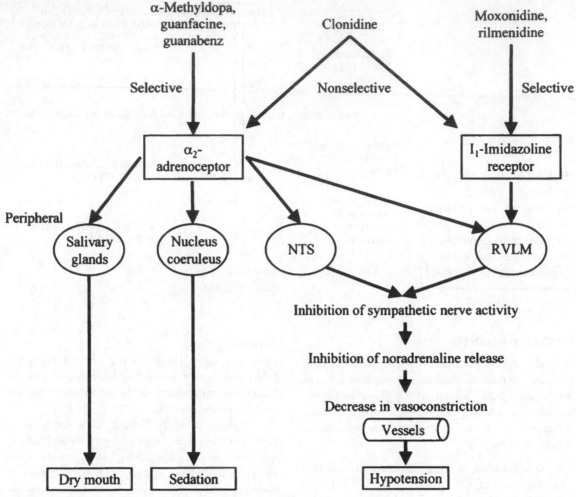

FIGURE 7-6   Central antihypertensive mechanisms of various types of centrally acting antihypertensive drugs. NTS, nucleus tractus solitarii; RVLM, rostral ventrolateral medulla. (Modified from van Zwieten PA. The renaissance of centrally acting antihypertensive drugs. *J Hypertens* 1999;17(Suppl. 3):S15–S21.)

of serious hepatotoxicity were reported by 1975 (Rodman et al., 1976), with diffuse parenchymal injury similar to autoimmune chronic active hepatitis (Lee, 1995).

An impairment of psychometric performance (Johnson et al., 1990) and a selective loss of upper airway motor activity (Lahive et al., 1988) may not be obvious until the drug is stopped. Overall, in large surveys, the number and range of the adverse reactions to methyldopa are impressive (Webster & Koch, 1996). In view of its unique and potentially serious side effects, other central α-agonists should be used in place of methyldopa. In the United States, it remains a favored drug only for the treatment of hypertension during pregnancy (see Chapter 15).

Guanabenz

Guanabenz, an aminoguanidine, works like clonidine and methyldopa and causes similar side effects. Therapy should begin with 4 mg twice per day, with increments up to a total of 64 mg per day.

The side effects mimic those seen with other central α2-agonists and a withdrawal syndrome may occur if the drug is stopped abruptly (Ram et al., 1979).

Guanfacine

Another selective central α2-agonist, guanfacine appears to enter the brain more slowly and to maintain its antihypertensive effect longer then guanabenz, translating into a once-per-day dosage and perhaps fewer CNS side effects (Lewin et al., 1990). Withdrawal symptoms are less common than with clonidine (Wilson et al., 1986). These characteristics make it the most attractive of this group of centrally acting α_2-agonists.

Clonidine

Clonidine acts centrally on both α_2-receptors and imidazoline receptors (Fig. 7-6). When taken orally, the BP begins to fall within 30 minutes, with the greatest effect occurring between 2 and 4 hours. The duration of effect is from 8 to 12 hours.

The starting dose may be as little as 0.075 mg twice daily (Clobass Study Group, 1990), with a maximum of 1.2 mg per day. Repeated hourly doses of 0.1 to 0.2 mg have been used to lower markedly elevated BP (Houston, 1986).

A transdermal preparation that delivers clonidine continuously over a 7-day interval is effective and causes milder side effects than oral therapy (Giugliano et al., 1998), but it may cause considerable skin irritation and side effects similar to those seen with the oral drug (Langley & Heel, 1988), including rebound hypertension when discontinued (Metz et al., 1987). It is available in doses of 0.1, 0.2, and 0.3 mg per day.

Side Effects

Clonidine shares the two most common side effects, sedation and dry mouth with methyldopa but not the autoimmune hepatic and hematologic derangements. Depression of sinus and atrioventricular (AV) nodal function may be common, and a few cases of severe bradycardia have been reported (Byrd et al., 1988).

Rebound and Discontinuation Syndromes

If any antihypertensive therapy is inadvertently stopped abruptly, various discontinuation syndromes may occur: (a) a rapid asymptomatic return of the BP to pretreatment levels which occurs in the majority of patients; (b) a rebound of the BP plus symptoms and signs of sympathetic overactivity; and (c) an overshoot of the BP above pretreatment levels.

A discontinuation syndrome has been reported, more frequently with clonidine (Neusy & Lowenstein, 1989), likely reflecting a rapid return of catecholamine secretion that had been suppressed during therapy. Those who had been on a combination of a central adrenergic inhibitor, e.g., clonidine, and a β-blocker may be particularly susceptible if the central inhibitor is withdrawn while the β-blocker is continued (Lilja

et al., 1982). This leads to a sudden surge in plasma catecholamines in a situation in which peripheral α-receptors are left unopposed to induce vasoconstriction because the β-receptors are blocked and cannot mediate vasodilation.

If a discontinuation syndrome appears, clonidine should be restarted, and the symptoms will likely recede rapidly. If needed, labetalol will effectively lower a markedly elevated BP (Mehta & Lopez, 1987).

Other Uses

Clonidine has been reported to be useful in numerous conditions that may accompany hypertension, including:

- Restless legs syndrome (Wagner et al., 1996)
- Opiate withdrawal (Bond, 1986)
- Menopausal hot flashes (Pandya et al., 2000)
- Diarrhea due to diabetic neuropathy (Fedorak et al., 1985)
- Sympathetic nervous hyperactivity in patients with alcoholic cirrhosis (Esler et al., 1992)
- Perioperative protection for patients at high risk of coronary events (Wallace et al., 2004)

Imidazoline Receptor Agonists

Not available in the United States but used elsewhere, monoxidine and rilmenidine are two centrally acting drugs that have as their primary site of action the imidazoline receptor located in the rostral ventrolateral medulla oblongata, wherein α_2-receptors are less abundant (Fig. 7-6) (van Zwieten, 1999). They effectively reduce sympathetic activity (Esler et al., 2004) and may diminish insulin resistance so they are being used for patients with metabolic syndrome (Sharma et al., 2004), with less of the sedation and dry mouth seen with clonidine and selective α_2-agonists.

Peripheral Adrenergic Inhibitors

Reserpine

First reported to be an effective antihypertensive in the 1940s (Bhatia, 1942), reserpine became a popular drug in the 1960s and 1970s but has been used less and less because, being an inexpensive generic, it has no constituency pushing for its use, and when used in high doses, it has caused depression, earning it a bad reputation.

Reserpine, one of the many alkaloids of the Indian snakeroot *Rauwolfia serpentina*, is absorbed readily from the gut, is taken up rapidly by lipid-containing tissue, and binds to sites involved with storage of biogenic amines. Its effects start slowly and persist, so only one dose per day is needed.

Reserpine blocks the transport of NE into its storage granules so that less of the neurotransmitter is available when the adrenergic nerves are stimulated, resulting in a decrease of peripheral vascular resistance. Catecholamines also are depleted in the brain, which may account for the sedative and depressant effects of the drug, and in the myocardium, which may decrease cardiac output and induce a slight bradycardia.

Antihypertensive Efficacy

By itself, reserpine has limited antihypertensive potency, resulting in an average decrease of only 3/5 mm Hg; when combined with a thiazide, the reduction averaged 14/11 mm Hg (VA Cooperative Study, 1962). It works as well as other drugs (Krönig et al., 1997) and induces significant regression of LVH (Horn et al., 1997). With a diuretic, as little as 0.05 mg once daily will provide most of the antihypertensive effect of 0.25 mg and is associated with less lethargy and impotence (Participating VA Medical Centers, 1982).

Side Effects

Side effects, which are relatively infrequent at appropriately low doses (Prisant et al., 1991), include nasal stuffiness, increased gastric acid secretion, which rarely may activate an ulcer, and CNS depression, which may simply tranquilize an apprehensive patient and is rarely severe enough to lead to serious depression.

Guanethidine

Guanethidine at one time was frequently used because it requires only one dose per day and has a steep dose-response relationship, thus producing an effect in almost every patient. The BP is reduced somewhat in the supine position but much more so when the patient is upright, because the normal vasoconstrictive response to posture is blunted (Goldberg & Raftery, 1976). As other effective drugs with fewer side effects became available, the use of guanethidine has virtually disappeared.

Guanadrel Sulfate

A close relative of guanethidine, guanadrel sulfate has almost all the attributes of that drug with a shorter onset and offset of action, which diminish the frequency of side effects and make it more tolerable (Owens & Dunn, 1988).

α-Adrenergic Receptor Blockers

Selective α_1-blockers have had a relatively small share of the overall market for antihypertensive drugs in the United States and as a consequence of the ALLHAT trial (ALLHAT Officers, 2000), their use in the United States is now almost exclusively for relief of prostatism.

Mode of Action

The nonselective α-blockers phenoxybenzamine and phentolamine are used almost exclusively in the medical management of pheochromocytoma, because they are only minimally effective in primary hypertension (see Chapter 12).

After recognition of the two major subtypes of α-receptors—the α_1 postsynaptic and the α_2 presynaptic, prazosin was recognized to act as a competitive antagonist of postsynaptic α_1-receptors, an effect shared by doxazosin and terazosin (Fig. 7-7). These agents block the activation of postsynaptic α_1-receptors by circulating or neurally released catecholamines, reducing peripheral resistance without major changes in cardiac output.

The presynaptic α_2-receptors remain open, capable of binding neurotransmitter and thereby inhibiting the release of additional NE through a direct negative-feedback mechanism. This inhibition of NE release explains the lesser frequency of tachycardia, increased cardiac output, and rise in renin levels that characterize the response to drugs that block both the presynaptic

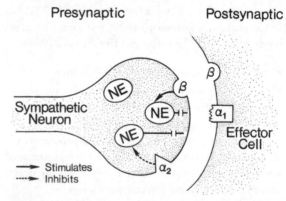

FIGURE 7-7 Schematic view of the action of selective postsynaptic α_1-blockers. By blocking the α_1-adrenergic receptor on the vascular smooth muscle, catecholamine-induced vasoconstriction is inhibited. The α_2-adrenergic receptor on the neuronal membrane is not blocked; therefore, inhibition of additional NE release by the short feedback mechanism is maintained.

α_2-receptor and the postsynaptic α_1-receptor (e.g., phentolamine). Despite this selective blockade, neurally mediated responses to stress and exercise are unaffected, and the baroreceptor reflex remains active.

Accompanying these desirable attributes may be other actions that lessen the usefulness of α-adrenergic blockers: They relax the venous bed as well and, at least initially, may affect the visceral vascular bed more than the peripheral vascular bed. The subsequent pooling of blood in the viscera may explain the propensity to first-dose hypotension seen with the fast-acting prazosin (Saxena & Bolt, 1986). Volume retention is common, perhaps because renin and aldosterone levels are less suppressed than they are with other adrenergic-inhibiting drugs (Webb et al., 1987).

Prazosin is rapidly absorbed, reaches maximal blood levels at 2 hours, and has a plasma half-life of approximately 3 hours. Terazosin and doxazosin are less lipid-soluble and have half, or less, of the affinity for α_1-receptors as compared with prazosin. Therefore, they induce a slower and less profound initial fall in BP, particularly after standing, than does prazosin.

Tamsulosin produces a lesser blockade of the α_1-receptors on blood vessels than in the prostate (Harada et al., 2000). It is not approved for treatment of hypertension. It has been associated with serious opthalmic adverse effects (Bell et al., 2009).

Antihypertensive Efficacy

The antihypertensive efficacy of doxazosin and terazosin is equivalent to that of diuretics, β-blockers, ACEIs, and CCBs (Achari et al., 2000). The drugs work equally well in black and in nonblack patients (Batey et al., 1989) and in the elderly (Cheung et al., 1989). The addition of doxazosin was shown in the ASCOT Trial to control hypertension effectively in patients resistant to two or more other agents (Chapman et al., 2008).

The initial dose should be 1 mg, slowly titrated upward to achieve the desired fall in BP, with a total daily dose of up to 20 mg. α-Blockers can be given at bedtime to provide a greater nocturnal fall in BP in and blunting of the morning surge that is involved in the increased incidence of cardiovascular events at that time (Matsui et al., 2008).

Other Uses
Genitourinary Function

Doxazosin, tamsulosin, and terazosin have been found to provide excellent relief from the obstructive symptoms of benign prostatic hypertrophy (Schwinn et al., 2004). The combination of doxazosin and the 5α-reductace inhibitor finasteride slowed the clinical progression of BPH better than either drug alone (McConnell et al., 2003).

In the TOMHS trial of a representative from each of the five major classes of antihypertensives, only doxazosin reduced the incidence of impotence below that seen with placebo (Grimm et al., 1997).

Metabolic Benefits

α_1-Blockers have been repeatedly found to improve the lipid profile (Hirano et al., 2001) and insulin sensitivity (Lithell, 1996).

The ALLHAT Experience

Despite these generally attractive features, the termination of the doxazosin arm of the ALLHAT Trial (ALLHAT Officers, 2000) because of a higher incidence of heart failure has reduced the use of α-blockers (Stafford et al., 2004). Neither cardiovascular nor all-cause mortality was increased in the doxazosin group, suggesting that the twofold increased numbers of heart failure likely were not of severe degree.

The ALLHAT experience indicates the need to use a diuretic with an α blocker for the treatment of hypertension, particularly in those with LVH or other risk factors for congestive heart failure (CHF) (Matsui et al., 2008). α-Blockers remain useful as add-on therapy in patients with resistant hypertension and the preferred initial therapy for many hypertensives with benign prostatic hypertrophy.

Side Effects

Postural hypotension developing in 30 to 90 minutes may be seen particularly in volume-depleted patients given the shorter-acting prazosin. The problem generally can be avoided by initiating therapy with a small dose and ensuring that the patient is not volume-depleted as a result of diuretic therapy. Urinary incontinence in women may be caused by α-blockers (Marshall & Beevers, 1996).

β-Adrenergic Receptor Blockers

For many years, β-adrenergic blocking agents were the second most popular antihypertensive drugs after diuretics. Although they are no more effective than other antihypertensive agents and may on occasion induce serious side effects, they offer the special advantage of relieving a number of concomitant diseases. In view of their proven ability to provide secondary cardioprotection after an acute MI, it was hoped that they would provide special primary protection against initial coronary events as well. This hope remains unfulfilled. To the contrary, β-blockers have failed to reduce heart attacks better than other classes while providing less protection against stokes (Liu et al., 2009). In the words of Messerli et al. as far back as 1998: "The time has come to admit that beta-blockers should no longer be considered appropriate first-line therapy of uncomplicated hypertension." This is particularly true for the most popular, atenolol (Lindholm et al., 2005).

Nonetheless, the proven benefits of β-blockers in patients with either coronary disease (particularly after an acute MI) or CHF ensure that these drugs will continue to be widely used.

Mode of Action

These agents are chemically similar to β-agonists and to each other (Fig. 7-8). The competitive inhibition of β-blockers on β-adrenergic receptors produces numerous effects on functions that regulate the BP, including a reduction in cardiac output, a diminution of renin release, perhaps a decrease in central sympathetic nervous outflow, and a presynaptic blockade that inhibits catecholamine release. The hemodynamic effects appear to change over time. Cardiac output usually falls acutely (except with high-ISA [intrinsic sympathomimetic activity] pindolol) and remains lower chronically; peripheral resistance, on the other hand, usually rises

acutely but falls toward, if not to, normal with time (Man in't Veld et al., 1988).

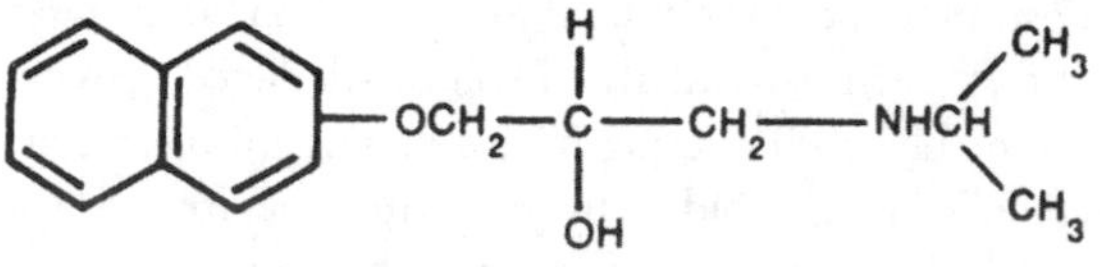

Pharmacologic Differences

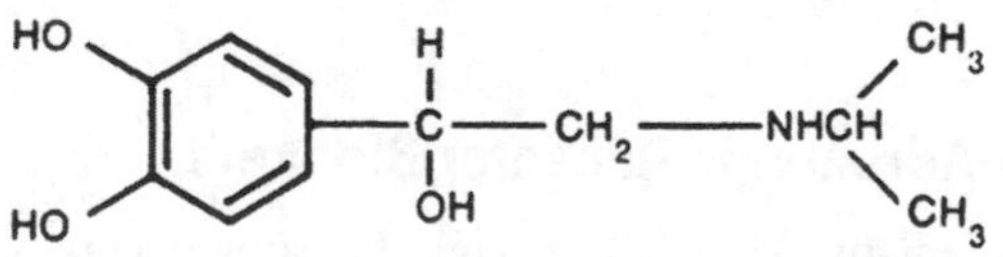

Since the introduction of propranolol in 1964 (Black et al., 1964), a number of similar drugs have been synthesized, approximately 20 being marketed throughout the world, 12 in the United States. The various β-blockers can be conveniently classified by their relative selectivity for the β_1-receptors (primarily in the heart) and presence of ISA, also referred to as *partial agonist activity* and their *lipid solubility* (Fig. 7-9) (Table 7-4). In addition, two agents (labetalol, carvedilol) have both α- and β-blocking effects and one (nebivolol) vasodilates by increasing nitric oxide. They are considered separately.

Lipid Solubility

Those that are more lipid-soluble (lipophilic) tend to be taken up and metabolized extensively by the liver. As an example, with oral propranolol and metoprolol, up to 70% is removed on the first pass of portal blood through the liver. The bioavailability of these β-blockers is, therefore, less after oral than after intravenous administration.

Those such as nadolol, which is much less lipid-soluble (lipophobic), escape hepatic metabolism and are mainly excreted by the kidneys, unchanged. As a result, its plasma half-life and duration of action is much longer.

β_1-Receptor Cardioselectivity

All currently available β-blockers antagonize cardiac β_1-receptors competitively, but they vary in their degree of β_2-receptor blockade in extracardiac tissues. The assumption that an agent with relative cardioselectivity is automatically less likely to cause side effects must be tempered by these considerations: recognizing that no β-blocker is purely cardioselective, particularly in large doses, and when high endogenous catechol levels are needed, as during an attack of asthma, even minimal degrees of β_2-blockade from a cardioselective drug such as bisoprolol may cause trouble (Haffner et al., 1992).

On the other hand, in the presence of certain concomitant diseases, such as migraine and tremor, a nonselective β_2-antagonist effect may be preferable.

Intrinsic Sympathomimetic Activity

Of the β-blockers now available in the United States, pindolol and, to a lesser degree, acebutolol have ISA,

FIGURE 7-8 Structure of propranolol and the β-agonist isoproterenol.

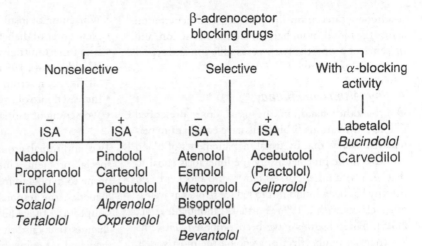

FIGURE 7-9 Classification of β-adrenoreceptor blockers based on cardioselectivity and ISA. Drugs not approved for use in the United States for the treatment of hypertension are in italics. ISA, intrinsic sympathomimetic activity.

implying that even in concentrations that fully occupy the β-receptors, the biologic effect is less than that seen with a full agonist.

In commenting on studies of patients with heart failure given different β-blockers (Go et al., 2008; Kramer et al., 2008), Pitt (2008) states: "Many clinicians may be tempted to consider BBs as a class and to use the least expensive one. It should, however, be emphasized that the differences between various BBs are far greater than for other agents shown to be effective in HF, such as ACE inhibitors, ARBs, or aldosterone blockers. These include selectivity for the B_2 and

TABLE 7.4   Pharmacologic Properties of Some β-Blockers

Drug	β₁-Selectivity	Intrinsic Sympathomimetic Activity	α-Blockage	Lipid Solubility	Usual Daily Dosage (Frequency)
Acebutolol	+	+	−	+	200–1,200 mg (1)
Atenolol	++	−	−	−	25–100 mg (2)
Betaxolol	++	−	−	−	5–40 mg (1)
Bisoprolol	+++	−	−	+	2.5–20 mg (1)
Bucindolol	−	−	−	+	50–200 mg
Carteolol	−	+	−	−	2.5–10 mg (1)
Carvedilol[a]	−	−	+	+++	12.5–50 mg (2)
Celiprolol	++	+	−	−	200–400 mg (1)
Esmolol	++	−	−	−	25–300 µg/kg/min iv
Labetalol[a]	−	−	+	++	200–1,200 mg (2)
Metoprolol	++	−	−	++	50–200 mg (2, 1)
Nadolol	−	−	−	−	20–240 mg (1)
Nebivolol[a]	++	−	−	++	5–10 mg (1)
Penbutolol	−	+	−	+++	10–20 mg (1)
Pindolol	−	+++	−	++	10–60 (2)
Propranolol	−	−	−	+++	40–240 mg (2, 1)
Timolol	−	−	−	++	10–40 mg (2)

[a] Vasodilating.

+, ++, and +++ signs indicate the magnitude of the effect on various properties; − sign indicates no effect.

α-adrenergic receptor, lipophilicity, and penetration across the blood-brain barrier, duration of action, and presence of properties such as vasodilation and type 3 antiarrhythmic activity."

Antihypertensive Efficacy

On the other hand, in the usual doses prescribed (Table 7-4), various β-blockers have equal antihypertensive efficacy, that by usual measurements of blood pressure at the brachial artery (peripheral) is equal to that seen with other classes. However β-blocker based therapy has been found not to reduce strokes as well as other classes with a 19% shortfall (Lindholam et al., 2005). Three reasons have been proposed. First the less than 24 hours effect of atenolol, the most widely used β-blocker, but given only once daily in all of the trials. The 2nd and 3rd reasons relate to the higher central (aortic) pressure with β-blockers than with vasodilating agents, i.e. all other classes of antihypertensive drugs, despite their equal effect as measured at the periphery. The 2nd culprit is the bradycardia increasing cardiac work to maintain total cardiac output (Bangalore et al., 2008). The 3rd relates to the peripheral vasoconstriction induced by the β2 blocking action, causing the reflected pulse wave to strike the heart during systolic, further increasing cardiac work to overcome the higher central pressure. With vasodilators, the pulse wave returns even slower, bringing higher pressure during diastole, increasing coronary perfusion without increasing cardiac work. This difference was documented in the CAFE substudy of the ASCOT trial (CAFE Investigators, 2006) and has been further validated (Mackenzie et al., 2009).

Other Uses

- Coronary disease (Snow et al., 2004)
- Postmyocardinal infarction (Bangalore et al., 2007a)
- Heart failure from LV systolic dysfunction (Kramer et al., 2008)
- Hypertrophic cardiomyopathy (Spirito et al., 1997)
- Severe mitral regurgitation (Varadarajan et al., 2008)
- Therapy with direct vasodilators (Zacest et al., 1972)
- Anxiety and stress (Fogari et al., 1992)

Side Effects

These have been reported to be more common in patients receiving β-blockers:

- Fatigue (Ko et al., 2002)
- Diminished exercise ability (Vanhees et al., 2000)
- Weight gain (Messerli et al., 2007)

- Worsening of insulin sensitivity (Lithell,1996)
- New onset of diabetes (Gress et al., 2000)
- Rise in serum triglycerides, fall in HDL-cholesterol (Kasiske et al., 1995)
- Slight rise in serum potassium (Traub et al., 1980)
- Increased rate of suicide (Sørensen et al., 2001)
- Worsening of psoriasis (Savola et al., 1987)

Two additional groups of patients may experience special problems: insulin-taking diabetics who are prone to hypoglycemia and coronary patients. As for diabetics, the responses to hypoglycemia—both the symptoms and the counterregulatory hormonal changes that raise the blood sugar level—are largely mediated by epinephrine, particularly in those who are insulin-dependent because they usually are also deficient in glucagon. If these patients become hypoglycemic, β-blockade delays the return of the blood sugar. The only symptom of hypoglycemia may be sweating, which may be enhanced by the presence of a β-blocker (Molnar et al., 1974).

Patients with coronary disease who discontinue chronic β-blocker therapy may experience a discontinuation syndrome of increasing angina, infarction, or sudden death (Teichert et al., 2007). These ischemic episodes likely reflect the phenomenon of supersensitivity: an increased number of β-receptors appear in response to the functional blockade of receptors by the β-blocker; when the β-blocker is discontinued and no longer occupies the receptors, the increased number of receptors are suddenly exposed to endogenous catecholamines, resulting in a greater α-agonist response for a given level of catechols. Hypertensives, with a high frequency of underlying coronary atherosclerosis, may be particularly susceptible to this type of withdrawal syndrome; thus, when the drugs are discontinued, their dosage should be cut by half every 2 or 3 days, and the drugs stopped after the third reduction.

The following side effects have *not* been consistently or significantly found to be more common with β-blocker use:

- Depression (Ko et al., 2002)
- Sexual dysfunction (Ko et al., 2002)
- Cognitive loss (Pérez-Stable et al., 2000)
- Worsening of peripheral vascular disease (Radack & Deck, 1991)
- Worsening of mild to moderate reactive airway disease or obstructive lung disease (Prichard & Vallance, 2004).

Moveover, on the positive side, β-blockers may reduce urine calcium excretion (Lind et al., 1994) and thereby decrease the risk of fractures (Schlienger et al., 2004).

Vasodilating β-Blockers

In this category are one old drug (labetalol) whose vasodilatory properties come from its high level of α-blockade, one newer drug (carvedilol) with some α-blocking activity, but primarily a direct vasodilatory action, and one (nebivolol) that is a highly selective $β_1$-blocker that works by generating NO.

Labetalol

Labetalol is a nonselective $β_1$- and $β_2$-receptor blocker combined with α-blocking action in a 4:1 ratio. It is an effective antihypertensive when given twice daily, maintaining good 24-hour control and blunting the early morning surges in pressure (Ruilope, 1994). The usual starting doses are 100 mg b.i.d. The maximal daily dose is 1,200 mg.

Labetalol has been used both orally and intravenously to treat hypertensive emergencies, including postoperative hypertension (Lebel et al., 1985) and acute aortic dissection (Grubb et al., 1987). It has been successfully used to treat hypertension during pregnancy (Pickles et al., 1992).

Side Effects

Symptomatic orthostatic hypotension is the most common side effect, seen most often during initial therapy with larger doses. Other side effects include intense scalp itching, ejaculatory failure (Goa et al., 1989), and bronchospasm (George et al., 1985). An increased titer of antinuclear and antimitochondrial antibodies develops in some patients; although a systemic lupus syndrome has not been reported, lichenoid skin eruptions have been (Goa et al., 1989).

Perhaps the most serious side effect of labetalol is hepatotoxicity: At least three deaths have been reported (Clark et al., 1990). As a result, a warning has been added to its label in the United States, stating, "Hepatic injury may be slowly progressive despite minimal symptomatology. Appropriate laboratory testing should be done at the first symptom or sign of liver dysfunction."

In keeping with its α-blocking effect, labetalol has less adverse effect on lipids as do β-blockers (Lardinois & Neuman, 1988).

Carvedilol

This "third" generation nonselective β-blocker with only one-tenth as much α-blocking activity has been used mainly for treatment of heart failure. It is also approved for the treatment of hypertension.

Beyond its slight α-blocking effect, carvedilol vasodilates by increasing generation of endogenous NO from endothelial cells (Kalinowski et al., 2003). As with labetalol, BP falls without a fall in cardiac output but rather a decrease in peripheral resistance (Dupont et al., 1987).

In doses starting at 6.25 mg twice a day and proceeding up to 25 mg b.i.d, carvedilol is equal to 50 up to 200 mg of metoprolol b.i.d (Bakris et al., 2004). A once-a-day formulation is now available.

Carvedilol has been found to provide additional survival benefit in patients with varying grades of CHF than metoprolol (Poole-Wilson et al., 2003) even in those with low systolic pressure (Rouleau et al., 2004) while better preserving renal function (Di Lenarda et al., 2005).

Unlike traditional β-blockers, carvedilol does not worsen insulin sensitivity or have as much of an adverse effect on lipids (Bakris et al., 2004; Torp-Pedersen et al., 2007).

Nebivolol

This drug, only recently approved for use in the United States, is the most selective $β_1$-blocker of this family of drugs and exerts its effect by generating and releasing NO while having a complimentary antioxidant effect (Ignarro, 2004).

Nebivolol may be particularly effective in the treatment of elderly patients with isolated systolic hypertension. In addition to reducing aortic stiffness, as do other β-blockers, it also reduces the amplification of central systolic pressure by reducing wave reflection from the periphery (Dhakam et al., 2008; Mahmud & Feely, 2008).

DIRECT VASODILATORS

In this category, we have added nitrates to those agents which vasodilate by entering vascular smooth muscle cells. This is in contrast to those that vasodilate in other ways—by inhibiting hormonal vasoconstrictor mechanisms (e.g., ACEIs), by preventing calcium entry into the cells that initiate constriction (e.g., CCBs), or by blocking α-receptor–mediated vasoconstriction (e.g., $α_1$-blockers). The various vasodilators

TABLE 7.5 Vasodilator Drugs Used to Treat Hypertension

Drug	Relative Action on Arteries (A) or Veins (V)
Direct	
Hydralazine	A >> V
Minoxidil	A >> V
Nitroprusside	A + V
Diazoxide	A > V
Nitroglycerin	V > A
CCBs	A >> V
ACEIs	A > V
α-Blockers	A + V

>, greater than; >>, much greater than; +, equal or both.

differ considerably in their power, mode of action, and relative activities on arteries and veins (Table 7-5). The intravenous direct vasodilators are covered in Chapter 8.

Hydralazine

Hydralazine was introduced in the early 1950s (Freis et al., 1953) but was little used because of its activation of the sympathetic nervous system. Its use increased in the 1970s when the rationale for triple therapy—a diuretic, an adrenergic inhibitor, and a direct vasodilator—was demonstrated (Zacest et al., 1972). However, its use receded again with the advent of the newer vasodilating drugs.

Hydralazine acts directly to relax the smooth muscle in the walls of peripheral arterioles, the resistance vessels more so than the capacitance vessels, thereby decreasing peripheral resistance and BP (Saxena & Bolt, 1986). Coincidental to the peripheral vasodilation, the heart rate, stroke volume, and cardiac output rise, reflecting a baroreceptor-mediated reflex increase in sympathetic discharge (Lin et al., 1983) and direct stimulation of the heart (Khatri et al., 1977). In addition, the sympathetic overactivity and the fall in BP increase renin release, further counteracting the vasodilator's effect and likely adding to the reactive sodium retention that accompanies the fall in BP (Fig. 7-10). Therefore, it is given along with a β-blocker and a diuretic in the treatment of more severe hypertension.

Hydralazine should usually be started at 25 mg two times per day. The maximal dose should be limited to 200 mg per day to lessen the likelihood of a lupuslike syndrome and because higher doses seldom provide additional benefit.

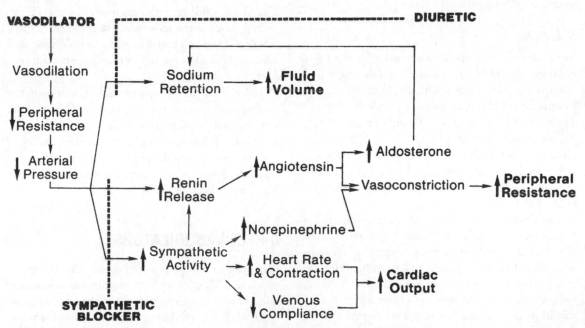

FIGURE 7-10 Primary and secondary effects of vasodilator therapy in essential hypertension and the manner by which diuretic and β-adrenergic blocker therapy can overcome the undesirable secondary effects. (Modified from Koch-Weser J. Vasodilator drugs in the treatment of hypertension. *Arch Intern Med* 1974;133:1017–1027.)

The inactivation of hydralazine involves acetylation in the liver by the enzyme *N*-acetyltransferase. The level of this enzyme activity is genetically determined, and rapid acetylators require larger doses than do slow acetylators to achieve an equivalent effect (Ramsay et al., 1984). Perry (1973) showed that patients who develop a lupuslike toxicity tend to be slow acetylators and thus are exposed to the drug longer.

Side Effects

Three kinds of side effects are seen: those due to reflex sympathetic activation, those due to a lupuslike reaction, and those due to nonspecific problems. Headaches, flushing, and tachycardia should be anticipated and prevented by concomitant use of adrenergic inhibitors. The drug should be given with caution to patients with coronary artery disease (CAD) and should be avoided in patients with a dissecting aortic aneurysm or recent cerebral hemorrhage, in view of its propensity to increase cardiac output and cerebral blood flow (CBF).

The lupuslike reaction was first described by Perry (1973). An early, febrile reaction resembling serum sickness was seen in 11 patients; late toxicity developed in 44 resembling systemic lupus erythematosus or rheumatoid arthritis. These symptoms almost invariably go away when the drug is stopped or the dosage is lowered. The lupuslike syndrome is clearly dose dependent. (Cameron & Ramsay, 1984).

Other side effects of hydralazine include anorexia, nausea, vomiting, and diarrhea; less common effects are paresthesias, tremor, and muscle cramps. An additional potential disadvantage of hydralazine and other direct vasodilators is their failure when given alone to regress LVH, presumably because of their marked stimulation of sympathetic nervous activity (Leenen et al., 1987).

Minoxidil

More potent than hydralazine, minoxidil has become a mainstay in the therapy of severe hypertension associated with renal insufficiency (see Chapter 9). Its propensity to grow hair precludes its use in many women, but this effect has led to its use as a topical ointment for male pattern baldness.

Minoxidil induces smooth muscle relaxation by opening cardiovascular ATP-sensitive potassium channels, a mechanism apparently unique among vasodilators currently available in the United States but similar to the mode of action of various potassium channel openers (e.g., nicorandil) (Ito et al., 2004).

Because minoxidil is both more potent and longer lasting than hydralazine, it turns on the various reactions to direct arteriolar vasodilation to an even greater degree. Therefore, large doses of potent loop diuretics and adrenergic blockers will be needed in most patients (see Fig. 7-10).

When used with diuretics and adrenergic inhibitors, minoxidil controls hypertension in more than 75% of patients whose disease was previously resistant to multiple drugs (Sica, 2004b). It can be given once daily in a range of 2.5 to 80 mg.

Side Effects

The most common side effect, seen in nearly 80% of patients, is hirsutism, beginning with fairly fine hair on the face and then with coarse hair increasing everywhere. It is apparently related to the vasodilation produced by the drug and not to hormonal effects. The hair gradually disappears when the drug is stopped (Kidwai & George, 1992).

Beyond generalized volume expansion, pericardial effusions appear in approximately 3% of patients who receive minoxidil (Martin et al., 1980).

Nitrates

Nitrates, both nitroglycerin (Willmot et al., 2006) and oral isosorbide nitrate (Stokes et al., 2005), by their vasodilating properties as exogenous endothelium-derived relaxing factor (NO), can also be used as antihypertensives. Stokes et al. (2005) found isosorbide mononitrate to lower systolic BP by an average of 16 mm Hg without significant effect on diastolic BPM in 16 elderly patients with resistant systolic hypertension. The pulse pressure fell by 13 mm Hg and the augmentation index, a measure of pulse wave reflection, fell by 25%. Tolerance did not seem to develop.

Despite the attractiveness of this approach for treatment of systolic hypertension, the lack of a commercial sponsor for testing a generic drug in a large clinical trial makes it unlikely that a currently available nitrate will be approved as an antihypertensive drug.

CALCIUM CHANNEL BLOCKERS

CCBs were introduced as antianginal agents in the 1970s and as antihypertensives in the 1980s. Their use grew rapidly so that they became the second most popular group of drugs used by US practitioners for the treatment of hypertension in the early 2000s.

Mode of Action

Three types of CCBs are now available. All interact with the same calcium channel: the L-type voltage-gated plasma membrane channel, but they have major differences in their structure and cardiovascular effects (Eisenberg et al., 2004) (Table 7-6).

Diltiazem, a benzothiazepine, and *verapamil*, a phenylalkylamine, the currently available nondihydropyridine (non-DHP), are rate slowing: At equivalent concentrations, they induce vasodilation, depress cardiac contractility, and inhibit AV conduction.

Dihydropyridines (DHPs) are predominantly vasodilators and improve endothelial function (Sugiura et al., 2008). The first generation, exemplified by nifedipine, had modest effects on cardiac contractility. The second generation, such as amlodipine, felodipine, and nicardipine, has more effect on vascular dilation than on myocardial contractility or cardiac conduction. A number of other DHPs are not yet approved in the United States but are being used elsewhere; these include benidipine, cilnidipine, efonidipine, lacidipine, lercanidipine, manidipine, and nitrendipine. Although the major differences are between non-DHP and the DHP-CCBs, there are enough differences between the multiple DHP-CCBs so that "caution should be exercised in assuming that all DHP CCBs licensed for once-daily administration are equivalent in their durations of action and overall antihypertensive efficacy" (Meredith & Elliott, 2004).

Surprisingly, some CCBs (felodipine, nimodipine, nifedipine, and, too a lesser extent, amlodipine) have been found to provide mineralocorticoid receptor antagonist activity (Dietz et al., 2008). Neither diltrazem nor verapamil had such activity. Most of the data are in vitro and with fairly high doses of the CCBs, so their relevance to the antihypertensive effect of CCBs in clinical practice remains uncertain.

Sympathetic Activation

One pharmacologic feature that may explain some of the initial side effects of CCBs and has been incriminated as a possible contributor to adverse cardiovascular effects of short-acting agent is their activation of the sympathetic nervous system (Lindqvist et al., 2007).

Grassi et al. (2003) found marked increases in heart rate, plasma NE, and muscle sympathetic nerve traffic on the first day of intake of two long-acting DHP-CCBs, felodipine and lercanidipine, which lowered BP equally. After 8 weeks of daily therapy, which continued to provide similar BP reductions, the effects on heart rate, plasma NE, and muscle nerve traffic were markedly attenuated.

Duration of Action

One of the major differences between CCBs is their duration of action. As shown in Table 7-7, some of these, such as the formulation of verapamil that affords 24-hour effectiveness, are provided by special delivery

TABLE 7.6	**Cardiovascular Profile of CCBs**			
	Nidefipine	**Amlodipine**	**Diltiazem**	**Verapamil**
Heart rate	↑	↑/0	↓	↓
Sinoatrial node conduction	0	0	↓↓	↓
AV node conduction	0	0	↓	↓
Myocardial contractility	↓/0	↓/0	↓	↓↓
Neurohormonal activation	↑	↑/0	↑	↑
Vascular dilatation	↑↑	↑↑	↑	↑
Coronary flow	↑	↑	↑	↑

↓, decrease; 0, no change; ↑, increase.
Adapted from Eisenberg MJ, Brox A, Bestawros AN. Calcium channel blockers: An update. *Am J Med* 2004;116:35–43.

TABLE 7.7	CCBs Approved for Use in the Treatment of Hypertension in the United States		
Drug	Form and Dose	Time to Peak Effect (h)	Elimination Half-Life (h)
Amlodipine	Tablet; 2.5–10 mg	6–12	30–50
Diltiazem[a]	Immediate-release tablet; dose varies	0.5–1.5	2–5
	Sustained-release tablet; 180–480 mg	6–11	2–5
Felodipine	Sustained-release tablet; 2.5–10 mg	2.5–5	11–16
Isradipine	Tablet; 2.5–10 mg	1.5	8–12
Nicardipine[a]	Immediate-release tablet; 20–40 mg	0.5–2.0	8
	Sustained-release tablet; 60–120 mg	?	8
Nifedipine	Immediate-release capsule; dose varies	0.5	2
	Sustained-release tablet; 30–120 mg	6	7
Nisoldipine	Sustained-release tablet; 20–40 mg	6–12	7–12
Verapamil[a]	Immediate-release tablet; dose varies	0.5–1.0	4.5–12
	Sustained-release tablet; 120–480 mg	4–6	4.5–12

[a]Also available in an intravenous formation, with a time to peak effect ranging from 5 to 15 minutes after administration.

systems; others, such as amlodipine, have intrinsically long durations of action. The slow onset and long duration of action of amlodipine provide continued effects even if daily doses are missed (Elliott et al., 2002).

On the other hand, short-acting agents may induce abrupt falls in BP, which may incite coronary ischemia (Burton & Wilkinson, 2008). Such effects are not seen with long-acting agents, which lower the BP gradually and smoothly (Eisenberg et al., 2004).

Antihypertensive Efficacy

The currently available CCBs seem comparable in their antihypertensive potency. The relative effectiveness in protecting against major cardiovascular events of various types of CCBs—short- and long-acting, DHP and non-DHP—has been tested in 12 randomized controlled trials (RCTs) against three of the other major classes of antihypertensives: diuretics or β-blockers or ACEIs (Eisenberg et al., 2004). As seen in Table 7-8, various types of CCBs have proven to be equally effective as other classes with the exception of short-acting agents, which have been minimally less

effective. However, they have provided *less* protection against heart failure, but *more* protection against stroke than other classes (Angeli et al., 2004).

Determinants of Efficacy
Age

An apparently greater antihypertensive effectiveness of CCBs in the elderly may reflect pharmacokinetic changes that increase the bioavailability of various CCBs, providing more active drug at any given dose than in younger patients (Lernfelt et al., 1998).

Race

In blacks, the response of the BP to monotherapy with CCBs is better than to ACEIs, ARBs, or β-blockers and equal to the response to diuretics (Brewster et al., 2004).

Additive Effect of Diuretic or Low Sodium Intake

Two factors that increase the efficacy of other classes of antihypertensive drugs—dietary sodium reduction and concomitant use of a diuretic—may not add to the efficacy of CCBs.

TABLE 7.8	Major Cardiovascular Events with CCBs Versus Other Antihypertensive Drugs			
		Major Cardiovascular Events[a] **No. Events/No. Patients (%)**		
CCB Formulation	**Number of Trials**	*CCBs*	*Others*	**Relative Risk (95% CI)**
Short-acting	7	1,222/9,351 (13.1)	1,768/11,691 (15.1)	1.09 (1.00–1.18)
Long-acting	5	2,567/31,934 (8.0)	3,546/38,278 (9.3)	1.01 (0.96–1.07)
Non-DHP	4	1,359/25,625 (5.3)	1,365/25,848 (5.3)	1.00 (0.93–1.09)
DHP	8	2,430/15,630 (15.5)	3,949/24,121 (16.4)	1.05 (0.99–1.11)

[a]Major cardiovascular events included myocardial infarction, heart failure, stroke, and cardiovascular mortality, except in ALLHAT, where composite coronary heart disease included death from coronary heart disease, nonfatal myocardial infarction, coronary revascularization procedures, and angina requiring hospitalization, and in INVEST, where the primary outcome was cardiovascular mortality.
Composed from Eisenberg MJ, Brox A, Bestawros AN. Calcium channel blockers: An update. *Am J Med* 2004;116:35–43.

Numerous studies have examined these relationships. In general, the findings support the view that dietary sodium restriction may reduce (but not abolish) the antihypertensive effect of CCBs, whereas high sodium intake may enhance (or not diminish) their efficacy (Luft et al., 1991). The explanation may be simple: CCBs have a mild natriuretic effect (Krekels et al., 1997); this effect would be more obvious in the presence of a higher sodium diet so that the BP would fall more. With a low sodium intake, this natriuretic effect would not be as pronounced, so the BP would diminish less. This explanation fits with the observation that the fall in BP with a CCB is greater in more sodium-sensitive patients (Damasceno et al., 1999).

On the other hand, most well-controlled studies have shown an additional antihypertensive effect when diuretics are combined with CCBs (Stergiou et al., 1997). The combination of a diuretic with a CCB has been shown to provide additive effects equal to those seen when a diuretic is added to a β-blocker (Thulin et al., 1991) or to an ACEI (Elliott et al., 1990).

Renal Effects
The mild natriuretic action of DHP-CCBs likely reflects their unique ability, unlike other vasodilators, to maintain or increase effective renal blood flow, glomerular filtration rate (GFR), and renal vascular resistance, which has been attributed to their selective vasodilative action on the renal afferent arterioles (Delles et al., 2003). On the surface, this preferential vasodilation of afferent arterioles with increases in GFR, renal blood flow, and natriuresis appears to favor the use of CCBs as a way of maintaining good renal function. However, a large body of experimental data suggests that increased renal plasma flow and GFR may accelerate the progression of glomerulosclerosis by increasing intraglomerular pressure (Griffin et al., 1995).

In hypertensive patients with renal damage, as manifested by proteinuria, DHP-CCBs do not reduce proteinuria, whereas verapamil and diltiazem do about as well as ACEIs (Hart & Bakris, 2008). In the African American Study of Kidney Disease and Hypertension, amlodipine did not slow the rate of decline of renal function in hypertensive blacks with renal insufficiency and heavy proteinuria as well as did the ACEI ramipril (Agodoa et al., 2001). Therefore, DHP-CCBs should only be added to an ACEI or ARB if needed to control hypertension in patients with renal insufficiency. On the other hand, as shown in the RENAAL trial, the addition of a DHP-CCB does not diminish the benefits of an ACEI or ARB on the slowing of progression of nephropathy (Bakris et al., 2003).

Other Uses

- Coronary artery disease (Nissen et al., 2004)
- LVH (Klingbeil et al., 2003) (Fig. 7-11)
- Tachyarrhythmias (non-DHP-CCBs) (Abernethy & Schwartz, 1999)
- Hypertrophic cardiomyopathy (Roberts & Sigwart, 2001)
- Aortic regurgitation (Levine & Gaasch, 1996)
- Vasospasm after subarachnoid hemorrhage (nimodipine) (Rinkel & Kliju, 2009)
- Peripheral vascular disease (Baggar et al., 1997)
- Raynaud phenomenon (Wigley et al., 2002)
- Dementia (Forette et al., 2002)

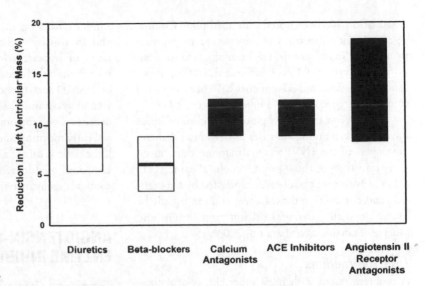

FIGURE 7-11 Change in LV mass index (as percentage from baseline) with antihypertensive treatment by drug class. Mean values and 95% confidence intervals, adjusted for change in diastolic blood pressure and treatment duration, are given. ACE, angiotensin-converting enzyme. (Modified from Klingbeil AU, Schneider M, Martus P, et al. A meta-analysis of the effects of treatment on left ventricular mass in essential hypertension. *Am J Med* 2003;115.41–46.)

Side Effects

Serious consequences of the use of short-acting CCBs were reported in retrospective observational studies. Multiple prospective RCTs comparing CCBs against placebo and other classes of antihypertensive drugs (Table 7-8) clearly show that the observational studies were largely invalid with the possible exception of an increased risk of coronary ischemia with short-acting CCBs (Eisenberg et al., 2004).

More common

Relatively mild but sometimes bothersome side effects will preclude the use of these drugs in perhaps 10% of patients. Most side effects—headaches, flushing, local

ankle edema—are related to the vasodilation for which drugs are given. With slow-release and longer-acting formulations, vasodilative side effects are reduced. The side effects of the three major classes of CCBs differ considerably (Table 7-9). Dependent edema is related to localized vasodilation and not generalized fluid retention and is not prevented or relieved by diuretics (van der Heijden et al., 2004). If the pedal edema is bothersome, either a non-DHP-CCB should be substituted (Weir et al., 2001) or the DHP-CCB combined with an ACEI to reduce the edema (Gradman et al., 1997).

Other Side Effects

Gingival hyperplasia may occur with DHPs (Missouris et al., 2000). Eye pain, possibly due to ocular

TABLE 7.9	Relative Frequency of Side Effects of CCBs		
Effect	**Verapamil**	**Diltiazem**	**Dihydropyridines**
Cardiovascular system			
Hypotension	+	+	++
Flush	+	–	++
Headache	+	+	++
Ankle edema	+	+	++
Palpitation	–	–	+
Conduction disturbances	++	+	–
Bradycardia	++	+	–
Gastrointestinal tract			
Nausea	+	+	+
Constipation	++	(+)	–

+, increase; –, no effect.

vasodilation, has been noted with nifedipine (Coulter, 1988). A wide spectrum of adverse cutaneous reactions, some quite serious, has been reported to occur rarely with various CCBs (Garijo et al., 2005). Impotence seems rare, but 31 patients have been reported to develop gynecomastia (Tanner & Bosco, 1988).

No adverse effects on glucose, insulin, or lipids have been seen and fewer cases of new onset diabetes developed in the INVEST trials among those given verapamil than in those given atenolol (Pepine et al., 2003). Overdoses usually are manifested by hypotension and conduction disturbances and can usually be overcome with parenteral calcium and insulin and glucose (Salhanick & Shannon, 2003).

Drug Interactions

A problem noted with most other classes of antihypertensive drugs—interference from NSAIDs—is usually not seen with CCBs (Celis et al., 2001). Another interaction has been noted with the DHPs felodipine and nifedipine but not with amlodipine (Vincent et al., 2000): an increased plasma level and duration of action when taken along with large amounts of grapefruit juice (Bailey et al., 2000) or Seville orange juice (Malhotra et al., 2001). Most other drug interactions with CCBs are of little consequence (Abernethy & Schwartz, 1999), except the possible major cost savings represented by the lower doses of cyclosporine needed with concomitant CCB therapy (Valantine et al., 1992).

Perspective on Use

CCBs have been found to reduce the risk of coronary disease equally, stroke more, but heart failure less, than other antihypertensive therapies while having similar effects on overall mortality. They work well and are usually well tolerated across the entire spectrum of hypertensives. They have some particular niches: the elderly, coexisting angina, and cyclosporine or NSAID use. If chosen, an inherently long-acting, second-generation DHP seems the best choice, because it will maintain better BP control in the critical early morning hours and on through the next day if the patient misses a daily dose. Rate-slowing CCBs, verapamil or diltiazem, may be preferable with concomitant tachyarrhythmias or heavy proteinuria.

ANGIOTENSIN-CONVERTING ENZYME INHIBITORS

There are four ways to reduce the activity of the renin-angiotensin system in humans (Fig. 7-12). The first way, the use of β-blockers to reduce renin release from the juxtaglomerular (J-G) cells, has been covered. The second way, direct inhibition of the activity of renin, has recently become clinically feasible. The third way is to inhibit the activity of the angiotensin-converting enzyme (ACE), which converts the inactive decapeptide angiotensin I (AI) to the potent hormone angiotensin II (AII); i.e., ACEIs. The fourth way is to use a competitive antagonist that attaches to the AII receptors and blocks the attachment of the native hormone, i.e., angiotensin receptor blockers (ARBs). Multiple ARBs are now available and all remain patent-protected. Nonetheless, their higher cost seems not to have slowed their acceptance.

Multiple studies have documented an equal antihypertensive efficacy between the multiple ACEIs and ARBs now available with no consistent differences in the outcomes associated with their use (Matchar

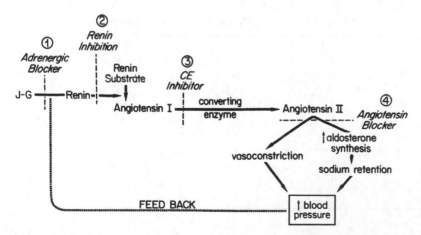

FIGURE 7-12 The renin-angiotensin system and four sites where its activity may be inhibited. CE, converting enzyme; J-G, juxtaglomerular.

et al., 2008). Using data from 26 large-scale trials, the Blood Pressure Trialist (2007) conclude that "there are similar blood pressure-dependent effects of ACEI and ARB for the risks of stroke, CHD, and heart failure. For ACEI, but not for ARB, there is evidence of blood pressure-independent effects [of approximately 9%] on the risk of major coronary disease events." In an even more recent meta-analysis, ACEIs and ARBs were equally protective against MI and mortality, but ARBs had an 8% lower incidence of strokes (Reboldi et al., 2008).

DRIs are likely equivalent to both ACEIs and ARBs, but outcome data remain inadequate to prove this.

As will be noted at the end of this chapter, renin-angiotensin inhibitors have been used in trials of prevention of hypertension.

Before advancing, we will briefly address the relationship of the preexisting level of renin-angiotensin activity and the response to these four classes of drugs that block the system at some site. Laragh (1993) has long supported a clear separation between those drugs that primarily reduce volume, e.g., diuretics, and those drugs that primarily reduce vasoconstriction, e.g., all other classes of antihypertensives, save β-blockers, which reduce renin-angiotensin activity and vasodilate. Most clinical data on responses to various antihypertensive drugs support this separation, but only partially. None have shown a clear connection between renin levels and response to any drug. Nonetheless, as will be described later in this chapter, patients who are younter or nonblack (and tend to have higher levels of renin activity) respond somewhat better to renin-blocking drugs while those who are older or black (and tend to have lower levels of renin activity) respond somewhat better to drugs that do not primarily block renin, i.e., diuretics and CCBs.

However, this clinical separation does not require measurements of renin activity and can be based on the age and race of the patient (Preston et al., 1998). Therefore, whereas broad distinctions are possible, older and black patients may respond well to renin-blocking drugs and their use need not be predicated on their level of renin activity (Canzanello et al., 2008).

This section examines the use of ACEIs. Thereafter, the use of ARBs and DRIs will be described.

Mode of Action

Peptides from the venom of the Brazilian viper *Bothrops jararaca* were discovered to potentiate the effects of bradykinin by inhibiting its degradation (Ferreira, 1965). Soon thereafter, Ng and Vane (1967) recognized that the same enzyme from the carboxypeptidase family could be responsible for both the conversion of AI to AII and the degradation of bradykinin. The nature of this ACE was identified by Erdös and coworkers in 1970 (Yang et al., 1970). Biochemists at the Squibb laboratories fashioned the first inhibitor for the ACE enzyme, teprotide or SQ20881 (Ondetti et al., 1971), which was shown to lower BP when given intravenously (Gavras et al., 1974). The Squibb group then identified the active site on the ACE and developed the first orally effective ACEI, captopril (Ondetti et al., 1977).

Three chemically different classes of ACEIs have been developed, classified by the ligand of the zinc ion of ACE: sulfhydryl, carboxyl, and phosphoryl (Table 7-10). Their different structures influence their tissue distribution and routes of elimination (Brown & Vaughan, 1998), differences that could alter their effects on various organ functions beyond their shared ability to lower the BP by blocking the circulating renin-angiotensin mechanism.

Pharmacokinetics

As seen in Table 7-10, most ACEIs are prodrugs, esters of the active compounds that are more lipid-soluble, so that they are more quickly and completely absorbed. Although there are large differences in bioavailability, these seem to make little difference in their clinical effects. Most ACEIs, except fosinopril and spirapril, are eliminated through the kidneys, having undergone variable degrees of metabolism. Fosinopril has a balanced route of elimination, with increasingly more of the drug removed through the liver as renal function decreases (Hui et al., 1991).

Pharmacodynamics

As seen in Figure 7-12, the most obvious manner by which ACEIs lower the BP is to reduce the circulating levels of AII markedly, thereby removing the direct vasoconstriction induced by this peptide. However, with usual doses of ACEIs, plasma angiotensin II levels begin to "escape" after a few hours, in part because of the release of more renin, freed from its feedback suppression (Azizi & Ménard, 2004).

Although the presence of the complete renin-angiotensin system within various tissues, including vessel walls, heart, and brain, is certain, the role of these tissue renin-angiotensin systems in

TABLE 7.10	Characteristics of ACEIs				
Drug	Zinc Ligand	Prodrug	Rate of Elimination	Duration of Action, h	Dose Range, mg
Benazepril	Carboxyl	Yes	Renal	24	5–40
Captopril	Sulfhydryl	No	Renal	6–12	25–150
Cilazapril	Carboxyl	Yes	Renal	24+	2.5–5.0
Enalapril	Carboxyl	Yes	Renal	18–24	5–40
Fosinopril	Phosphoryl	Yes	Renal-hepatic	24	10–40
Lisinopril	Carboxyl	No	Renal	24	5–40
Moexipril	Carboxyl	Yes	Renal	12–18	7.5–30
Perindopril	Carboxyl	Yes	Renal	24	4–16
Quinapril	Carboxyl	Yes	Renal	24	5–80
Ramipril	Carboxyl	Yes	Renal	24	1.25–20
Spirapril	Carboxyl	Yes	Hepatic	24	12.5–50
Trandolapril	Carboxyl	Yes	Renal	24+	1–8

pathophysiology remains uncertain, as does the contribution of inhibition of tissue ACE to the antihypertensive effects of ACEIs (Re, 2004).

Moreover, nonclassical pathways may be involved in the elaboration of AII, involving either nonrenin effects on angiotensinogen or non-ACE effects on AI (Fig. 7-13). Because ACEIs block only AII production via the classical pathway, there could then be additional effects of both ARBs and DRIs. On the other hand, some of the effects of ACEIs may be mediated via their inhibition of the breakdown of bradykinin (Erdös et al., 1999), with an additional contribution from kinin stimulation of nitric oxide production (Burnier & Brunner, 2000). NSAIDs clearly reduce the antihypertensive effect of ACEIs, likely by inhibiting vasodilatory prostaglandin production (Polónia et al., 1995).

Effect of ACEI

Regardless of the contributions of various other mechanisms beyond the reduction in AII levels, the lower AII levels certainly play a major role. In addition to the relief of vasoconstriction, multiple other effects may contribute to their antihypertensive effect, including these:

- A decrease in aldosterone secretion that may not be persistent (Sato & Saruta, 2003).
- An increase in bradykinin which in turn increases release of tissue plasminogen activator (tPA) (Labinjoh et al., 2001).
- An increase in the activity of the 11β-hydroxysteroid dehydrogenase-2 enzyme, which could increase renal

sodium excretion by protecting the nonselective mineralocorticoid receptor from cortisol (Ricketts & Stewart, 1999).

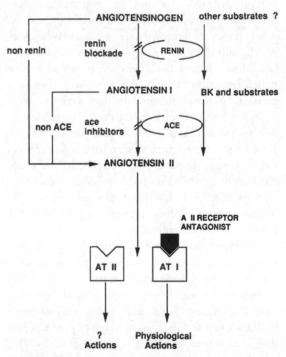

FIGURE 7-13 Theoretic biochemical and physiologic consequences of blocking the renin-angiotensin system at different steps in the pathway. ACE, angiotensin-converting enzyme; AT, angiotensin; BK, bradykinin. (Modified from Johnston CI, Burrell LM. Evolution of blockade of the renin-angiotensin system. *J Hum Hypertens* 1995;9:375–380.)

- Blunting of the expected increase in sympathetic nervous system activity typically seen after vasodilation (Lyons et al., 1997). As a result, heart rate is not increased and cardiac output does not rise, as is seen with direct vasodilators such as hydralazine.
- Suppression of endogenous endothelin secretion (Brunner & Kukovetz, 1996).
- Improvement in endothelial dysfunction (Ghiadoni et al., 2003).
- Reduction in oxidative stress by reducing production of reactive oxygen species (Hamilton et al., 2004) and inflammatory factors (Sattler et al., 2005).
- Stimulation of endothelial progenitor cells (Bahlmann et al., 2005).

As a consequence of these multiple effects, ACEI results in a dampening of arterial wave reflections and increased aortic distensibility that provide a greater fall in central aortic pressure (Morgan et al., 2004). These hemodynamic improvements contribute to the reversal of hypertrophy both in the heart and vasculature. As will be noted, ACEIs lower the BP in a manner that tends to protect the function of two vital organs—heart and the kidneys. In addition, ACEIs may reduce the incidence of new-onset diabetes via multiple mechanisms (Jandeleit-Dahm, 2005). However, in the largest trial to closely examine this effect, the ACEI ramipril did not reduce the incidence of diabetes (Dream Trial Investigators, 2006).

ACEIs are also venodilators (Zarnke & Feldman, 1996), which may be responsible for their ability to reduce the accumulation of ankle edema seen with CCBs when the two agents are combined (Gradman et al., 1997).

Monotherapy
An immediate fall in BP occurs in approximately 70% of patients given captopril, and the decrease is sometimes rather precipitous (Postma et al., 1992). Such a dramatic fall is more likely in those with high renin levels. Black or elderly hypertensives, with lower renin levels as a group, respond less well to ACEIs than do white or younger patients (Brewster et al., 2004).

As expected, patients with high-renin hypertension from renal artery stenosis may respond particularly well to ACEIs, but the removal of AII's support of perfusion to the ischemic kidney may precipitously reduce renal function, particularly in those with bilateral stenoses (see Chapter 10). If such patients are excluded, ACEIs are usually effective and well tolerated in patients with renal insufficiency. An initial decline of 25% to 30% in renal function after starting ACEI therapy in patients with mild to moderate renal insufficiency was found to be associated with a *better* long-term renoprotection (Apperloo et al., 1997), presumably reflecting a beneficial dilation of efferent arterioles which reduces intraglomerular pressure and filtration (Bakris & Weir, 2000).

Combination Therapy
The addition of a diuretic, even in as low a dose as 6.25 mg HCTZ, will enhance the efficacy of an ACEI (Cheng & Frishman, 1998), normalizing the BP of another 20% to 25% of patients with mild to moderate hypertension more effectively than would raising the dose of the ACEI (Townsend & Holland, 1990). The marked additive effect of a diuretic likely reflects the ACEI blunting of the reactive rise of AII that usually occurs with diuretic use and that opposes the antihypertensive effect of the diuretic. The combination of an ACEI and a CCB provided greater benefit than seen with an ACEI plus diuretic (Jamerson et al., 2008). The combination of an ACEI and an ARB has been increasingly used to presumably reduce proteinuria to a greater degree than seen with either agent alone (Kunz et al., 2008) but the combination was associated with more hypotension and renal insufficiency in the ONTARGET trial (ONTARGET Investigators, 2008) and adverse effects in patients with heart failure (Phillips et al., 2007), so the practice will likely be curtailed.

Effectiveness in Reducing Morbidity and Mortality
In their analysis, including all large trials completed by the end of 2004, the Blood Pressure Lowering Treatment Trialists Collaboration (2007) found that treatment with ACEI-based regimens provided a 19% reduction in stroke risk, a 16% reduction in CHD risk, and a 27% reduction in CHF risk for each 5 mm Hg reduction in BP. Moreover, ACEI-based therapy provided an additional 9% reduction in CHD risk at zero BP reduction, i.e., an independent effect that was not seen with ARB-based therapy.

When compared against diuretic/β-blocker-based therapy, ACEI-based therapy provided equal protection against stroke, CHD, and CHF. When compared against CCB-based therapy, ACEI-therapy was 10% better for CHF risk, suggesting "a BP-independent adverse effect of CCBs, rather than a BP-independent protective effect of ACEI" (Blood Pressure Trialist, 2007).

Other Uses

Heart Diseases

With these impressive results of ACEI-based therapy, an ACEI is now widely accepted as indicated for patients with CHD, post-MI or CHF.

The first large trial that documented the benefit of an ACEI in patients with known coronary disease, the HOPE Trial (Heart Outcomes, 2000), used ramipril as the ACEI. In a follow-up of 43,316 patient treated with an ACEI for heart failure, mortality was the same with all except captopril and enalapril which were associated with a 10% to 15% *higher* mortality (Pilote et al., 2008).

With the excellent results of the HOPE Trial in mind, the same protocol was expanded to compare ramipril against an ARB, telmisartan, and the combination of the ACEI + ARB (ONTARGET Investigators, 2008). The effects of the individual drugs were virtually identical, whereas the combination was no better and caused more adverse renal effects.

For treatment of CHF, an ACEI, usually a shorter-acting one such as captopril, is started in a low dose to minimize hypotension and azotemia. If tolerated, the dose is gradually increased to a full dose of a once-daily ACEI.

Cerebrovascular Diseases

As noted by the Blood Pressure Trialist (2007), ACEI-based therapy has been effective for primary stroke prevention. There is, however, controversy that ARBs may be better. This will be covered in the next section on ARBs.

The PROGRESS trial (PROGRESS Collaborative Group, 2001) tested the efficacy of the ACEI perindopril for secondary stroke prevention, i.e., in patients who had survived a stroke. By itself, the ACEI had no benefit, but when a diuretic, indapamide, was added, the BP fell further and excellent protection, a 43% relative risk reduction, was noted.

Renal Diseases

Renin-angiotensin inhibitors preferentially dilate the renal efferent arteriole, reducing intraglomerular pressure and restraining glomerulosclerosis, podocyte damage, and proteinuria (Lassila et al., 2004). The clinical consequences of the use of ACEIs in patients with kidney diseases have been examined using four end points:

• The incidence of proteinuria in diabetic patients has been reduced by 40% (Strippoli et al., 2006),

most impressively in a study of 1,204 type 2 diabetes free of proteinuria who took one of four regimens for 3 or more years (Remuzzi et al., 2006). The incidence of microalbuminuria was reduced from 10% with placebo to 6% with the ACEI trandolapril alone or in combination with the non-DHP-CCB verapamil, whereas those on the CCB alone had an 11.1% incidence.

• Reduction of existing proteinuria has been documented both in diabetics and in nondiabetics (Kunz et al., 2008).

• Slowing of the progress of renal damage has been noted both in diabetic (Sarafidis et al., 2008) and nondiabetic (Kent et al., 2007) nephropathies. However, no benefit has been reported in nondiabetic nephropathy with proteinuria less than 500 mg per day (Kent et al., 2007) nor in normoalbuminuria type 1 diabetics (Mauer et al., 2009).

• Overall mortality has not been reduced in 20 trials of patients with diabetic nephropathy despite a significant reduction in the incidence of ESRD.

Despite the absence of survival benefit, these data have been used to support, almost to demand, the use of an ACEI (or an ARB) in those prone to develop nephropathy, i.e., diabetics, and in those who have proteinuria alone or in concert with reduced renal function, in particular to reduce proteinuria (Berl, 2008).

However, two issues have been raised which may dampen the overall enthusiasm for use of ACEIs in patients with chronic kidney disease (CKD). The first is the argument that most, if not all, of the renoprotective effects of ACEIs are provided not by their special properties but by their lowering of BP (Casas et al., 2005; Griffin & Bidani, 2006).

The second issue is more alarming: two reports suggesting that the use of ACEIs may be responsible for progressive renal failure. The first involved five patients, of whom four were diabetic, with progressive worsening of renal function while on an ACEI (in four) or ARB (in one) and with prompt improvement in renal function when the ACEI or ARB was stopped (Onuigbo & Onuigbo, 2005). The second report is even more incriminating, but retrospective. Suissa et al. (2006) performed a nested case-control analysis comparing 102 diabetic patients who entered ESRD after having been on antihypertensive therapy for an average of 7.8 years, against 4,129 cohort members who could be matched to the ESRD patients by age, type, duration, and form of therapy for diabetes. They found the adjusted rate of ESRD associated with use of ACEIs to be 2.5 relative to thiazide use, whereas it was below 1.0 for those on β-blockers or CCBs. The rate of ESRD associated with ACEIs rose after 3 years of therapy to 4.2 relative to thiazide use.

These reports are obviously of concern. Adding to this concern is the recognition that ACEI therapy given to 608 African Americans with hypertensive renal disease failed to prevent the progression of their CKD, with a 10-year cumulative incidence of 54% of the outcomes of doubling of serum creatinine progression to ESRD, or death (Appel et al., 2008)

Worriesome as the concerns may be, the guidelines of expert groups recommend the use of ACEIs and ARBs for both prevention and relief of progressive kidney disease (American Diabetes Association, 2008; Crowe et al., 2008; KDOQI, 2007).

Other Uses

ACEI therapy is associated with a reduced risk of rupture of abdominal aortic aneurysms, an effect not seen in patients taking diuretics, β-blockers, α-blockers, CCBs, or ARBs (Hackam et al., 2006).

ACEIs have been found to ameliorate altitude polycythemia (Plata et al., 2002), diminish hypertriglyceridemia in nephrotic patients (Ruggenenti et al., 2003), and ameliorate migraine (Schrader et al., 2001).

All of this good is only partly countered by an increased sensitivity to pain (Guasti et al., 2002).

Side Effects

The recognized side effects of ACEIs can be divided into three types: (a) those anticipated from their specific pharmacologic actions, (b) those probably related to their chemical structure, and (c) nonspecific effects, as seen with any drug that lowers the BP.

Effects Anticipated from Pharmacologic Actions
First-Dose Hypotension

An immediate fall in mean arterial BP of more than 30% was seen in 3.3% of 240 hypertensive patients given 25 mg captopril (Postma et al., 1992). The likelihood of such an abrupt fall is less with other ACEIs which are prodrugs and have a slower onset of action (Table 7-10).

Hyperkalemia

Hyperkalemia occurs in about 10% of patients taking an ACEI (Palmer, 2004). The reasons are multiple (Table 7-11), mostly reflecting diminished renal perfusion, decreased aldosterone, and reduced renal tubular function (Palmer, 2004). If recognized, the problem can usually be managed by deleting drugs

TABLE 7.11	**Risk Factors for Hyperkalemia with the Use of Drugs that Interfere with the Renin-Angiotensin-Aldosterone System**

CKD, particularly with GFR < 30
Bilateral renal artery stenosis
DM
Volume depletion
Advanced age
Drugs used concomitantly that interfere in renal potassium excretion
    Nonsteroidal anti-inflammatory drugs
    β-blockers
    Calcineurin inhibitors: cyclosporine, tacrolimus
    Heparin
    Ketoconazole
    Potassium-sparing diuretics: spironolactone, eplerenone, amiloride, triamterine
    Trimethoprim
    Pentamidine
Potassium supplements, including salt substitutes and certain herbs

Modified from Palmer BF. Managing hyperkalemia caused by inhibitors of the renin-angiotensin-aldosterone system. *N Engl J Med* 2004;351:585–592.

that further increase potassium load or interfere with its excretion.

Hypoglycemia

Perhaps as a reflection of increased insulin sensitivity, ACEI use has been accompanied by hypoglycemia both in insulin-dependent and non–insulin-dependent diabetics (Herings et al., 1995).

Interference with Erythropoietin

Angiotensin II enhances erythrocytosis and ACEIs may interefere with the action of erythropoieten in correcting the anemia of CKD patients but also to reduce secondary erythrocytosis as after transplantation (Fakhouri et al., 2004).

Deterioration of Renal Function

Most reports of acute loss of renal function involve preexisting renal hypoperfusion: patients with CHF, volume depletion, or renal artery stenoses, either bilaterally or to a solitary kidney. Rarely, acute renal failure may occur, usually associated with vomiting- and/or diarrhea-induced marked volume depletion (Stirling et al., 2003). However, acute increases of serum creatinine of up to 30% that stabilize within the first 2 months of ACEI therapy are associated with *better* long-term renoprotection (Bakris & Weir, 2000), and so such rises need not lead to withdrawal of ACEI therapy.

Pregnancy

ACEIs are contraindicated during pregnancy, including the first trimester, because they cause fetal injury and death (Cooper et al., 2006).

Cough and Bronchospasm

A dry, hacking, nonproductive, and sometimes intolerable cough is the most frequent side effect of ACEI therapy; bronchospasm may be the second most frequent. In a controlled cohort study of 1,013 patients on an ACEI and 1,017 on lipid-lowering drugs, cough developed in 12.3% and bronchospasm in 5.5% of patients on an ACEI versus 2.7% and 2.3%, respectively, in those on the lipid-lowering drugs (Wood, 1995).

Either problem may begin soon after the start of therapy but, in Wood's (1995) study, bronchospasm was not usually associated with cough. An increase in bradykinin has been assumed to be the mechanism for the cough (Yeo et al., 1995), and a genetic polymorphism of the bradykinin β_2-receptor has been found in a higher proportion of patients who have an ACEI-related cough (Mukae et al., 2000).

Cough is more common in older patients, women, and blacks (Morimoto et al., 2004) and was reported in almost half of Chinese patients (Woo & Nicholls, 1995). It usually goes away in a few weeks after the drug is withdrawn and usually recurs with reexposure to an ACEI. The easiest way to resolve the problem is to replace the ACEI with an ARB.

Angioedema

Angioedema occurs in 0.2% of patients given an ACEI, usually within days but sometimes after prolonged use (Miller et al., 2008). The rate is fourfold higher in blacks, and 5-fold higher in patients taking glitin drug (Brown et al., 2009) 50% higher in women. Fatal airway obstruction has been reported, so that it is mandatory that patients with angioedema on an ACEI never be given an ACEI again. Switching to an ARB should be done very cautiously if at all (Sica & Black, 2002). Two patients with localized penile angioedema have been reported (McCabe et al., 2008).

Effects Related to Chemical Structure

Effects related to chemical structure may be more common with captopril than with the nonsulfhydryl ACEIs. These include loss of taste (Doty et al., 2008), a maculopapular rash and very rarely serious skin reactions, and leukopenia. Most patients who experience one of these reactions while on captopril can be safely crossed over to another ACEI (Jackson et al., 1988).

Nonspecific Side Effects

ACE activity is present in intestinal brush border, and adverse GI effects have been reported with ACEI use (Jacobs et al., 1994). Other rare effects include pancreatitis (Roush et al., 1991) and cholestatic jaundice (Nissan et al., 1996).

ACEIs that cross the blood-brain brarrier slow decline of congnitive function; those that do not (benazapril, enalapril, moexipril, quinapril) may has ten decline (Sink et al., 2009). ACEIs are "lipid-neutral" (Kasiske et al., 1995). Headache, dizziness, fatigue, diarrhea, and nausea are listed in reviews but are seldom problems. Sudden withdrawal does not usually lead to a rebound. Overdose causes hypotension that should be easily managed with fluids and, if needed, dopamine (Lip & Ferner, 1995).

Perspective on Use

Captopril, when first introduced for use in severe hypertensives and in high doses, earned a bad reputation that was quickly overcome. As appropriately lower doses were used and found to be as effective as other drugs, often with fewer side effects, captopril and then enalapril became increasingly popular. Over the last few years, many more ACEIs have been marketed, most with the added advantage of longer duration of action, allowing for once-daily dosing.

As ACEIs have been used in various situations, three places have been recognized wherein they provide special benefits beyond those provided by other agents: relief of acute and chronic heart failure, prevention of remodeling and progressive ventricular dysfunction after MI, and slowing of glomerular sclerosis in diabetic and other nephropathies. Even as ACEIs became increasingly popular, their popularity was threatened by the introduction of ARBs, agents that act at a more distal site of the renin-angiotensin system (Fig. 7-13). The encroachment of ARBs would have been even greater but for the increasing cost differential between ACEIs as they became generic while almost all ARBs remained patent-protected.

ANGIOTENSIN II RECEPTOR BLOCKERS

Even before ACEIs were available, a peptidic antagonist of AII receptors, saralasin, was shown to lower BP. However, its use was limited by the need for intravenous administration and its pressor effect in low-renin patients resulting from its partial agonist effects. Subsequently, the AII receptor was found to have at least two major subtypes, with the type 1 (AT_1) receptor mediating most of the physiologic roles of AII. The signaling mechanisms and functions of these receptor subtypes are different, and they may exert opposite effects on cell growth and BP regulation (Nickenig, 2004) (Fig. 7-14). Agents that selectively block the AT_1 receptor have been synthesized and marketed for the treatment of hypertension. Losartan was the first, and now six more have been approved for use in the United States (Table 7-12).

Mode of Action

ARBs displace AII from its specific AT_1 receptor, antagonizing all of its known effects and resulting in a dose-dependent fall in peripheral resistance and little change in heart rate or cardiac output (Burnier, 2001). As a consequence of the competitive displacement, circulating levels of AII increase while at the same time the blockade of the renin-angiotensin mechanism is more complete, including any AII that

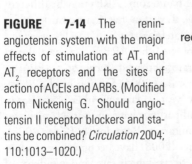

FIGURE 7-14 The renin-angiotensin system with the major effects of stimulation at AT_1 and AT_2 receptors and the sites of action of ACEIs and ARBs. (Modified from Nickenig G. Should angiotensin II receptor blockers and statins be combined? *Circulation* 2004; 110:1013–1020.)

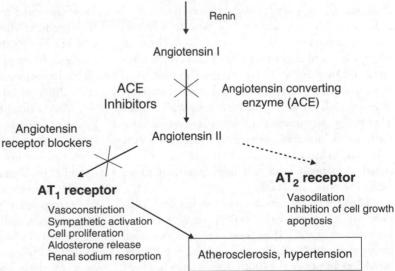

TABLE 7.12	Angiotensin II Receptor Blockers			
Drug	**Trade Name**	**Half-Life (h)**	**Active metabolite**	**Daily Dosage (mg)**
Candesartan	Atacand (Astra)	3–11	Yes	8–32 in 1 dose
Eprosartan	Tevetan (Smith Kline)	5–7	No	400–800 in 1–2 doses
Irbesartan	Avapro (BMS, Sanofi)	11–15	No	150–300 in 1 dose
Losartan	Cozaar (Merck)	2 (6–9)	Yes	50–100 in 1–2 doses
Olmesartan	Benicar (Sankyo)	13	Yes	20–40 in 1 dose
Telmisartan	Micardis (BI)	24	No	40–80 in 1 dose
Valsartan	Diovan (Novartis)	9	No	80–320 in 1 dose

is generated through pathways that do not involve the ACE (Fig. 7-13). No obvious good or bad effects of the increased AII levels have been proven but, in experimental animals, chronic stimulation of AT_2 receptors exerts a hypertrophic and antiangiogenic influence that, if seen in humans, could lead to cardiac hypertrophy, vascular fibrosis, and a decrease in neovascularization in hypoxic tissues (Levy, 2004). On the other hand, chronic stimulation of AT_2 receptors has been found in experimental models to provide neuroprotection (Thöne-Reineke et al., 2004), an issue which will receive attention later in this section.

Differences Between ARBs and ACEIs

Since their introduction, the major obvious difference between ARBs and ACEIs has been thought to be the absence of an increase in kinin levels with the ARB, increases that may be responsible for some of the beneficial effects of ACEIs and likely even more of their side effects, such as cough. However, Campbell et al. (2005) have found twofold increases in blood levels of bradykinin after 4 weeks use of losartan 50 mg a day and slightly smaller increases with eprosartan 600 mg a day. These increases are similar to those seen with ACEIs but they did not find increases in blood kallidin levels which are seen with ACEIs. They believe the absence of this rise is responsible for the lesser incidence of angioedema with ARBs. In the TRANSEND trial, the ARB telmisartan was well tolerated in patients who had been intolerant to an ACEI (Telmisartan, 2008).

Direct comparisons between ACEIs and ARBs show little difference in antihypertensive efficacy (Matchar et al., 2008) or long-term renoprotection (Kunz et al., 2008). Although cough is not provoked by ARBs (Tanser et al., 2000), angioedema has been seen (Sica & Black, 2002) and ageusia reported with losartan (Doty et al., 2008). The ARBs valsartan

(Fogari et al., 2004) and candesartan (Saxby et al., 2008) improved some cognitive functions in elderly hypertensives.

As seen with ACEIs, ARBs have been found to improve endothelial dysfunction and correct the altered structure of resistance arteries in patients with hypertension (Smith et al., 2008). Major anti-inflammatory effects of various ARBs have been reported in experimental models (Ando et al., 2004), human cells (Dandona et al., 2003), and hypertensive patients (Koh et al., 2003). These effects include suppression of reactive oxygen species and a variety of inflammatory cytokines (Fliser et al., 2004). These effects have been translated into attenuation of nitrate tolerance (Hirai et al., 2003) and stabilization of atherosclerotic plaques (Cipollone et al., 2004).

Differences Between ARBs

To gain position in a crowded market of ARBs (and ACEIs), pharmaceutical marketers have expended a lot of effort and money to provide a special niche for their product. Most of these studies show little difference in efficacy with comparable doses but a definitely longer duration of action for those with a longer half-life: telmisartan acts longer than losartan (Neutel et al., 2005) or valsartan (White et al., 2004).

On the other hand, some ARBs may be different in other respects. Losartan has a uricosuric effect (Dang et al., 2006); telmisartan and, to a lesser extent, irbesartan but not the other ARBs act as partial peroxisome proliferator-activated receptor-γ (PPARγ) agonists (Benson et al., 2004; Schupp et al., 2004). Over the past few years, a large number of studies in cells, animals, and patients have supported "pleiotropic" effects of telmisartan (Benndorf & Böger, 2008). Kurtz and Pravenec (2008) have been persistent advocates of these effects which are independent of blockade of the angiotensin receptor. However, telmisartan was no more effective in preventing new-onset diabetes than the ACEI ramipril in the ONTARGET trial (ONTARGET Investigators, 2008), so proof of special benefits of telmisartan beyond its long duration of action remains elusive.

Antihypertensive Efficacy

In the recommended doses (Table 7-12), all seven currently available ARBs have comparable antihypertensive efficacy and all are potentiated by addition of a diuretic (Conlin et al., 2000). The dose-response curve is fairly flat for all, although increasing doses of valsartan provide greater reductions in albuminuria (Hollenberg et al., 2007).

As noted, a single daily dose of 50 mg losartan does not provide as complete 24-hour efficacy as do single daily doses of the other ARBs (Xi et al., 2008). However, either the 100-mg dose or the combination of losartan with HCTZ may provide full 24-hour efficacy (Weber et al., 1995). In an analysis of 36 publications wherein 24 hour ABPM was performed, most of the ARBs were found to maintain good antihypertensive efficacy at the end of the 24-hour interval (Fabia et al., 2007).

ARBs may be combined with other agents for additive effects. Multiple studies have shown additive effects when submaximal doses of an ARB are added to submaximal doses of an ACEI but the only convincing evidence now available for additive effects of presumably maximal doses of an ARB and an ACEI is in reduction of proteinuria (Kunz et al., 2008). However, in the ONTARGET trial, the combination was associated with more renal dysfunction than seen with the individual drugs (Mann et al., 2008).

Other Uses

Renal Diseases

ARBs have been shown to be renoprotective in three placebo-controlled trials in type II diabetics with nephropathy (Brenner et al., 2001; Lewis et al., 2001; Parving et al., 2001), two using irbesartan, the third losartan, all three showing 20% to 30% reductions in progression of renal damage. However, ARBs did not reduce mortality in those trials, a problem also noted with the use of ACEIs in patients with diabetic nephropathy (Sarafidis et al., 2008).

Cerebrovascular Disease

As previously noted, numerous trials have shown protective effects of ARBs on stroke, CHD, and heart failure, all appearing to be mostly dependent on BP lowering (Blood PressureTrialists, 2007). However,

controversy has arisen on the relative benefits of ARBs versus ACEIs and other drugs in the prevention of stroke.

The issue of stroke points to an advantage of ARBs over other drugs, in particular ACEIs (Reboldi et al., 2008). What has become known as the Fournier hypothesis was presaged by Brown and Brown (1986), who postulated that "angiotensin II could protect against stroke by causing vasoconstriction of the proximal cerebral arteries, thereby preventing Charcot-Bouchard aneurysms from rupturing." This 1986 hypotheses preceded the identification of two major angiotensin II receptors, AT_1 and AT_2, both restrained by ACEIs which lower circulating angiotensin II, whereas only the AT_1 receptor is blocked by the ARBs, leaving the AT_2 receptor even more stimulated by higher levels of circulating angiotensin II. Whereas stimulation of AT_1 receptors evokes vasoconstriction and vascular damage, stimulation of AT_2 receptors, at least experimentally, evokes a number of helpful effects including vasodilation, anti-inflammation, and regeneration of neuronal tissues (Thöne-Reineke et al., 2004).

Fournier et al. (2004) evaluated the reduction of strokes reported in 11 RCTs and found that drugs which activate the AT_2 receptors, i.e., diuretics, CCBs, and ARBs, were consistently more effective in reducing strokes than drugs which did not activate AT_2 receptors, i.e., β-blockers and ACEIs, despite equal falls in systemic BP with all drugs. Animal experimentation supports neuroprotection by ARBs (Anderson, 2008; Faure et al., 2008). Further clinical support comes from a meta-analysis of 26 RCTs including over 200,000 patients in whom a total of 7,108 strokes occurred (Boutite et al., 2007). In keeping with the hypothesis, stroke risk was reduced by only 13% with AII-decreasing drugs (that do not stimulate the AT_2 receptor), but by 33% with AII-increasing drugs (which stimulate the AT_2 receptor).

All of this looks clear: ARBs seem to be neuroprotective. However, a prospective RCT involving 20,332 stroke survivors, the PROFESS (Prevention Regimen for Effectively Avoiding Second Strokes) trial, reported that 8.7% of patients on the ARB telmisartan had a second stroke compared to 9.2% on placebo, a statistically insignificant ($p = 0.23$) difference (Yusuf et al., 2008).

The issue remains unsettled. ARBs have not been as effective for primary prevention of stroke as the CCB amlodipine (Wang et al., 2007a), though CCBs are also included as AT_2 stimulating drugs by Boutite et al. (2007). Moreover, in the ONTARGET trial, the ACEI ramipril was equally stroke-protective as the ARB telmisartan (ONTARGET Investigators, 2008). We are left with a plausible hypothesis, supported by both experimental and some clinical data. However the hypothesis needs further clinical proof.

Cardiac Diseases

In their 2007 meta-analysis, the Blood Pressure Trialists reported that ARB-based therapy reduced coronary events and heart failure in accordance with its BP lowering effects, whereas ACEIs also had an additional 9% reduction that was BP independent. Of the trials, LIFE has been extensively reported in multiple publications of subgroup analyses as evidence that the ARB losartan was better than the β-blocker atenolol among hypertensives with LVH in multiple ways including regression of LVH, cardiovascular morbidity and mortality (Dahlöf et al., 2002). It should be noted that atenolol is a less effective drug and therefore a good one to compare against (Carlberg et al., 2004), that almost 80% of patients who remained on therapy in the LIFE trial were also taking a diuretic and that 25% of patients were off the study drugs by the end of the study.

ARBs have been extensively studied in patients with chronic heart failure or post-MI and found to be equally effective as ACEIs (Lee et al., 2004). However, in an RCT of 341 patients with diastolic dysfunction, valsartan was not significantly better than placebo in improving diastolic function (Solomon et al., 2007).

A reduced incidence of atrial fibrillation (AF) with ARB-based therapy was claimed (Aksnes et al., 2007a) but not seen in a large RCT with Valsartan (G1551-AF, 2009). In a small cohort study of 18 patients with Marfan syndrome, ARB therapy significantly slowed the rate of progression of aortic-root dilation (Brooke et al., 2008).

Side Effects

In virtually every trial of ARBs given to hypertensive patients, they have been better tolerated than other classes of antihypertensives, usually causing no more symptoms than placebo with no increase in cough as seen with ACEIs although angioedema may still occur (Mancia et al., 2003). Such tolerability is likely responsible for the higher maintenance of therapy with ARBs than with other antihypertensives (Conlin et al., 2001).

ARBs, like ACEIs, are contraindicated in pregnancy (Chen et al., 2004). The rare occurrence of a rash and even rarer acute nephritis with candesartan

have been reported from Australia (Morton et al., 2004).

Perspective on Use

ARBs have rapidly taken their place as excellent drugs for the treatment of hypertension, proteinuric renal diseases, and heart failure, in general equal to but no better than the effects of ACEIs except for the potential for better neuroprotection. Their major current advantage is their better tolerability over other classes, in particular the absence of the cough seen in about 10% of ACEI users.

Since generic ACEIs are less expensive than patent-protected ARBs, the argument can be made to use ACEIs and switch to an ARB if a cough develops, or the patient is taking a glitin (Brown et al., 2009).

The combination of an ACEI and an ARB has been quickly adopted by nephrologists for use in proteinuric patients. The combination has not proven to be better in patients with hypertension or heart failure and may lead to more renal dysfunction.

Meanwhile, as always seems to happen in clinical medicine, something even better may now be available.

DIRECT RENIN INHIBITORS

A DRI, aliskerin (Texturna) has been approved for treatment of hypertension. Despite its limited absorption and bioavailability (3%), aliskerin works because of its high aqueous solubility, high specificity for the enzymatically active site of human renin, and long half-life (40 hours), and because it is minimally metabolized (Brown, 2008; Luft & Weinberger, 2008; Shafiq et al., 2008). Aliskerin binds to intracellularly stored renin, thereby inhibiting renin's activity before its secretion (Krop et al., 2008).

Now that aliskerin has been marketed, other orally effective DRIs are sure to follow.

Mechanism of Action

As detailed in Chapter 3, the renal J-G apparatus secretes prorenin which is enzymatically converted to the active renin, largely in the kidney. Renin cleaves the ten amino acid angiotensin I from the protein substrate angiotensinogen. Aliskerin blocks renin's catalytic site, reducing the formation of angiotensin I and its generation of angiotensin II, resulting in a fall of BP. The lower levels of angiotensin I and II remove the normal inhibition of prorenin secretion from the J-G apparatus so that levels of prorenin and renin are markedly increased. According to conventional wisdom, as long as aliskerin blocks the catalytic action of prorenin and renin, the BP will fall.

How ever, prorenin is now recognized to attach to its own receptor in various tissues where it exerts profibrotic effects, without interference from aliskerin (Feldt et al., 2008; Schefe et al., 2008). Therefore the eventual benefits and potential dangers of a DRI remain uncertain. Sealey and Laragh (2007) have argued that the reactive renin secretion may limit the antihypertensive effects of aliskerin particularly in patients who start with low levels of renin activity. Whether or not there are hazards from prorenin acting on its own receptor without interference from aliskerin will hopefully be fully understood in the near future.

Antihypertensive Efficacy

Aliskerin lowers BP (Jordan et al., 2007; Oh et al., 2007). Moreover, its combination with ARBs appears to provide additional antihypertensive effect and end-organ protection. The rationale for the combination is the potential of nonrenin enzymes, e.g., cathepsin D and chymase to generate AI and AII which will not be inhibited by DRIs.

In the first published large trial, aliskerin was combined wth the ARB valsartan in 1797 hypertensive patients (Oparil et al., 2007). The combination lowered mean sitting diastolic BP by 12.2 mm Hg, significantly more than with aliskerin (–9.0 mm Hg), valsartan (–9.7 mm Hg), or placebo (–4.1 mm Hg). There was at least a transient increase of serum potassium to above 5.5 mmol/L in 4% of the combination treated.

Renoprotective Effect

The combination of aliskerin with the ARB losartan was examined in a RCT of 599 patients with hypertension and type 2 diabetic nephropathy (Parving et al., 2008). The patients already had good BP control with other classes of drugs, and the combination of aliskerin plus losartan lowered BP by only 2/1 mm Hg. At the end of the 24th week, mean urinary albumin excretion had fallen from the baseline level of 495 µg/minute by 18% in those on aliskerin versus a slight rise in the placebo group. A reduction of 50% or more in albuminuria occurred in 25% of those on aliskerin versus 12% of those on placebo. Transient hyper-

kalemia of 6.0 mmol/L or higher was seen in 4.7% of the aliskerin group and 1.7% of the placebo group.

Parving et al. (2008) concluded that "Aliskerin may have renoprotective effects that are independent of its blood pressure-lowering effect in patients with hypertension, type 2 diabetes, and nephropathy, who are receiving the recommended renoprotective treatment." More data are needed to know if a DRI is more renoprotective than an ACEI or ARB.

It should be noted that diabetics have high levels of prorenin, as observed by Luetscher et al. (1985). Experimental data support a role of prorenin in the pathogenisis of both diabetic nephropathy and retinopathy (Satofuka et al., 2006; Takahashi et al., 2007), so there may be a particular advantage for DRIs in the treatment of diabetic patients.

Adverse Effects

Save for transient (and not unexpected) rises in serum potassium, aliskerin has been as benign as ARBs. However, as Brown (2008) noted: "It appears to be safe, but this statement is made with the obvious qualification for any novel drug or class that rare, or long-term, adverse events may take time to become apparent."

As with ACEIs and ARBs, DRIs are contraindicated during pregnancy.

Place in Therapy of Hypertension

There is great enthusiasm over aliskerin, the only new antihypertensive agent introduced in over a decade. But the enthusiasm remains cautious. In the words of two (old) wise hypertensive experts, "No new class of antihypertensive agents should make it to routine use without hard outcome data. That necessity applies even more to dual inhibition of the renin system, which exposes patients to hyperkalemia and renal insufficiency" (Birkenhäger & Staessen, 2007).

Time will tell, but for now, more caution and less enthusiasm may be appropriate.

DRUGS UNDER INVESTIGATION

Angiotensin II Immunization

In a Phase IIa RCT, 72 hypertensives were given either one or two doses of a vaccine based on a virus-like particle that targets angiotensin II or a placebo (Tissot et al., 2008). The larger dose reduced the early morning BP surge compared to placebo by 25/13 mm

Hg and, at week 14, the mean ABPM daytime BP was reduced by 9/4 mm Hg.

Vasopeptidase Inhibitors

Vasopeptidase inhibitors are single molecules that simultaneously inhibit the ACE and the neutral endopeptidase (NEP) enzymes, which normally degrade a number of endogenous natriuretic peptides so that decreases in AII and increases in bradykinin are combined with increases in natriuretic peptides (Burnett, 1999). The most widely studied of these agents was omapatrilat (Vanlev) (Kostis et al., 2004).

The obvious attraction of the combined ACE and NEP inhibitors is the ability to have effects on both high and low renin states while providing a natriuresis without activating the renin system as do traditional diuretics. Unfortunately, the high levels of bradykinin induced by these agents presumably led to a disturbing incidence of severe angioedema, so that the approval of omapatrilat was rejected in 2002 (Pickering, 2002).

Endothelin Antagonists

As noted in Chapter 3, endothelin may have a role in the pathogenesis of hypertension. Drugs to block one or both endothelin receptors, ET_A and ET_B, have been developed and one, bosentan, has been approved for treatment of pulmonary hypertension.

Darusentan (Enseleit et al., 2008) and atrasentan (Raichlin et al., 2008) have been used to treat systemic hypertension. They work, but with so many side effects, including facial edema in as many as 50%, it seems unlikely that one will be developed for clinical use (Sica, 2008a).

Possible Drugs for the Far Future

- Agents that reduce uric acid levels (Feig et al., 2008a)
- Tetrahydrodiopterin, a cofactor for the nitric oxide synthase enzyme (Porkert et al., 2008)
- Stimulants of calcitonin gene-related peptide synthesis (Deng et al., 2004)
- Inhibitors of endogenous cannabinoid breakdown (Batkai et al., 2004)
- Aminopeptidase A inhibitors of the brain renin-angiotensin system (Bodineau et al., 2008)
- Activators of ACE 2 (Hernández Prada et al., 2008)
- Inhibitors of aldosterone synthase (Mulder et al., 2008)
- Gene therapy (Rubattu et al., 2008)

Conclusion

A number of different drugs are under investigation. Time—and, in the United States, the U.S. Food and Drug Administration (FDA)—will tell which of them will be available for clinical use. More drugs will be available, probably in rate-controlled forms, so that a single capsule or a patch may provide smooth control over many days. In the meantime, proper use of what is available will control BP in virtually every hypertensive patient and whether new drugs will necessarily improve our ability to do so is questionable.

GENERAL GUIDELINES FOR DRUG CHOICES

We will put our current knowledge about the drugs available to treat hypertension into a useful clinical context, proceeding to considerations of the appropriate choices for multiple types of hypertensive patients.

Before proceeding, it should be noted that the current nonsystem of health care in the United States provides a control rate of about 33% for adult hypertensives. This is not much better than seen in the similarly developed countries of Western Europe, despite the spending of twice as much money per person for health care in the United States. With the same drugs, Canada, which also spends much less than the United States, has achieved a control rate of 66% (Leenen et al., 2008), thereby obtaining a fall in hypertension-related mortality (Tu et al., 2008a), despite a significant increase in the incidence of the disease (Tu et al., 2008b).

As will become apparent, our past and current obsession of choosing the "best" drug for initial therapy is rapidly giving way to the realization that most patients require two or more drugs for adequate control. Now the search is for the "best" combinations.

Comparisons Between Drugs: Efficacy

The individual practitioner's choice of drug is often based on perceived differences in efficacy in lowering BP and the likelihood of side effects. In fact, overall antihypertensive efficacy varies little between the various available drugs. To gain U.S. FDA approval for marketing in the United States, the drug must have been shown to be effective in reducing the BP in a large portion of the 1,500 or more patients given the drug during its clinical investigation and to have equal efficacy as currently available drugs. Moreover, the dose and formulation of drug are chosen so as not to lower the BP too much or too fast, to avoid hypotensive side effects. Virtually, all oral drugs are designed to do the same thing: lower the BP at least 10% in the majority of patients with mild to moderate hypertension.

When comparisons between various drugs are made, they almost always come out close to one another. The best such comparison was performed in the TOMHS study (Neaton et al., 1993) with random allocation of five drugs (chlorthalidone, acebutolol, doxazosin, amlodipine, and enalapril), each given to almost 200 mild hypertensives, while another group took a placebo and all patients remained on a nutritional hygienic program. The overall antihypertensive efficacy of the five drugs over 4 years was virtually equal (Neaton et al., 1993).

Despite the fairly equal overall efficacy of various antihypertensive drugs, individual patients may vary considerably in their response to different drugs, often for no obvious reason (Senn, 2004). However, some of this variability can be accounted for by patient characteristics, including age and race. This was seen in a VA cooperative 1-year trial in which 1,292 men were randomly given one of six drugs from each major class: Overall, the CCB was most effective, but the ACEI was best in younger whites and the β-blocker was best in older whites (Materson et al., 1993; 1995). Similarly, in a randomized crossover trial of elderly patients with isolated systolic hypertension given a representative of four major classes—ACEI, β-blocker, CCB, and diuretic—each for 1 month, the diuretics and CCB were more effective than the β-blocker or ACEI (Morgan et al., 2001). In similarly designed trials of younger patients with combined systolic and diastolic hypertension, the ACEI and β-blocker were more effective than the CCB or diuretic (Deary et al., 2002; Dickerson et al., 1999). These different effects, which are at least partly related to the level of renin-angiotensin activity, resulted in the AB/CD concept (Fig. 7-15). This concept is now incorporated in the guidelines of the British Hypertension Society (Williams et al., 2004) to be more fully covered later in this chapter.

Comparisons Between Drugs: Reductions in Morbidity and Mortality

The critical issue is not efficacy in lowering BP but rather effectiveness in reducing morbidity and mortality. As detailed in Chapter 5, all major classes of antihypertensive drugs except α-blockers have been shown to reduce mortality and morbidity in large RCTs and there are few differences between them (Blood PressureTrialists, 2007; Task Force, 2007).

In virtually every trial, the benefits reflect not the type of drug, but its efficacy in lowering BP.

As noted, the issue of determining which one drug is best is irrelevant. As the need to achieve lower goals of therapy has become obvious, the need to use more than one drug in the majority of hypertensives

FIGURE 7-15 Steps 1 and 2 are monotherapy, with the order influence by the patient's renin status. This is partly determined by the patient's age and ethnic group, permitting initial selection of treatment without actual renin measurements. Steps 3 and 4 are combination treatment. Progress to each step is indicated by failure to meet the treatment target. *A*, ACEI; *B*, β-blocker; *C*, CCB; *D*, diuretic. (Modified form Dickerson JE, Hingorani AD, Ashby MJ, et al. Optimisation of antihypertensive treatment by crossover rotation of four major classes. *Lancet* 1999;353:2008–2013.)

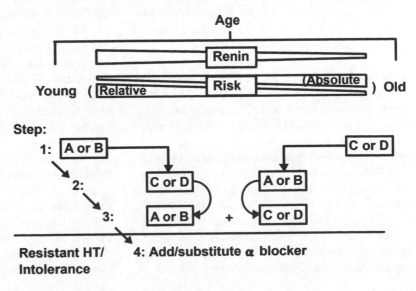

has also become obvious. Therefore, the best combination of agents, usually to include a low dose of diuretic, will be a more pertinent object of trials in the future.

Comparisons Between Drugs: Adverse Effects

As to the issue of differences in adverse effects among different agents, two points are obvious: First, no drug that causes dangerous adverse effects beyond a rare idiosyncratic reaction when given in usual doses will remain on the market, even if it slips by the approval process, as witnessed by the CCB mibefradil. Second, drugs that cause frequent bothersome although not dangerous adverse effects, such as guanethidine, will likely no longer be used now that so many other choices are available.

The various antihypertensive agents vary significantly, both in the frequency of adverse effects and, to an even greater degree, in their nature. The only currently available comparisons of a representative drug from all major classes given as monotherapy to sizable numbers of patients are TOMHS (Neaton et al., 1993) and the VA Cooperative Study (Materson et al., 1993; 1995). Side effects differed between the drugs, but no one drug was markedly more or less acceptable than the others. The differences may include sexual dysfunction. Impotence was twice as common in men in the TOMHS study given the diuretic chlorthalidone than in those given a placebo, whereas less impotence was seen among those given the α-blocker doxazosin (Grimm et al., 1997).

Neither ARBs nor DRIs were available for those previous trials, but equivalence in antihypertensive effect has been seen when one of them was compared against another (Oparil et al., 2007).

Quality of Life

A number of studies have examined the side effects of antihypertensive agents on QOL using various questionnaires and scales. The results show that, although 10% to 20% of patients will experience bothersome adverse effects from most antihypertensive drug (ARBs and DRIs not included), the overall impact of therapies on QOL over 2 to 6 months of observation is positive (Weir et al., 1996; Wiklund et al., 1999).

The most important component of QOL is cognitive function. The best available evidence for the ability to delay dementia remains the Syst-Eur trial which found that CCB-based therapy reduced the

incidence by 55% over a mean follow-up of 3.9 years (Forette et al., 2002).

Apparent Intolerance to All Drugs

Some patients have adverse effects from every drug they take, often bringing to the office a long list of what they have been unable to tolerate. In a few, this may reflect successful reduction in BP below the threshold of cerebral autoregulation by usual doses of drugs so that the patient appears to be intolerant to all medications. Some of these highly susceptible patients can be treated with very small doses of an appropriate agent, because they may be to the far left of the curve of responsiveness. More likely, such patients have psychiatric morbidity that sometimes can respond to behavioral cognitive therapy or antidepressants (Davies et al., 2003).

Serious Side Effects

In addition to these QOL issues, more serious problems have been blamed on various classes of antihypertensive drugs. Virtually, all these claims have come from noncontrolled, often retrospective, observational case-control studies, and most of them have been subsequently proved to be wrong.

Cancer from Reserpine, Calcium Channel Blockers, and Diuretics

The first and perhaps most egregious claim was that the use of reserpine was associated with a twofold to fourfold increased risk of breast cancer in women (Armstrong et al., 1974). As subsequently shown by Feinstein (1988), these studies were all contaminated by the bias of excluding women at high risk for cancer from the control groups.

More recently, Pahor et al. (1996) reported a twofold greater risk for cancer in elderly patients taking short-acting CCBs as compared to users of β-blockers. Multiple subsequent reports of much larger populations in which drug use was appropriately ascertained have found no increase in cancer among users of CCBs (Kizer & Kimmel, 2001).

On the other hand, there may be an association between diuretic use and cancers arising in renal cells (Grossman et al., 2001) or colon (Tenenbaum et al., 2001). The association with renal cell cancers has been repeatedly observed and could reflect conversion of thiazides to mutagenic nitroso derivatives in the stomach. These claims must all be balanced against the multiple observations that the rates of cancer are increased among untreated hypertensives as well as obese patients (Yuan et al., 1998).

Coronary Disease from Calcium Channel Blockers

Psaty et al. (1995) reported a 60% increase in the risk of acute MI among patients taking short-acting CCBs. This report coincided with republication of a meta-analysis of the adverse effects of high doses of short-acting CCBs in the immediate post-MI period (Furberg et al., 1995). Psaty et al. (1995) and Furberg et al. (1995) strongly suggested that their claims against short-acting CCBs also carried over to the longer-acting agents. In fact, the multiple RCTs comparing long-acting CCBs against placebo show a *decrease* in coronary morbidity and mortality in the CCB users whereas comparisons between CCBs and other drugs show no differences (Blood Pressure Lowering Treatment Trialists' Collaboration, 2003; Task Force, 2007).

Dose-Response Relationships

Need to Avoid Overdosing

Beyond the individual variabilities in response to drugs, there is a more generalized problem with the use of antihypertensive agents: They often are prescribed in doses that are too high. The problem of overdosing has been obvious with virtually every new drug introduced, wherein the initial recommended doses have been gradually reduced because, after widespread clinical experience, they proved to be too high (Johnston, 1994). The obvious solution to this problem is for practitioners to start patients with doses that will not be fully effective and to titrate the dose gradually to the desired response.

Need to Lower the Pressure Gradually

While it may be true that more rapid reduction in BP is needed to protect high-risk hypertensives as seen in the VALUE trial (Julius et al., 2004b), the "quick fix" is inappropriate for most patients, who are at low to moderate risk. In a large trial with an ACEI, slower dose escalation (every 6 weeks) was shown to provide higher BP control rates and fewer serious adverse events than more rapid escalation (every 2 weeks) (Flack et al., 2000). These results are in keeping with what is known about the autoregulation of CBF supporting the need for a slow and gradual fall in BP to maintain blood flow to the brain. Normally, CBF remains relatively constant at approximately 50 mL/minute/100 g of brain (Strandgaard & Paulson, 1996). When the systemic BP falls, the vessels dilate; when the BP rises, the vessels constrict. The limits of cerebral autoregulation in normal people are between mean arterial BPs of about 60 and 120 mm Hg (e.g., 80/50 to 160/100 mm Hg) (Strandgaard & Haunsø, 1987).

In hypertensives without neurologic deficits, the CBF is not different from that found in normotensives (Eames et al., 2003). This constancy of the CBF reflects a shift in the range of autoregulation to the right to a range of mean BP from approximately 100 to 180 mm Hg (e.g., 130/85 to 240/150 mm Hg). As seen in Figure 7-16 this shift maintains a normal CBF despite the higher BP but makes the hypertensive vulnerable to cerebral ischemia when the BP falls to a level that is well tolerated by normotensives.

Note that the lower limit of autoregulation capable of preserving CBF in hypertensive patients shown in Figure 7-16 is at a mean BP of nearly 110 mm Hg. Thus, acutely lowering the BP from 160/100 mm Hg (mean, 127 mm Hg) to 140/85 mm Hg (mean,

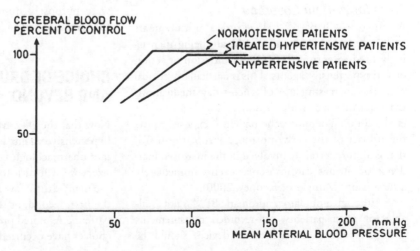

FIGURE 7-16 Autoregulation of CBF. Mean CBF autoregulation curves from normotensive, severely hypertensive, and effectively treated hypertensive patients are shown. (Modified from Strandgaard S, Haunsø S. Why does antihypertensive treatment prevent stroke but not myocardial infarction? *Lancet* 1987;2:658–661.)

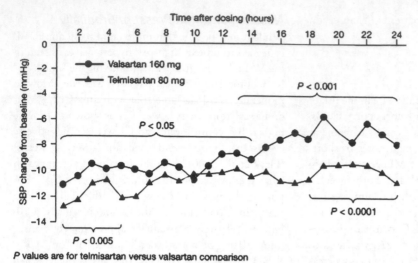

FIGURE 7-17 Changes in SBP control in the 24 hours after a missed dose of telmisartan 80 mg or valsartan 160 mg in patients with mild-to-moderate hypertension. SBP, systolic blood pressure. (Reproduced from McInnes G. 24-hour powerful blood pressure-lowering: Is there a clinical need? *J Am Soc Hypertens* 2008;2:S16–S22, with permission.)

102 mm Hg) may induce cerebral hypoperfusion, although hypotension in the usual sense has not been induced. This likely explains why many patients experience manifestations of cerebral hypoperfusion (weakness, easy fatigability, and postural dizziness) at the start of antihypertensive therapy, even though BP levels do not seem inordinately low.

Fortunately, with slow and effective control of the BP by medication, the curve drifts back toward normal, explaining the eventual ability of hypertensive patients to tolerate falls in BP to levels that initially produced symptoms of cerebral ischemia. In a study of elderly hypertensives treated for 6 months, reduction of systolic BP to less than 140 mm Hg with various drugs resulted in increases in CBF velocity and carotid distensibility, decreases in cerebrovascular resistance, and unimpaired cerebral autoregulation (Lipsitz et al., 2005).

Need for 24-Hour Coverage

As noted in Chapter 2, self-recorded measurements and ambulatory automatic BPM are being increasingly used to ensure the 24-hour duration of action of antihypertensive agents. This is particularly critical with the increasing use of once-a-day medications that often do not provide 24-hour efficacy (Lacourcière et al., 2000). Therefore, the patient is exposed to the full impact of the early morning, abrupt rise in BP that is almost certainly involved in the increased incidence of various cardiovascular events immediately after arising (Munger & Kenney, 2000).

Although ambulatory automatic BPM is not available for most patients, self-recorded measurements with inexpensive semiautomatic devices should be possible for most, thereby ensuring the adequacy of control throughout the waking hours—particularly the early morning hours. As noted earlier, this may require taking medications in the evening or bedtime rather than the usually recommended early a.m.

Value of Greater than 24-Hour Efficacy

Drugs that continue to work beyond 24 hours are even more attractive to prevent loss of control in the considerable number of patients who skip a dose at least once weekly, as documented in 30% or more of patients with hypertension (Rudd, 1995). Among those currently available drugs that likely will maintain good efficacy on a missed day are the diuretic chlorthalidone, the CCB amlodipine, the ACEIs perindopril and trandolapril, and the ARB telmisartan (Lacourciere et al., 2004). In the study shown in Figure 7-17, when the daily doses of the two ARBs were purposely missed, telmisartan maintained its full effect for the 24 hours, valsartan did not.

CHOICE OF DRUGS: FIRST, SECOND, AND BEYOND

Now that the effectiveness and safety of various antihypertensive agents have been compared and important pharmacologic considerations have been emphasized, we will turn to the practical issue of which of the many drugs now available (Table 7-13) should be the first, second, or subsequent choices in individual patients. As noted previously, major changes in these choices have occurred.

TABLE 7.13	Oral Antihypertensive Drugs Available in the United States *(Continued)*

Drug	Usual Dose Range, Total mg (Frequency per Day)[a]	Selected Side Effects and Comments[b]
Diuretics (partial list)		
Chlorthalidone[c]	12.5–50 (1)	High doses: ↑ cholesterol, ↑ glucose,
Hydrochlorothiazide[c]	1.25–2.5 (1)	↓ potassium, ↑ uric acid, ↑ calcium, ↓ magnesium
Indapamide[c]	0.5–1.0 (1)	Rare: blood dyscrasias, photosensitivity, pancreatitis
Metolazone	2.5–10 (1)	
Loop Diuretics		No hypercalcemia
Bumetanide[c]	0.5–4 (2–3)	
Ethacrynic acid	25–100 (2–3)	(Only nonsulfonamide diuretic)
Furosemide[c]	20–240 (2–3)	
Torsemide	2.5–100 (2)	
Potassium-sparing agents		Hyperkalemia
Amiloride[c]	5–10 (1)	
Triamterene[c]	25–100 (1)	
Aldosterone blockers		
Eplerenone[c]	50–100 (1)	
Spironolactone[c]	25–100 (1)	(Gynecomastia)
Adrenergic inhibitors		
Peripheral-acting		
Guanadrel[b,c]	10–75 (2)	(Postural hypotension, diarrhea)
Guanethidine	10–150 (1)	(Same as above)
Reserpine[c]	0.05–0.25 (1)	(Nasal congestion, sedation, depression)
Centrally acting a-agonists		Sedation, dry mouth, withdrawal hypertension
Clonidine[c]	0.2–1.2 (2–3)	
Guanabenz[c]	8–32 (2)	
Guanfacine[c]	1–3 (1)	
Methyldopa[c]	500–3,000 (2)	(Autoimmune disorders)
α-Blockers		Postural hypotension
Doxazosin	1–16 (1)	
Prazosin[c]	2–30 (2–3)	
Terazosin	1–20 (1)	
β-Blockers		Bronchospasm, fatigue, bradycardia, heart failure,
Acebutolol	20–1,200 (1)	masking of insulin-induced hypoglycemia; decreased
Atenolol[c]	25–100 (1–2)	exercise tolerance, hypertriglyceridemia
Betaxolol	5–40 (1)	
Bisoprolol	2.5–20 (1)	
Metoprolol[c]	50–200 (2,1)	
Nadolol[c]	20–240 (1)	
Penbutolol[c]	10–20 (1)	
Pindolol[c]	10–60 (2)	
Propanolol[c]	40–240 (2,1)	
Timolol[c]	10–40 (2)	
Vasodilating -Blockers		Postural hypotension, bronchospasm
Carvedilol	12.5–50 (2,1)	
Labetalolc	200–1,200 (2)	
Nebivolol	5–40 (1)	
Direct vasodilators		Headaches, fluid retention, tachycardia
Hydralazine	50–300 (2)	(Lupus syndrome)
Minoxidil	5–100 (1)	(Hirsutism)

(continued)

TABLE 7.13	Oral Antihypertensive Drugs Available in the United States (Continued)	
Drug	**Usual Dose Range, Total mg (Frequency per Day)[a]**	**Selected Side Effects and Comments[b]**
CCBs		
Nondihydropyridines		Conduction defects
Diltiazem	120–480 (1,2)	
Verapamilc	90–480 (2)	(Constipation)
	120–480 (1)	
Dihydropyridines		Ankle edema, flushing, headache, gingival hyperplasia
Amlodipinec	2.5–10 (1)	
Felodipinec	2.5–20 (1)	
Isradipinec	5–20 (2, 1)	
Nicardipinec	60–120 (2)	
Nifedipinec	30–120 (1)	
Nisoldipinec	20–40 (1)	
Angiotensin converting enzyme inhibitors		Common: cough
Benazeprilc	5–40 (1)	Rare: angioedema,
Captoprilc	25–150 (2–3)	hyperkalemia, rash, loss of taste,
Enalaprilc	5–40 (2)	leucopenia, fetal toxicity
Fosinopril	10–40 (1)	
Lisinoprilc	5–40 (1)	
Moexipril	7.5–30 (2)	
Perindopril	4–16 (1)	
Quinapril	5–80 (1)	
Ramipril	1.25–20 (1)	
Trandolapril	1–4 (1)	
Angiotensin II- receptor blockers		Angioedema, Hyperkalemia, fetal toxicity
Candesartan	8–32 (1)	
Eprosartan	400–800 (1)	
Irbesartan	150–300 (1)	
Losartan	50–100 (1–2)	
Olmesartan	20–40 (1)	
Telmisartan	40–80 (1)	
Valsartan	80–320 (1)	
Direct renin inhibitor		Hyperkalemia, fetal toxicity
Aliskerin	150–300 (1)	

[a] These dosages may vary from those listed in the Physicians' Desk Reference, which may be consulted for additional information. The listing of side effects is not all-inclusive, and clinicians are urged to refer to the package insert for more detailed listing.
[b] Parentheses are individual drug effects. All others are class effects.
[c] Generic available.

Before proceeding into the specifics, we need to recall the overriding issue: to lower the BP to reduce cardiovascular risk maximally without decreasing (and perhaps even improving) the enjoyment of life.

One impediment is threatening to interfere with clinicians' ability to use the therapy of their choice: restrictive formularies that often provide only the least expensive drugs even if they are not the most appropriate for patients' needs. Care must be taken to ensure that formularies provide long-acting, once-a-day preparations of at least one member of each major class of antihypertensive.

Choice of First Drug

As more patients with less severe hypertension are being treated with drugs, the choices of therapy, particularly for the first choice, should be made with care.

Comparative Trials

As reviewed in Chapter 5, multiple RCTs have compared the long-term ability of six classes of antihypertensive drugs—diuretics, β-blockers, α-blockers, ACEIs, ARBs, and CCBs—to protect patients from overall and cardiovascular morbidity and mortality, the only meaningful criterion. Only in a few trials are the differences in outcome significant and, for the most of these, the differences are attributed to differences in BP reduction (Mancia, 2008).

Expert Committee Recommendations

According to the 2003 JNC-7 algorithm, as seen in Figure 7-18, if there are no specific indications for another type of drug, a diuretic is recommended because numerous RCTs have shown a reduction in morbidity and mortality with diuretic based therapy (Chobanian et al., 2003). Until now, HCTZ in doses of 12.5 to 25 mg has been the overwhelming choice and is the diuretic combined with various β-blockers, ACEIs, ARBs, and the DRI that are now available with the exception of atenolol combined with chlorthalidone. However, HCTZ in these doses has not been shown to reduce morbidity or mortality. On the other hand, chlorthalidone 12.5 to 25 mg has been the diuretic in the NIH sponsored trials (MRFIT, SHEP, ALLHAT) that have shown benefit. After many years of apparent denial, chlorthalidone is increasing being recommended to be the appropriate diuretic (Ernst et al., 2009; Messerli & Bangladore, 2009).

The other recent expert guidelines take different approaches:

• The European Hypertension Society-European Society of Cardiology recommend any of the five major classes (Task Force, 2007).
• The British Hypertension Society (Williams et al., 2004) and the British National Institute for Clinical Excellence (2006) both recommend that the choice be based on age and race, the A/CD algorithm (see Fig. 7-15 with the B [β-blocker] removed).
• The Canadian Hypertension Education Program recommends any one of the five drug classes but "initial therapy should include thiazide diuretics" (Khan et al., 2008).

Obviously, disagreements persist but diuretics are included in all.

Once-Daily Therapy

One point agreed upon by all expert guidelines is the need for long-acting, once-a-day therapy. As noted in Table 7-13, choices that are either inherently or artificially long-acting are available in every category. Some may work to reduce the early morning surge of BP if taken in the evening or at bedtime. That requires home BPM which, hopefully, will be done by more and more patients.

Compelling Indications

Another point of agreement is the need for certain drugs for those compelling indications which have shown to respond better to them. Table 7-14 is the listing shown in JNC-7. A more liberal listing is shown in Table 7-15 with a number of combinations matched to choices that seem logical but that have not been adequately tested in RCTs.

Other Factors
Characteristics of the Patient

Individual patient's characteristics may affect the likelihood of a good response to various classes of drugs. As shown in crossover rotations of the four major classes (Deary et al., 2002; Dickerson et al., 1999; Morgan et al., 2001), younger, white patients will usually respond better to either an ACEI/ARB or a β-blocker, perhaps because they tend to have higher renin levels, whereas older and black patients will respond better to diuretics and CCBs, perhaps because they have lower renin levels. From these results, the AB/CD (now A/CD) algorithm was proposed. These differences apply to monotherapy; with a low-dose of a diuretic as part of the regimen, responses to all other agents are largely equalized. Moreover, for the individual patient, any drug may work well or poorly, and there is no set formula that can be used to predict certain success without side effects (Senn, 2004).

Plasma Renin Levels

The differences in BP response between younger versus older and blacks versus nonblacks could reflect differences in the activity of the renin-angiotensin system, as measured by PRA. Laragh and coworkers, as far back as 1972 (Bühler et al., 1972), have used the level of PRA to guide the choice of initial therapy. As attractive as the concept is, in practice it often does not work: Donnelley et al. (1992) found that pretreatment PRA accounted for considerably less than 10% of the variability in response to treatement.

Genomic Associations

Slowly growing evidence shows associations between genetic makeup and response to various drugs. The

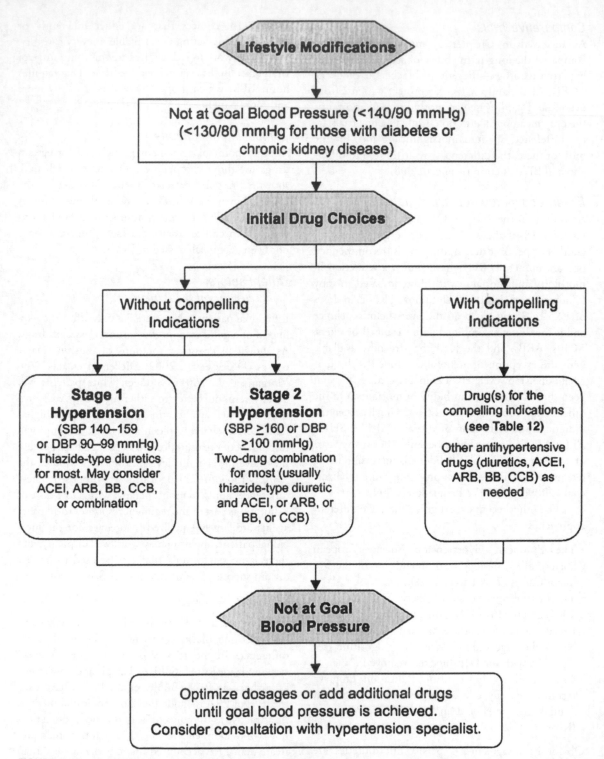

FIGURE 7-18 The JNC-7 algorithm. BP, blood pressure; ACE, angiotensin-converting enzyme; ARB, angiotenin-receptor blocker; CCB, calcium channel blocker. (From Chobanian AV, Bakris GL, Black HR et al. The Seventh Report of the Joint National Committee on Prevention, Detection, Evaluation, and Treatment of High Blood Pressure: The JNC 7 report. *JAMA* 2003;289:2560–2572.)

TABLE 7.14	Clinical Trial and Guideline Basis for Compelling Indications for Individual Drug Classes

	Recommended Drugs					
Compelling Indication	*Diuretic*	*βB*	*ACEI*	*ARB*	*CCB*	*Aldo Ant*
Heart failure	•	•	•	•	•	•
Post-MI		•	•			•
High coronary disease risk	•	•	•		•	
Diabetes	•	•	•	•	•	
CKD			•	•		
Recurrent stroke prevention	•		•			

βB, beta-blocker; ACEI, angiotensin-converting enzyme inhibitor; ARB, angiotensin receptor blocker; CCB, calcium channel blocker; Aldo Ant, aldosterone antagonist.
Modified from Chobanian AV, Bakris GL, Black HR, et al. Seventh report of the Joint National Committee on Prevention, Detection, Evaluation, and Treatment of High Blood Pressure. *Hypertension* 2003;42:1206–1252.

TABLE 7.15	Considerations for Individualizing Antihypertensive Drug Therapy[a]

May Have Favorable Effects on Comorbid Conditions		May Have Unfavorable Effects on Comorbid Conditions[b]	
Condition	*Drug*	*Condition*	*Drug*
Angina	β-Blockers, CCB	Bronchospasic disease	β-Blockers
Atrial tachycardia and fibrillation	β-Blockers CCB (non-DHP)	2° or 3° heart block	β-Blockers CCB (non-DHP)
Cough from ACEI	ARB	Depression	Central α-agonists
Cyclosporine-induced hypertension	CCB	Dyslipidemia	Reserpine[c] β-Blockers (non-ISA)
DM, particularly with proteinuria	ACEI, ARB, low-dose diuretics, CCBs, β-blockers	Gout heart failure hyperkalemia	Diuretics (high-dose) Diuretics CCB[b] ACEI, ARB, DRI,
Dyslipidemia	α-Blockers		aldo-blockers
Essential tremor	β-Blockers (non-CS)		
Heart failure	ACEI, ARB, Carvedilol,	Liver disease	Labetalol
Hyperthyroidism	β-blockers, diuretics		Methyldopa[c]
Migraine	β-Blockers β-Blockers (non-CS) CCB Thiazides	Peripheral vascular disease Pregnancy	β-Blockers[b] ACEI[c], ARB[c], DRI[c]
		Renal insufficiency	Potassium-sparing agents,
Osteoporosis			aldo-blockers[b]
Preoperative hypertension	β-Blockers		
Prostatism	α-Blockers	Renovascular disease, bilateral	ACEI, ARB, DRI
Renal insufficiency	ACEI, ARB, loop diuretic		
		Type I and II diabetes	β-Blockers
Systolic hypertension in elderly	Diuretics, CCB		High-dose diuretics

[a]Conditions and drugs are listed in alphabetical order.
[b]These drugs may be used with special monitoring, unless contraindicated.
[c]Contraindicated.
ACEI, angiotensin-converting enzyme inhibitor; Aldo, aldosterone; ARB, angiotensin II receptor blocker; CCB, calcium channel blocker;DRI, direct renin inhibitor; DHP, dihydropyridine; non-CS, non-cardioselective; non-ISA, non-intrinsic sympathomimetic activity.

data include polymorphisms on chromosome 12 loci and the response to thiazides diuretics (Turner et al., 2008); CYP11B2 gene polymorphisms and the response to ACEIs (Yu et al., 2006); β-adrenergic gene polymorphisms and the outcomes to treatment with β-blockers (Pacanowski et al., 2008). Eventually, pharmacogenetics may play an important role in the choice of drugs, but this is not likely before the next edition of this book.

Overall Risk Status

The higher the risk of the patient, the greater the protection to be achieved with treatments that correct the risk. As noted in Chapter 5, this means that treating the higher risk elderly will provide more short-term benefit than treating the lower-risk young. And, as new risk factors are identified, e.g., albuminuria, the higher the risks are the more benefit will be provided with therapy, e.g., ACEIs and ARBs, that correct them (Boersma et al., 2008).

Characteristics of the Drug

The five major classes differ in their characteristics that play a role in their advantages and disadvantages. Some agents—such as the direct-acting smooth-muscle vasodilators, central α_2-agonists, and peripheral-acting adrenergic antagonists—are not well suited for initial monotherapy because they produce annoying adverse effects in a large number of patients. However, as repeatedly documented, if they effectively lower BP, all drugs provide protection from cardiovascular events.

Cost of the Drug

There is clear evidence of an overall cost-effectiveness of the treatment of hypertension, as reviewed in Chapter 1. Multiple studies have shown a cost-benefit of starting effective therapy before the advent of expected complications (Coyle et al., 2007) and using more effective therapies, even if they are more expensive (Boersma et al., 2007; Heidenreich et al., 2008). Rather obviously, if two classes are equally effective, e.g., ACEIs and ARBs, using less expensive generic ACEIs first rather than more expensive patent-protected ARBs will save money (Yokoyama et al., 2007).

For even greater cost-benefit, the provision of a Polypill (Law et al., 2009) to all high-risk people in 23 low- and middle-income countries is estimated to avert 18 million cardiovascular deaths over a 10-year interval, while costing $1.08 yearly per person (Lim et al., 2007).

Combinations as Initial Therapy

Another possible way to reduce the costs of antihypertensive care is to use those combination tablets that cost less than their separate ingredients.

As JNC-7 and all other guidelines recognize, most patients will end up on two or more drugs to achieve adequate control. Therefore, the idea of starting with two drugs is gaining currency, in the JNC-7 for all with BP above 160/100 mm Hg.

A number of combination tablets are available. These are mostly of a low dose of the diuretic HCTZ with a β-blocker, ACEI, ARB, or DRI. More and more combinations of one of these renin-suppressing drugs with a CCB are appearing, particularly with amlodipine which is no longer patent-protected.

Such fixed-dose combinations will be more likely taken by patients than will be separate drugs (Bangalore et al., 2007b). However, if they include a patent-protected drug, the total cost to the patient may exceed that of two generics.

An increasing number of trials are comparing different combinations. It should be remembered that in every trial comparing single drugs against another, additional drugs were always added to achieve the preset goal. As an example, in the LIFE trial, comparing the ARB losartan against the β-blocker atenolol, 80% of both groups were also given HCTZ by the end of the trial (Dahlöf et al., 2002). The need for a diuretic to be combined with an ACEI was demonstrated in the PROGRESS trial wherein stroke survivors had no benefit from the ACEI alone, but a 43% reduction in recurrent stroke when the diuretic indapamide was combined with the ACEI (PROGRESS Collaborative Group, 2001). Subsequently, the ASCOT trial showed superiority of a CCB-ACEI combination over a β-blocker-diuretic combination (Dahlöf et al., 2005). More recently, the ACCOMPLISH trial found better BP control and cardiovascular protection with an ACEI-CCB combination than an ACEI-HCTZ combination (Jamerson et al., 2008). This greater benefit may be ascribable to the short duration of the effect of HCTZ particularly in the average daily dose of 19 mg (Chobanian, 2008).

One combination particularly favored by nephrologists to reduce proteinuria is an ACEI + ARB. This advantage, however, was negated in the large ONTARGET trial, where an ACEI + ARB was associated with more hypotension and worse major renal outcomes than seen with either the ACEI or ARB alone (Mann et al., 2008).

The Polypill

The initial proposal of simplifying treatment by giving a polypill to all people over age 55 and younger people already afflicted with vascular disease (Wald & Law, 2003) was met with some doubt. In the ensuing years, however, the concept has received considerable support, both as therapeutically sound (Hippisley-Cox & Coupland, 2005; Mahmud & Feely, 2007) and as exceedingly cost-effective for low- and middle-income countries (Gaziano et al., 2006; Lim et al., 2007).

Choice of Second Drug

If a moderate dose of the first choice is well tolerated and effective but not enough to bring the BP down to the desired level, a second drug can be added, and thereby control will likely be better achieved than by increasing the dose of the first drug (White et al., 2008). A logical overall algorithm for the use of a diuretic plus K$^+$-sparer as first choice and the choice of second drug based upon some of the compelling indications is shown in Figure 7-19.

Choice of Third or Fourth Drug

Various combinations usually work. The key, as with two drugs, is to combine agents with different mechanisms of action. The most rational is a diuretic, an ACEI or ARB, and a CCB.

Few patients should need more than three drugs, particularly if the various reasons for resistance to therapy are considered. For those who do, the JNC-7 recommends considering consultation with a hypertension specialist (Chobanian et al., 2003). In the ASCOT trial, either an α-blocker or spironolactone was chosen (Chapman et al., 2007; 2008).

Reduction or Discontinuation of Therapy

Once a good response has occurred and has been maintained for a year or longer, medications may be

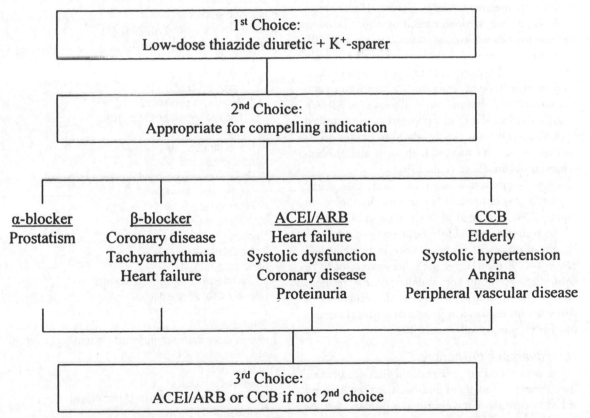

FIGURE 7-19   A treatment algorithm based on JNC-7 and certain compelling indications for different classes.

reduced or discontinued. However, in a closely monitored group of over 6,200 hypertensives who had been successfully controlled, only 18% were able to remain normotensive after stopping therapy (Nelson et al., 2003). The characteristics that make withdrawal more likely to be successful were lower levels of BP before and after therapy, fewer and lower doses of medication needed to control hypertension, and patient's willingness to follow lifestyle modifications.

Whether it is worth the trouble to stop successful drug therapy completely is questionable. The more sensible approach in well-controlled patients would be first to decrease the dose of whatever is being used. If this succeeds, withdrawal may be attempted with continued close surveillance of the BP.

RESISTANT HYPERTENTION

Causes

Ten percent of adult hypertensives will not be controlled to a BP less than 140/90 mm Hg with three drugs, i.e., they are resistant. The reasons for an inadequate response are numerous (Table 7-16); the most likely is volume overload caused by either excessive sodium intake, inadequate diuretic (Graves, 2000), or higher than expected aldosterone levels (Gaddam et al., 2008). Resistance is found more often in those who are elderly, obese, diabetic, black, or women and those with renal dysfunction (Calhoun et al., 2008). In a disadvantaged minority population, uncontrolled hypertension is most closely related to limited access to care, noncompliance with therapy, and alcohol-related problems (Shea et al., 1992).

An appropriate diagnostic and therapeutic approach to resistant hypertension is shown in Figure 7-20, patterned after Calhoun et al. (2008). The first need is to establish the presence of resistance by out-of-office BP readings, since as many as half above 140/90 mm Hg in the office may actually be controlled by home or ambulatory BP readings (Brown et al., 2001). Moreover, the prognosis of patients with resistance is provided by ABPM but not by office readings (Salles et al., 2008)

Nonadherence to Therapy

Often patients do not take their medications because they cannot afford them and because they have no access to consistent and continuous primary care. As noted earlier in this chapter, there are ways to simplify the regimen and improve access. Recall as well

the evidence that patients may appear to be resistant only because their physicians simply do not keep increasing their therapy (Amar et al., 2003).

Drug-Related Causes

In a survey of 1,377 hypertensives over 9 months, 75% had some potential interaction with their antihypertensive drugs and in 35% the interaction was considered highly significant (Carter et al., 2004).

TABLE 7.16	Causes of Inadequate Responsiveness to Therapy

Pseudo-resistance
   White coat or office elevations
   Pseudohypertension in the elderly
Nonadherence to therapy
   Side effects or costs of medication
   Lack of consistent and continuous primary care
   Inconvenient and chaotic dosing schedules
   Instructions not understood
   Organic brain syndrome (e.g., memory deficit)
Drug-related causes
   Doses too low
   Inappropriate combinations
   Rapid inactivation (e.g., hydralazine)
   Drug actions and interactions
      NSAIDS
      Sympathomimetics
         Nasal decongestants
         Appetite suppressants
         Cocaine and other street drugs
         Caffeine
      Oral contraceptives
      Adrenal steroids
      Licorice (as may be found in chewing tobacco)
      Cyclosporine, tacrolimus
      Erythropoietin
Associated conditions
   Smoking
   Increased obesity
   Sleep apnea
   Insulin resistance or hyperinsulinemia
   Ethanol intake >1 oz a day
   Anxiety-induced hyperventilation or panic attacks
   Chronic pain
   Intense vasoconstriction (Raynaud phenomenon, arteritis)
Identifiable causes of hypertension
Volume overload
   Excess sodium intake
   Progressive renal damage (nephrosclerosis)
   Fluid retention from reduction of BP
   Inadequate diuretic therapy

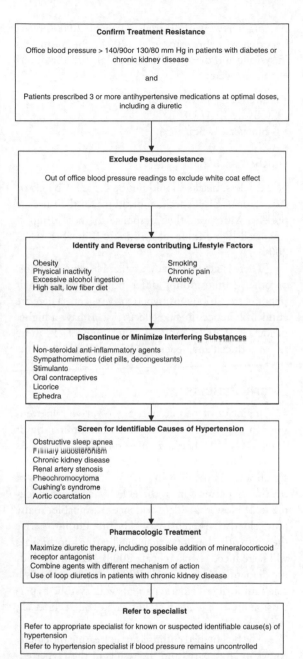

Confirm Treatment Resistance

Office blood pressure > 140/90or 130/80 mm Hg in patients with diabetes or chronic kidney disease

and

Patients prescribed 3 or more antihypertensive medications at optimal doses, including a diuretic

Exclude Pseudoresistance

Out of office blood pressure readings to exclude white coat effect

Identify and Reverse contributing Lifestyle Factors

Obesity   Smoking
Physical inactivity   Chronic pain
Excessive alcohol ingestion Anxiety
High salt, low fiber diet

Discontinue or Minimize Interfering Substances

Non-steroidal anti-inflammatory agents
Sympathomimetics (diet pills, decongestants)
Stimulants
Oral contraceptives
Licorice
Ephedra

Screen for Identifiable Causes of Hypertension

Obstructive sleep apnea
Primary aldosteronism
Chronic kidney disease
Renal artery stenosis
Pheochromocytoma
Cushing's syndrome
Aortic coarctation

Pharmacologic Treatment

Maximize diuretic therapy, including possible addition of mineralocorticoid receptor antagonist
Combine agents with different mechanism of action
Use of loop diuretics in patients with chronic kidney disease

Refer to specialist

Refer to appropriate specialist for known or suspected identifiable cause(s) of hypertension
Refer to hypertension specialist if blood pressure remains uncontrolled

FIGURE 7-20 Diagnosis and management of patients with resistant hypertension. (Adapted from Calhoun DA, Jones C, Textor S, et al. Resistant hypertension: Diagnosis, evaluation, and treatment. *Hypertension* 2008;51:1403–1419.)

The most common of these in the United States is likely the interference with the antihypertensive effect of virtually all agents save CCBs by nonsteroidal anti-inflammatory drugs (NSAIDs). This effect likely involves inhibition of the cyclooxygenase-2 (COX-2) enzyme in the kidneys, thereby reducing sodium excretion and increasing intravascular volume (White, 2007). There is a common misconception of a sharp difference between NSAIDs that also block the COX-1 enzyme of the gut (nonselective NSAIDs such as naproxen) and those which spare the COX-1 enzyme (such as Celecoxib). In fact, all NSAIDs must block COX-2 to reduce inflammation and pain and therefore all may raise BP (Warner & Mitchell, 2008). Large doses of aspirin also pose a problem but 80 mg a day does not (Zanchetti et al., 2002).

A number of other drug interactions may be seen, mostly reducing the effectiveness of one or both drugs, although some increase the duration or degree of action, e.g., large amounts of grapefruit juice or Seville oranges (Lilja et al., 2004) inhibit the activity of the cytochrome P450 isoenzyme CYP3A4 which is involved in the metabolism of many drugs and can raise the blood levels of some statins, CCBs, and immunesuppressive drugs (Medical Letter, 2004).

In these days of increasing use of herbal remedies, which in the United States are totally unregulated because of Senator Hatch's bill prohibiting FDA surveillance of these agents, a number of herb-drug interactions are seen. More about such interactions which can raise BP is provided in Chapter 14.

Associated Conditions

Nicotine transiently raises BP but the effect is often not recognized because the BP is almost ways taken in a no-smoking environment. The combination of abdominal and generalized obesity, insulin resistance, and sleep apnea is an increasingly common cause of resistant hypertension (Calhoun et al., 2008).

Identifiable Causes of Hypertension

These are covered in Chapters 9 through 15. Recently, a possibly higher prevalence of primary aldosteronism than previously recognized has been reported and the presence of a low plasma renin level in a resistant hypertensive can be the tip-off for the condition (Calhoun et al., 2008).

Treatment

The need for adequate diuretic is obvious. The need for blockade of high or even "normal" levels of aldosterone, whether or not associated with autonomous hypersecretion, has become increasingly documented by impressive relief of resistance with even low doses of spironolactone (Chapman et al., 2007). The potent vasodilator, minoxidil, may work when nothing else does (Black et al., 2007). Two invasive procedures are being tested: an implantable electric activation of the carotid baroreflex (Scheffers et al., 2008), and catheter-based renal sympathetic nerve denervation (Krum et al., 2009).

A careful search of the cause(s) and appropriate antihypertensive therapy almost always can correct resistance. If not, consultation with a hypertension specialist should be obtained.

SPECIAL CONSIDERATIONS IN THE CHOICE OF THERAPY

Children are covered in Chapter 16; women who are pregnant or on estrogens are covered in Chapter 15.

Women

In the United States, women who are hypertensive are much more likely to be treated but are less likely to achieve good control (Gu et al., 2008). Compared to men, women have been found to have higher vascular reactivity (Lipsitz et al., 2005) and to have less regression of LVH on equivalent antihypertensive therapy (Okin et al., 2008). Moreover in the Second Australian National Blood Pressure Study, women randomly assigned to an ACEI derived no reduction in the hazard ratio for cardiovascular events or mortality, whereas the men on an ACEI had a 17% reduction in hazard despite equal and substantial reductions of BP in both groups (Wing et al., 2003).

Blacks and Other Ethnic Groups

As noted in Chapter 4, black hypertensives have many distinguishing characteristics, some of which could affect their responses to antihypertensive therapy. However, when they achieve adequate control, blacks usually respond as whites do and experience similar reductions in the incidences of cardiovascular disease as do whites (Brewster et al., 2004). However, in the LIFE trial, the small number of blacks (n = 533) did not receive the cardiovascular protection from an ARB than did the larger number of whites (n = 8,660) despite equal reductions in BP (Julius et al., 2004a).

Blacks respond less well to monotherapy with drugs that suppress the angiotensin-renin system, i.e., β-blockers, ARBs, ACEIs, and DRIs perhaps because they tend to have lower renin levels, and equally as well to diuretics and CCBs (Wright et al., 2005). In a

systematic review of 30 trials involving 20,006 black hypertensives (Brewster et al., 2004), the mean falls in systolic and diastolic BP (mm Hg) with the different agents were:

- Diuretics ... 11.8/8.1
- CCBs ... 12.1/9.4
- β-blockers ... 3.5/5.4
- ACEIs ... 7.0/3.8
- ARBs ... 3.6/2.1

Nonetheless, blacks should not be denied β-blockers, ARBs, or ACEIs if special indications for their use are present. Moreover, their response to these drugs is equalized by addition of a diuretic (Libhaber et al., 2004).

There is no good evidence that Hispanics, Asians, or other ethnic groups differ from whites in their responses to various antihypertensive agents. There are ethnic differences in side effects: Asians have a higher incidence of ACEI-induced cough, and blacks more ACEI-induced angioedema (McDowell et al., 2006).

Elderly Patients

The majority of people over age 65 have hypertension; in most, the hypertension is predominantly or purely systolic because of arterial stiffness. As described in Chapter 4, the risks for such patients are significant. As detailed in Chapter 5, the benefits of treating hypertension in the elderly have been documented. Now that such evidence is available, many more elderly hypertensives will be brought into active therapy with the hope that debilitating morbidities will be reduced (Beckett et al., 2008), possibly including dementia (Hanon et al., 2008). At present, only a small minority of elderly patients with systolic hypertension are being adequately treated (Borzecki et al., 2006).

The heightened enthusiasm for treating the elderly comes in large part from the results of the Hypertension in the Very Elderly Trial (HYVET) (Beckett et al., 2008). In HYVET, 3,845 subjects over age 80 (mean age 84) were allocated to placebo on therapy starting with the diuretic indapamide and adding the ACEI perindopril if the target BP of less than 150/80 mm Hg was not reached. It should be noted that only 33% of these subjects had isolated systolic hypertension, with the overall mean BP of 173/91 mm Hg. Moreover, they were healthier than most 80-plus-year-old hypertensives with only 12% having had a prior cardiovascular event. Therefore, application of the HYVET results to the overall elderly hypertensive population may be inappropriate (Mann, 2009).

Nonetheless, the results of HYVET are impressive. After only 2 years, total mortality was reduced by 21%, stroke by 30%, and heart failure by 64% in those on active therapy.

Before beginning drug therapy, the evidence described in Chapter 2 showing that white-coat hypertension is even more common in the elderly than in younger patients should be remembered (Pickering, 2004). Therefore, before making the diagnosis, out-of-office readings should be obtained, if possible.

Regardless of age, as long as the patient appears to have a reasonable life expectancy, active therapy is appropriate for all who have a systolic level above 160 mm Hg, with or without an elevated diastolic pressure. No published RCTs have involved elderly patients with systolic BP between 140 and 160 mm Hg so the decision to treat should be based on overall risk. Those at high risk (e.g., diabetics or smokers) should be started on therapy at systolic levels above 140 mm Hg.

Table 7-17 lists factors often present in the elderly that may complicate their therapy. Because the elderly may have sluggish baroreceptor and sympathetic nervous responsiveness as well as impaired cerebral autoregulation, therapy should be gentle and gradual, avoiding drugs that are likely to cause postural hypotension. Nonetheless, treatment should not be delayed if it is indicated, since the elderly are inherently at greater risk (Staessen et al., 2004) and hypertension hastens cell senescence (Westhoff et al., 2008).

Lifestyle Modifications

Before beginning drug therapy, the multiple benefits of nondrug therapies that were described in Chapter 6 should also be remembered. The ability of lifestyle changes to lower BP in the elderly has been well documented (Pickering, 2004). In particular, dietary sodium should be moderately restricted down to 100 to 120 mmol per day because the pressor effect of sodium excess and the antihypertensive efficacy of sodium restriction progressively increase with age (Geleijnse et al., 1994; Weinberger & Fineberg, 1991). However, the elderly may have at least two additional hurdles to overcome in achieving this goal: First, their taste sensitivity may be lessened, so they may ingest more sodium to compensate; and second, they may depend more on processed, prepackaged foods that are high in sodium rather than fresh foods that are low in sodium.

Postural Hypotension

Defined as a fall in BP of either 20 mm Hg systolic or 10 mm Hg diastolic upon unsupported standing from the supine position, postural or orthostatic hypotension is found in 10% to 30% of ambulatory hypertensives over age 60 and as many as 50% of those in a geriatric ward (Gupta & Lipsitz, 2007). It is often associated with postprandial hypotension induced by splanchnic pooling. It is more common in diabetics and is a marker of increased mortality. As noted in Figure 7-21, numerous causes may be responsible, including arterial stiffness and baroreceptor insensitivity (Mattace-Rasso et al., 2007). Postural hypotension is often found with supine hypertension, may be delayed beyond ten minutes on standing, and is a component of more severe syndromes of autonomic failure (Freeman, 2008).

Postural hypotension must be recognized before antihypertensive therapy is begun to avoid traumatic falls when the BP is lowered further. Fortunately, the physical therapies listed in Figure 7-21 can usually

TABLE 7.17	**Factors that Might Contribute to Complications from Pharmacologic Treatment of Hypertension in the Elderly**
Factors	**Potential Complications**
Diminished baroreceptor activity	Orthostatic hypotension
Impaired cerebral autoregulation	Cerebral ischemia with small falls in systolic pressure
Decreased intravascular volume	Orthostatic hypotension
	Volume depletion, hyponatremia
Sensitivity to hypokalemia	Arrhythmia, muscular weakness
Decreased renal and hepatic function	Drug accumulation
Polypharmacy	Drug interaction
CNS changes	Depression, confusion

manage the problem but various medications have been tried with limited success, including the sodium-retaining fludrocortisone and the sympathomimetic midodrine (Freeman, 2008; Low & Singer, 2008).

Choice of Drugs for the Elderly

Conventional practice has largely adopted the British A/CD scheme, indicating diuretic or CCB as initial therapy of the elderly. However, a meta-analysis of the results of 31 RCTs including over 190,000 patients showed equal and significant benefit from diuretics, CCBs, ACEIs, and ARBs in those younger than or in those older than age 65 (Table 7-18) (Blood Pressure Trialists, 2008). Beyond the ACEI or CCB versus placebo trials shown in Table 7-18, the remainder of the trials compared one class of drug versus another class; here again, there were no significant differences in the benefits between the under age 65 or over age 65 subjects.

Therapy should begin with small doses and then should be slowly increased: Start low and go slow. Small doses may be fully effective. Even more so than in younger patients, the elderly do better with long-acting (once-daily), smoothly working agents since they may have trouble following complicated dosage schedules, reading the labels, and opening bottles

CAUSAL FACTOR	PATHOPHYSIOLOGY	THERAPY
Rapid rising	Pooling of blood in lower body	Slow rising, particularly from sleep
Vasodilation	Venous pooling Splanchnic pooling Sympatholytic drugs	Supportive panty hose Avoid large meals Avoid such agents
Volume depletion	Low cardiac output - diuretic - very low sodium intake	Maintain intravascular volume by avoiding over-diuresis and sleeping with head of bed elevated
Baroreflex dysfunction	Loss of normal vasoconstriction by sympathetic stimulation	Drinking 16 oz water before arising Various drugs: - sympathomimetics - volume expanders Isometric exercise
Cerebrovascular disease	Low cerebral perfusion	Avoid overtreatment of hypertension Correct dyslipidemia Stop smoking

FIGURE 7-21 Summary of the pathophysiologic events that occur during the development of symptoms of postural hypotension **(middle column)** and the interaction of exacerbating factors **(left column)** and remedial measures **(right column)** with these events.

TABLE 7.18	RCTs on Treatment of Hypertensives Under Age 65 Versus over Age 65	
Drug	**Difference in SBP/DBP (mm Hg)**	**Relative Risk (95% CI)**
ACEI vs Placebo		
Age < 65	−4.6/−2.1 0	0.76 (0.66–0.88)
Age > 65	−4.2/−2.0	0.83 (0.74–0.94)
CCB vs Placebo		
Age < 65	−7.2/−2.9	0.84 (0.54–1.31)
Age > 65	−9.3/−3.8	0.74 (0.59–0.92)

Data from Blood Pressure Trialist. Effects of different regimens to lower blood pressure on major cardiovascular events in older and younger adults: Meta-analysis of randomised trials. *Br Med J* 2008;336:1121–1123.

with safety caps. Home BP recording may be particularly useful, first in overcoming the white-coat effect which is quantitatively greater in the elderly and second, in ensuring that therapy is enough but not too much. The white-coat effect in the doctor's office may conceal considerable overtreatment.

Goal of Therapy

The question of how far to lower BP is covered in Chapter 5. As previously written (Kaplan, 2000), "There may very well be a J-curve of increasing cardiovascular disease when the diastolic pressure is lowered below the level needed to maintain perfusion to vital organs…. Therefore, caution is advised in treating those with [isolated systolic hypertension], who obviously start with already low diastolic blood pressures."

On the other hand, no J-curve for systolic BP has been documented. The investigators of the HYVET trial of patients aged 80 or older recommend a target BP of 150/80 mm Hg, the target reached in almost half of their patients (Beckett et al., 2008).

Effect on Cognitive Decline and Dementia

There is evidence that lowering of BP with antihypertensive therapy will reduce the incidence of cognitive decline and dementia (Forette et al., 2002; Hanon et al., 2008; Khachaturian et al., 2006; Skoog et al., 2005; Yasar et al., 2008). However, no such benefit was seen in the HYVET trial over 2 years in patients 80 years or older (Peters et al., 2008).

Most of these trials, in particular HYVET, may have been too little, too late. There are experimental data supporting a neuroprotective effect of lowering BP in rats (Elewa et al., 2007) and data in humans showing plasticity of cerebral hemodynamics to preserve or improve CBF when BP is lowered (Lipsitz et al., 2005; Zhang et al., 2007). Therefore, the

least that can now be said is that appropriate antihypertensive therapy will do no harm and may provide protection from cognitive decline.

Obesity and the Metabolic Syndrome

Visceral or abdominal obesity, easily identified by tape measurement of waist circumference, is associated with the Metabolic Syndrome (Wildman et al., 2008) and, in particular, with hypertension (Redon et al., 2008). With the marked increase in obesity worldwide, the syndrome will increase in prevalence, reaching down into childhood (Hudley et al., 2004) and up into the elderly (Sloan et al., 2008). In managing the hypertension, care must be taken not to worsen the other components of the syndrome.

Lifestyle Modifications

The major focus must be prevention of obesity. Failing that, weight loss and increased physical activity will slow the onset of diabetes, as described in Chapter 6. A Mediterranean-style diet, even with little weight loss, reduced the prevalence of the syndrome by more than half (Esposito et al., 2004).

Antihypertensive Drug Therapy

High doses of diuretics and, even more, β-blockers should be avoided in those who are prone to develop or who have the Metabolic Syndrome (Mason et al., 2005; Messerli et al., 2008a). The incidence of new-onset diabetes in multiple RCTs has been reduced significantly with therapy based on ACEIs, ARBs, and CCBs compared to therapy based on diuretics, β-blockers, or their combination (Aksnes et al., 2008a). Of these, ACEIs or ARBs are least likely to induce diabetes (Lam & Owen, 2007). In the LIFE trial, new-onset diabetes was less likely with either the β-blocker or the ARB if regression of LVH occurred, so more may be involved than the type of drug alone (Okin et al., 2007).

Insulin Sensitizers and Other Drugs

Thiazolidinediones are the most effective insulin sensitizers (Yki-Järvinen, 2004) and lower the BP by about 4 mm Hg (Raji et al., 2003). Metformin reduced the appearance of diabetes in the Diabetes Prevention Program (Knowler et al., 2002) and acarbose improved multiple features of the Metabolic Syndrome (Chiasson et al., 2003).

Diabetes

Diabetes markedly increases cardiovascular risk and must be treated intensively. Unfortunately, few hypertensive diabetics have both conditions adequately treated (Lonati et al., 2008), despite the recognition that tighter control of both is needed (American Diabetes Association, 2008).

Before addressing treatment, a misconception over the risk of medication-induced, new-onset diabetes needs correction. In the ALLHAT trial (2002), the new onset of diabetes was more frequent in those whose therapy was based on the diuretic chlorthalidone (11.6%) versus the CCB amlodipine (9.8%) or the ACEI lisinopril (8.6%). During the average duration of follow-up of 4.9 years (1,788 days), no excess in cardiovascular morbidity or mortality was seen among those who developed diabetes while on the diuretic (Wright et al., 2008). This apparent

paradox has been explained as a reflection of the greater antihypertensive effect of diuretic-based therapy, so that "the benefit of blood pressure reduction outweighs any risk associated with development of DM [diabetes mellitus]" (Phillips, 2006). The ALLHAT investigators propose that "thiazide-induced DM is a different and benign disease entity compared with either de novo DM or that which develops in the context of other antihypertensive agents" (Phillips, 2006).

The apparent benignity of diuretic-induced DM was also seen in the SHEP trial, even after 14 years of follow-up (Kostis et al., 2005). However, the ALLHAT data suffer from a short duration of observation. In the VALUE trial, 1,298 patients had new-onset diabetes (Aksnes et al., 2007b). As seen in Figure 7-22, those patients had a slightly greater incidence of heart failure than seen in those who did not develop diabetes over the first 5 years of follow-up, but a sharply increased incidence after 2,000 days or 5.5 years, to a level equal to those with diabetes on entry into the study. Verdecchia et al. (2007), in their commentary about the data shown in Figure 7-22, conclude "New-onset diabetes, regardless of its determinants, remains an adverse prognostic marker." Therefore, prevention of diabetes is necessary. If it appears, treatment must be intensive.

Lifestyle Modifications

The same principles apply as with the Metabolic Syndrome: weight loss and physical activity are critical (see Chapter 6). Considering the need for tight

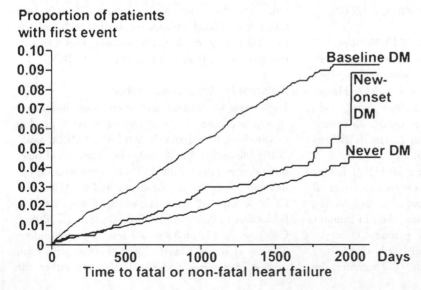

Proportion of patients with first event

FIGURE 7-22 CHF (fatal and non-fatal) in the three groups. DM, diabetes mellitus. (Reproduced from Aksnes TA, Kjeldsen SE, Rostrup M, et al. Impact of new-onset diabetes mellitus on cardiac outcomes in the Valsartan Antihypertensive Long-term Use Evaluation (VALUE) trial population. *Hypertension* 2007b; 50:467–473, with permission.)

control of hypertension to a level of 130/80 mm Hg, the ADA advises use of lifestyle therapy alone for a maximum of 3 months (American Diabetes Association, 2008).

Antihypertensive Drug Therapy

Therapy should be started at levels of BP above 130/80 mm Hg and intensified enough to keep the BP below 130/80 mm Hg. Such therapy will save the patient misery and the health care system money even better than will glycemic or lipid control (CDC Diabetes Cost-Effectiveness Group, 2002).

The best drugs to achieve control are, in order, ACEIs, ARBs, diuretics, and CCBs (American Diabetes Association, 2008). As stated in the ADA guidelines: "Although evidence for distinct advantages of renin-angiotensin system (RAS) inhibitors on cardiovascular disease outcomes in diabetes remains conflicting.... The compelling benefits of RAS inhibitors in diabetic patients with albuminuria or renal insufficiency provide additional rationale for their use." The last point relates to the need to prevent diabetic nephropathy, the leading cause of end-stage renal disease in the United States (Burgess, 2008). The management of diabetic nephropathy is covered in Chapter 9.

Whichever drug is chosen as first, almost all diabetic hypertensives will need 2, 3, or 4 to accomplish the goal of 130/80 mm Hg. If that goal is even approximated, marked protection against most diabetic complications can be provided (Gaede et al., 2008). To reach the goal, a diuretic will almost always be needed (Arroll et al., 2008).

Lipid-Lowering Therapy

Diabetics have more atherogenic lipid patterns than nondiabetics (Sam et al., 2008), and a strong argument has been made for routine use of a statin in all diabetics regardless of lipid levels (Howard et al., 2008). In a study of 2,838 type 2 diabetics, those given atorvastatin 10 mg a day had a 37% reduction in major cardiovascular risk compared to those given placebo and the protection was almost the same in those without elevated lipids as in those with dyslipidemia (Colhoun et al., 2004).

Other Drugs

The same benefits of thiazolidinediones (Sarafidis et al., 2004) and metformin (Manzella et al., 2004) have been seen in diabetes as with the Metabolic Syndrome.

Recall the 5-fold increase in angioedema when an ACEI is combined with a gliptin (Brown et al., 2009).

Dyslipidemia

Although other drugs are sometimes needed, statins are the mainstay of therapy for dyslipidemia. The protection against coronary disease provided by statins is in keeping with the known close association between dyslipidemia and coronary atherosclerosis. However, the almost equal protection against stroke, 21% in a meta-analysis (Amarenco et al., 2004), was unexpected since dyslipidemia is so much less of a risk factor for stroke. One possibility is that statins lower BP. In a meta-analysis of 20 trials with statins including 828 patients, the mean fall in BP was –1.9/–0.9 mm Hg but –4.0/–1.2 in those with hypertension (Strazzullo et al., 2007). However, Trompet et al. (2008) found no effect on BP in the PROSPER trial whereas atorvastatin was markedly effective in the ASCOT trial (Sever et al., 2009).

Since hypertensives are, by definition, at higher risk, an argument can be made that virtually all should receive a statin or other therapy to improve their lipid profile, regardless of what it is. In a meta-analysis of 14 large trials, the cardiovascular benefits of statins were shown to be the same in hypertensives as in normotensives (Messerli et al., 2008b).

Patients with Existing Cardiovascular-Renal Disease

Left Ventricular Hypertrophy

Whether detected by electrocardiography or more sensitive echocardiography, LVH is a significant risk factor. There is now convincing evidence that the risks are reduced by regression of LVH (Okin et al., 2004; Verdecchia et al., 2003; Wachtell et al., 2007). For unknown reasons, women achieve less regression with antihypertensive therapy (Okin et al., 2008).

Any drug that reduces BP will regress LVH except for naked direct vasodilators. Better and equal results have been seen with ACEIs, ARBs, and CCBs, whereas less regression has been seen with diuretics and β-blockers (Klingbeil et al., 2003). Beyond regression of LVH, the persistence of wall motion abnormalities during treatment increases the risk of cardiovascular events (Cicala et al., 2008).

Coronary Artery Disease

The 2007 guidelines from an expert committee of the American Heart Association covered the various presentations of CAD (Rosendorff et al., 2007). These are the recommended targets for BP: less than 140/90 mm Hg for general CAD prevention; less than 130/80 mm Hg for high CAD risk, including stable angina; less than 120/80 mm Hg for left ventricular dysfunction or heart failure.

Heart Failure

Elderly hypertensives have a high prevalence of LV diastolic dysfunction, present in 25.8% of 2545 patients studied in Italy (Zanchetti et al., 2007). There are inadequate data on the benefits of treating LV diastolic dysfunction, but the evidence for treatment of systolic dysfunction is unequivocal. Long-acting ACEIs are more beneficial than either captopril or enalapril (Pilote et al., 2008). Aldosterone blockade is particularly indicated for post-MI patients with LV dysfunction (Pitt et al., 2008).

Atrial Fibrillation

The most common cardiac arrhythmia, AF, is even more common in hypertensive patients. Novo et al. (2008) state: "Although many studies and meta-analyses have supported the advantage of RAS blockade in preventing AF recurrence, it is premature to recommend the use of ACEIs and ARBs specifically for the prevention of AF." Valsartan has been shown to be in effective (GISSI-AF, 2009).

Cerebrovascular Disease

Stroke is becoming more common as people live longer and develop systolic hypertension, as noted in Chapter 4. Fortunately, antihypertensive therapy has its greatest protective effect against stroke, as noted in Chapter 5. However, as with all hypertension-related conditions, the strong evidence has elicited only a weak response: many stroke survivors, known to be at very high risk for recurrence are not being adequately protected (Touzé et al., 2008).

Since the pathogenesis of stroke and the overall value of lowering BP have been covered in Chapters 4 and 5, we will provide only reminders about primary preventive measures and focus on treatment in the acute phase and long-term secondary prevention.

Prevention

Adoption of a healthy lifestyle is beneficial. In a large observational study, those who adhered to a healthy lifestyle, composed of five features—not smoking, nonobese, physically active, moderate alcohol consumption, and a lower fat, higher fruit and vegetable diet—had a phenomenally lower risk of stroke, 79% lower for women, 69% lower for men, compared to those who had none of these features (Chiuve et al., 2008).

Beyond lifestyle changes, hypertension must be adequately controlled (Pedelty & Gorelick, 2008). There remains controversy as to how best to treat for primary prevention of stroke. Most believe that a lower BP, regardless of how it is lowered, is the primary protector (Wang et al., 2007a). However, as described earlier in this chapter, a rather persuasive argument has been presented that drugs which *increase* blood angiotensin II levels are better than those which *decrease* blood AII levels (Boutite et al., 2007).

Despite some experimental evidence in support of the position of Boutite et al. (Li et al., 2008), the results of the ONTARGET trial weaken their argument, since an ACEI ramipril, was equally effective in reducing stroke as an ARB, telmisartan (ONTARGET Investigators, 2008). Moreover, an ARB was not better than a placebo in the PROFESS trial of stroke survivors who where intolerant to ACEIs (Yusuf et al., 2008).

Statin therapy reduces the risk of stroke (Nassief & Marsh, 2008) without, as feared, an increase in intracranial hemorrhage (FitzMaurice et al., 2008).

Acute Stroke

Once a stroke begins, outcomes are improved with rapid hospitalization in a facility with brain-imaging equipment and a stroke unit, where thrombolysis with intra-arterial or intravenous tPA is available (Adams et al., 2007; Swain et al., 2008).

More than 60% of stroke patients have an acute hypertensive response above premorbid levels within the first 24 hours (Qureshi, 2008). Guidelines for treatment to lower this acutely elevated pressure have been very conservative because of concern that immediate lowering of BP may increase the extent of brain damage (Adams et al., 2007). However, this hesitation is relieved if the patient is a candidate for thrombolysis since the persistence of BP above 185/110 mm Hg is a contraindication to thrombolysis (Qureshi, 2008) (Fig. 7-23).

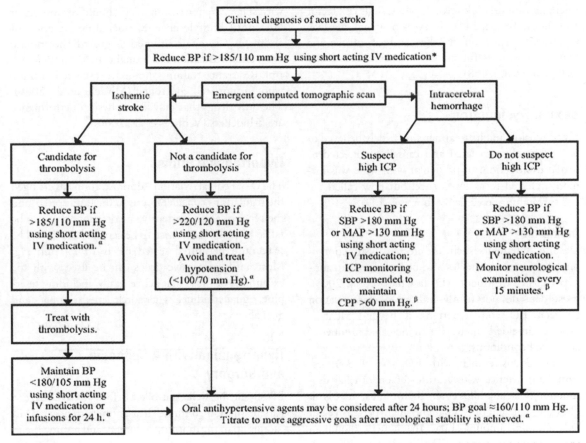

FIGURE 7-23   Algorithm for treatment of acute hypertensive response among patients with stroke and stroke subtypes. IV indicates intravenous; SBP, systolic BP; DBP, diastolic BP; and CPP, cerebral perfusion pressure. (Reproduced from Quershi. Acute hypertensive responses in patients with stroke. *Circulation* 2008;118:176–187, with permission.)

Sare et al. (2008) state that "There is little existing evidence that antihypertensive agents reduce cerebral blood flow in spite of their effects on lowering blood pressure." Therefore, careful but persistent lowering of elevated BP has been performed acutely in patients with both ischemic and hemorrhagic stroke with generally positive results (Adams et al., 2009; Eveson et al., 2007).

A large number of ongoing trials are examining this issue and others in the management of acute stroke (see the journal *Stroke* for a listing).

Poststroke Management

The evidence for secondary prevention of recurrent stroke by antihypertensive therapy is strong. The HYVET Trial found that such protection extends to those over age 80 (Beckett et al., 2008). In addition, aspirin, statins, and control of other risk factors are recommended (Sacco et al., 2006). Although markers of poor prognosis are being proposed (Ovbiagele et al., 2008; Yip et al., 2008), they seem to be unnecessary. All patients with prior TIA or stroke should be intensively treated and carefully followed.

Peripheral Vascular Disease

Because ACEIs, ARBs, and CCBs have been shown to normalize endothelial dysfunction and vascular remodeling in arteries from hypertensive patients (Park & Schiffrin, 2000), they are the logical choices in patients with concomitant peripheral vascular disease.

Renal Disease

Because there are so many facets to hypertension in renal disease, Chapter 9 covers that combination in depth. Two points seem worth mentioning here: first, the presence of renal dysfunction complicates the treatment of hypertension (Sica, 2008b), and second, microalbuminuria is known to be a serious risk factor and should be looked for in every new hypertensive; if present, reduction in the level of proteinuria may serve as a useful marker of successful therapy (Jefferson et al., 2008).

Sexual Dysfunction

Hypertension and its treatment are widely believed to be commonly associated and causally connected to sexual dysfunction, in particular with what was formerly referred to as impotence, but now called the less threatening "erectile dysfunction (ED)."

Incidence

Despite statements such as "erectile dysfunction is one of the major obstacles for noncompliance in antihypertensive treatment" (Della Chiesa et al., 2003), most data do not firmly indicate a close relation between ED and hypertension beyond what is expected in elderly men with an increased number of comorbid conditions.

Hypertensive men with ED have thicker, less compliant arteries with features of endothelial dysfunction (Vlachopoulos et al., 2008). Thus, there is no question that a lot of ED patients are hypertensive but only a modest amount of data that hypertension is an independent predictor of ED (Russell et al., 2004).

Treatment

If an antihypertensive drug is thought to induce ED (perhaps by further lowering arterial pressure into the sclerotic genital vessels), that drug should be stopped and another from a different class given in small dose to gradually lower BP.

If no reversible cause is found, a phosphodiesterase-5 inhibitor can be safely given with an expectation of return of erectile function in 50% to 70% (Kloner, 2004). Caution about hypotension is needed if nitrates or α-blockers are being used.

Competitive Athletes

Competitive athletes may be anxious during their precompetition exam, and therefore may have "white-coat hypertension." If found to be hypertensive, they should obtain out-of-office readings. Those with persistent stage 1 hypertension should have a more complete workup perhaps to include an echocardiogram, but need not be limited in their training or competition (Kaplan et al., 2005). Those

with stage 2 hypertension likely should be limited, at least until lifestyle changes (including cessation of androgens, sympathomimetics, growth hormones, etc.), and medication has brought the BP under control. Resistance training should be restricted in those who are not well controlled (Miyachi et al., 2004). The only drugs that may limit physical performance are β-blockers (Vanhees et al., 2000).

Hypertensive Pilots

The U.S. Federal Aviation Administration has changed the regulations considerably as to the limits of BP and the types of antihypertensive medications that can be taken by people who wish to be certified as pilots. The maximum permitted seated BP is 155/95 mm Hg. Most antihypertensive drugs can be used, with the exceptions of those that act centrally, including reserpine, guanethidine, guanadrel, methyldopa, and guanabenz.

Hypertension with Anesthesia and Surgery

BP should be well controlled before elective surgery. Patients should continue their antihypertensive medications up to the morning of surgery and resume them, either orally or intravenously, as soon as possible postoperative (Auerback & Goldman, 2006). β-Blockers are often given preoperatively to patients at high risk for atherosclerotic disease. However, in a RCT of 8,351 such patients, the half given extended-release metoprolol 2 to 4 hours before surgery and for 30 days thereafter had fewer cardiac events but more strokes and more deaths (POISE Study Group, 2008). On the other hand, in a series of trials called DECREASE, a small dose of bisoprolol was started at least 7 days before surgery and titrated to achieve a heart rate of 50 to 65/minute. The results showed a decrease in perioperative cardiac events, but a slight increase in strokes (Fleisher & Poldermans, 2008). These authors recommend that a low dose of β-blocker titrated to full effect be started at least 7 days preoperative.

Caution is advised in patients taking an ACEI or ARB. Arora et al. (2008) found a 27.6% increased risk of acute kidney failure in a retrospective cohort study of 1,358 patients who underwent cardiac surgery soon after being on these drugs.

If hypertension needs to be treated during surgery, intravenous labetalol, nitroprusside, nicardipine, or esmolol can be used (see Chapter 8).

Postoperative hypertension is usually precipitated by volume overload, pain, or agitation. For those in need of postoperative BP reduction, parenteral forms of various agents, including the short-acting β-blocker esmolol, labetalol, or nicardipine can be used. Special problems in postoperative patients after coronary bypass surgery, trauma, and burns are covered in Chapter 14. Anesthetic considerations in patients with pheochromocytoma are covered in Chapter 12.

Postoperatively, significant lowering of BP may occur as a nonspecific response to surgery and may persist for months (Volini & Flaxman, 1939). Do not be deceived by what appears to be an improvement in the patient's hypertension: Anticipate a gradual return to preoperative levels.

PREVENTION OF HYPERTENSION

Two trials have examined the ability to prevent progression of high-normal BP (130 to 139/85 to 89 mm Hg) to above 140/90 mm Hg (Julius et al., 2006; Luders et al., 2008). In these trials the BP was lowered with an ARB (candesartan) by Julius et al. and an ACEI (ramipril) by Luders et al. In both trials, the BP remained below 140/90 mm Hg during the time of drug intake but in most subjects followed after the drug was stopped, it rose to above 140/90 mm Hg.

Prevention of future hypertension has been shown in spontaneously hypertensive rats (who all become hypertensive after 20 weeks of age) by giving them an ACEI for as short a time of 2 weeks but only if they were treated before 20 weeks of age (Smallegange et al., 2004). That would translate into treating humans during adolescence to prevent future hypertension. Waiting until the subjects are in their 40s to 70s as done by Julius et al. and Luders et al. may be much too late. Such a study in humans young enough to be protected may not be feasible.

CONCLUSION

The large numbers of drugs now available can be used to treat virtually every hypertensive patient successfully under most any circumstance. Perhaps of even greater eventual value will be the treatment of prehypertensives to prevent the onset of hypertension, only now being examined. Meanwhile, even those at highest risk—the few who develop a hypertensive emergency—can be effectively treated, as is described in the next chapter.

REFERENCES

Abernethy DR, Schwartz JB. Calcium-antagonist drugs. *N Engl J Med* 1999;341:1447–1457.

Achari R, Hosmane B, Bonacci E, et al. The relationship between terazosin dose and blood pressure response in hypertensive patients. *J Clin Pharmacol* 2000;40:1166–1172.

Adams HP Jr, del ZG, Alberts MJ, et al. Guidelines for the early management of adults with ischemic stroke. *Stroke* 2007;38: 1655–1711.

Agodoa LY, Appel L, Bakris GL, et al. Effect of ramipril vs amlodipine on renal outcomes in hypertensive nephrosclerosis. *JAMA* 2001;285:2719–2728.

Ahmed A, Husain A, Love TE, et al. Heart failure, chronic diuretic use, and increase in mortality and hospitalization: An observational study using propensity score methods. *Eur Heart J* 2006;27:1431–1439.

Aksnes TA, Flaa A, Strand A, et al. Prevention of new-onset atrial fibrillation and its predictors with angiotensin II-receptor blockers in the treatment of hypertension and heart failure. *J Hypertens* 2007a;25.15–23.

Aksnes TA, Kjeldsen SE, Rostrup M, et al. Impact of new-onset diabetes mellitus on cardiac outcomes in the Valsartan Antihypertensive Long-term Use Evaluation (VALUE) trial population. *Hypertension* 2007b;50:467–473.

Aksnes TA, Kjeldsen SE, Rostrup M, et al. Predictors of new-onset diabetes mellitus in hypertensive patients: The VALUE trial. *J Hum Hypertens* 2008;22:520–527.

Aksnes N, Wahlgren N, Brainin M, et al. Relationship of blood pressure, antihypertensive therapy, and outcome in ischemic stroke treated with intravenous thrombolysis: retrospective analysis from Safe Implementation of Thrombolysis in Stroke-International Stroke Thrombolysis Register (SITS-ISTR). *Stroke* 2009;40:2442–2449.

ALLHAT Officers and Coordinators for the ALLHAT Collaborative Research Group. Major cardiovascular events in hypertensive patients randomized to doxazosin vs chlorthalidone. *JAMA* 2000;283:1967–1975.

ALLHAT Officers and Coordinators for the ALLHAT Collaborative Research Group. The Antihypertensive and Lipid-Lowering Treatment to Prevent Heart Attack Trial. Major outcomes in high-risk hypertensive patients randomized to angiotensin-converting enzyme inhibitor or calcium channel blocker vs diuretic: The Antihypertensive and Lipid-Lowering Treatment to Prevent Heart Attack Trial (ALLHAT). *JAMA* 2002;288: 2981–2997.

Almgren T, Wilhelmsen L, Samuelsson O, et al. Diabetes in treated hypertension is common and carries a high cardiovascular risk: Results from a 28-year follow-up. *J Hypertens* 2007;25: 1311–1317.

Amar J, Cambou JP, Touze E, et al. Comparison of hypertension management after stroke and myocardial infarction: Results from ECLAT1—a French nationwide study. *Stroke* 2004; 35: 1579–1583.

Amar J, Chamontin B, Genes N, et al. Why is hypertension so frequently uncontrolled in secondary prevention? *J Hypertens* 2003;21:1199–1205.

Amarenco P, Labreuche J, Lavallee P, et al. Statins in stroke prevention and carotid atherosclerosis: Systematic review and up-to-date meta-analysis. *Stroke* 2004;35:2902–2909.

American Diabetes Association. Standards of medical care in diabetes-2008. *Diabetes Care* 2008;31:524–526.

Anderson C. Neuroprotection by angiotensin receptor blockers? *J Hypertens* 2008;26:853.

Anderson J, Godfrey BE, Hill DM, et al. A comparison of the effects of hydrochlorothiazide and of furosemide in the treatment of hypertensive patients. *QJM* 1971;40:541–560.

Ando H, Zhou J, Macova M, et al. Angiotensin II AT1 receptor blockade reverses pathological hypertrophy and inflammation in brain microvessels of spontaneously hypertensive rats. *Stroke* 2004;35:1726–1731.

Andrén L, Weiner L, Svensson A, et al. Enalapril with either a "very low" or "low" dose of hydrochlorothiazide is equally effective in essential hypertension. *J Hypertens* 1983;1: 384–386.

Angeli F, Verdecchia P, Reboldi GP, et al. Calcium channel blockade to prevent stroke in hypertension: A meta-analysis of 13 studies with 103, 793 subjects. *Am J Hypertens* 2004;17: 817–822.

Appel LJ, Wright JT Jr, Greene T, et al. Long-term effects of renin-angiotensin system-blocking therapy and a low blood pressure goal on progression of hypertensive chronic kidney disease in African Americans. *Arch Intern Med* 2008;168: 832–839.

Apperloo AJ, de Zeeuw D, de Jong PE. A short-term antihypertensive treatment-induced fall in glomerular filtration rate predicts long-term stability of renal function. *Kidney Int* 1997;51: 793–797.

Armstrong B, Stevens N, Doll R. Retrospective study of the association between use of rauwolfia derivatives and breast cancer in English women. *Lancet* 1974;21;672–675.

Arora P, Rajagopalam S, Ranjan R, et al. Preoperative use of angiotensin-converting enzyme inhibitors/angiotensin receptor blockers is associated with increased risk for acute kidney injury after cardiovascular surgery. *Clin J Am Soc Nephrol* 2008;3:1266–1273.

Arroll B, Kenealy T, Elley CR. Should we prescribe diuretics for patients with prediabetes and hypertension? *Br Med J* 2008; 337:a679.

Auerbach A, Goldman L. Assessing and reducing the cardiac risk of noncardiac surgery. *Circulation* 2006;113:1361–1376.

Azizi M, Menard J. Combined blockade of the renin-angiotensin system with angiotensin-converting enzyme inhibitors and angiotensin II type 1 receptor antagonists. *Circulation* 2004;109:2492–2499.

Bagger JP, Helligsoe P, Randsback F, et al. Effect of verapamil in intermittent claudication. *Circulation* 1997;95:411–414.

Bahlmann FH, de Groot K, Mueller O, et al. Stimulation of endothelial progenitor cells: A new putative therapeutic effect of angiotensin II receptor antagonists. *Hypertension* 2005;45: 526–529.

Bailey DG, Dresser GK, Kreeft JH, et al. Grapefruit-felodipine interaction. *Clin Pharmacol Ther* 2000;68:468–477.

Baker EH, Duggal A, Dong Y, et al. Amiloride, a specific drug for hypertension in black people with T594M variant? *Hypertension* 2002;40:13–17.

Bakris GL, Fonseca V, Katholi RE, et al. Metabolic effects of carvedilol vs metoprolol in patients with type 2 diabetes mellitus and hypertension: A randomized controlled trial. *JAMA* 2004;292:2227–2236.

Bakris GL, Weir MR. Angiotensin-converting enzyme inhibitor-associated elevations in serum creatinine. *Arch Intern Med* 2000;160:685–693.

Bakris GL, Weir MR, Shanifar S, et al. Effects of blood pressure level on progression of diabetic nephropathy: Results from the RENAAL study. *Arch Intern Med* 2003;163:1555–1565.

Bangalore S, Messerli FH, Cohen JD, et al. Verapamil-sustained release-based treatment strategy is equivalent to atenolol-based treatment strategy at reducing cardiovascular events in patients with prior myocardial infarction: An INternational VErapamil SR-Trandolapril (INVEST) substudy. *Am Heart J* 2008a;156: 241–247.

Bangalore S, Messerli FH, Kostis JB, et al. Cardiovascular protection using beta-blockers: A critical review of the evidence. *J Am Coll Cardiol* 2007a;50:563–572.

Bangalore S, Sawhney S, Messerli FH. Relation of beta-blocker-induced heart rate lowering and cardioprotection in hypertension. *J Am Coll Cardiol* 2008b;52:1482–1489.

Bangalore S, Shahane A, Parkar S, et al. Compliance and fixed-dose combination therapy. *Hypertension* 2007b;49:272–275.

Batey DM, Nicolich MJ, Lasser VI, et al. Prazosin versus hydrochlorothiazide as initial antihypertensive therapy in black versus white patients. *Am J Med* 1989;86:74–78.

Batkai S, Pacher P, Osei-Hyiaman D, et al. Endocannabinoids acting at cannabinoid-1 receptors regulate cardiovascular function in hypertension. *Circulation* 2004;110:1996–2002.

Bautista LE. Predictors of persistence with antihypertensive therapy: Results from the NHANES. *Am J Hypertens* 2008;21: 183–188.

Beckett NS, Peters R, Fletcher AE, et al. Treatment of hypertension in patients 80 years of age or older. *N Engl J Med* 2008;358: 1887–1898.

Bell CM, Hatch WV, Fischer HD, et al. Association between tamsulosin and serious ophthalmic adverse events in older men follwing cataract surgery. *JAMA* 2009;301:1991–1996.

Benndorf RA, Boger RH. Pleiotropic effects of telmisartan: Still more to come? *J Hypertens* 2008;26:854–856.

Benson SC, Pershadsingh HA, Ho CI, et al. Identification of telmisartan as a unique angiotensin II receptor antagonist with selective PPARgamma-modulating activity. *Hypertension* 2004;43: 993–1002.

Berl T. Maximizing inhibition of the renin-angiotensin system with high doses of converting enzyme inhibitors or angiotensin receptor blockers. *Nephrol Dial Transplant* 2008;23:2443–2447.

Bhatia BB. On the use of rauwolfia serpentina in high blood pressure. *J Ind Med Assoc* 1942;11:262–265.

Birkenhäger WH, Staessen JA. Dual inhibition of the renin system by aliskiren and valsartan. *Lancet* 2007;370:195–196.

Black HR. Evolving role of aldosterone blockers alone and in combination with angiotensin-converting enzyme inhibitors or angiotensin II receptor blockers in hypertension management: A review of mechanistic and clinical data. *Am Heart J* 2004;147: 564–572.

Black HR, Davis B, Barzilay J, et al. Metabolic and clinical outcomes in nondiabetic individuals with the metabolic syndrome assigned to chlorthalidone, amlodipine, or lisinopril as initial treatment for hypertension: A report from the Antihypertensive and Lipid-Lowering Treatment to Prevent Heart Attack Trial (ALLHAT). *Diabetes Care* 2008;31:353–360.

Black JW, Crowther AF, Shanks RG, et al. A new adrenergic beta-receptor antagonist. *Lancet* 1964;2:1080–1081.

Black RN, Hunter SJ, Atkinson AB. Usefulness of the vasodilator minoxidil in resistant hypertension. *J Hypertens* 2007;25: 1102–1103.

Blood Pressure Lowering Treatment Trialists' Collaboration. Effects of different blood-pressure-lowering regimens on major cardiovascular events: Results of prospectively-designed overviews of randomised trials. *Lancet* 2003;362:1527–1535.

Blood Pressure Trialist. Blood pressure-dependent and independent effects of agents that inhibit the renin-angiotensin system. *J Hypertens* 2007;25:951–958.

Blood Pressure Trialist. Effects of different regimens to lower blood pressure on major cardiovascular events in older and younger adults: Meta-analysis of randomised trials. *Br Med J* 2008;336: 1121–1123.

Bodineau L, Frugiere A, Marc Y, et al. Orally active aminopeptidase A inhibitors reduce blood pressure: A new strategy for treating hypertension. *Hypertension* 2008;51:1318–1325.

Boersma C, Carides GW, Atthobari J, et al. An economic assessment of losartan-based versus atenolol-based therapy in patients with hypertension and left-ventricular hypertrophy: Results from the Losartan Intervention For Endpoint reduction (LIFE) study adapted to the Netherlands. *Clin Ther* 2007;29:963–971.

Boersma C, Postma MJ, Visser ST, et al. Baseline albuminuria predicts the efficacy of blood pressure-lowering drugs in preventing cardiovascular events. *Br J Clin Pharmacol* 2008;65: 723–732.

Bond WS. Psychiatric indications for clonidine. *J Clin Psychopharmacol* 1986;6:81–87.

Borzecki AM, Glickman ME, Kader B, et al. The effect of age on hypertension control and management. *Am J Hypertens* 2006;19: 520–527.

Bosworth HB, Olsen MK, Oddone EZ. Improving blood pressure control by tailored feedback to patients and clinicians. *Am Heart J* 2005;149:795–803.

Boutitie F, Oprisiu R, Achard JM, et al. Does a change in angiotensin II formation caused by antihypertensive drugs affect the risk of stroke? A meta-analysis of trials according to treatment with potentially different effects on angiotensin II. *J Hypertens* 2007;25:1543–1553.

Brater DC. Pharmacokinetics and pharmacodynamics of torasemide in health and disease. *J Cardiovasc Pharmacol* 1993; 22(Suppl. 3):S24–S31.

Brater DC. Pharmacology of diuretics. *Am J Med Sci* 2000;319: 38–50.

Brater DC, Chennavasin P, Day B, et al. Bumetanide and furosemide. *Clin Pharm Ther* 1983;34:207–213.

Brenner BM, Cooper ME, de Zeeuw D, et al. Effects of losartan on renal and cardiovascular outcomes in patients with type 2 diabetes and nephropathy. *N Engl J Med* 2001;345: 861–869.

Brewster LM, van Montfrans GA, Kleijnen J. Systematic review: Antihypertensive drug therapy in black patients. *Ann Intern Med* 2004;141:614–627.

Brooke BS, Habashi JP, Judge DP, et al. Angiotensin II blockade and aortic-root dilation in Marfan's syndrome. *N Engl J Med* 2008;358:2787–2795.

Brown MA, Buddle ML, Martin A. Is resistant hypertension really resistant? *Am J Hypertens* 2001;14:1263–1269.

Brown MJ. Aliskiren. *Circulation* 2008;118:773–784.

Brown MJ, Brown J. Does angiotensin-II protect against strokes? *Lancet* 1986;2:427–429.

Brown MJ, Cruickshank JK, Dominiczak AF, et al. Better blood pressure control: How to combine drugs. *J Hum Hypertens* 2003;17:81–86.

Brown NJ, Byiers S, Carr D, et al. Dipeptidyl peptidase-IV inhibitor use associated with increased risk of ACE inhibitor-associated angioedema. *Hypertension* 2009;54:514–523.

Brown NJ, Vaughan DE. Angiotensin-converting enzyme inhibitors. *Circulation* 1998;97:1411–1420.

Brunner F, Kukovetz WR. Postischemic antiarrhythmic effects of angiotensin-converting enzyme inhibitors. *Circulation* 1996; 94:1752–1761.

Bühler FR, Laragh JH, Baer L, et al. Propranolol inhibition of renin secretion. *N Engl J Med* 1972;287:1209–1214.

Burgess E. Slowing the progression of kidney disease in patients with diabetes. *J Am Soc Hypertens* 2008;2:S30–S37.

Burnett JC Jr. Vasopeptidase inhibition: A new concept in blood pressure management. *J Hypertens* 1999;17(Suppl. 1): S37–S43.

Burnier M. Angiotensin II type 1 receptor blockers. *Circulation* 2001;103:904–912.

Burnier M, Brunner HR. Angiotensin II receptor antagonists. *Lancet* 2000;355:637–645.

Burton TJ, Wilkinson IB. The dangers of immediate-release nifedipine in the emergency treatment of hypertension. *J Hum Hypertens* 2008;22:301–302.

Byrd BF III, Collins HW, Primm RK. Risk factors for severe bradycardia during oral clonidine therapy for hypertension. *Arch Intern Med* 1988;148:729–733.

Calhoun DA, Jones C, Textor S, et al. Resistant hypertension: Diagnosis, evaluation, and treatment. *Hypertension* 2008;51: 1403–1419.

Cameron HA, Ramsay LE. The lupus syndrome induced by hydralazine. *Br Med J* 1984;289:410–412.

Campbell DJ, Krum H, Esler MD. Losartan increases bradykinin levels in hypertensive humans. *Circulation* 2005;111:315–320.

Canzanello VJ, Baranco-Pryor E, Rahbari-Oskoui F, et al. Predictors of blood pressure response to the angiotensin receptor blocker candesartan in essential hypertension. *Am J Hypertens* 2008;21:66.

Carlberg B, Samuelsson O, Lindholm LH. Atenolol in hypertension: Is it a wise choice? *Lancet* 2004;364:1684–1689.

Carlsen JE, Køber L, Torp-Pedersen C, et al. Relation between dose of bendrofluazide, antihypertensive effect, and adverse biochemical effects. *Br Med J* 1990;300:974–978.

Carter BL, Bergus GR, Dawson JD, et al. A cluster randomized trial to evaluate physician/pharmacist collaboration to improve blood pressure control. *J Clin Hypertens (Greenwich)* 2008a;10: 260–271.

Carter BL, Einhorn PT, Brands M, et al. Thiazide-induced dysglycemia: Call for research from a working group from the national heart, lung, and blood institute. *Hypertension* 2008b; 52:30–36.

Carter BL, Lund BC, Hayase N, et al. A longitudinal analysis of antihypertensive drug interactions in a Medicaid population. *Am J Hypertens* 2004;17:421–427.

Casas JP, Chua W, Loukogeorgakis S, et al. Effect of inhibitors of the renin-angiotensin system and other antihypertensive drugs on renal outcomes: Systematic review and meta-analysis. *Lancet* 2005;366:2026–2033.

CDC Diabetes Cost-effectiveness Group. Cost-effectiveness of intensive glycemic control, intensified hypertension control, and serum cholesterol level reduction for type 2 diabetes. *JAMA* 2002;287:2542–2551.

Celis H, Thijs L, Staessen JA, et al. Interaction between nonsteroidal anti-inflammatory drug intake and calcium-channel blocker-based antihypertensive treatment in the Syst-Eur trial. *J Hum Hypertens* 2001;15:613–618.

Chapman AB, Schwartz GL, Boerwinkle E, et al. Predictors of antihypertensive response to a standard dose of hydrochlorothiazide for essential hypertension. *Kidney Int* 2002;61: 1047–1055.

Chapman N, Chang CL, Dahlof B, et al. Effect of doxazosin gastrointestinal therapeutic system as third-line antihypertensive therapy on blood pressure and lipids in the Anglo-Scandinavian Cardiac Outcomes Trial. *Circulation* 2008;118:42–48.

Chapman N, Dobson J, Wilson S, et al. Effect of spironolactone on blood pressure in subjects with resistant hypertension. *Hypertension* 2007;49:839–845.

Chen Y, Lasaitiene D, Gabrielsson BG, et al. Neonatal losartan treatment suppresses renal expression of molecules involved in cell-cell and cell-matrix interactions. *J Am Soc Nephrol* 2004;15:1232–1243.

Cheng A, Frishman WH. Use of angiotensin-converting enzyme inhibitors as monotherapy and in combination with diuretics and calcium channel blockers. *J Clin Pharmacol* 1998;38:477–491.

Cheng HF, Harris RC. Cyclooxygenases, the kidney, and hypertension. *Hypertension* 2004;43:525–530.

Cherry DK, Hing E, Woodwell DA. *National Ambulatory Medical Care Survey 2006 Summary. National Health Statistics Reports; No. 3.* Hyattsville, MD: National Center for Health Statistics; 2008.

Cheung DG, Hoffman CA, Ricci ST, et al. Mild hypertension in the elderly. *Am J Med* 1989;86:87–90.

Chiasson JL, Josse RG, Gomis R, et al. Acarbose treatment and the risk of cardiovascular disease and hypertension in patients with impaired glucose tolerance: The STOP-NIDDM trial. *JAMA* 2003;290:486–494.

Chillon JM, Baumbach GL. Effects of indapamide, a thiazide-like diuretic, on structure of cerebral arterioles in hypertensive rats. *Hypertension* 2004;43:1092–1097.

Chiuve SE, Rexrode KM, Spiegelman D, et al. Primary prevention of stroke by healthy lifestyle. *Circulation* 2008;118:947–954.

Chobanian AV. Does it matter how hypertension is controlled? *N Engl J Med* 2008;359:2485–2485.

Chobanian AV, Bakris GL, Black HR, et al. Seventh report of the Joint National Committee on Prevention, Detection, Evaluation, and Treatment of High Blood Pressure. *Hypertension* 2003;42:1206–1252.

Chun TY, Bankir L, Eckert GJ, et al. Ethnic differences in renal responses to furosemide. *Hypertension* 2008;52:241–248.

Cicala S, de SG, Wachtell K, et al. Clinical impact of "in-treatment" wall motion abnormalities in hypertensive patients with left ventricular hypertrophy: The LIFE study. *J Hypertens* 2008;26:806–812.

Cipollone F, Fazia M, Iezzi A, et al. Blockade of the angiotensin II type 1 receptor stabilizes atherosclerotic plaques in humans by inhibiting prostaglandin E2-dependent matrix metalloproteinase activity. *Circulation* 2004;109:1482–1488.

Clark JA, Zimmerman HJ, Tanner LA. Labetalol hepatotoxicity. *Ann Intern Med* 1990;113:210–213.

Clobass Study Group. Low-dose clonidine administration in the treatment of mild or moderate essential hypertension. *J Hypertens* 1990;8:539–546.

Coca SG, Perazella MA, Buller GK. The cardiovascular implications of hypokalemia. *Am J Kidney Dis* 2005;45:233–247.

Cohen DL, Townsend RR. Should we be treating blood pressure more aggressively and earlier after acute stroke? *J Clin Hypertens (Greenwich)* 2008;10:504–505.

Cohn JN, Anand IS, Latini R, et al. Sustained reduction of aldosterone response in response to the angiotensin receptor blocker valsartan in patients with chronic heart failure: Results of the Valsartan Heart Failure Trial. *Circulation* 2003;108:1306–1309.

Colhoun HM, Betteridge DJ, Durrington PN, et al. Primary prevention of cardiovascular disease with atorvastatin in type 2 diabetes in the Collaborative Atorvastatin Diabetes Study (CARDS): Multicentre randomised placebo-controlled trial. *Lancet* 2004;364:685–696.

Conlin PR, Gerth WC, Fox J, et al. Four-year persistence patterns among patients initiating therapy with the angiotensin II receptor antagonist losartan versus other artihypertensive drug classes. *Clin Ther* 2001;23:1999–2010.

Conlin PR, Spence JD, Williams B, et al. Angiotensin II antagonists for hypertension: Are there differences in efficacy? *Am J Hypertens* 2000;13:418–426.

Conway J, Lauwers P. Hemodynamic and hypotensive effects of long-term therapy with chlorothiazide. *Circulation* 1960; 21:21–26.

Cooper WO, Hernandez-diaz S, Arbogast PG, et al. Major congenital malformations after first-trimester exposure to ACE inhibitors. *N Engl J Med* 2006;354:2443–2451.

Coulter DM. Eye pain with nifedipine and disturbance of taste with captopril. *Br Med J* 1988;296:1086–1088.

Coyle D, Rodby R, Soroka S, et al. Cost-effectiveness of irbesartan 300 mg given early versus late in patients with hypertension and a history of type 2 diabetes and renal disease: A Canadian perspective. *Clin Ther* 2007;29:1508–1523.

Cranston WI, Juel-Jensen BE, Semmence AM, et al. Effects of oral diuretics on raised arterial pressure. *Lancet* 1963;2:966–970.

Crowe E, Halpin D, Stevens P. Early identification and management of chronic kidney disease: Summary of NICE guidance. *Br Med J* 2008;337:a1530.

Cutler J, Sorlie P, Wolz M, et al. Trends in hypertension prevalence, awareness, treatment, and control rates in US adults between 1988–1994 and 1999–2004. *Hypertension* 2008;52:818–827.

Dahlöf B, Devereux RB, Kjeldsen SE, et al. Cardiovascular morbidity and mortality in the Losartan Intervention For Endpoint reduction in hypertension study (LIFE): A randomised trial against atenolol. *Lancet* 2002;359:995–1003.

Dahlöf B, Sever PS, Poulter NR, et al. Prevention of cardiovascular events with an antihypertensive regimen of amlodipine adding perindopril as required versus atenolol adding bendroflumethiazide as required, in the Anglo-Scandinavian Cardiac Outcomes Trial-Blood Pressure Lowering Arm (ASCOT-BPLA): A multicentre randomised controlled trial. *Lancet* 2005;366:895–906.

Damasceno A, Santos A, Pestana M, et al. Acute hypotensive, natriuretic, and hormonal effects of nifedipine in salt-sensitive and salt-resistant black normotensive and hypertensive subjects. *J Cardiovasc Pharmacol* 1999;34:346–353.

Dandona P, Kumar V, Aljada A, et al. Angiotensin II receptor blocker valsartan suppresses reactive oxygen species generation in leukocytes, nuclear factor-kappa B, in mononuclear cells of normal subjects: Evidence of an antiinflammatory action. *J Clin Endocrinol Metab* 2003;88:4496–4501.

Dang A, Zhang Y, Liu G, et al. Effects of losartan and irbesartan on serum uric acid in hypertensive patients with hyperuricaemia in Chinese population. *J Hum Hypertens* 2006;20:45–50.

Davies SJ, Jackson PR, Ramsay LE, et al. Drug intolerance due to nonspecific adverse effects related to psychiatric morbidity in hypertensive patients. *Arch Intern Med* 2003;163:592–600.

Davis BR, Piller LB, Cutler JA, et al. Role of diuretics in the prevention of heart failure: The Antihypertensive and Lipid-Lowering Treatment to Prevent Heart Attack Trial. *Circulation* 2006;113:2201–2210.

Deary AJ, Schumann AL, Murfet H, et al. Double-blind, placebo-controlled crossover comparison of five classes of antihypertensive drugs. *J Hypertens* 2002;20:771–777.

Della Chiesa A, Pfiffner D, Meier B, et al. Sexual activity in hypertensive men. *J Hum Hypertens* 2003;17:515–521.

Delles C, Klingbeil AU, Schneider MP, et al. Direct comparison of the effects of valsartan and amlodipine on renal hemodynamics in human essential hypertension. *Am J Hypertens* 2003;16:1030–1035.

Deng PY, Ye F, Cai WJ, et al. Stimulation of calcitonin gene-related peptide synthesis and release: Mechanisms for a novel antihypertensive drug, rutaecarpine. *J Hypertens* 2004;22:1819–1829.

Dhakam Z, Yasmin, McEniery CM, et al. A comparison of atenolol and nebivolol in isolated systolic hypertension. *J Hypertens* 2008;26:351–356.

Di Lenarda A, Remme WJ, Charlesworth A, et al. Exchange of beta-blockers in heart failure patients. Experiences from the poststudy phase of COMET investors. *Eur J Heart Fail* 2005;7(4):640–649.

Dickerson JE, Hingorani AD, Ashby MJ, et al. Optimisation of antihypertensive treatment by crossover rotation of four major classes. *Lancet* 1999;353:2008–2013.

Dietz JD, Du S, Bolten CW, et al. A number of marketed dihydropyridine calcium channel blockers have mineralocorticoid receptor antagonist activity. *Hypertension* 2008;51:742–748.

Diffey BL, Langtry J. Phototoxic potential of thiazide diuretics in normal subjects. *Arch Dermatol* 1989;125:1354–1358.

Donnelly R, Elliott HL, Meredith PA. Antihypertensive drugs: Individualized and clinical relevance of kinetic dynamic relationships. *Pharmacol Ther* 1992;53:67–79.

Doran T, Fullwood C, Gravelle H, et al. Pay-for-performance programs in family practices in the United Kingdom. *N Engl J Med* 2006;355:375–384.

Doty RL, Philip S, Reddy K, et al. Influences of antihypertensive and antihyperlipidemic drugs on the senses of taste and smell: A review. *J Hypertens* 2003;21:1805–1813.

Doty RL, Shah M, Bromley SM. Drug-induced taste disorders. *Drug Safety* 2008;31:199–215.

Dream Trial Investigators. Effect of ramipril on the incidence of diabetes. *N Engl J Med* 2006;355:1551–1562.

Dunn CJ, Fitton A, Brogden RN. Torasemide. *Drugs* 1995;49: 121–142.

Dupont AG, Van der Niepen P, Taeymans Y, et al. Effect of carvedilol on ambulatory blood pressure, renal hemodynamics, and cardiac function in essential hypertension. *J Cardiovasc Pharmacol* 1987;10(Suppl. 11):S130–S136.

Dykman D, Simon EE, Avioli LV. Hyperuricemia and uric acid nephropathy. *Arch Intern Med* 1987;147:1341–1345.

Eames PJ, Blake MJ, Panerai RB, et al. Cerebral autoregulation indices are unimpaired by hypertension in middle aged and older people. *Am J Hypertens* 2003;16:746–753.

Eisenberg MJ, Brox A, Bestawros AN. Calcium channel blockers: An update. *Am J Med* 2004;116:35–43.

Elewa HF, Kozak A, Johnson MH, et al. Blood pressure lowering after experimental cerebral ischemia provides neurovascular protection. *J Hypertens* 2007;25:855–859.

Elliott HL, Elawad M, Wilkinson R, et al. Persistence of antihypertensive efficacy after missed doses: Comparison of amlodipine and nifedipine gastrointestinal therapeutic system. *J Hypertens* 2002;20:333–338.

Elliott WJ, Polascik TB, Murphy MB. Equivalent antihypertensive effects of combination therapy using diuretic + calcium antagonist compared with diuretic + ACE inhibitor. *J Hum Hypertens* 1990;4:717–723.

Ellison DH. Diuretic resistance: Physiology and therapeutics. *Semin Nephrol* 1999;19:581–597.

Emeriau JP, Knauf H, Pujadas JO, et al. A comparison of indapamide SR 1.5 mg with both amlodipine 5 mg and hydrochlorothiazide 25 mg in elderly hypertensive patients. *J Hypertens* 2001;19:343–350.

Enseleit F, Luscher TF, Ruschitzka F. Darusentan: A new perspective for treatment of resistant hypertension? *Expert Opin Investig Drugs* 2008;17:1255–1263.

Erdös EG, Deddish PA, Marcic BM. Potentiation of bradykinin actions by ACE inhibitors. *Trends Endocrinol Metab* 1999;10:223–229.

Eriksson JW, Jansson PA, Carlberg B, et al. Hydrochlorothiazide, but not Candesartan,aggravates insulin resistance and causes visceral and hepatic fat accumulation: the mechanisms for the diabetes preventing effect of Candesartan (MEDICA) study. *Hypertension* 2008;52:1030–1037.

Ernst ME, Carter BL, Basile JN. All thiazide-like diuretics are not chlorthalidone: Putting the ACCOMPLISH study into perspective. *J Clin Hypertens* 2009;11:5–10.

Ernst ME, Carter BL, Goerdt CJ, et al. Comparative antihypertensive effects of hydrochlorothiazide and chlorthalidone on ambulatory and office blood pressure. *Hypertension* 2006;47: 352–358.

Esler M, Dudley F, Jennings G, et al. Increased sympathetic nervous activity and the effects of its inhibition with clonidine in alcoholic cirrhosis. *Ann Intern Med* 1992;116:446–455.

Esler M, Lux A, Jennings G, et al. Rilmenidine sympatholytic activity preserves mental stress, orthostatic sympathetic responses and adrenaline secretion. *J Hypertens* 2004;22:1529–1534.

Esposito K, Marfella R, Ciotola M, et al. Effect of a Mediterranean-style diet on endothelial dysfunction and markers of vascular inflammation in the metabolic syndrome: A randomized trial. *JAMA* 2004;292:1440–1446.

Eveson DJ, Robinson TG, Potter JF. Lisinopril for the treatment of hypertension within the first 24 hours of acute ischemic stroke and follow-up. *Am J Hypertens* 2007;20:270–277.

Fabia MJ, Abdilla N, Oltra R, et al. Antihypertensive activity of angiotensin II AT1 receptor antagonists: A systematic review of studies with 24 h ambulatory blood pressure monitoring. *J Hypertens* 2007;25:1327–1336.

Fakhouri F, Grunfeld JP, Hermine O, et al. Angiotensin-converting enzyme inhibitors for secondary erythrocytosis. *Ann Intern Med* 2004;140:492–493.

Faure S, Bureau A, Oudart N, et al. Protective effect of candesartan in experimental ischemic stroke in the rat mediated by AT2 and AT4 receptors. *J Hypertens* 2008;26:2008–2015.

Fedorak RN, Field M, Chang EB. Treatment of diabetic diarrhea with clonidine. *Ann Intern Med* 1985;102:197–199.

Feig DI, Kang Duk-Hee, Johnson RJ. Uric acid and cardiovascular risk. *N Engl J Med* 2008a;359:1811–1821.

Feig DI, Soletsky B, Johnson RJ. Effect of allopurinol on blood pressure of adolescents with newly diagnosed essential hypertension: A randomized trial. *JAMA* 2008b;300:924–932.

Feinstein AR. Scientific standards in epidemiologic studies of the menace of daily life. *Science* 1988;242:1257–1263.

Feldt S, Batenburg WW, Mazak I, et al. Prorenin and renin-induced extracellular signal-regulated kinase 1/2 activation in monocytes is not blocked by aliskiren or the handle-region peptide. *Hypertension* 2008;51:682–688.

Ferreira SH. A bradykinin-potentiating factor (BPF) present in the venom of *Bothrops jararaca*. *Br J Pharmacol* 1965;24: 163–169.

Finnerty FA Jr, Davidov M, Mroczek WJ, Gavrilovich L. Influence of extracellular fluid volume on response to anti-hypertensive drugs. *Circ Res* 1970;26(suppl 1):71–80.

Finkielman JD, Schwartz GL, Chapman AB, et al. Lack of agreement between office and ambulatory blood pressure responses to hydrochlorothiazide. *Am J Hypertens* 2005;18:398–402.

FitzMaurice E, Wendell L, Snider R, et al. Effect of statins on intracerebral hemorrhage outcome and recurrence. *Stroke* 2008;39:2151–2154.

Flack JM, Yunis C, Preisser J, et al. The rapidity of drug dose escalation influences blood pressure response and adverse effects burden in patients with hypertension. *Arch Intern Med* 2000;160:1842–1847.

Fleisher LA, Poldermans D. Perioperative beta blockade: Where do we go from here? *Lancet* 2008;371:1813–1814.

Fliser D, Buchholz K, Haller H. Antiinflammatory effects of angiotensin II subtype 1 receptor blockade in hypertensive patients with microinflammation. *Circulation* 2004;110: 1103–1107.

Flynn MA, Nolph GB, Baker AS, et al. Total body potassium in aging humans: A longitudinal study. *Am J Clin Nutr* 1989;50: 713–717.

Fogari R, Mugellini A, Zoppi A, et al. Effects of valsartan compared with enalapril on blood pressure and cognitive function in elderly patients with essential hypertension. *Eur J Clin Pharmacol* 2004;59:863–868.

Fogari R, Zoppi A, Tettamanti F, et al. Effects of nifedipine and indomethacin on cough induced by angiotensin-converting enzyme inhibitors. *J Cardiovasc Pharmacol* 1992;19:670–673.

Forette F, Seux ML, Staessen JA, et al. The prevention of dementia with antihypertensive treatment: New evidence from the Systolic Hypertension in Europe (Syst-Eur) study. *Arch Intern Med* 2002;162:2046–2052.

Fournier A, Messerli FH, Achard JM, et al. Cerebroprotection mediated by angiotensin II: A hypothesis supported by recent randomized clinical trials. *J Am Coll Cardiol* 2004;43: 1343–1347.

Franse LV, Pahor M, Di Bari M, et al. Hypokalemia associated with diuretic use and cardiovascular events in the Systolic Hypertension in the Elderly Program. *Hypertension* 2000;35:1025–1030.

Frassetto LA, Nash E, Morris RC Jr, et al. Comparative effects of potassium chloride and bicarbonate on thiazide-induced reduction in urinary calcium excretion. *Kidney Int* 2000; 58:748–752.

Frazier L, Turner ST, Schwartz GL, et al. Multilocus effects of the rennin-angiotensin-aldosterone system genes on blood pressure response to a thiazide diuretic. *Pharmacogenomics J.* 2004; 4:17–23.

Freeman R. Clinical practice. Neurogenic orthostatic hypotension. *N Engl J Med* 2008;358:615–624.

Freis ED, Reda DJ, Materson BJ. Volume (weight) loss and blood pressure response following thiazide diuretics. *Hypertension* 1988;12:244–250.

Freis ED, Rose JC, Higgins TF, et al. The hemodynamic effects of hypotensive drugs in man. IV. 1-hydrazinophthalazine. *Circulation* 1953;8:199.

Friedman PA, Bushinsky DA. Diuretic effects on calcium metabolism. *Semin Nephrol* 1999;19:551–556.

Frishman WH, Bryzinski BS, Coulson LR, et al. A multifactorial trial design to assess combination therapy in hypertension. *Arch Intern Med* 1994;154:1461–1468.

Fu Q, Zhang R, Witkowski S, et al. Persistent sympathetic activation during chronic antihypertensive therapy: A potential mechanism for long term morbidity? *Hypertension* 2005;45: 513–521.

Funder JW. New biology of aldosterone, and experimental studies on the selective aldosterone blocker eplerenone. *Am Heart J* 2002;144(Suppl. 5):S8–S11.

Furberg CD, Psaty BM, Meyer JV. Nifedipine. Dose-related increase in mortality in patients with coronary heart disease. *Circulation* 1995;92:1326–1331.

Gaddam KK, Nishizaka MK, Pratt-Ubunama MN, et al. Characterization of resistant hypertension: Association between resistant hypertension, aldosterone, and persistent intravascular volume expansion. *Arch Intern Med* 2008;168:1159–1164.

Gaede P, Lund-Andersen H, Parving HH, et al. Effect of a multifactorial intervention on mortality in type 2 diabetes. *N Engl J Med* 2008;358:580–591.

Garijo GMA, Perez Caderon R, Fernandez-Duran de A, Rangel Mayoral JF. Cutaneous reactions to diltiazem and cross reactivity with other calcium channel blockers. Allergol Immunopathol (Madr) 2005;33:238–240.

Gavras H, Brunner HR, Laragh JH, et al. An angiotensin converting-enzyme inhibitor to identify and treat vasoconstrictor and volume factors in hypertensive patients. *N Engl J Med* 1974; 291:817–821.

Gaziano TA, Opie LH, Weinstein MC. Cardiovascular disease prevention with a multidrug regimen in the developing world: A cost-effectiveness analysis. *Lancet* 2006;368:679–686.

Geleijnse JM, Witteman JC, Bak AA, et al. Reduction in blood pressure with a low sodium, high potassium, high magnesium salt in older subjects with mild to moderate hypertension. *Br Med J* 1994;309:436–440.

George RB, Light RW, Hudson LD, et al. Comparison of the effects of labetalol and hydrochlorothiazide on the ventilatory function of hypertensive patients with asthma and propranolol sensitivity. *Chest* 1985;88:814–818.

Ghiadoni L, Magagna A, Versari D, et al. Different effect of antihypertensive drugs on conduit artery endothelial function. *Hypertension* 2003;41:1281–1286.

GISSI-AF Investigators. Valsartan for prevention of recurrent ratial fibrillation. *N Engl J Med* 2009;360:1606–1617.

Giugliano D, Acampora R, Marfella R, et al. Hemodynamic and metabolic effects of transdermal clonidine in patients with hypertension and non-insulin-dependent diabetes mellitus. *Am J Hypertens* 1998;11:184–189.

Go AS, Yang J, Gurwitz JH, et al. Comparative effectiveness of different beta-adrenergic antagonists on mortality among adults with heart failure in clinical practice. *Arch Intern Med* 2008;168:2415–2421.

Goa KL, Benfield P, Sorkin EM. Labetalol. *Drugs* 1989;37: 583–627.

Goldberg AD, Raftery EB. Patterns of blood-pressure during chronic administration of postganglionic sympathetic blocking drugs for hypertension. *Lancet* 1976;2:1052–1054.

Gosse P, Sheridan DJ, Zannad F, et al. Regression of left ventricular hypertrophy in hypertensive patients treated with indapamide SR 1.5 mg versus enalapril 20 mg. *J Hypertens* 2000;18:1465–1475.

Gradman AH, Cutler NR, Davis PJ, et al. Combined enalapril and felodipine extended release (ER) for systemic hypertension. *Am J Cardiol* 1997;79:431–435.

Grandi AM, Imperiale D, Santillo R, et al. Aldosterone antagonist improves diastolic function in essential hypertension. *Hypertension* 2002;40:647–652.

Grassi G, Seravalle G, Turri C, et al. Short-versus long-term effects of different dihydropyridines on sympathetic and baroreflex function in hypertension. *Hypertension* 2003;41:558–562.

Graves JW. Management of difficult to control hypertension. *Mayo Clin Proc* 2000;75:278–284.

Green BB, Cook AJ, Ralston JD, et al. Effectiveness of home blood pressure monitoring, Web communication, and pharmacist care on hypertension control: A randomized controlled trial. *JAMA* 2008;299:2857–2867.

Gress TW, Nieto FJ, Shahar E, et al. Hypertension and antihypertensive therapy as risk factors for type 2 diabetes mellitus. *N Engl J Med* 2000;342:905–912.

Griffin KA, Bidani AK. Progression of renal disease: Renoprotective specificity of renin-angiotensin system blockade. *Clin J Am Soc Nephrol* 2006;1:1054–1065.

Griffin KA, Picken MM, Bidani AK. Deleterious effects of calcium channel blockade on pressure transmission and glomerular injury in rat remnant kidneys. *J Clin Invest* 1995;96: 793–800.

Grimm RH Jr, Grandits GA, Prineas RJ, et al. Long-term effects on sexual function of five antihypertensive drugs and nutritional hygienic treatment of hypertensive men and women. *Hypertension* 1997;29:8–14.

Grobbee DE, Hoes AW. Non-potassium-sparing diuretics and risk of sudden cardiac death. *J Hypertens* 1995;13:1539–1545.

Grossman E, Messerli FH, Goldbourt U. Antihypertensive therapy and the risk of malignancies. *Eur Hert J* 2001;22:1343–1352.

Grubb BP, Sirio C, Zelis R. Intravenous labetalol in acute aortic dissection. *JAMA* 1987;258:78–79.

Gu Q, Burt VL, Paulose-Ram R, et al. Gender differences in hypertension treatment, drug utilization patterns, and blood pressure control among US adults with hypertension: Data from the National Health and Nutrition Examination Survey 1999–2004. *Am J Hypertens* 2008;21:789–798.

Guasti L, Zanotta D, Diolisi A, et al. Changes in pain perception during treatment with angiotensin converting enzyme-inhibitors and angiotensin II type 1 receptor blockade. *J Hypertens* 2002;20:485–491.

Gulmez SE, Lassen AT, Aalykke C, et al. Spironolactone use and the risk of upper gastrointestinal bleeding: A population-based case-control study. *Br J Clin Pharmacol* 2008;66:294–299.

Gumieniak O, Williams GH. Mineralocorticoid receptor antagonists and hypertension: Is there a rationale? *Curr Hypertens Rep* 2004;6:279–287.

Gupta V, Lipsitz LA. Orthostatic hypotension in the elderly: Diagnosis and treatment. *Am J Med* 2007;120:841–847.

Gutierrez-Macias A, Lizarralde-Palacios E, Martinez-Odriozola P, et al. Fatal allopurinol hypersensitivity syndrome after treatment of asymptomatic hyperuricaemia. *Br Med J* 2005; 331:623–624.

Hackam DG, Thiruchelvam D, Redelmeier DA. Angiotensin-converting enzyme inhibitors and aortic rupture: A population-based case-control study. *Lancet* 2006;368:659–665.

Haffner CA, Horton RC, Lewis HM, et al. A metabolic assessment of the beta$_1$ selectivity of bisoprolol. *J Hum Hypertens* 1992;6:397–400.

Hamilton CA, Miller WH, Al-Benna S, et al. Strategies to reduce oxidative stress in cardiovascular disease. *Clin Sci (Lond)* 2004;106:219–234.

Hanon O, Berrou JP, Negre-Pages L, et al. Effects of hypertension therapy based on eprosartan on systolic arterial blood pressure and cognitive function: Primary results of the Observational Study on Cognitive function And Systolic Blood Pressure Reduction open-label study. *J Hypertens* 2008;26: 1642–1650.

Harada K, Kawaguchi A, Ohmori M, et al. Antagonistic activity of tamsulosin against human vascular α_1-adrenergic receptors. *Clin Pharmacol Ther* 2000;67:405–412.

Harper R, Ennis CN, Heaney AP, et al. A comparison of the effects of low- and conventional-dose thiazide diuretic on insulin action in hypertensive patients with NIDDM. *Diabetologia* 1995;38:853–859.

Hart P, Bakris GL. Calcium antagonists: Do they equally protect against kidney injury? *Kidney Int* 2008;73:795–796.

Hawkins RG. Is population-wide diuretic use directly associated with the incidence of end-stage renal disease in the United States? *Curr Hypertens Rep* 2006;8:219–225.

Healy JJ, McKenna TJ, Canning B, et al. Body composition changes in hypertensive subjects on long-term diuretic therapy. *Br Med J* 1970;1:716–719.

Heart Outcomes Prevention Evaluation (HOPE) Study Investigators. Effects of an angiotensin-converting-enzyme inhibitor, ramipril, on cardiovascular events in high-risk patients. *N Engl J Med* 2000;342:145–153.

Hebert PR, Coffey CS, Byrne DW, et al. Treatment of elderly hypertensive patients with epithelial sodium channel inhibitors combined with a thiazide diuretic reduces coronary mortality and sudden cardiac death. *J Am Soc Hypertens* 2008;2: 355–365.

Hedley AA, Ogden CL, Johnson CL, et al. Prevalence of overweight and obesity among US children, adolescents, and adults, 1999–2002. *JAMA* 2004;291:2847–2850.

Heidenreich PA, Davis BR, Cutler JA, et al. Cost-effectiveness of chlorthalidone, amlodipine, and lisinopril as first-step treatment for patients with hypertension: An analysis of the Antihypertensive and Lipid-Lowering Treatment to Prevent Heart Attack Trial (ALLHAT). *J Gen Intern Med* 2008;23: 509–516.

Herings RM, de Boer A, Stricker BH, et al. Hypoglycemia associated with use of inhibitors of angiotensin converting enzyme. *Lancet* 1995;345:1194–1198.

Hernández Prada JA, Ferreira AJ, Katovich MJ, et al. Structure-based identification of small-molecule angiotensin-converting enzyme 2 activators as novel antihypertensive agents. *Hypertension* 2008;51:1312–1317.

Hernández-Díaz S, Werler MM, Walker AM, et al. Folic acid antagonists during pregnancy and the risk of birth defects. *N Engl J Med* 2000;343:1608–1614.

Hiitola P, Enlund H, Kettunen R, et al. Postural changes in blood pressure and the prevalence of orthostatic hypotension among home-dwelling elderly aged 75 years or older. *J Hum Hypertens* 2009;23:33–39.

Hippisley-Cox J, Coupland C. Effect of combinations of drugs on all cause mortality in patients with ischaemic heart disease: Nested case-control analysis. *Br Med J* 2005;330: 1059–1063.

Hirai N, Kawano H, Yasue H, et al. Attenuation of nitrate tolerance and oxidative stress by an angiotensin II receptor blocker in patients with coronary spastic angina. *Circulation* 2003; 108:1446–1450.

Hirano T, Yoshino G, Kashiwazaki K, et al. Doxazosin reduces prevalence of small dense low density lipoprotein and remnant-like particle cholesterol levels in nondiabetic and diabetic hypertensive patients. *Am J Hypertens* 2001;14: 908–913.

Ho PM, Magid DJ, Shetterly SM, et al. Importance of therapy intensification and medication nonadherence for blood pressure control in patients with coronary disease. *Arch Intern Med* 2008;168:271–276.

Hoes AW, Grobbee DE, Lubsen J, et al. Diuretics, beta-blockers, and the risk for sudden cardiac death in hypertensive patients. *Ann Intern Med* 1995;123:481–487.

Holland OB, Gomez-Sanchez CE, Kuhnert LV, et al. Antihypertensive comparison of furosemide with hydrochlorothiazide for black patients. *Arch Intern Med* 1979;139:1014–1021.

Hollenberg NK, Parving HH, Viberti G, et al. Albuminuria response to very high-dose valsartan in type 2 diabetes mellitus. *J Hypertens* 2007;25:1921–1926.

Horn HJ, Detmar K, Pittrow DB, et al. Impact of a low-dose reserpine/thiazide combination on left ventricular hypertrophy assessed with magnetic resonance tomography and echocardiography. *Clin Drug Invest* 1997;14:109–116.

Houston MC. Treatment of hypertensive emergencies and urgencies with oral clonidine loading and titration. *Arch Intern Med* 1986;146:586–589.

Howard BV, Roman MJ, Devereux RB, et al. Effect of lower targets for blood pressure and LDL cholesterol on atherosclerosis in diabetes: The SANDS randomized trial. *JAMA* 2008;299: 1678–1689.

Hui KK, Duchin KL, Kripalani KJ, et al. Pharmacokinetics of fosinopril in patients with various degrees of renal function. *Clin Pharmacol Ther* 1991;49:457–467.

Ignarro J. Experimental evidence of nitric oxide-dependent vasodilatory activity of nebivolol, a third generation beta-blocker. *Blood Press Suppl* 2004;1:2–16.

Ito I, Hayashi Y, Kawai Y, et al. Prophylactic effect of intravenous nicorandil on perioperative myocardial damage in patients undergoing off-pump coronary artery bypass surgery. *J Cardiovasc Pharmacol* 2004;44:501–506.

Jackson B, McGrath BP, Maher D, et al. Lack of cross sensitivity between captopril and enalapril. *Aust N Z J Med* 1988; 18: 21–27.

Jacobs RL, Hoberman LJ, Goldstein HM. Angioedema of the small bowel caused by an angiotensin-converting enzyme inhibitor. *Am J Gastroenterol* 1994;89:127–128.

Jamerson K, Weber MA, Bakris GL, et al. Benazepril plus amlodipine or hydrochlorothiazide for hypertension in high-risk patients. *N Engl J Med* 2008;359:2417–2428.

Jandeleit-Dahm KA, Tikellis C, Reid CM, et al. Why blockade of the renin-angiotensin system reduces the incidence of new-onset diabetes. *J Hypertens* 2005;23:463–473.

Jefferson JA, Shankland SJ, Pichler RH. Proteinuria in diabetic kidney disease: A mechanistic viewpoint. *Kidney Int* 2008; 74:22–36.

Jeunemaitre X, Kreft-Jais C, Chatellier G, et al. Long-term experience of spironolactone in essential hypertension. *Kidney Int* 1988;34:S14–S17.

Johnson B, Hoch K, Errichetti A, et al. Effects of methyldopa on psychometric performance. *J Clin Pharmacol* 1990;30: 1102–1105.

Johnson RJ, Feig DI, Herrera-Acosta J, et al. Resurrection of uric acid as a causal risk factor in essential hypertension. *Hypertension* 2005;45:18–20.

Johnston GD. Selecting appropriate antihypertensive drug dosages. *Drugs* 1994;47:567–575.

Jordan J, Engeli S, Boye SW, et al. Direct renin inhibition with aliskiren in obese patients with arterial hypertension. *Hypertension* 2007;49:1047–1055.

Julius S, Alderman MH, Beevers G, et al. Cardiovascular risk reduction in hypertensive black patients with left ventricular hypertrophy: The LIFE study. *J Am Coll Cardiol* 2004a; 43:1047–1055.

Julius S, Kjeldsen SE, Weber M, et al. Outcomes in hypertensive patients at high cardiovascular risk treated with regimens based on valsartan or amlodipine: The VALUE randomised trial. *Lancet* 2004b;363:2022–2031.

Julius S, Nesbitt SD, Egan BM, et al. Feasibility of treating prehypertension with an angiotensin-receptor blocker. *N Engl J Med* 2006;354:1685–1697.

Juurlink DN, Mamdani MM, Lee DS, et al. Rates of hyperkalemia after publication of the Randomized Aldactone Evaluation Study. *N Engl J Med* 2004;351:543–551.

Kakar SM, Paine MF, Stewart PW, et al. 6 7 -Dihydroxybergamottin contributes to the grapefruit juice effect. *Clin Pharmacol Ther* 2004;75:569–579.

Kalinowski L, Dobrucki LW, Szczepanska-Konkel M, et al. Third-generation beta-blockers stimulate nitric oxide release from endothelial cells through ATP efflux: A novel mechanism for antihypertensive action. *Circulation* 2003;107:2747–2752.

Kaplan NM. Renin profiles. The unfulfilled promises. *JAMA* 1977;238:611–613.

Kaplan NM. New issues in the treatment of isolated systolic hypertension. *Circulation* 2000;102:1079–1081.

Kaplan NM, Carnegie A, Raskin P, et al. Potassium supplementation in hypertensive patients with diuretic-induced hypokalemia. *N Engl J Med* 1985;312:746–749.

Kaplan NM, Gidding SS, Pickering TG, et al. Task Force 5: Systemic hypertension. *J Am Coll Cardiol* 2005;45:1346–1348.

KDOQI. Diabetes and chronic kidney disease. *Am J Kidney Dis* 2007;49:S13–S41.

Kasiske BL, Ma JZ, Kalil RS, et al. Effects of antihypertensive therapy on serum lipids. *Ann Intern Med* 1995;122:133–141.

Keenan K, Hayen A, Neal BC, et al. Long term monitoring in patients receiving treatment to lower blood pressure: Analysis of data from placebo controlled randmised controlled trial. *BMJ* 2009;338:b1492.

Kelton JG. Impaired reticuloendothelial function in patients treated with methyldopa. *N Engl J Med* 1985;313:596–600.

Kent DM, Jafar TH, Hayward RA, et al. Progression risk, urinary protein excretion, and treatment effects of angiotensin-converting enzyme inhibitors in nondiabetic kidney disease. *J Am Soc Nephrol* 2007;18:1959–1965.

Kerr EA, Zikmund-Fisher BJ, Klamerus ML, et al. The role of clinical uncertainty in treatment decisions for diabetic patients with uncontrolled blood pressure. *Ann Intern Med* 2008;148:717–727.

Kesselheim AS, Misono AS, Lee JL, et al. Clinical equivalence of generic and brand-name drugs used in cardiovascular disease: A systematic review and meta-analysis. *JAMA* 2008;300:2514–2526.

Khachaturian AS, Zandi PP, Lyketsos CG, et al. Antihypertensive medication use and incident Alzheimer disease: The Cache County Study. *Arch Neurol* 2006;63:686–692.

Khan NA, Hemmelgarn B, Herman RJ, et al. The 2008 Canadian Hypertension Education Program recommendations for the management of hypertension: Part 2—therapy. *Can J Cardiol* 2008;24:465–475.

Khatri I, Uemura N, Notargiacomo A, et al. Direct and reflex cardiostimulating effects of hydralazine. *Am J Cardiol* 1977; 40: 38–42.

Kidwai BJ, George M. Hair loss with minoxidil withdrawal. *Lancet* 1992;340:609–610.

Kizer JR, Kimmel SE. Epidemiologic review of the calcium channel blocker drugs. *Arch Intern Med* 2001;161:1145–1158.

Klingbeil AU, Schneider M, Martus P, et al. A meta-analysis of the effects of treatment on left ventricular mass in essential hypertension. *Am J Med* 2003;115:41–46.

Kloner RA. Cardiovascular effects of the 3 phosphodiesterase-5 inhibitors approved for the treatment of erectile dysfunction. *Circulation* 2004;110:3149–3155.

Knowler WC, Barrett-Connor E, Fowler SE, et al. Reduction in the incidence of type 2 diabetes with lifestyle intervention or metformin. *N Engl J Med* 2002;346:393–403.

Ko DT, Hebert PR, Coffey CS, et al. Adverse effects of beta-blocker therapy for patients with heart failure: A quantitative overview of randomized trials. *Arch Intern Med* 2002;164:1389–1394.

Koh KK, Ahn JY, Han SH, et al. Pleiotropic effects of angiotensin II receptor blocker in hypertensive patients. *J Am Coll Cardiol* 2003;42:905–910.

Kopyt N, Dalal F, Narins RG. Renal retention of potassium in fruit. *N Engl J Med* 1985;313:582–583.

Kostis JB, Packer M, Black HR, et al. Omapatrilat and enalapril in patients with hypertension: The Omapatrilat Cardiovascular Treatment vs. Enalapril (OCTAVE) trial. *Am J Hypertens* 2004;17:103–111.

Kostis JB, Wilson AC, Freudenberger RS, et al. Long-term effect of diuretic-based therapy on fatal outcomes in subjects with isolated systolic hypertension with and without diabetes. *Am J Cardiol* 2005;95:29–35.

Kramer JM, Curtis LH, Dupree CS, et al. Comparative effectiveness of beta-blockers in elderly patients with heart failure. *Arch Intern Med* 2008;168:2422–2428.

Krekels MM, Gaillard CA, Viergever PP, et al. Natriuretic effect of nitrendipine is preceded by transient systemic and renal hemodynamic effects. *Cardiovasc Drugs Ther* 1997;11:33–38.

Kripalani S, Henderson LE, Jacobson TA, et al. Medication use among inner-city patients after hospital discharge: Patient-reported barriers and solutions. *Mayo Clin Proc* 2008;83:529–535.

Kripalani S, Yao X, Haynes RB. Interventions to enhance medication adherence in chronic medical conditions: A systematic review. *Arch Intern Med* 2007;167:540–550.

Krönig B, Pittrow DB, Kirch W, et al. Different concepts in first-line treatment of essential hypertension. Comparison of a low-dose reserpine-thiazide combination with nitrendipine monotherapy. *Hypertension* 1997;29:651–658.

Krop M, Garrelds IM, de Bruin RJ, et al. Aliskiren accumulates in Renin secretory granules and binds plasma prorenin. *Hypertension* 2008;52:1076–1083.

Krum H, Schlaich M, Whitbourn R, et al. Catheter-based renal sympathetic denervation for resistant hypertension: A multicentre safety and proof-of-principle cohort study. *Lancet* 2009;373:1275–1281.

Kunz R, Friedrich C, Wolbers M, et al. Meta-analysis: Effect of monotherapy and combination therapy with inhibitors of the renin angiotensin system on proteinuria in renal disease. *Ann Intern Med* 2008;148:30–48.

Kurtz TW, Pravenec M. Molecule-specific effects of angiotensin II-receptor blockers independent of the renin-angiotensin system. *Am J Hypertens* 2008;21:852–859.

Labinjoh C, Newby DE, Pellegrini MP, et al. Potentiation of bradykinin-induced tissue plasminogen activator release by angiotensin-converting enzyme inhibition. *J Am Coll Cardiol* 2001; 38:1402–1408.

Lacourcière Y, Krzesinski JM, White WB, et al. Sustained antihypertensive activity of telmisartan compared with valsartan. *Blood Press Monit* 2004;9:203–210.

Lacourcière Y, Poirier L, Lefebvre J. A comparative review of the efficacy of antihypertensive agents on 24 h ambulatory blood pressure. *Can J Cardiol* 2000;16:1155–1166.

Lahive KC, Weiss JW, Weinberger SE. Alpha-methyldopa selectively reduces alae nasi activity. *Clin Sci* 1988;74:547–551.

Lam SK, Owen A. Incident diabetes in clinical trials of antihypertensive drugs. *Lancet* 2007;369:1513–1514.

Langley MS, Heel RC. Tansdermal clonidine. *Drugs* 1988;35: 123–142.

Laragh JH. Renin profiling for diagnosis, risk assessment, and treatment of hypertension. *Kidney Int* 1993;44:1163–1175.

Lardinois CK, Neuman SL. The effects of antihypertensive agents on serum lipids and lipoproteins. *Arch Intern Med* 1988; 148:1280–1288.

Lassila M, Cooper ME, Jandeleit-Dahm K. Antiproteinuric effect of RAS blockade: New mechanisms. *Curr Hypertens Rep* 2004;6:383–392.

Law MR, Wald NJ, Morris JK, et al. Value of low dose combination treatment with blood pressure lowering drugs: Analysis of 354 randomised trials. *Br Med J* 2003;326:1427.

Law MR, Morris JK, Wald NJ. Use of blood pressure lowering drugs in the prevention of cardiovascular disease: Meta-analysis of 147 randomised trials in the context of expectations from prospective epidemiological studies. *BMJ* 2009;338. b1665.

Lebel M, Langlois S, Belleau LJ, et al. Labetalol infusion in hypertensive emergencies. *Clin Pharmacol Ther* 1985;37: 614–618.

Lee W. Drug-induced hepatotoxicity. *N Engl J Med* 1995;17: 1118–1127.

Lee VC, Rhew DC, Dylan M, et al. Meta-analysis: Angiotensin-receptor blockers in chronic heart failure and high-risk acute myocardial infarction. *Ann Intern Med* 2004;141: 693–704.

Leenen FH, Dumais J, McInnis NH, et al. Results of the Ontario survey on the prevalence and control of hypertension. *CMAJ* 2008;178:1441–1449.

Leenen FH, Smith DL, Farkas RM, et al. Vasodilators and regression of left ventricular hypertrophy. *Am J Med* 1987;82:969–978.

Lenzer J. Underinsurance threatens physical and financial wellbeing of US families. *Br Med J* 2008;336:1399.

Lernfelt B, Landahl S, Johansson P, et al. Haemodynamic and renal effects of felodipine in young and elderly patients. *Eur J Clin Pharmacol* 1998;54:393–601.

Levine HJ, Gaasch WH. Vasoactive drugs in chronic regurgitant lesions of the mitral and aortic valves. *J Am Coll Cardiol* 1996;28:1083–1091.

Levine SR, Coull BM. Potassium depletion as a risk factor for stroke: Will a banana a day keep your stroke away? *Neurology* 2002;59:302–303.

Levy BI. Can angiotensin II type 2 receptors have deleterious effects in cardiovascular disease? Implications for therapeutic blockade of the renin-angiotensin system. *Circulation* 2004; 109:8–13.

Lewin A, Alderman MH, Mathur P. Antihypertensive efficacy of guanfacine and prazosin in patients with mild to moderate essential hypertension. *J Clin Pharmacol* 1990;30:1081–1087.

Lewis EJ, Hunsicker LG, Clarke WR, et al. Renoprotective effect of the angiotensin-receptor antagonist irbesartan in patients with nephropathy due to type 2 diabetes. *N Engl J Med* 2001;345:851–860.

Li JM, Mogi M, Iwanami J, et al. Temporary pretreatment with the angiotensin II type 1 receptor blocker, valsartan, prevents ischemic brain damage through an increase in capillary density. *Stroke* 2008;39:2029–2036.

Libhaber EN, Libhaber CD, Candy GP, et al. Effect of slow-release indapamide and perindopril compared with amlodipine on 24-hour blood pressure and left ventricular mass in hypertensive patients of African ancestry. *Am J Hypertens* 2004;17:428–432.

Lilja JJ, Juntti-Patinen L, Neuvonen PJ. Orange juice substantially reduces the bioavailability of the beta-adrenergic-blocking agent celiprolol. *Clin Pharmacol Ther* 2004;75:184–190.

Lilja M, Jounela AJ, Juustila HJ, et al. Abrupt and gradual change from clonidine to beta blockers in hypertension. *Acta Med Scand* 1982;211:374–380.

Lim LS, Fink HA, Kuskowski MA, et al. Loop diuretic use and increased rates of hip bone loss in older men: The Osteoporotic Fractures in Men Study. *Arch Intern Med* 2008;168: 735–740.

Lim SS, Gaziano TA, Gakidou E, et al. Prevention of cardiovascular disease in high-risk individuals in low-income and middle-income countries: Health effects and costs. *Lancet* 2007;370: 2054–2062.

Lin MS, McNay JL, Shepherd AM, et al. Increased plasma norepinephrine accompanies persistent tachycardia after hydralazine. *Hypertension* 1983;5:257–263.

Lind L, Hänni A, Hvarfner A, et al. Influences of different antihypertensive treatments on indices of systemic mineral metabolism. *Am J Hypertens* 1994;7:302–307.

Lindholm LH, Carlberg B, Samuelsson O. Should beta blockers remain first choice in the treatment of primary hypertension? A meta-analysis. *Lancet* 2005;366:1545–1553.

Lindqvist M, Kahan T, Melcher A, et al. Long-term calcium antagonist treatment of human hypertension with mibefradil or amlodipine increases sympathetic nerve activity. *J Hypertens* 2007;25:169–175.

Lip GY, Ferner RE. Poisoning with anti-hypertensive drugs: Angiotensin converting enzyme inhibitors. *J Hum Hypertens* 1995; 9:711–715.

Lip GY, Ferner RE. Diuretic therapy for hypertension: A cancer risk? *J Hum Hypertens* 1999;13:421–423.

Lipsitz LA, Gagnon M, Vyas M, et al. Antihypertensive therapy increases cerebral blood flow and carotid distensibility in hypertensive elderly subjects. *Hypertension* 2005;45:216–221.

Lithell HO. Hyperinsulinemia, insulin resistance, and the treatment of hypertension. *Am J Hypertens* 1996;9:150S–154S.

Liu PH, Hu FC, Wang JD. Differential risks of stroke in pharmacotherapy on uncomplicated hypertensive patients? *J Hypertens* 2009;27:174–180.

Lonati C, Morganti A, Comarella L, et al. Prevalence of type 2 diabetes among patients with hypertension under the care of 30 Italian clinics of hypertension: Results of the (Iper)tensione and (dia)bete study. *J Hypertens* 2008;26:1801–1808.

Lottermoser K, Hertfelder HJ, Vetter H, et al. Fibrinolytic function in diuretic-induced volume depletion. *Am J Hypertens* 2000;13:359–363.

Low PA, Singer W. Management of neurogenic orthostatic hypotension: An update. *Lancet Neurol* 2008;7:451–458.

Luders S, Schrader J, Berger J, et al. The PHARAO study: Prevention of hypertension with the angiotensin-converting enzyme inhibitor ramipril in patients with high-normal blood pressure: A prospective, randomized, controlled prevention trial of the German Hypertension League. *J Hypertens* 2008;26: 1487–1496.

Luetscher JA, Kraemer FB, Wilson DM, et al. Increased plasma inactive renin in diabetes mellitus. A marker of microvascular complications. *N Engl J Med* 1985;312:1412–1417.

Luft FC, Fineberg NS, Weinberger MH. Long-term effect of nifedipine and hydrochlorothiazide on blood pressure and sodium homeostasis at varying levels of salt intake in mildly hypertensive patients. *Am J Hypertens* 1991;4:752–760.

Luft FC, Weinberger MH. Antihypertensive therapy with aliskiren. *Kidney Int* 2008;73:679–683.

Lyons D, Roy S, O'Byrne S, et al. ACE inhibition: Postsynaptic adrenergic sympatholytic action in men. *Circulation* 1997; 96:911–915.

Ma J, Lee KV, Stafford RS. Changes in antihypertensive prescribing during US outpatient visits for uncomplicated hypertension between 1993 and 2004. *Hypertension* 2006;48:846–852.

Mackenzie IS, McEniery CM, Dhakam Z, et al. Comparison of the effects of antihypertensive agents on central blood pressure and arterial stiffness in isolated systolic hypertension. *Hypertension* 2009;54:409–413.

Madkour H, Gadallah M, Riveline B, et al. Comparison between the effects of indapamide and hydrochlorothiazide on creatinine clearance in patients with impaired renal function and hypertension. *Am J Nephrol* 1995;15:251–255.

Mahmud A, Feely J. Low-dose quadruple antihypertensive combination: More efficacious than individual agents—a preliminary report. *Hypertension* 2007;49:272–275.

Mahmud A, Feely J. Beta-blockers reduce aortic stiffness in hypertension but nebivolol, not atenolol, reduces wave reflection. *Am J Hypertens* 2008;21:663–667.

Maitland-van der Zee A-H, Turner ST, Chapman AB, et al. Multifocus approach to the pharmacogenetics of thiazide diuretics [Abstract]. *Circulation* 2004;110:III-428.

Malhotra S, Bailey DG, Paine MF, et al. Seville orange juice-felodipine interaction. *Clin Pharmacol Ther* 2001;69:14–23.

Man in't Veld AJ, Van den Meiracker AH, Schalekamp MA. Do beta-blockers really increase peripheral vascular resistance? *Am J Hypertens* 1988;1:91–96.

Mancia G. The broadening landscape for hypertension management. *J Am Soc Hypertens* 2008;2:S3–S9.

Mancia G, Grassi G. Systolic and diastolic blood pressure control in antihypertensive drug trials. *J Hypertens* 2002;20:1461–1464.

Mancia G, Seravalle G, Grassi G. Tolerability and treatment compliance with angiotensin II receptor antagonists. *Am J Hypertens* 2003;16:1066–1073.

Mann JF. What's new in hypertension 2008? *Nephrol Dial Transplant* 2009;24:38–42.

Mann JF, Schmieder RE, McQueen M, et al. Renal outcomes with telmisartan, ramipril, or both, in people at high vascular risk (the ONTARGET study): A multicentre, randomised, double-blind, controlled trial. *Lancet* 2008;372:547–553.

Mann SJ. The silent epidemic of thiazide-induced hyponatremia. *J Clin Hypertens (Greenwich)* 2008;10:477–484.

Manzella D, Grella R, Esposito K, et al. Blood pressure and cardiac autonomic nervous system in obese type 2 diabetic patients: Effect of metformin administration. *Am J Hypertens* 2004;17:223–227.

Marre M, Puig JG, Kokot F, et al. Equivalence of indapamide SR and enalapril on microalbuminuria reduction in hypertensive patients with type 2 diabetes: The NESTOR Study. *J Hypertens* 2004;22:1613–1622.

Marshall HJ, Beevers DG. α-adrenoceptor blocking drugs and female urinary incontinence. *Br J Clin Pharmacol* 1996;42:507–509.

Martin WB, Spodick DH, Zins GR. Pericardial disorders occurring during open-label study of 1,869 severely hypertensive patients treated with minoxidil. *J Cardiovasc Pharmacol* 1980;2:S217–S227.

Mason JM, Dickinson HO, Nicolson DJ, et al. The diabetogenic potential of thiazide-type diuretic and beta-blocker combinations in patients with hypertension. *J Hypertens* 2005;23:1777–1781.

Matchar DB, McCrory DC, Orlando LA, et al. Systematic review: Comparative effectiveness of angiotensin-converting enzyme inhibitors and angiotensin II receptor blockers for treating essential hypertension. *Ann Intern Med* 2008;148:16–29.

Materson BJ, Reda DJ, Cushman WC, et al. Single-drug therapy for hypertension in men. *N Engl J Med* 1993;328:914–921.

Materson BJ, Reda DJ, Cushman WC. Department of Veterans Affairs single-drug therapy of hypertension study. *Am J Hypertens* 1995;8:189–192.

Mathew TH, Boyd IW, Rohan AP. Hyponatraemia due to the combination of hydrochlorothiazide and amiloride (Moduretic). *Med J Aust* 1990;152:308–309.

Matsui Y, Eguchi K, Shibasaki S, et al. Effect of doxazosin on the left ventricular structure and function in morning hypertensive patients: The Japan Morning Surge 1 study. *J Hypertens* 2008;26:1463–1471.

Mattace-Raso FU, van den Meiracker AH, Bos WJ, et al. Arterial stiffness, cardiovagal baroreflex sensitivity and postural blood pressure changes in older adults: The Rotterdam Study. *J Hypertens* 2007;25:1421–1426.

Mauer M, Zinman B, Gardiner R, et al. Renal and retinal effects of enalapril and losartan in type 1 diabetes. *N Engl J Med* 2009;361:40–51.

McCabe J, Stork C, Mailloux D, et al. Penile angioedema associated with the use of angiotensin-converting-enzyme inhibitors and angiotensin II receptor blockers. *Am J Health Syst Pharm* 2008;65:420–421.

McConnell JD, Roehrborn CG, Bautista OM, et al. The long-term effect of doxazosin, finasteride, and combination therapy on the clinical progression of benign prostatic hyperplasia. *N Engl J Med* 2003;349:2387–2398.

McDowell SE, Coleman JJ, Ferner RE. Systematic review and meta-analysis of ethnic differences in risks of adverse reactions to drugs used in cardiovascular medicine. *Br Med J* 2006;332:1177–1181.

McWilliams JM, Meara E, Zaslavsky AM, et al. Differences in control of cardiovascular disease and diabetes by race, ethnicity, and education: U.S. trends from 1999 to 2006 and effects of medicare coverage. *Ann Intern Med* 2009;150:505–515.

Medical Letter. Drug interactions with grapefruit juice. *Medical Letter* 2004;46:2–4.

Medical Research Council Working Party on Mild Hypertension. Adverse reactions to bendrofluazide and propranolol for the treatment of mild hypertension. *Lancet* 1981;2:539–543.

Mehta JL, Lopez LM. Rebound hypertension following abrupt cessation of clonidine and metoprolol. *Arch Intern Med* 1987;147:389–390.

Mena-Martin FJ, Martin-Escudero JC, Simal-Blanco F, et al. Health-related quality of life of subjects with known and unknown hypertension: Results from the population-based Hortega study. *J Hypertens* 2003;21:1283–1289.

Meredith PA, Elliott HL. Dihydropyridine calcium channel blockers: Basic pharmacological similarities but fundamental therapeutic differences. *J Hypertens* 2004;22:1641–1648.

Messerli FH, Bangalore S. Antihypertensive efficacy of aliskeren: Is hydrochlorothiazide and appropriate benchmark? *Circulation* 2009;119:371–373.

Messerli FH, Bangalore S, Julius S. Should β-Blockers and diuretics remain as first-line therapy for hypertension? *Circulation* 2008a;117:2706–2715.

Messerli FH, Bell DS, Fonseca V, et al. Body weight changes with beta-blocker use: Results from GEMINI. *Am J Med* 2007;120:610–615.

Messerli FH, Grossman E, Goldbourt U. Are beta-blockers efficacious as first-line therapy for hypertension in the elderly? A systematic review. *JAMA* 1998;279:1903–1907.

Messerli FH, Pinto L, Tang SS, et al. Impact of systemic hypertension on the cardiovascular benefits of statin therapy—a meta-analysis. *Am J Cardiol* 2008b;101:319–325.

Metz S, Klein C, Morton N. Rebound hypertension after discontinuation of transdermal clonidine therapy. *Am J Med* 1987;82:17–19.

Miller DR, Oliveria SA, Berlowitz DR, et al. Angioedema incidence in US veterans initiating angiotensin-converting enzyme inhibitors. *Hypertension* 2008;51:1624–1630.

Miller RP, Woodworth JR, Graves DA, et al. Comparison of three formulations of metolazone. *Curr Ther Res* 1988;43:1133–1142.

Missouris GG, Kalaitzidis RG, Cappuccio FP, et al. Gingival hyperplasia caused by calcium channel blockers. *J Hum Hypertens* 2000;14:155–156.

Miyachi M, Kawano H, Sugawara J, et al. Unfavorable effects of resistance training on central arterial compliance: A randomized intervention study. *Circulation* 2004;110:2858–2863.

Molnar GW, Read RC, Wright FE. Propranolol enhancement of hypoglycemic sweating. *Clin Pharmacol Ther* 1974;15: 490–496.

Morgan T, Lauri J, Bertram D, et al. Effect of different antihypertensive drug classes on central aortic pressure. *Am J Hypertens* 2004;17:118–123.

Morgan TO, Anderson AIE, MacInnis RJ. ACE inhibitors, beta-blockers, calcium blockers, and diuretics for the control of systolic hypertension. *Am J Hypertens* 2001;14:241–247.

Morimoto T, Gandhi TK, Fiskio JM, et al. Development and validation of a clinical prediction rule for angiotensin-converting enzyme inhibitor-induced cough. *J Gen Intern Med* 2004; 19:684–691.

Morisky DE, Ang A, Krousel-Wood M, et al. Predictive validity of a medication adherence measure in an outpatient setting. *J Clin Hypertens (Greenwich)* 2008;10:348–354.

Morton A, Muir J, Lim D. Rash and acute nephritic syndrome due to candesartan. *Br Med J* 2004;328:25.

Mosenkis A, Townsend RR. What time of day should I take my antihypertensive medications? *J Clin Hypertens* 2004;6: 593–594.

Mukae S, Aoki S, Itoh S, et al. Bradykinin B$_2$ receptor gene polymorphism is associated with angiotensin-converting enzyme inhibitor related cough. *Hypertension* 2000;36:127–131.

Mulder P, Mellin V, Favre J, et al. Aldosterone synthase inhibition improves cardiovascular function and structure in rats with heart failure: A comparison with spironolactone. *Eur Heart J* 2008;29:2171–2179.

Multiple risk factor intervention trial research group. Mortality after 10½ years for hypertensive participants in the Multiple Risk Factor Intervention Trial. *Circulation* 1990;82: 1616–1628.

Munger MA, Kenney JK. A chronobiologic approach to the pharmacotherapy of hypertension and angina. *Ann Pharmacother* 2000;34:1313–1319.

Nassief A, Marsh JD. Statin therapy for stroke prevention. *Stroke* 2008;39:1042–1048.

National Institute for Clinical Excellance. Hypertension: Management in adults in primary care: Pharmacological update. 2006. Available at: www.nice.org.uk

Neaton JD, Grimm RH Jr, Prineas RJ, et al. Treatment of mild hypertension study (TOMHS). *JAMA* 1993;270:713–724.

Nelson MR, Reid CM, Krum H, et al. Short-term predictors of maintenance of normotension after withdrawal of antihypertensive drugs in the second Australian National Blood Pressure Study (ANBP2). *Am J Hypertens* 2003;16:39–45.

Neusy AJ, Lowenstein J. Blood pressure and blood pressure variability following withdrawal of propranolol and clonidine. *J Clin Pharmacol* 1989;29:18–24.

Neutel JM, Littlejohn TW, Chrysant SG, et al. Telmisartan/Hydrochlorothiazide in comparison with losartan/hydrochlorothiazide in managing patients with mild-to-moderate hypertension. *Hypertens Res* 2005;28:555–563.

Neuvonen PJ, Kivistö KT. The clinical significance of food-drug interactions. *Med J Aust* 1989;150:36–40.

Ng KFF, Vane JR. Conversion of angiotensin I to angiotensin II. *Nature* 1967;216:762–766.

Nickenig G. Should angiotensin II receptor blockers and statins be combined? *Circulation* 2004;110:1013–1020.

Nissan A, Spira RM, Seror D, et al. Captopril-associated "Pseudocholangitis." *Arch Surg* 1996;131:670–671.

Nissen SE, Tuzcu EM, Libby P, et al. Effect of antihypertensive agents on cardiovascular events in patients with coronary disease and normal blood pressure. The CAMELOT study: A randomized controlled trial. *JAMA* 2004;292:2217–2225.

Nørgaard A, Kjeldsen K. Interrelation of hypokalaemia and potassium depletion and its implications. *Clin Sci* 1991;81: 449–455.

Novo G, Guttilla D, Fazio G, et al. The role of the renin-angiotensin system in atrial fibrillation and the therapeutic effects of ACE-Is and ARBS. *Br J Clin Pharmacol* 2008;66:345–351.

Obermayr RP, Temml C, Gutjahr G, et al. Elevated uric acid increases the risk for kidney disease. *J Am Soc Nephrol* 2008;19:2407–2413.

Oh BH, Mitchell J, Herron JR, et al. Aliskiren, an oral renin inhibitor, provides dose-dependent efficacy and sustained 24-hour blood pressure control in patients with hypertension. *J Am Coll Cardiol* 2007;49:1157–1163.

Okin PM, Devereux RB, Harris KE, et al. In-treatment resolution or absence of electrocardiographic left ventricular hypertrophy is associated with decreased incidence of new-onset diabetes mellitus in hypertensive patients: The Losartan Intervention for Endpoint Reduction in Hypertension (LIFE) Study. *Hypertension* 2007;50:984–990.

Okin PM, Devereux RB, Jern S, et al. Regression of electrocardiographic left ventricular hypertrophy during antihypertensive treatment and the prediction of major cardiovascular events. *JAMA* 2004;292:2343–2349.

Okin PM, Gerdts E, Kjeldsen SE, et al. Gender differences in regression of electrocardiographic left ventricular hypertrophy during antihypertensive therapy. *Hypertension* 2008;52:100–106.

Ondetti MA, Rubin B, Cushman DW. Design of specific inhibitors of angiotensin-converting enzyme. *Science* 1977;196: 441–444.

Ondetti MA, Williams NJ, Sabo EF, et al. Angiotensin-converting enzyme inhibitors from the venom of Bothrops jararaca. *Biochemistry* 1971;10:4033–4039.

ONTARGET Investigators. Telmisartan, ramipril, or both in patients at high risk for vascular events. *N Engl J Med* 2008;358;1547–1559.

Onuigbo MA, Onuigbo NT. Late onset renal failure from angiotensin blockade (LORFFAB): A prospective thirty-month Mayo Health System clinic experience. *Med Sci Monit* 2005;11:CR462–CR469.

Oparil S, Yarows SA, Patel S, et al. Efficacy and safety of combined use of aliskiren and valsartan in patients with hypertension: A randomised, double-blind trial. *Lancet* 2007;370: 221–229.

Osterberg L, Blaschke T. Adherence to medication. *N Engl J Med* 2005;353:487–497.

Ouzan J, Pérault C, Lincoff AM, et al. The role of spironolactone in the treatment of patients with refractory hypertension. *Am J Hypertens* 2002;15:333–339.

Ovbiagele B, Starkman S, Teal P, et al. Serum calcium as prognosticator in ischemic stroke. *Stroke* 2008;39:2231–2236.

Owens SD, Dunn MI. Efficacy and safety of guanadrel in elderly hypertensive patients. *Arch Intern Med* 1988;148:1514–1518.

Pacanowski MA, Gong Y, Cooper-Dehoff RM, et al. β-Adrenergic receptor gene polymorphisms and β-Blocker treatment outcomes in hypertension. *Clin Pharmacol Ther* 2008;84:715–721.

Pahor M, Guralnik JM, Ferrucci L, et al. Calcium-channel blockade and incidence of cancer in aged populations. *Lancet* 1996; 348:493–497.

Pak CYC. Correction of thiazide-induced hypomagnesemia by potassium-magnesium citrate from review of prior trials. *Clin Nephrol* 2000;54:271–275.

Palmer BF. Managing hyperkalemia caused by inhibitors of the renin-angiotensin-aldosterone system. *N Engl J Med* 2004;351: 585–592.

Pandya KJ, Raubertas RF, Flynn PJ, et al. Oral clonidine in postmenopausal patients with breast cancer experiencing tamoxifen-induced hot flashes. *Ann Intern Med* 2000;132:788–793.

Parati G, Omboni S, Albini F, et al. Home blood pressure telemonitoring improves hypertension control in general practice. The TeleBPCare study. *J Hypertens* 2009;27:198–203.

Park JB, Schiffrin EL. Effects of antihypertensive therapy on hypertensive vascular disease. *Curr Hypertens Rep* 2000;2: 280–288.

Participating VA Medical Centers. Low doses v standard dose of reserpine. *JAMA* 1982;248:2471–2477.

Parving HH, Persson F, Lewis JB, et al. Aliskiren combined with losartan in type 2 diabetes and nephropathy. *N Engl J Med* 2008;358:2433–2446.

Parving H-H, Lehnert H, Bröchner-Mortensen J, et al. The effect of irbesartan on the development of diabetic nephropathy in patients with type 2 diabetes. *N Engl J Med* 2001;345: 870–878.

Paton RR, Kane RE. Long-term diuretic therapy with metolazone of renal failure and the nephrotic syndrome. *J Clin Pharm* 1977;17:243–251.

Pedelty L, Gorelick PB. Management of hypertension and cerebrovascular disease in the elderly. *Am J Med* 2008;121: S23–S31.

Pepine CJ, Handberg EM, Cooper-DeHoff RM, et al. A calcium antagonist vs a non-calcium antagonist hypertension treatment strategy for patients with coronary artery disease. The International Verapamil-Trandolapril Study (INVEST): A randomized controlled trial. *JAMA* 2003;290:2805–2816.

Pérez-Stable E, Halliday R, Gardiner PS, et al. The effects of propranolol on cognitive function and quality of life. *Am J Med* 2000;108:359–365.

Perry HM Jr. Late toxicity to hydralazine resembling systemic lupus erythematosus or rheumatoid arthritis. *Am J Med* 1973; 54:58–72.

Peters R, Beckett N, Forette F, et al. Incident dementia and blood pressure lowering in the Hypertension in the Very Elderly Trial cognitive function assessment (HYVET-COG): A double-blind, placebo controlled trial. *Lancet Neurol* 2008;7: 683–689.

Phillips CO, Kashani A, Ko DK, et al. Adverse effects of combination angiotensin II receptor blockers plus angiotensin-converting enzyme inhibitors for left ventricular dysfunction: A quantitative review of data from randomized clinical trials. *Arch Intern Med* 2007;167:1930–1936.

Phillips LS, Twombly JG. It's time to overcome clinical inertia. *Ann Intern Med* 2008;148:783–785.

Phillips RA. New-onset diabetes mellitus less deadly than elevated blood pressure? Following the evidence in the administration of thiazide diuretics. *Arch Intern Med* 2006;166:2174–2176.

Pickering TG. Effects of stress and behavioral interventions in hypertension: The rise and fall of omapatrilat. *J Clin Hypertens* 2002;4:371–373.

Pickering TG. Treatment of hypertension in the elderly. *J Clin Hypertens (Greenwich)* 2004;6:18–23.

Pickles CJ, Pipkin FB, Symonds EM. A randomised placebo controlled trial of labetalol in the treatment of mild to moderate pregnancy induced hypertension. *Br J Obstet Gynaecol* 1992; 99:964–968.

Piepho RW, Beal J. An overview of antihypertensive therapy in the 20th century. *J Clin Pharmacol* 2000;40:967–977.

Pilote L, Abrahamowicz M, Eisenberg M, et al. Effect of different angiotensin-converting-enzyme inhibitors on mortality among elderly patients with congestive heart failure. *CMAJ* 2008; 178:1303–1311.

Pitt B. Comparative effectiveness of β-blockers in elderly patients with heart failure: Invited commentary. *Arch Intern Med* 2008;168(22):2431–2432.

Pitt B, Ahmed A, Love TE, et al. History of hypertension and eplerenone in patients with acute myocardial infarction complicated by heart failure. *Hypertension* 2008;52:271–278.

Pitt B, Remme W, Zannad F, et al. Eplerenone, a selective aldosterone blocker, in patients with left ventricular dysfunction after myocardial infarction. *N Engl J Med* 2003; 348:1309–1321.

Pitt B, White H, Nicolau J, et al. Eplerenone reduces mortality 30 days after randomization following acute myocardial infarction in patients with left ventricular systolic dysfunction and heart failure. *J Am Coll Cardiol* 2005;46:425–431.

Pitt B, Zannad F, Remme WJ, et al. The effect of spironolactone of morbidity and mortality in patients with severe heart failure. *N Engl J Med* 1999;341:709–717.

Plata R, Cornejo A, Arratia C, et al. Angiotensin-converting-enzyme inhibition therapy in altitude polycythaemia: A prospective randomised trial. *Lancet* 2002;359:663–666.

POISE Study Group. Effects of extended-release metoprolol succinate in patients undergoing non-cardiac surgery (POISE trial): A randomised controlled trial. *Lancet* 2008;371: 1839–1847.

Polonia J, Boaventura I, Gama G, et al. Influence of non-steroidal anti-inflammatory drugs in renal function and 24 hr ambulatory blood pressure-reducing effects of enalapril and nifedipine gastrointestinal therapeutic system in hypertensive patients. *J Hypertens* 1995;13:924–931.

Poole-Wilson PA, Swedberg K, Cleland JG, et al. Comparison of carvedilol and metoprolol on clinical outcomes in patients with chronic heart failure in the Carvedilol Or Metoprolol European Trial (COMET): Randomised controlled trial. *Lancet* 2003;362:7–13.

Porkert M, Sher S, Reddy U, et al. Tetrahydrobiopterin: A novel antihypertensive therapy. *J Hum Hypertens* 2008;22:401–407.

Postma CT, Dennesen PJW, de Boo T, et al. First dose hypotension after captopril; can it be predicted? *J Hum Hypertens* 1992;6:204–209.

Preston RA, Materson BJ, Reda DJ, et al. Age-race subgroup compared with renin profile as predictors of blood pressure response to antihypertensive therapy. Department of Veterans Affairs Cooperative Study Group on Antihypertensive Agents. *JAMA* 1998;280:1168–1172.

Prichard BN, Vallance P. ESH/ESC guidelines. *J Hypertens* 2004;22:859–861.

Prisant LM, Spruill WJ, Fincham JE, et al. Depression associated with antihypertensive drugs. *J Fam Pract* 1991;33:481–485.

PROGRESS Collaborative Group. Randomised trial of a perindopril-based blood-pressure-lowering regimen among 6105 individuals with previous stroke or transient ischaemic attack. *Lancet* 2001;358:1033–1041.

Psaty BM, Heckbert Sr, Koepsell TD, et al. The risk of myocardial infarction associated with antihypertensive drug therapies. *JAMA* 1995;274:620–625.

Psaty BM, Lumley T, Furberg CD, et al. Health outcomes associated with various antihypertensive therapies used as first-line agents. *JAMA* 2003;289:2534–2544.

Psaty BM, Smith NL, Heckbert SL, et al. Diuretic therapy, the alpha-adducin gene variant,and the risk of myocardial infarction or stroke in persons with treated hypertension. *JAMA* 2002;287:1680–1689.

Puschett JB. Diuretics and the therapy of hypertension. *Am J Med Sci* 2000;319:1–9.

Quereda C, Orte L, Sabater J, et al. Urinary calcium excretion in treated and untreated essential hypertension. *J Am Soc Nephrol* 1996;7:1058–1065.

Qureshi AI. Acute hypertensive response in patients with stroke: Pathophysiology and management. *Circulation* 2008;118: 176–187.

Radack K, Deck C. Beta-adrenergic blocker therapy does not worsen intermittent claudication in subjects with peripheral arterial disease. *Arch Intern Med* 1991;151:1769–1776.

Raichlin E, Prasad A, Mathew V, et al. Efficacy and safety of atrasentan in patients with cardiovascular risk and early atherosclerosis. *Hypertension* 2008;52:522–528.

Raji A, Seely EW, Bekins SA, et al. Rosiglitazone improves insulin sensitivity and lowers blood pressure in hypertensive patients. *Diabetes Care* 2003;26:172–178.

Ram CVS, Garrett BN, Kaplan NM. Moderate sodium restriction and various diuretics in the treatment of hypertension. *Arch Intern Med* 1981;141:1014–1019.

Ram CVS. Antihypertensive efficacy of angiotensin receptor blockers in combination with hydrochlorothiazide: A review of the factorial-design studies. *J Clin Hypertens* 2004;6: 569–577.

Ram CVS, Holland OB, Fairchild C, et al. Withdrawal syndrome following cessation of guanabenz therapy. *J Clin Pharmacol* 1979;19:148–150.

Ramsay LE, Silas JH, Ollerenshaw JD, et al. Should the acetylator phenotype be determined when prescribing hydralazine for hypertension? *Eur J Clin Pharmacol* 1984;26:39–42.

Re RN. Tissue renin angiotensin systems. *Med Clin North Am* 2004;88:19–38.

Reboldi G, Angeli F, Cavallini C, et al. Comparison between angiotensin-converting enzyme inhibitors and angiotensin receptor blockers on the risk of myocardial infarction, stroke and death: A meta-analysis. *J Hypertens* 2008;26:1282–1289.

Redon J, Cea-Calvo L, Moreno B, et al. Independent impact of obesity and fat distribution in hypertension prevalence and control in the elderly. *J Hypertens* 2008;26:1757–1764.

Rédon J, Roca-Cusachs A, Mora-Maciá J. Uncontrolled early morning blood pressure in medicated patients: The ACAMPA study. Analysis of the control of blood pressure using ambulatory blood pressure monitoring. *Blood Press Monit* 2002;7: 111–116.

Remuzzi G, Macia M, Ruggenenti P. Prevention and treatment of diabetic renal disease in type 2 diabetes: The BENEDICT study. *J Am Soc Nephrol* 2006;17:S90–S97.

Reyes AJ, Taylor SH. Diuretics in cardiovascular therapy. *Cardiovasc Drugs Ther* 1999;13:371–398.

Ricketts ML, Stewart PM. Regulation of 11beta hydroxysteroid dehydrogenase type 2 by diuretics and the renin-angiotensin-aldosterone axis. *Clin Sci* 1999;96:669–675.

Rinkel GL, Klijn CJ. Prevention and treatment of medical and neurological complications in patients with aneurysmal subarachnoid haemorrhage. *Pract Neurol* 2009;9:195–209.

Roberts R, Sigwart U. New concepts in hypertrophic cardiomyopathies, part II. *Circulation* 2001;104:2249–2252.

Rodman JS, Deutsch DJ, Gutman SI. Methyldopa hepatitis. *Am J Med* 1976;60:941–948.

Rosamond W, Flegal K, Furie K, et al. Heart disease and stroke statistics—2008 update: A report from the American Heart Association Statistics Committee and Stroke Statistics Subcommittee. *Circulation* 2008;117:e25–e146.

Rosendorff C, Black HR, Cannon CP, et al. Treatment of hypertension in the prevention and managment of ischemic heart disease. *Hypertension* 2007;50:e28–e55.

Rouleau JL, Roecker EB, Tendera M, et al. Influence of pretreatment systolic blood pressure on the effect of carvedilol in patients with severe chronic heart failure: The Carvedilol Prospective Randomized Cumulative Survival (COPERNICUS) study. *J Am Coll Cardiol* 2004;43:1423–1439.

Roumie CL, Elasy TA, Greevy R, et al. Improving blood pressure control through provider education, provider alerts, and patient education: A cluster randomized trial. *Ann Intern Med* 2006;145:165–175.

Rubattu S, Sciarretta S, Valenti V, et al. Natriuretic peptides: An update on bioactivity, potential therapeutic use, and implication in cardiovascular diseases. *Am J Hypertens* 2008;21: 733–741.

Rudd P. Clinicians and patients with hypertension. *Am Heart J* 1995;130:572–578.

Ruggenenti P, Mise N, Pisoni R, et al. Diverse effects of increasing lisinopril doses on lipid abnormalities in chronic nephropathies. *Circulation* 2003;107:586–592.

Ruilope LM. Comparison of a new vasodilating beta-blocker, carvedilol, with atenolol in the treatment of mild to moderate essential hypertension. *Am J Hypertens* 1994;7:129–136.

Russell ST, Khandheria BK, Nehra A. Erectile dysfunction and cardiovascular disease. *Mayo Clin Proc* 2004;79:782–794.

Sacco RL, Adams R, Albers G, et al. Guidelines for prevention of stroke in patients with ischemic stroke or transient ischemic attack. *Circulation* 2006;113:e409–e449.

Saito F, Kimura G. Antihypertensive mechanism of diuretics based on pressure-natriuresis relationship. *Hypertension* 1996;27: 914–918.

Sakhaee K, Alpern R, Jacobson HR, et al. Contrasting effects of various potassium salts on renal citrate excretion. *J Clin Endocrinol Metab* 1991;72:396–400.

Salhanick SD, Shannon MW. Management of calcium channel antagonist overdose. *Drug Saf* 2003;26:65–79.

Salles GF, Cardoso CR, Muxfeldt ES. Prognostic influence of office and ambulatory blood pressures in resistant hypertension. *Arch Intern Med* 2008;168:2340–2346.

Sam S, Haffner S, Davidson MH, et al. Relationship of abdominal visceral and subcutaneous adipose tissue with lipoprotein particle number and size in type 2 diabetes. *Diabetes* 2008;57: 2022–2027.

Sarafidis PA, Lasaridis AN, Nilsson PM, et al. Ambulatory blood pressure reduction after rosiglitazone treatment in patients with type 2 diabetes and hypertension correlates with insulin sensitivity increase. *J Hypertens* 2004;22:1769–1777.

Sarafidis PA, Stafylas PC, Kanaki AI, et al. Effects of renin-angiotensin system blockers on renal outcomes and all-cause mortality in patients with diabetic nephropathy: An updated meta-analysis. *Am J Hypertens* 2008;21:922–929.

Sare GM, Gray LJ, Bath PM. Effect of antihypertensive agents on cerebral blood flow and flow velocity in acute ischaemic stroke: Systematic review of controlled studies. *J Hypertens* 2008; 26:1058–1064.

Sato A, Hayashi K, Naruse M, et al. Effectiveness of aldosterone blockade in patients with diabetic nephropathy. *Hypertension* 2003;41:64–68.

Sato A, Saruta T. Aldosterone breakthrough during angiotensin-converting enzyme inhibitor therapy. *Am J Hypertens* 2003; 16:781–788.

Satofuka S, Ichihara A, Nagai N, et al. Suppression of ocular inflammation in endotoxin-induced uveitis by inhibiting nonproteolytic activation of prorenin. *Invest Ophthalmol Vis Sci* 2006;47:2686–2692.

Sattler KJE, Woodrum JE, Galili O, et al. Concurrent treatment with renin-angiotensin system blockers and acetylsalicylic acid reduces nuclear factor κB activation and C-reactive protein expression in human carotid artery plaques. *Stroke* 2005;36:14–20.

Savola J, Vehviäinen O, Väätäinen NJ. Psoriasis as a side effect of beta blockers. *Br Med J* 1987;295:637.

Sawyer N, Gabriel R. Progressive hypokalaemia in elderly patients taking three thiazide potassium-sparing diuretic combinations for thirty-six months. *Postgrad Med J* 1988;64:434–437.

Saxby BK, Harrington F, Wesnes KA, et al. Candesartan and cognitive decline in older patients with hypertension: A substudy of the SCOPE trial. *Neurology* 2008;70:1858–1866.

Saxena PR, Bolt GR. Haemodynamic profiles of vasodilators in experimental hypertension. *Trends Pharmacol Sci* 1986;7: 501–506.

Schefe JH, Neumann C, Goebel M, et al. Prorenin engages the (pro)renin receptor like renin and both ligand activities are unopposed by aliskiren. *J Hypertens* 2008;26:1787–1794.

Scheffers IJ, Kroon AA, Tordoir JH, et al. Rheos Baroreflex Hypertension Therapy System to treat resistant hypertension. *Expert Rev Med Devices* 2008;5:33–39.

Schiffrin EL. Effects of aldosterone on the vasculature. *Hypertension* 2006;47:312–318.

Schlienger RG, Kraenzlin ME, Jick SS, et al. Use of beta-blockers and risk of fractures. *JAMA* 2004;292:1326–1332.

Schnaper HW, Freis ED, Friedman RG, et al. Potassium restoration in hypertensive patients made hypokalemic by hydrochlorothiazide. *Arch Intern Med* 1989;149:2677–2681.

Schoofs MW, van der Klift M, Hofman A, et al. Thiazide diuretics and the risk for hip fracture. *Ann Intern Med* 2003;139: 476–482.

Schrader H, Stovner LJ, Helde G, et al. Prophylactic treatment of migraine with angiotensin converting enzyme inhibitor (lisinopril). *Br Med J* 2001;322:19–22.

Schupp M, Janke J, Clasen R, et al. Angiotensin type 1 receptor blockers induce peroxisome proliferator-activated receptor-gamma activity. *Circulation* 2004;109:2054–2057.

Schwinn DA, Price DT, Narayan P. Alpha1-adrenoceptor subtype selectivity and lower urinary tract symptoms. *Mayo Clin Proc* 2004;79:1423–1434.

Sealey JE, Laragh JH. Aliskiren, the first renin inhibitor for treating hypertension: Reactive renin secretion may limit its effectiveness. *Am J Hypertens* 2007;20:587–597.

Senn S. Individual response to treatment: Is it a valid assumption? *Br Med J* 2004;329:966–968.

Sever PS, Poulter NR, Dahlof B, et al. Antihypertensive therapy and the benefits of atorvastatin in the Anglo-Scandinavian Cardiac Outcomes Trail: Lipid-lowering arm extension. *J Hypertens* 2009;27:947–954.

Shafiq MM, Menon DV, Victor RG. Oral direct renin inhibition: Premise, promise, and potential limitations of a new antihypertensive drug. *Am J Med* 2008;121:265–271.

Shah NC, Pringle SD, Donnan PT, et al. Spironolactone has antiarrhythmic activity in ischaemic cardiac patients without cardiac failure. *J Hypertens* 2007;25:2345–2351.

Sharma AM, Wagner T, Marsalek P. Moxonidine in the treatment of overweight and obese patients with the metabolic syndrome: A postmarketing surveillance study. *J Hum Hypertens* 2004; 18:669–675.

Shea S, Misra D, Ehrlich MH, et al. Predisposing factors for severe, uncontrolled hypertension in an inner-city minority population. *N Engl J Med* 1992;327:776–781.

Shimosawa T, Takano K, Ando K, Fujita T. Magnesium inhibits norepinephrine release by blocking N-type calcium channels at peripheral sympathetic nerve endings. *Hypertension* 2004; 44:897–902.

Shrank WH, Hoang T, Ettner SL, et al. The implications of choice: Prescribing generic or preferred pharmaceuticals improves medication adherence for chronic conditions. *Arch Intern Med* 2006;166:332–337.

Sica DA. Current concepts of pharmacotherapy in hypertension. Thiazide-type diuretics: Ongoing considerations on mechanism of action. *J Clin Hypertens* 2004a;6:661–664.

Sica DA. Minoxidil: An underused vasodilator for resistant or severe hypertension. *J Clin Hypertens* 2004b;6:283–287.

Sica DA. Endothelin receptor antagonism: What does the future hold? *Hypertension* 2008a;52:460–461.

Sica DA. The kidney and hypertension: Causes and treatment. *J Clin Hypertens (Greenwich)* 2008b;10:541–548.

Sica DA, Black HR. Current concepts of pharmacotherapy in hypertension. ACE inhibitor-related angioedema: Can angiotensin-receptor blockers be safely used? *J Clin Hypertens* 2002;4:375–380.

Siegel D, Lopez J, Meier J. Antihypertensive medication adherence in the Department of Veterans Affairs. *Am J Med* 2007; 120: 26–32.

Sink KM, Leng X, Williamson J, et al. Angiotensin-converting enzyme inhibitors and cognitive decline in older adults with hypertension: Results from the cardiovascular health study. *Arch Intern Med* 2009;169:1195–1202.

Siscovick DS, Raghunathan TE, Wicklund KG, et al. Diuretic therapy for hypertension and the risk of primary cardiac arrest. *N Engl J Med* 1994;330:1852–1857.

Skoog I, Lithell H, Hansson L, et al. Effect of baseline cognitive function and antihypertensive treatment on cognitive and cardiovascular outcomes: Study on COgnition and Prognosis in the Elderly (SCOPE). *Am J Hypertens* 2005;18: 1052–1059.

Sloan FA, Bethel MA, Ruiz D Jr, et al. The growing burden of diabetes mellitus in the US elderly population. *Arch Intern Med* 2008;168:192–199.

Smallegange C, Hale TM, Bushfield TL, et al. Persistent lowering of pressure by transplanting kidneys from adult spontaneously hypertensive rats treated with brief antihypertensive therapy. *Hypertension* 2004;44:89–94.

Smith RD, Yokoyama H, Averill DB, et al. Reversal of vascular hypertrophy in hypertensive patients through blockade of angiotensin II receptors. *J Am Soc Hypertens* 2008;2: 165–172.

Snow V, Barry P, Fihn SD, et al. Primary care management of chronic stable angina and asymptomatic suspected or known coronary artery disease: A clinical practice guideline from the American College of Physicians. *Ann Intern Med* 2004;141: 562–567.

Solomon SD, Janardhanan R, Verma A, et al. Effect of angiotensin receptor blockade and antihypertensive drugs on diastolic function in patients with hypertension and diastolic dysfunction: A randomised trial. *Lancet* 2007;369:2079–2087.

Sørensen HT, Mellemkjær L, Olsen JH. Risk of suicide in users of beta-adrenoceptor blockers, calcium channel blockers and angiotensin converting enzyme inhibitors. *Br J Clin Pharmacol* 2001;52:313–318.

Sörgel F, Ettinger B, Benet LZ. The true composition of kidney stones passed during triamterene therapy. *J Urol* 1985;134: 871–873.

Spirito P, Seidman CE, McKenna WJ, et al. The management of hypertrophic cardiomyopathy. *N Engl J Med* 1997;336: 774–785.

Staessen JA, Thijisq L, Fagard R, et al. Effects of immediate versus delayed antihypertensive therapy on outcome in the Systolic Hypertension in Europe Trial. *J Hypertens* 2004;22: 847–857.

Stafford RS, Furberg CD, Finkelstein SN, et al. Impact of clinical trial results on national trends in alpha-blocker prescribing, 1996–2002. *JAMA* 2004;291:54–62.

Steinman MA, Fischer MA, Shlipak MG, et al. Clinician awareness of adherence to hypertension guidelines. *Am J Med* 2004; 117:747–754.

Stergiou GS, Malakos JS, Achimastos AD, et al. Additive hypotensive effect of a dihydropyridine calcium antagonist to that produced by a thiazide diuretic. *J Cardiovasc Pharmacol* 1997; 29:412–416.

Stirling C, Houston J, Robertson S, et al. Diarrhoea, vomiting and ACE inhibitors: An important cause of acute renal failure. *J Hum Hypertens* 2003;17:419–423.

Stokes GS, Bune AJ, Huon N, et al. Long term effectiveness of extended-release nitrate for the treatment of systolic hypertension. *Hypertension* 2005;45:380–384.

Strandgaard S, Haunsø S. Why does antihypertensive treatment prevent stroke but not myocardial infarction? *Lancet* 1987; 2:658–661.

Strandgaard S, Paulson OB. Antihypertensive drugs and cerebral circulation. *Eur J Clin Invest* 1996;26:625–630.

Strazzullo P, Kerry SM, Barbato A, et al. Do statins reduce blood pressure?: A meta-analysis of randomized, controlled trials. *Hypertension* 2007;49:792–798.

Strippoli GF, Craig MC, Schena FP, et al. Role of blood pressure targets and specific antihypertensive agents used to prevent diabetic nephropathy and delay its progression. *J Am Soc Nephrol* 2006;17:S153–S155.

Sugiura T, Kondo T, Kureishi-Bando Y, et al. Nifedipine improves endothelial function: Role of endothelial progenitor cells. *Hypertension* 2008;52:491–498.

Suissa S, Hutchinson T, Brophy JM, et al. ACE-inhibitor use and the long-term risk of renal failure in diabetes. *Kidney Int* 2006;69:913–919.

Sun Z, Zheng L, Detrano R, et al. The accelerating epidemic of hypertension among rural Chinese women: Results from Liaoning Province. *Am J Hypertens* 2008;21:784–788.

Svensson P, de Faire U, Sleight P, et al. Comparative effects of ramipril on ambulatory and office blood pressures: A HOPE Substudy. *Hypertension* 2001;38:E28–E32.

Swain S, Turner C, Tyrrell P, et al. Diagnosis and initial management of acute stroke and transient ischaemic attack: Summary of NICE guidance. *Br Med J* 2008;337:a786.

Takahashi H, Ichihara A, Kaneshiro Y, et al. Regression of nephropathy developed in diabetes by (pro)renin receptor blockade. *J Am Soc Nephrol* 2007;18:2054–2061.

Tanner LA, Bosco LA. Gynecomastia associated with calcium channel blocker therapy. *Arch Intern Med* 1988;148:379–380.

Tannergren C, Engman H, Knutson L, et al. St John's wort decreases the bioavailability of R- and S-verapamil through induction of the first-pass metabolism. *Clin Pharmacol Ther* 2004;75:298–309.

Tanser PH, Campbell LM, Carranza J, et al. Candesartan cilexetil is not associated with cough in hypertensive patients with enalapril-induced cough. *Am J Hypertens* 2000;13:214–218.

Task Force. The Task Force for the Management of Arterial Hypertension of the European Society of Hypertension (ESH) and of the European Society of Cardiology (ESC). *J Hypertens* 2007;25:1105–1187.

Teichert M, de Smet PAGM, Hoffman A, et al. Discontinuation of β-blockers and the risk of myocardial infarction in the elderly. *Drug Saf* 2007;30:541–549.

Telmisartan Randomised AssesmeNt Study in ACE iNtolerant subjects with cardiovascular disease (TRANSCEND) Investigators. Effects of the angiotensin-receptor blocker telmisartan on cardiovascular events in high-risk patients intolerant to angiotensin-converting enzyme inhibitors: A randomised controlled trial. *Lancet* 2008;372:1174–1183.

Tenenbaum A, Motro M, Jones M, et al. Is diuretic therapy associated with an increased risk of colon cancer? *Am J Med* 2001; 110:143–145.

Thöne-Reineke C, Zimmermann M, Neumann C, et al. Are angiotensin receptor blockers neuroprotective? *Curr Hypertens Rep* 2004;6:257–266.

Thulin T, Hedneer T, Gustafsson S, et al. Diltiazem compared with metoprolol as add-on-therapies to diuretics in hypertension. *J Hum Hypertens* 1991;5:107–114.

Tissot AC, Maurer P, Nussberger J, et al. Effect of immunisation against angiotensin II with CYT006-AngQb on ambulatory blood pressure: A double-blind, randomised, placebo-controlled phase IIa study. *Lancet* 2008;371:821–827.

Toner JM, Brawn LA, Yeo WW, et al. Adequacy of twice daily dosing with potassium chloride and spironolactone in thiazide treated hypertensive patients. *Br J Clin Pharmacol* 1991;31: 457–461.

Torp-Pedersen C, Metra M, Charlesworth A, et al. Effects of metoprolol and carvedilol on pre-existing and new onset diabetes in patients with chronic heart failure: Data from the Carvedilol Or Metoprolol European Trial (COMET). *Heart* 2007;93: 968–973.

Touze E, Coste J, Voicu M, et al. Importance of in-hospital initiation of therapies and therapeutic inertia in secondary stroke

prevention: IMplementation of Prevention After a Cerebrovascular evenT (IMPACT) Study. *Stroke* 2008;39:1834–1843.

Townsend RR, Holland OB. Combination of converting enzyme inhibitor with diuretic for the treatment of hypertension. *Arch Intern Med* 1990;150.1171–1103.

Traub YM, Rabinov M, Rosenfeld JB, et al. Elevation of serum potassium during beta blockade. *Clin Pharmacol Ther* 1980; 28:764–768.

Trompet S, Jukema JW, Ford I, et al. Statins and blood pressure. *Arch Intern Med* 2008;168:2383.

Tu K, Chen Z, Lipscombe LL. Mortality among patients with hypertension from 1995 to 2005: A population-based study. *CMAJ* 2008a;178:1436–1440.

Tu K, Chen Z, Lipscombe LL. Prevalence and incidence of hypertension from 1995 to 2005: A population-based study. *CMAJ* 2008b;178:1429–1435.

Turner ST, Bailey KR, Fridley BL, et al. Genomic association analysis suggests chromosome 12 locus influencing antihypertensive response to thiazide diuretic. *Hypertension* 2008;52:359–365.

Valantine H, Keogh A, McIntosh N, et al. Cost containment: Coadministration of diltiazem with cyclosporine after heart transplantation. *J Heart Lung Transplant* 1992;11:1–8.

van Brummelen P, Man in't Veld AJ, Schalekamp MA. Hemodynamic changes during long-term thiazide treatment of essential hypertension in responders and nonresponders. *Clin Pharmacol Ther* 1980;27:328–336.

van Wieren-de Wijer DB, Maitland-van der Zee AH, de Boer A, et al. Interaction between the Gly460Trp alpha-adducin gene variant and diuretics on the risk of myocardial infarction. *J Hypertens* 2009;27:61–68.

van Zwieten PA. The renaissance of centrally acting antihypertensive drugs. *J Hypertens* 1999;17(Suppl. 3):S15–S21.

Vanhees L, Defoor JG, Schepers D, et al. Effect of bisoprolol and atenolol on endurance exercise capacity in healthy men. *J Hypertens* 2000;18.35–43.

Varadarajan P, Joshi N, Appel D, et al. Effect of Beta-blocker therapy on survival in patients with severe mitral regurgitation and normal left ventricular ejection fraction. *Am J Cardiol* 2008; 102:611–615.

Vasan RS, Evans JC, Larson MG, et al. Serum aldosterone and the incidence of hypertension in nonhypertensive persons. *N Eng J Med* 2004;351:33–41.

Vasavada N, Saha C, Agarwal R. A double-blind randomized crossover trial of two loop diuretics in chronic kidney disease. *Kidney Int* 2003;64:632–640.

Verdecchia P, Angeli F, Borgioni C, et al. Changes in cardiovascular risk by reduction of left ventricular mass in hypertension: A meta-analysis. *Am J Hypertens* 2003;16:895–899.

Verdecchia P, Angeli F, Reboldi G. New-onset diabetes, antihypertensive treatment, and outcome. *Hypertension* 2007;50:459–460.

Veterans Administration (VA) Cooperative Study on Antihypertensive Agents. Double blind control study of antihypertensive agents, II: Further report on the comparative effectiveness of reserpine, reserpine and hydralazine, and three ganglion blocking agents, chlorisondamine, mecamylamine, and pentolinium tartrate. *Arch Intern Med* 1962;110:222–229.

Victor RG, Leonard D, Hess P, et al. Factors associated with hypertension awareness, treatment, and control in Dallas County, Texas. *Arch Intern Med* 2008;168:1285–1293.

Victor RG, Ravenell JE, Freeman A, et al. A barber-based intervention for hypertension in African American men: Design of a group randomized trial. *Am Heart J* 2009;157:30–36.

Vincent J, Harris SI, Foulds G, et al. Lack of effect of grapefruit juice on the pharmacokinetics and pharmacodynamics of amlodipine. *Br J Clin Pharmacol* 2000;50:455–463.

Vlachopoulos C, Aznaouridis K, Ioakeimidis N, et al. Arterial function and intima-media thickness in hypertensive patients with erectile dysfunction. *J Hypertens* 2008;26:1829–1836.

Volini IF, Flaxman N. The effect of nonspecific operations on essential hypertension. *JAMA* 1939;112:2126–2128.

Vrijens B, Vincze G, Kristanto P, et al. Adherence to prescribed antihypertensive drug treatments: Longitudinal study of electronically compiled dosing histories. *Br Med J* 2008;336:1114–1117.

Wachtell K, Okin PM, Olsen MH, et al. Regression of electrocardiographic left ventricular hypertrophy during antihypertensive therapy and reduction in sudden cardiac death: The LIFE Study. *Circulation* 2007;116:700–705.

Wagner ML, Walters AS, Coleman RG, et al. Randomized, double-blind, placebo-controlled study of clonidine in restless legs syndrome. *Sleep* 1996;19:52–58.

Wald NJ, Law MR. A strategy to reduce cardiovascular disease by more than 80%. *Br Med J* 2003;326:1419.

Wallace AW, Galindez D, Salahieh A, et al. Effect of clonidine on cardiovascular morbidity and mortality after noncardiac surgery. *Anesthesiology* 2004;101:284–293.

Wang JG, Li Y, Franklin SS, et al. Prevention of stroke and myocardial infarction by amlodipine and Angiotensin receptor blockers: A quantitative overview. *Hypertension* 2007a;50: 181–188.

Wang PS, Avorn J, Brookhart MA, et al. Effects of noncardiovascular comorbidities on antihypertensive use in elderly hypertensives. *Hypertension* 2005;46:273–279.

Wang YR, Alexander GC, Stafford RS. Outpatient hypertension treatment, treatment intensification, and control in Western Europe and the United States. *Arch Intern Med* 2007b;167:141–147.

Warner TD, Mitchell JA. COX-2 selectivity alone does not define the cardiovascular risks associated with non-steroidal anti-inflammatory drugs. *Lancet* 2008;371:270–273.

Webb DJ, Fulton JD, Leckie BJ, et al. The effect of chronic prazosin therapy on the response of the renin-angiotensin system in patients with essential hypertension. *J Hum Hypertens* 1987;1:194–200.

Weber MA, Byyny RL, Pratt H, et al. Blood pressure effects of the angiotensin II receptor blocker, losartan. *Arch Intern Med* 1995;155:405–411.

Webster J, Koch H-F. Aspects of tolerability of centrally acting antihypertensive drugs. *J Cardiovasc Pharmacol.* 1996;27:S49-S54.

Weir MR, Moser M. Diuretics and beta-blockers: Is there a risk for dyslipidemia. *Am Heart J* 2000;139:174–184.

Weir MR, Prisant LM, Papademmetriou V, et al. Antihypertensive therapy and quality of life. *Am J Hypertens* 1996;9:854–859.

Weir MR, Rosenberger C, Fink JC. Pilot study to evaluate a water displacement technique to compare effects of diuretics and ACE inhibitors to alleviate lower extremity edema due to dihydropyridine calcium antagonists. *Am J Hypertens* 2001;14:963–968.

Weirnberger MH. The use of selective aldosterone antagonists. *Curr Hypertens Rep.* 2004;6:342–345.

Weinberger MH, Fineberg NS. Sodium and volume sensitivity of blood pressure. *Hypertension* 1991;18:67–71.

Westhoff JH, Hilgers KF, Steinbach MP, et al. Hypertension induces somatic cellular senescence in rats and humans by induction of cell cycle inhibitor p16INK4a. *Hypertension* 2008;52:123–129.

Whang R, Flink EB, Dyckner T, et al. Magnesium depletion as a cause of refractory potassium repletion. *Arch Intern Med* 1985;145:1686–1689.

White WB. Cardiovascular effects of the cyclooxygenase inhibitors. *Hypertension* 2007;49:408–418.

White WB, Calhoun DA, Samuel R, et al. Improving blood pressure control: Increase the dose of diuretic or switch to a fixed-dose angiotensin receptor blocker/diuretic? The valsartan hydrochlorothiazide diuretic for initial control and titration to achieve optimal therapeutic effect (Val-DICTATE) trial. *J Clin Hypertens (Greenwich)* 2008;10:450–458.

White WB, Lacourciere Y, Davidai G. Effects of the antiotensin II receptor blockers telmisartan versus valsartan on the circadian variation of blood pressure: Impact of the early morning period. *Am J Hypertens* 2004;17:347–353.

Widmer P, Maibach R, Knzi UP, et al. Diuretic-related hypokalaemia. *Eur J Clin Pharmacol* 1995;49:31–36.

Wigley FM. Raynaud's phenomenon. *N Engl J Med* 2002;347:1001–1008.

Wiklund I, Halling K, Ryden-Bergsten T, et al. What is the effect of lowering the blood pressure on quality of life? *Arch Mal Coeur Vaiss* 1999;92:1079–1082.

Wilcox CS. Metabolic and adverse effects of diuretics. *Semin Nephrol* 1999;19:557–568.

Wilcox CS, Mitch WE, Kelly RA, et al. Response of the kidney to furosemide. I. Effects of salt intake and renal compensation. *J Lab Clin Med* 1983;102:450–458.

Wildman RP, Muntner P, Reynolds K, et al. The obese without cardiometabolic risk factor clustering and the normal weight with cardiometabolic risk factor clustering: Prevalence and correlates of 2 phenotypes among the US population (NHANES 1999–2004). *Arch Intern Med* 2008;168:1617–1624.

Williams B, Poulter NR, Brown MJ, et al. British Hypertension Society guidelines for hypertension management 2004 (BHS-IV): Summary. *Br Med J* 2004;328:634–640.

Williams TA, Mulatero P, Filigheddu F, et al. Role of HSD11B2 polymorphisms in essential hypertension and the diuretic response to thiazides. *Kidney Int* 2005;67:631–637.

Willmot M, Ghadami A, Whysall B, et al. Transdermal glyceryl trinitrate lowers blood pressure and maintains cerebral blood flow in recent stroke. *Hypertension* 2006;47:1209–1215.

Wilson IM, Freis ED. Relationship between plasma and extracellular fluid volume depletion and the antihypertensive effect of chlorothiazide. *Circulation* 1959;20:1028–1036.

Wilson MF, Haring O, Lewin A, et al. Comparison of guanfacine versus clonidine for efficacy, safety and occurrence of withdrawal syndrome in step-2 treatment of mild to moderate essential hypertension. *Am J Cardiol* 1986;57:43E–49E.

Winer BM. The antihypertensive mechanisms of salt depletion induced by hydrochlorothiazide. *Circulation* 1961;24:788–796.

Wing LM, Reid CM, Ryan P, et al. A comparison of outcomes with angiotensin-converting-enzyme inhibitors and diuretics for hypertension in the elderly. *N Engl J Med* 2003;348:583–592.

Woo KS, Nicholls MG. High prevalence of persistent cough with angiotensin converting enzyme inhibitors in Chinese. *Br J Clin Pharmacol* 1995;40:141–144.

Wood R. Bronchospasm and cough as adverse reactions to the ACE inhibitors captopril, enalapril and lisinopril. *Br J Clin Pharmacol* 1995;39:264–270.

Wood DA, Kotseva K, Connolly S, et al. Nurse-coordinated multidisciplinary, family-based cardiovascular disease prevention programme (EUROACTION) for patients with coronary heart disease and asymptomatic individuals at high risk of cardiovascular disease: A paired, cluster-randomised controlled trial. *Lancet* 2008;371:1999–2012.

Wright JT Jr, Dunn JK, Cutler JA, et al. Outcomes in hypertensive black and nonblack patients treated with chlorthalidone, amlodipine, and lisinopril. *JAMA* 2005;293:1595–1608.

Wright JT Jr, Harris-Haywood S, Pressel S, et al. Clinical outcomes by race in hypertensive patients with and without the metabolic syndrome: Antihypertensive and Lipid-Lowering Treatment to Prevent Heart Attack Trial (ALLHAT). *Arch Intern Med* 2008;168:207–217.

Wu JY, Leung WY, Chang S, et al. Effectiveness of telephone counselling by a pharmacist in reducing mortality in patients receiving polypharmacy: Randomised controlled trial. *Br Med J* 2006;333:522.

Wu Y, Tai ES, Heng D, et al. Risk factors associated with hypertension awareness, treatment, and control in a multi-ethnic Asian population. *J Hypertens* 2009;27:190–197.

Xi GL, Cheng JW, Lu GC. Meta-analysis of randomized controlled trials comparing telmisartan with losartan in the treatment of patients with hypertension. *Am J Hypertens* 2008;21: 546–552.

Yang HYT, Erdös EG, Levin YA. Dipeptidyl carboxypeptidase that converts angiotensin I and inactivates bradykinin. *Biochim Biophys Acta* 1970;214:374–376.

Yasar S, Zhou J, Varadhan R, et al. The use of angiotensin-converting enzyme inhibitors and diuretics is associated with a reduced incidence of impairment on cognition in elderly women. *Clin Pharmacol Ther* 2008;84:119–126.

Yeo WW, Chadwick IG, Kraskiewics M, et al. Resolution of ACE inhibitor cough. *Br J Clin Pharmacol* 1995;40:423–429.

Yip HK, Chang LT, Chang WN, et al. Level and value of circulating endothelial progenitor cells in patients after acute ischemic stroke. *Stroke* 2008;39:69–74.

Yki-Järvinen H. Thiazolidinediones. *N Engl J Med* 2004;351: 1106–1118.

Yokoyama K, Yang W, Preblick R, et al. Effects of a step-therapy program for angiotensin receptor blockers on antihypertensive medication utilization patterns and cost of drug therapy. *J Manag Care Pharm* 2007;13:235–244.

Yu HM, Lin SG, Liu GZ, et al. Associations between CYP11B2 gene polymorphisms and the response to angiotensin-converting enzyme inhibitors. *Clin Pharmacol Ther* 2006;79. 581–589.

Yuan J-M, Castelao JE, Gago-Dominguez M, et al. Hypertension, obesity and their medications in relation to renal cell carcinoma. *Br J Cancer* 1998;77:1508–1513.

Yusuf S, Diener HC, Sacco RL, et al. Telmisartan to prevent recurrent stroke and cardiovascular events. *N Engl J Med* 2008; 359:1225–1237.

Zacest R, Gilmore E, Koch-Weser J. Treatment of essential hypertension with combined vasodilation and beta-adrenergic blockade. *N Engl J Med* 1972;286:617–622.

Zanchetti A, Cuspidi C, Comarella L, et al. Left ventricular diastolic dysfunction in elderly hypertensives: Results of the APROS-diadys study. *J Hypertens* 2007;25:2158–2167.

Zanchetti A, Hansson L, Leonetti G, et al. Low-dose aspirin does not interfere with the blood pressure-lowering effects of antihypertensive therapy. *J Hypertens* 2002;20:1015–1022.

Zarnke KB, Feldman RD. Direct angiotensin converting enzyme inhibitor-mediated venodilation. *Clin Pharmacol Ther* 1996; 59:559–568.

Zhang R, Witkowski S, Fu Q, et al. Cerebral hemodynamics after short- and long-term reduction in blood pressure in mild and moderate hypertension. *Hypertension* 2007;49:1149–1155.

Zhu Z, Zhu S, Liu D, et al. Thiazide-like diuretics attenuate agonist-induced vasoconstriction by calcium desensitization linked to rho kinase. *Hypertension* 2005;45:233–239.

Zillich AJ, Garg J, Basu S, et al. Thiazide diuretics, potassium, and the development of diabetes: A quantitative review. *Hypertension* 2006;48:219–224.

Zimlichman R, Shargorodsky M, Wainstein J. Prolonged treatment of hypertensive patients with low dose HCTZ improves arterial elasticity but not if they have NIDDM or IFG. Treatment with full dose HCTZ (25 mg/d) aggravates metabolic parameters and arterial stiffness [Abstract]. *Am J Hypertens* 2004;17:138A.

Hypertensive Crises

A lthough only a small spot in the large panorama of hypertension, hypertensive crises represent, on one hand, the most immediate danger to those afflicted and, on the other, the most dramatic proof of the life-saving potential of antihypertensive therapy. Such crises are now less likely to be the end result of chronic hypertension but may be seen at any age, representing the manifestations of suddenly developing hypertension from such diverse causes as substance abuse, immunosuppressive drugs, and human immunodeficiency virus infection (Ewen et al., 2009).

DEFINITIONS

A *hypertensive emergency* is a situation that requires immediate reduction in blood pressure (BP) with parenteral agents because of acute or progressing target organ damage (Table 8-1).

A *hypertensive urgency* is a situation with markedly elevated BP but without severe symptoms or progressive target organ damage, wherein the BP should be reduced within hours, often with oral agents. Some of the circumstances listed in Table 8-1 may be urgencies rather than emergencies if of lesser severity, including some patients with accelerated-malignant hypertension, perioperative or rebound hypertension, less severe body burn, or epistaxis. The distinction between an emergency and an urgency is often ambiguous.

Accelerated-malignant hypertension represents markedly elevated BP with papilledema (grade 4 Keith-Wagener retinopathy) and/or hemorrhages and exudates (grade 3 Keith-Wagener retinopathy). The clinical features and prognosis are similar with grade 3 or grade 4 retinopathy. (Ahmed et al., 1986).

Hypertensive encephalopathy is a sudden, marked elevation of BP with severe headache and altered mental status, reversible by reduction of BP. Encephalopathy is more common in previously normotensive individuals whose pressures rise suddenly, such as during pregnancy with eclampsia; the accelerated-malignant course often appears without encephalopathy in individuals with more chronic hypertension whose pressures progressively rise.

ACCELERATED-MALIGNANT HYPERTENSION

Mechanisms

When BP reaches some critical level—in experimental animals at a mean arterial pressure of 150 mm Hg—lesions appear in arterial walls, and the syndrome of accelerated-malignant hypertension begins (Fig. 8-1). This may be provoked by one or more vasoactive factors, but the accelerated-malignant phase is likely to be a nonspecific consequence of very high BP (Beilin & Goldby, 1977). Any form of hypertension may progress to the accelerated-malignant phase, some without activation of the renin-angiotensin system or other known humoral mechanisms (Gavras et al., 1975).

Structural Changes

In animal models, the level of the arterial pressure correlates closely with the development of fibrinoid necrosis, the experimental hallmark of accelerated-malignant hypertension (Byrom, 1974). In humans, fibrinoid necrosis is rare, perhaps because those who die from an acute attack have not had time to develop the lesion and those who live with therapy are able to repair it. The typical lesions, best seen in the kidney, are hyperplastic arteriosclerosis and accelerated glomerular obsolescence (Kitiyakara & Guzman, 1998).

TABLE 8.1   Hypertensive Emergencies

Accelerated-malignant hypertension with papilledema

Cerebrovascular conditions

Hypertensive encephalopathy
Atherothrombotic brain infarction with severe hypertension
Intracerebral hemorrhage
Subarachnoid hemorrhage
Head trauma

Cardiac conditions

Acute aortic dissection
Acute left ventricular failure
Acute or impending myocardial infarction
After coronary bypass surgery

Renal conditions

Acute glomerulonephritis
Renovascular hypertension
Renal crises from collagen-vascular diseases
Severe hypertension after kidney transplantation

Excess circulating catecholamines

Pheochromocytoma crisis
Food or drug interactions with monoamine oxidase
   inhibitors
Sympathomimetic drug use (cocaine)
Rebound hypertension after sudden cessation of
   antihypertensive drugs
Automatic hyperreflexia after spinal cord injury

Eclampsia
Surgical conditions

Severe hypertension in patients requiring immediate
   surgery
Postoperative hypertension
Postoperative bleeding from vascular suture lines
Severe body burns
Severe epistaxis

Humoral Factors

There is support, however, for the involvement of factors besides the level of the BP in setting off the accelerated-malignant phase (Kincaid-Smith, 1991). As shown on the right side of Figure 8-1, in both rats (Gross et al., 1975) and dogs (Dzau et al., 1981) with unilateral renal artery stenosis, the accelerated-malignant phase was preceded by natriuresis that markedly activated the renin-angiotensin system. The progression was delayed by giving saline loads after the natriuresis.

Whether these animal models involving a major insult to renal blood flow are applicable to most human accelerated-malignant hypertension is uncertain; however, renal artery stenosis is a common cause of

accelerated-malignant hypertension in humans, found in 20% to 35% of patients with this form of hypertension (Davis et al., 1979; Webster et al., 1993).

Evidence for the pathway shown on the left side of Figure 8-1 includes the presence of circulating endothelial and platelet microparticles in patients with severe uncontrolled hypertension (Preston et al., 2003) and markers of endothelial dysfunction and platelet activation in patients with malignant hypertension (Lip et al., 2001).

Clinical Features

Accelerated-malignant hypertension may be accompanied by various symptoms and signs (Table 8-2). However, it is not uncommon to see patients, particularly young black men, who deny any prior symptoms when seen in the end stages of the hypertensive process, with their kidneys destroyed, heart failing, and brain function markedly impaired. Even in the elderly, hypertension may initially present in the accelerated-malignant phase (Lip et al., 2000).

Less common clinical presentations include:

• Aortic dissection with giant cell arteritis (Smulders & Verhagen, 2008)
• Fibrinoid necrosis within abdominal arteries producing major gastrointestinal tract infarction with an acute abdomen (Padfield, 1975)
• Rapidly progressive necrotizing vasculitis as a feature of lupus (Mitchell, 1994) or polyarteritis nodosa (Blaustein et al., 2004)
• Hematospermia or hematuria (Fleming et al., 2008)

Funduscopic Findings

The effects of the markedly elevated BP are displayed in the optic fundi (Fig. 8-2). Acute changes may include arteriolar spasm, either segmental or diffuse; retinal edema, with a sheen or ripples; retinal

TABLE 8.2   Clinical Characteristics of Accelerated-Malignant Hypertension

Blood pressure: usually >140 mm Hg diastolic
Funduscopic findings: hemorrhages, exudates, papilledema
Neurologic status: headache, confusion, somnolence,
   stupor, vision loss, focal deficits, seizures, coma
Renal status: oliguria, azotemia
Gastrointestinal status: nausea, vomiting

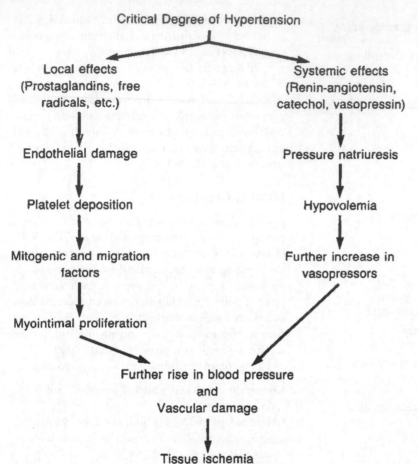

Critical Degree of Hypertension

Local effects
(Prostaglandins, free
radicals, etc.)

Systemic effects
(Renin-angiotensin,
catechol, vasopressin)

Endothelial damage

Pressure natriuresis

Platelet deposition

Hypovolemia

Mitogenic and migration
factors

Further increase in
vasopressors

Myointimal proliferation

Further rise in blood pressure
and
Vascular damage

Tissue ischemia

FIGURE 8-1   Scheme for initiation and progression of accelerated-malignant hypertension.

hemorrhages, either superficial and flame-shaped or deep and dot-shaped; retinal exudates, either hard and waxy from resorption of edema or with a raw cotton appearance from ischemia; and papilledema and engorged retinal veins (Foguet et al., 2008).

Similar retinopathy with hemorrhages and even papilledema rarely occurs in severe anemia, collagen diseases, and subacute bacterial endocarditis. Some patients have pseudopapilledema associated with congenital anomalies, hyaline bodies (drusen) in the disc, or severe farsightedness. Fluorescein fundus photography will distinguish between the true and the pseudo states. In addition, benign intracranial hypertension may produce real papilledema but is usually a minimally symptomatic and self-limited process (Jain & Rosner, 1992).

Evaluation

In addition to an adequate history and physical examination, a few laboratory tests should be done immediately to assess the patient's status (Table 8-3).

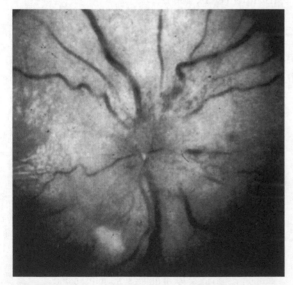

FIGURE 8-2   Funduscopic photography showing typical features of accelerated-malignant hypertension.

TABLE 8.3	Initial Evaluation of Patients with a Hypertensive Emergency

History

Prior diagnosis and treatment of hypertension
Intake of pressor agents: street drugs, sympathomimetics
Symptoms of cerebral, cardiac, and visual dysfunction

Physical examination

Blood pressure
Funduscopy
Neurologic status
Cardiopulmonary status
Body fluid volume assessment
Peripheral pulses

Laboratory evaluation

Hematocrit and blood smear
Urine analysis
Automated chemistry: creatinine, glucose, electrolytes
Electrocardiogram
Plasma renin activity and aldosterone (if primary aldosteronism is suspected)
Plasma renin activity before and 1 h after 25 mg captopril (if renovascular hypertension is suspected)
Spot urine or plasma for metanephrine (if pheochromocytoma is suspected)
Chest radiograph (if heart failure or aortic dissection is suspected)

Laboratory Findings

In 27% of patients with malignant hypertension, van den Born et al. (2008) found thrombotic microangiopathy, characterized by thromboses of small vessels, intravascular hemolysis with fragmented red blood cells, elevated lactic dehydrogenase, and consumption of platelets. They postulate that endothelial damage from high BP triggers release of the prothrombotic van Willebrand factor that activates factor which activates intravascular coagulation.

The urine contains protein and red cells. In a few patients, acute oliguric renal failure may be the presenting manifestation (Lip et al., 1997).

Various features of renal insufficiency may be present. Approximately half of patients have hypokalemia, reflecting secondary aldosteronism from increased renin secretion induced by intrarenal ischemia (Kawazoe et al., 1987). Hyponatremia is usual and can be extreme (Trivelli et al., 2005), in contrast to the hypernatremia found in primary aldosteronism.

The electrocardiogram usually displays evidence of left ventricular hypertrophy, strain, and lateral ischemia. Echocardiography may show incoordinate contractions with impaired diastolic function and delayed mitral valve opening (Shapiro & Beevers, 1983).

Evaluation for Identifiable Causes

Once causes for the presenting picture other than severe hypertension are excluded and necessary immediate therapy is provided, an appropriate evaluation for identifiable causes of the hypertension should be performed as quickly as possible. It is preferable to obtain necessary blood and urine samples for required laboratory studies before institution of therapies that may markedly complicate subsequent evaluation. None of these procedures should delay effective therapy.

Renovascular hypertension is by far the most likely secondary cause and, unfortunately, the one that may be least obvious by history, physical examination, and routine laboratory tests. It should be particularly looked for in older patients with extensive atherosclerosis (see Chapter 10).

If there are suggestive symptoms of phenochromocytoma, blood for a plasma metanephrine assay should be collected (see Chapter 12).

Primary aldosteronism should be considered, particularly if significant hypokalemia is noted on the initial blood test. A plasma renin and aldosterone level should be obtained. In most cases of primary aldosteronism presenting with malignant hypertension, plasma renin activity has initially been elevated, later being suppressed as the intrarenal necrotizing process subsides (Suzuki et al., 2002) (see Chapter 11).

Prognosis

If untreated, most patients with accelerated-malignant hypertension will die within 6 months. The 1-year survival rate was only 10% to 20% without therapy (Dustan et al., 1958). With current therapy, 5-year survival rates of greater than 70% are usual (Lip et al., 2000; Webster et al., 1993), clearly showing the major protection provided by antihypertensive therapy.

Many patients when first seen with accelerated-malignant hypertension have significant renal damage, which markedly worsens their prognosis (van den Born et al., 2005). In one series of 100 consecutive patients with malignant hypertension (Bing et al., 2004), the 5-year survival rate of those without renal impairment (serum creatinine <1.5 mg/dL) was 96%, no different from that of the general population. However, among those with renal impairment, 5-year survival fell to 65%. When vigorous antihypertensive therapy is begun, renal function often worsens transiently, but in nearly half of those with initial renal insufficiency, function remains invariant or improves (Lip et al., 1997). Of 54 patients with malignant hypertension requiring dialysis, 12 recovered sufficient renal function to allow withdrawal of dialysis (James et al., 1995).

HYPERTENSIVE ENCEPHALOPATHY

With or without the structural defects of accelerated-malignant hypertension, progressively higher BP can lead to hypertensive encephalopathy.

Pathophysiology

Breakthrough Vasodilation

With changes in BP, cerebral vessels dilate or constrict to maintain a relatively constant level of cerebral blood flow (CBF), the process of autoregulation that is regulated by sympathetic nervous activity (Tuor, 1992). Figure 8-3 shows direct measurements taken in cats, with progressive vasodilation as pressures are lowered and progressive vasoconstriction as pressures rise (MacKenzie et al., 1976). Note, however, that when mean arterial pressures reach a critical level, approximately 180 mm Hg, the previously constricted vessels, unable to withstand such high pressures, are stretched and dilated—first in areas with less muscular tone, producing irregular sausage-string patterns, and later diffusely, producing generalized vasodilation. This vasodilation allows a breakthrough of CBF, which hyperperfuses the brain under high pressure, with leakage of fluid into the perivascular tissue, leading to cerebral edema and the clinical syndrome of hypertensive encephalopathy (Strandgaard & Paulson, 1989).

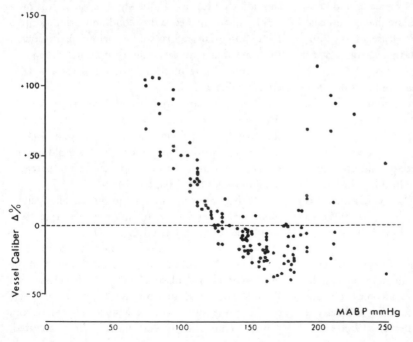

FIGURE 8-3 Observed change in the caliber of pial arterioles with a caliber of less than 50 mm in eight cats, calculated as a percentage of change from the caliber at a mean arterial blood pressure (MABP) of 135 mm Hg. The BP was raised by intravenous infusion of angiotensin II. (Reprinted from MacKenzie ET, Strandgaard S, Graham DI, et al. Effects of acutely induced hypertension in cats on pial arteriolar caliber, local cerebral blood flow, and the blood-brain barrier. *Circ Res* 1976;39:33, with permission.)

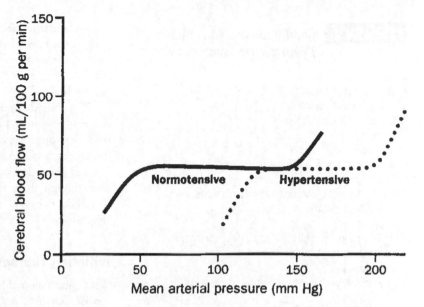

FIGURE 8-4 Idealized curves of CBF at varying levels of systemic BP in normotensive and hypertensive subjects. Rightward shift in autoregulation is shown with chronic hypertension. (Adapted from Strandgaard S, Olesen J, Skinhøj E, et al. Autoregulation of brain circulation in severe arterial hypertension. *Br Med J* 1973;1: 507–510.)

Breakthrough vasodilation has also been demonstrated in humans (Strandgaard et al., 1973). Figure 8-4 shows curves of autoregulation constructed by measuring CBF repetitively while arterial BP was lowered by vasodilators or raised by vasoconstrictors. CBF is constant between mean arterial pressures of 60 and 120 mm Hg in normotensive subjects. However, when pressure was raised beyond the limit of autoregulation, breakthrough hyperperfusion occurred.

Pressures such as these are handled without obvious trouble in chronic hypertensives, whose blood vessels adapt to the chronically elevated BP with structural thickening, presumably mediated by sympathetic nerves (Tuor, 1992). Thereby the entire curve of autoregulation is shifted to the right (Fig. 8-4). Even with this shift, breakthrough will occur if mean arterial pressures are markedly raised to levels beyond 180 mm Hg.

These findings explain a number of clinical observations. Previously normotensive people who suddenly become hypertensive may develop encephalopathy at relatively low levels of hypertension, which are nonetheless beyond their upper limit of autoregulation. These include children with acute glomerulonephritis and young women with eclampsia. On the other hand, chronically hypertensive patients less commonly develop encephalopathy and only at much higher pressures.

In regard to the lower portion of the curve, when the BP is lowered by antihypertensive drugs too quickly, chronic hypertensives often are unable to tolerate the reduction without experiencing cerebral hypoperfusion, manifested by weakness and dizziness.

These symptoms may appear at levels of BP that are still well within the normal range of autoregulation and well tolerated by normotensives. The reason is that the entire curve of autoregulation shifts, so that the lower end also is moved, with a falloff of CBF at levels of 100 to 120 mm Hg mean arterial pressure (Fig. 8-4). Moreover, chronic hypertensives may lose their ability to autoregulate, increasing their risk of cerebral ischemia when BP is lowered acutely (Jansen et al., 1987).

As detailed in Chapter 7, if the BP is lowered gradually, the curve can shift back toward normal so that greater reductions in pressure can eventually be tolerated. However, maneuvers that increase CBF further and thereby increase intracranial pressure, such as CO_2 inhalation or cerebral vasodilators (e.g., hydralazine and nitroprusside), may be harmful in patients with encephalopathy.

Central Nervous System Changes

Encephalopathic patients have many of the same laboratory findings seen in patients with malignant hypertension, but they have more central nervous system manifestations. The cerebrospinal fluid rarely shows pleocytosis (McDonald et al., 1993) but is usually under increased pressure. Computed tomography or magnetic resonance imaging shows a characteristic posterior leukoencephalopathy predominantly affecting the parietooccipital white matter, often the cerebellum and brainstem (Karampekios et al., 2004), and occasionally other areas as well (Vaughan & Delanty, 2000).

TABLE 8.4	Conditions that May Mimic a Hypertensive Emergency

Acute left ventricular failure
End-stage renal disease
Cerebrovascular accident
Subarachnoid hemorrhage
Brain tumor
Head injury
Reversible cerebral vasoconstriction syndromes
Epilepsy (postictal)
Collagen diseases, particularly systemic lupus, with cerebral vasculitis
Encephalitis
Drug ingestion: sympathomimetics (e.g., cocaine)
Acute intermittent porphyria
Hypercalcemia
Acute anxiety with hyperventilation syndrome or panic attack

Differential Diagnosis

There are clinical situations in which the BP is elevated and the patient has findings that suggest hypertension-induced target organ damage wherein the findings are unrelated to the elevated BP. Table 8-4 lists conditions that may mimic a hypertensive emergency. A less aggressive approach to lowering of the BP is indicated in such patients. Particular caution is warranted after a stroke, when a rapid decrease in BP may shunt blood away from the ischemic area and extend the lesion (Adams et al., 2007).

In addition to the two specific presentations of accelerated-malignant hypertension and hypertensive encephalopathy, hypertension may be life threatening when it accompanies other acute conditions wherein a markedly elevated BP contributes to the ongoing tissue damage (Table 8-1). The role of hypertension in most of these conditions is covered in Chapter 4, and some of the other specific circumstances (e.g., pheochromocytoma crises and eclampsia) are covered in their respective chapters.

THERAPY FOR HYPERTENSIVE EMERGENCIES

The majority of patients with the conditions shown in Table 8-1 require immediate reduction in BP. In those patients with hypertensive encephalopathy, if the pressure is not reduced, cerebral edema will

worsen and the lack of autoregulation in ischemic brain tissue may result in further increases in the volume of the ischemic tissue, which may cause either acute herniation or more gradual compression of normal brain.

On the other hand, the shift to the right of the curve of cerebral autoregulation in most patients who develop encephalopathy exposes them to the hazards of a fall in CBF when systemic pressure is lowered abruptly by more than approximately 25%, even though these levels are not truly hypotensive (Immink et al., 2004; Strandgaard & Paulson, 1996) (Fig. 8-4).

Initiating Therapy

With encephalopathy or evidence of progressive myocardial ischemia, no more than a very few minutes should be taken to admit a patient to an intensive care unit, set up intravenous access, and begin frequent monitoring of the BP, usually with an intra-arterial line. The initial blood and urine samples should be obtained, and antihypertensive therapy should begin immediately thereafter.

Monitoring Therapy

Abrupt falls in pressure should be avoided, and the goal of immediate therapy should be to lower the diastolic pressure only to approximately 110 mm Hg. The reductions may need to be even less if signs of tissue ischemia develop as the pressure is lowered. Most of the catastrophes seen with treatment of hypertensive emergencies were related to overly aggressive reduction of the BP (Jansen et al., 1987).

Particular care should be taken in elderly patients and in patients with known cerebrovascular disease, who are even more vulnerable to sudden falls in systemic BP (Fischberg et al., 2000). In patients with recent ischemic stroke, the American Stroke Association recommends cautious reduction of BP by 10% to 15% if systolic levels are above 220 mm Hg or diastolic above 120 mm Hg (Adams et al., 2007).

If the neurologic status worsens as treatment proceeds, urgent computed tomography of the brain should be obtained and, if potentially life-threatening cerebral edema is identified, osmotic diuresis with mannitol, often plus intravenous furosemide, can be effective (Brott & Bogousslavsky, 2000). It may be possible to monitor intracranial pressure and cerebral autoregulation noninvasively (Schmidt et al., 2003).

Parenteral Drugs

Table 8-5 lists the choices of parenteral therapy now available. All are capable of inducing hypotension, a risk that mandates careful monitoring of BP. They are covered in the order shown in Table 8-5.

Before examining the various parenteral agents, an important fact must be recognized: There are no

data to document which of these drugs is best or, more importantly, whether their use is followed by decrease in morbidity or mortality. As described by Perez and Musini (2008) in their Cochrane systematic review of 5,413 identified citations, only 15 were acceptable as a randomized control trial (RCT), and only one of these was of good quality. Perez and Musini (2008) could find no adequate evidence to ask the question, "Does antihypertensive therapy, as compared to placebo or no treatment, change mortality and morbidity in patients with hypertensive

TABLE 8.5	Parenteral Drugs for Treatment of Hypertensive Emergency				
Drug[a]	Dose	Onset of Action	Duration of Action	Adverse Effects[b]	Special Indications
Vasodilators					
Nitroprusside	0.25–10.00 µg/kg/min IV	Immediate	1–2 min	Nausea, vomiting, muscle twitching, thiocyanate and cyanide toxicity	Not preferred for most hypertensive emergencies
Nitroglycerin	5–100 µg/min	2–5 min	5–10 min	Headache, vomiting, methemoglobinemia, tolerance with prolonged use	Not preferred but may be useful with coronary ischemia
Fenoldopam (Corlopam)	0.1–0.6 µg/kg/min IV	4–5 min	10–15 min	Tachycardia, increased intraocular pressure,	May be indicated with renal insufficiency
Nicardipine[c] (Cardene IV)	5–15 mg/h	5–10 min	1–4 h	Headache, nausea, flushing, tachycardia	Most hypertensive emergencies
Clevidipine (Cleviprex)	1–2 mg IV, rapidly increasing dose to 16 mg maximum	2–4 min	5–15 min		Most hypertensive emergencies
Hydralazine	5–20 mg IV	10–20 min	1–4 h	Tachycardia, flushing, headache, vomiting, aggravation of angina	Eclampsia. Not for aortic dissection
	10–40 mg IM	20–30 min	4–6 h		
Adrenergic inhibitor					
Phentolamine	5–15 mg IV	1–2 min	3–10 min	Tachycardia, flushing, headache	Catecholamine excess
Esmolol (Brevibloc)	250–500 µg/kg/min for 4 min, then 50–300 µg/kg/min IV	1–2 min	10–20 min	Hypotension, nausea	Aortic dissection after surgery
Labetalol (Normodyne, Trandate)	20–80 mg IV bolus every 10 min	5–10 min	3–6 h	Vomiting, scalp tingling, burning in throat, dizziness, nausea, heart block, orthostatic hypotension	Most hypertensive emergencies except acute heart failure
	2 mg/min IV infusion				

[a]In order of rapidity of action.
[b]Hypotension may occur with any.
[c]Intravenous formulations of other CCBs are also available.

emergencies?… We feel it is important for physicians to know that this is one of the clinical settings where treatment is not supposed by RCT evidence."

The authors further note the absence of data to inform clinicians as to which drug class provides more benefit than harm. They state: "Neither did we find RCTs that compared different strategies to reduce blood pressure. Thus, how fast or how much blood pressure should be lowered in hypertensive emergencies remains unknown."

In the absence of evidence, clinicians must continue to administer parenteral drugs to lower markedly elevated BP in patients with hypertensive emergency. However, we must do so carefully, with close supervision, choosing drugs that allow for gradual reduction of BP, that have no inherent toxicity, and provide the ability to back down if target organ functions deteriorate.

With current criteria, the use of nitroprusside can no longer be defended though it was the first truly effective agent used in such patients (Gifford, 1959).

Nitroprusside

The BP always falls when nitroprusside is given, although it occasionally takes much more than the usual starting dose of 0.25 µg/kg/minute for a response. The antihypertensive effect disappears within minutes after the drug is stopped. Obviously, the drug should be used only with constant monitoring of the BP.

The nitric oxide that is part of the nitroprusside structure induces immediate arteriolar and venous dilation with no effects on the autonomic or central nervous system (Mansoor & Frishman, 2002). Nitroprusside is metabolized to cyanide by sulfhydryl groups in red cells, and the cyanide is rapidly metabolized to thiocyanate in the liver (Schulz, 1984). If high levels of thiocyanate (>10 mg/dL) remain for days, toxicity may be manifested as fatigue, nausea, disorientation, and psychosis. If cyanide toxicity is suspected because of metabolic acidosis and venous hyperoxemia, nitroprusside should be discontinued, and 4 to 6 mg of 3% sodium nitrite given intravenously over 2 to 4 minutes, followed by an infusion of 50 mL of 25% sodium thiosulfate (Friederich & Butterworth, 1995).

Beyond its inherent potential toxicity and the need for constant surveillance with its use, nitroprusside poses an even greater hazard: It reduces CBF while increasing intracranial pressure (Immink et al.,

2008). These effects are potentially detrimental in patients with hypertensive encephalopathy or after a stroke. As noted by Varon (2008): "considering the potential for severe toxicity with nitroprusside, this drug should be used only when other intravenous antihypertensive agents are not available and then, only in specific clinical circumstances in patients with normal renal and hepatic function."

Nitroglycerin

Nitroglycerin as a potent venodilator reduces BP, decreasing preload and cardiac output, both undesirable effects in patients with compromised cerebral perfusion (Varon, 2008). Therefore, it is not an acceptable first choice for hypertensive emergencies, but it may be helpful as an adjunct in patients with acute coronary ischemia.

Fenoldopam

Fenoldopam, a peripheral dopamine-I agonist, unlike other parenteral antihypertensive agents, maintains or increases renal perfusion while it lowers BP (Murphy et al., 2001). It maintains most of its efficacy for 48 hours of constant rate infusion without rebound hypertension when discontinued. Although theoretically attractive in maintaining renal perfusion, it was no better than nitroprusside when compared in a sequential study of 43 patients with hypertensive emergencies (Devlin et al., 2004).

Nicardipine

When given by continuous infusion, the intravenous formulations of various dihydropyridine calcium channel blockers (CCBs) produce a steady, progressive fall in BP with little change in heart rate and a small increase in cardiac output (Mansoor & Frishman, 2002). Nicardipine has been found to provide responses virtually equal to those seen with nitroprusside, with few side effects (Neutel et al., 1994).

Clevidipine

This dihydropyridine CCB has recently been approved for intravenous use in treating severe hypertension. Unlike nicardipine, clevidipine has a very fast onset of action and a short duration of action of about 15 minutes, as it is rapidly metabolized by red blood cell esterases. It reduces blood pressure by selective arterial dilation, reducing afterload without affecting cardiac filling pressure or causing a reflex tachycardia (Varon, 2008).

Hydralazine

The direct vasodilator hydralazine can be given by repeated intramuscular injections as well as intravenously with a fairly slow onset and prolonged duration of action, allowing for less intensive monitoring. Significant compensatory increases in cardiac output preclude its use as a sole agent except in young patients, as with preeclampsia, who can handle the increased cardiac work without the likelihood that coronary ischemia will be induced. Hydralazine's primary use is for severe hypertension during pregnancy, as noted in Chapter 15.

Phentolamine

The α-blocker phentolamine is specifically indicated for pheochromocytoma or tyramine-induced catecholamine crisis.

Esmolol

Esmolol, a relatively cardioselective β-blocker, is rapidly metabolized by blood esterases and has a short (approximately 9-minute) half-life and total duration of action (approximately 30 minutes). Its effects begin almost immediately, and it has found particular use during anesthesia to prevent postintubation hemodynamic perturbations (Oxorn et al., 1990).

Labetalol

The combined α- and β-blocker labetalol has been found to be both safe and effective when given intravenously either by repeated bolus (Huey et al., 1988) or by continuous infusion (Leslie et al., 1987). It starts acting within 5 minutes, and its effects last for 3 to 6 hours. Labetalol can likely be used in almost any situation requiring parenteral antihypertensive therapy, except when left ventricular dysfunction could be worsened by the predominant β-blockade. Caution is needed to avoid postural hypotension if patients are allowed out of bed. Nausea, itching, tingling of the skin, and β-blocker side effects may be noted.

Diuretic

A diuretic may be needed after other antihypertensives are used, because reactive renal sodium retention usually accompanies a fall in pressure and may blunt the efficacy of nondiuretic agents. On the other hand, if the patient is volume depleted from pressure-induced natriuresis and prior nausea and vomiting, additional diuresis could be dangerous, and volume expansion may be needed to restore organ perfusion and prevent an abrupt fall in BP when antihypertensives are given (Varon, 2008)

Criteria for Drug Selection

Because no clinical comparisons are available of the eventual outcome after the use of various agents, the choice of therapy is based on rapidity of action, ease of administration, and propensity for side effects. Although nitroprusside has been most widely used and continues to be preferred for most hypertensive emergencies by most authors, its propensity to increase intracranial pressure and the need for constant monitoring support the wider use of other effective parenteral agents such as labetalol, nicardipine, and fenoldopam.

The management of hypertensive emergencies in a number of special circumstances is considered in other chapters of this book: renal insufficiency, Chapter 9; pheochromocytoma, Chapter 12; drug abuse, Chapter 14; eclampsia, Chapter 15; and, in children and adolescents, Chapter 16.

THERAPY FOR HYPERTENSIVE URGENCIES

Hypertensive urgencies can usually be managed with oral therapy, including some cases of accelerated-malignant hypertension or perioperative or rebound hypertension. The management of the overwhelming majority of patients who are found to have a very high BP but who are asymptomatic and in little danger of rapidly progressive target organ damage, referred to as *uncontrolled severe hypertension* rather than a *hypertensive urgency*, is considered at the end of this chapter.

In particular, patients in a surgical recovery room or a nursing home whose BP is found to be above some arbitrary danger level such as 180/110 mm Hg should not automatically be given sublingual nifedipine or any other antihypertensive drug. This practice has been widespread. In a 2-month survey in three hospitals, 3.4% of all patients had been given sublingual nifedipine: 63% of the orders were given over the telephone for arbitrary and asymptomatic BP elevations and 98% with no bedside evaluation (Rehman et al., 1996).

Rather than such inappropriate prescribing, the proximate causes for abrupt increases in BP should be identified and managed (e.g., hypoxia, pain, or volume overload in the postoperative patient; a distended bladder, disturbed sleep, or arthritic pain in the nursing home patient). Only if the BP remains above 180/110 mm Hg after 15 to 30 minutes may there be a need for additional antihypertensive therapy but not for rapid and precipitous reduction of BP as induced by sublingual nifedipine. If such rises in BP are frequent, appropriate increases in long-term therapy may be indicated.

Choice of Oral Agents

Virtually, every available antihypertensive drug with a fairly short onset of action has been shown to be effective in patients with uncontrolled, severe hypertension. None is clearly better than the rest, and a combination will often be needed for long-term control. Those most widely used are listed in Table 8-6; complete information about them is provided in Chapter 7.

Nifedipine

The rapidly acting formulation of the CCB nifedipine has been widely used for the treatment of hypertensive urgencies (Grossman et al., 1996). Liquid nifedipine in a capsule will usually lower BP after a single 5- or 10-mg oral dose (Maharaj & van der Byl, 1992). The drug is effective even more quickly when the capsule is chewed and the contents are swallowed than when it is squirted under the tongue (van Harten et al., 1987).

As might be expected with any drug that induces such a significant and rapid fall in BP, with no way to titrate or overcome the response, occasional symptomatic hypotension can occur, resulting in severe cerebral or cardiac ischemia (Grossman et al., 1996). Grossman et al. (1996) therefore recommended that the use of short-acting nifedipine be abandoned. However, if taken in the unbroken capsule, it seems no more likely to cause a precipitous fall in BP than other short-acting agents (e.g., captopril). Certainly,

there is no place for such short-acting formulations in the chronic treatment of hypertension, but if the BP needs to be lowered over a few hours, short-acting nifedipine is an acceptable choice. Other slower and, therefore, possibly safer oral CCB formulations such as short-acting diltiazem, felodipine, or verapamil can be used (Shayne & Pitts, 2003).

Captopril

Captopril is the fastest acting of the oral ACEIs now available, and it can also be used sublingually in patients who cannot swallow (Angeli et al., 1991). As noted earlier in this chapter, an ACEI may be particularly attractive because it shifts the entire curve of cerebral autoregulation to the left, so CBF should be well maintained as the systemic BP falls (Barry, 1989).

Abrupt and marked first-dose hypotension after an ACEI has been rarely observed, usually in patients with an activated renin-angiotensin system (Postma et al., 1992). Caution is advised in patients who have significant renal insufficiency or who are volume depleted. Despite the small potential for hypotension, oral captopril may be the safest of nonparenteral agents for urgent hypertension.

Clonidine

Clonidine, a central α-agonist, has been widely used in repeated hourly doses to reduce very high BP safely and effectively (Jaker et al., 1989). Significant sedation is the major side effect that contraindicates its use in patients with central nervous system involvement. Because it has a greater proclivity than other drugs to cause rebound hypertension if it is suddenly discontinued, it should not be used by patients who have demonstrated poor compliance with therapy. Despite its past popularity, clonidine seems to be a most unattractive drug for such patients.

TABLE 8.6	Oral Drugs for Hypertensive Urgencies			
Drug	Class	Dose	Onset	Duration (h)
Captopril	Angiotensin-converting enzyme inhibitor	6.5–50.0 mg	15 min	4–6
Clonidine	Central α-agonist	0.2 mg initially, then 0.1 mg/h, up to 0.8 mg total	0.5–2.0 h	6–8
Furosemide	Diuretic	20–40 mg	0.5–1.0 h	6–8
Labetalol	α- and β-Blocker	100–200 mg	0.5–2.0 h	8–12
Nifedipine	Calcium channel blocker	5–10 mg	5–15 min	3–5
Propranolol	β-Blocker	20–40 mg	15–30 min	3–6

Labetalol

The α- and β-blocker labetalol has been given in hourly oral doses ranging from 100 to 200 mg. It has reduced elevated pressures as effectively as repeated doses of oral nifedipine; it works somewhat more slowly and, perhaps, more safely (McDonald et al., 1993).

Diuretics

Diuretics, specifically furosemide or bumetanide, often are needed in patients with hypertensive urgencies, both to lower the BP by getting rid of excess volume and to prevent the loss of potency from non-diuretic antihypertensives because of their tendency to cause fluid retention as they lower BP. However, volume depletion may be overdone, particularly in patients who start off with a shrunken fluid volume. Thereby, renin secretion may be further increased, producing more intensive vasoconstriction and worsening the hypertension.

Management After Acute Therapy

After the patient is out of danger, a careful search should continue for possible identifiable causes, as delineated earlier in the section "Evaluation" in this chapter. Identifiable causes, in particular renovascular hypertension, are much more likely in patients with severe hypertension.

After control of the acute presentation, most patients will likely require multiple drug therapy and chronic treatment should likely begin with a diuretic and an appropriate second agent. The guidelines delineated in Chapter 7 should be followed to ensure adherence to effective therapy.

UNCONTROLLED SEVERE HYPERTENSION

Most patients who are diagnosed and treated as a hypertensive urgency are not in the immediate danger of uncontrolled hypertension that this diagnosis connotes. Many such patients have come to an emergency department (ED) for unrelated acute problems, but whose BP is elevated in response to pain, anxiety, or an understandable white-coat effect from being in an inhospitable surrounding.

If there is no evidence of trouble from the elevated BP, additional readings should be obtained after the pain or anxiety is alleviated. If the BP remains above 180/115 mm Hg, an oral antihypertensive drug

should probably be given. The 180/115 mm Hg level is chosen with no basis for deciding that this is the "critical" level, but because it is the level used by neurologist to preclude thrombolysis for acute ischemic stroke, as valid a reason as any.

Thereafter, enough medication should be supplied to cover the time until appropriate follow-up can be obtained in a primary care facility. This will, at the least, relieve the ED physician from concern over not taking some action, as if such action could be lifesaving. However, as the American College of Emergency Physician Clinical Policy (Decker et al., 2006) states, "we could find no evidence demonstrating improved patient outcomes or decreased mortality or morbidity with acute management of elevated blood pressure in the ED." Their policy statement concludes with these three recommendations:

1. Initiating treatment for asymptomatic hypertension in the ED is not necessary when patients have follow up.
2. Rapidly lowering blood pressure in asymptomatic patients in the ED is unnecessary and may be harmful to some patient.
3. When ED treatment for asymptomatic hypertension in initiated, blood pressure management should attempt to gradually lower blood pressure and should not expect to be normalized during the initial ED visit.

We will now leave the realm of primary hypertension and examine the various identifiable (secondary) forms of hypertension, starting with the most common: renal parenchymal disease.

REFERENCES

Adams HP Jr, del ZG, Alberts MJ, et al. Guidelines for the early management of adults with ischemic stroke: A guideline from the American Heart Association/American Stroke Association Stroke Council, Clinical Cardiology Council, Cardiovascular Radiology and Intervention Council, and the Atherosclerotic Peripheral Vascular Disease and Quality of Care Outcomes in Research Interdisciplinary Working Groups: The American Academy of Neurology affirms the value of this guideline as an educational tool for neurologists. *Circulation* 2007;115: e478–e534.

Ahmed MEK, Walker JM, Beevers DG, et al. Lack of difference between malignant and accelerated hypertension. *Br Med J* 1986;292:235–237.

Angeli P, Chiesa M, Caregaro L, et al. Comparison of sublingual captopril and nifedipine in immediate treatment of hypertensive emergencies. A randomized, single-blind clinical trial. *Arch Intern Med* 1991;151:678–682.

Barry DI. Cerebrovascular aspects of antihypertensive treatment. *Am J Cardiol* 1989;63:14C–18C.

Beilin LJ, Goldby FS. High arterial pressure versus humoral factors in the pathogenesis of the vascular lesions of malignant hypertension. The case of pressure alone. *Clin Sci Mol Med* 1977; 52:111–117.

Bing BF, Heagerty AM, Russell GI et al. Prognosis in malignant hypertension. *J Hypertens* 2004;17:380–381.

Blaustein DA, Kumbar L, Srivastava M, et al. Polyarteritis nodosa presenting as isolated malignant hypertension. *Am J Hypertens* 2004;17:380–381.

Brott T, Bogousslavsky J. Treatment of acute ischemic stroke. *N Engl J Med* 2000;343:710–722.

Byrom FB. The evolution of acute hypertensive arterial disease. *Prog Cardiovasc Dis* 1974;17:31–37.

Davis BA, Crook JE, Vestal RE, et al. Prevalence of renovascular hypertension in patients with grade III or IV hypertensive retinopathy. *N Engl J Med* 1979;301:1273–1276.

Decker WW, Godwin SA, Hess EP, et al. Clinical policy: Critical issues in the evaluation and management of adult patients with asymptomatic hypertension in the emergency department. *Ann Emerg Med* 2006;47:237–249.

Devlin JW, Seta ML, Kanji S, et al. Fenoldopam versus nitroprusside for the treatment of hypertensive emergency. *Ann Pharmacother* 2004;38:755–759.

Dustan HP, Schneckloth RE, Corcoran AC, et al. The effectiveness of long-term treatment of malignant hypertension. *Circulation* 1958;18:644–651.

Dzau VJ, Siwek LG, Rosen S, et al. Sequential renal hemodynamics in experimental benign and malignant hypertension. *Hypertension* 1981;3(Suppl. 1):63–68.

Ewen E, Zhang Z, Kolm P et al. The risk of cardiovascular events in primary care patients following an episode of severe hypertension. *J Clin Hypertens* 2009;11:175–182.

Fischberg GM, Lozano E, Rajamani K, et al. Stroke precipitated by moderate blood pressure reduction. *J Emerg Med* 2000;19: 339–346.

Fleming JD, McSorley A, Bates KM. Blood, semen, and an innocent man. *Lancet* 2008;371:958.

Foguet Q, Rodriguez A, Saez M, et al. Usefulness of optic fundus examination with retinography in initial evaluation of hypertensive patients. *Am J Hypertens* 2008;21:400–405.

Friederich JA, Butterworth JF. Sodium nitroprusside: Twenty years and counting. *Anesth Analg* 1995;81:152–162.

Gavras H, Brunner HR, Laragh JH, et al. Malignant hypertension resulting from deoxycorticosterone acetate and salt excess. *Circ Res* 1975;36:300–310.

Gifford RW. Treatment of hypertensive emergencies, including use of sodium nitroprusside. *Mayo Clin Proc* 1959;34:387–394.

Gross F, Dietz R, Mast GJ, et al. Salt loss as a possible mechanism eliciting an acute malignant phase in renal hypertensive rats. *Clin Exp Pharmacol Physiol* 1975;2:323–333.

Grossman E, Messerli FH, Grodzicki T, et al. Should a moratorium be placed on sublingual nifedipine capsules given for hypertensive emergencies and pseudoemergencies? *JAMA* 1996;276: 1328–1331.

Huey J, Thomas JP, Hendricks DR, et al. Clinical evaluation of intravenous labetalol for the treatment of hypertensive urgency. *Am J Hypertens* 1988;1:284S–289S.

Immink RV, van den Born B-JH, van Montfrans GA, et al. Impaired cerebral autoregulation in patients with malignant hypertension. *Circulation* 2004;110:2241–2245.

Immink RV, van den Born BJ, van Montfrans GA, et al. Cerebral hemodynamics during treatment with sodium nitroprusside versus labetalol in malignant hypertension. *Hypertension* 2008;52:236–240.

Jain N, Rosner F. Idiopathic intracranial hypertension: Report of seven cases. *Am J Med* 1992;93:391–395.

Jaker M, Atkin S, Soto M, et al. Oral nifedipine vs oral clonidine in the treatment of urgent hypertension. *Arch Intern Med* 1989;149:260–265.

James SH, Meyers AM, Milne FJ, et al. Partial recovery of renal function in black patients with apparent end-stage renal failure due to primary malignant hypertension. *Nephron* 1995;71: 29–34.

Jansen PAF, Schulte BPM, Gribnau FWJ. Cerebral ischaemia and stroke as side effects of antihypertensive treatment; special danger in the elderly. A review of the cases reported in the literature. *Neth J Med* 1987;30:193–201.

Karampekios SK, Contopoulou E, Basta M, et al. Hypertensive encephalopathy with predominant brain stem involvement: MRI findings. *J Hum Hypertens* 2004;18:133–134.

Kawazoe N, Eto T, Abe I, et al. Pathophysiology in malignant hypertension: With special reference to the renin-angiotensin system. *Clin Cardiol* 1987;19:513–518.

Kincaid-Smith P. Malignant hypertension. *J Hypertens* 1991;9: 893–899.

Kitiyakara C, Guzman NJ. Malignant hypertension and hypertensive emergencies. *J Am Soc Nephrol* 1998;9:133–142.

Leslie JB, Kalayjian RW, Sirgo MA, et al. Intravenous labetalol for treatment of postoperative hypertension. *Anesthesiology* 1987; 67:413–416.

Lip GYH, Beevers M, Beevers DG. Do patients with de novo hypertension differ from patients with previously known hypertension when malignant phase hypertension occurs? *Am J Hypertens* 2000;13:934–939.

Lip GYH, Beevers M, Beevers DG. Does renal function improve after diagnosis of malignant phase hypertension? *J Hypertens* 1997;15:1309–1315.

Lip GY, Edmunds E, Hee FL, et al. A cross-sectional, diurnal, and follow-up study of platelet activation and endothelial dysfunction in malignant phase hypertension. *Am J Hypertens* 2001;14: 823–828.

MacKenzie ET, Strandgaard S, Graham DI, et al. Effects of acutely induced hypertension in cats on pial arteriolar caliber, local cerebral blood flow, and the blood-brain barrier. *Circ Res* 1976; 39:33–41.

Maharaj B, van der Byl K. A comparison of the acute hypotensive effects of two different doses of nifedipine. *Am Heart J* 1992;124: 720–725.

Mansoor GA, Frishman WH. Comprehensive management of hypertensive emergencies and urgencies. *Heart Dis* 2002;4: 358–371.

McDonald AJ, Yealy DM, Jacobson S. Oral labetalol versus oral nifedipine in hypertensive urgencies in the ED. *Am J Emerg Med* 1993;11:460–463.

Mitchell I. Cerebral lupus. *Lancet* 1994;343:579–582.

Murphy MB, Murray C, Shorten GD. Fenoldopam: A selective peripheral dopamine-receptor agonist for the treatment of severe hypertension. *N Engl J Med* 2001;345:1548–1557.

Neutel JM, Smith DHG, Wallin D, et al. A comparison of intravenous nicardipine and sodium nitroprusside in the immediate treatment of severe hypertension. *Am J Hypertens* 1994;7: 623–628.

Olsen KS, Svendsen LB, Larsen FS, et al. Effect of labetalol on cerebral blood flow, oxygen metabolism and autoregulation in healthy humans. *Br J Anaesth* 1995;75:51–54.

Oxorn D, Knox JWD, Hill J. Bolus doses of esmolol for the prevention of perioperative hypertension and tachycardia. *Can J Anaesth* 1990;37:206–209.

Padfield PL. Malignant hypertension presenting with an acute abdomen. *Br Med J* 1975;3:353–354.

Perez MI, Musini VM. Pharmacological interventions for hypertensive emergencies: A Cochrane systematic review. *J Hum Hypertens* 2008;22:596–607.

Postma CT, Dennesen PJW, de Boo T, Thien T. First dose hypotension after captopril: Can it be predicted? A study of 240 patients. *J Hum Hypertens* 1992;6:205–209.

Preston RA, Jy W, Jimenez JJ, et al. Effects of severe hypertension on endothelial and platelet microparticles. *Hypertension* 2003; 41:211–217.

Rehman F, Mansoor GA, White WB. "Inappropriate" physician habits in prescribing oral nifedipine capsules in hospitalized patients. *Am J Hypertens* 1996;9:1035–1039.

Schmidt B, Czosnyka M, Raabe A, et al. Adaptive noninvasive assessment of intracranial pressure and cerebral autoregulation. *Stroke* 2003;34:84–89.

Schulz V. Clinical pharmacokinetics of nitroprusside, cyanide, thiosulphate and thiocyanate. *Clin Pharmacokinet* 1984;9:239–251.

Shapiro LM, Beevers DG. Malignant hypertension: Cardiac structure and function at presentation and during therapy. *Br Heart J* 1983;49:477–484.

Shayne PH, Pitts SR. Severely increased blood pressure in the emergency department. *Ann Emerg Med* 2003;41:513–529.

Smulders YM, Verhagen DW. Giant cell arteritis causing aortic dissection and acute hypertension. *Br Med J* 2008;337:a426.

Strandgaard S, Olesen J, Skinhøj E, et al. Autoregulation of brain circulation in severe arterial hypertension. *Br Med J* 1973;1:507–510.

Strandgaard S, Paulson OB. Cerebral blood flow and its pathophysiology in hypertension. *Am J Hypertens* 1989;2:486–492.

Strandgaard S, Paulson OB. Antihypertensive drugs and cerebral circulation. *Eur J Clin Invest* 1996;26:625–630.

Suzuki H, Asano K, Eiro M, et al. Recovery from renal failure in malignant hypertension associated with primary aldosteronism: Effect of an ACE inhibitor. *Q JM* 2002;95:128–130.

Trivelli A, Ghiggeri GM, Canepa A, et al. Hyponatremic-hypertensive syndrome with extensive and reversible renal defects. *Pediatr Nephrol* 2005;20:101–104.

Tuor UI. Acute hypertension and sympathetic stimulation: Local heterogeneous changes in cerebral blood flow. *Am J Physiol* 1992;263.H1511–H518.

van den Born BJ, van der Hoeven NV, Groot E, et al. Association between thrombotic microangiopathy and reduced ADAMTS13 activity in malignant hypertension. *Hypertension* 2008;51:862–866.

van den Born BJH, Honnebier UPF, Koopmans RP, et al. Microangiographic hemolysis and renal failure in malignant hypertension. *Hypertension* 2005;45:246–251.

van Harten J, Burggraaf K, Danhof M, et al. Negligible sublingual absorption of nifedipine. *Lancet* 1987;2:1363–1365.

Varon J. Treatment of acute severe hypertension: current and newer agents. *Drugs* 2008;68:283–297.

Vaughan CJ, Delanty N. Hypertensive emergencies. *Lancet* 2000;356:411–417.

Webster J, Petrie JC, Jeffers TA, et al. Accelerated hypertension—patterns of mortality and clinical factors affecting outcome in treated patients. *Q JM* 1993;86:485–493.

Renal Parenchymal Hypertension

R enal parenchymal diseases are the most common secondary or reversible cause of hypertension and their incidence will continue to increase as the population grows older and fatter (Bakris & Ritz, 2009). Before covering them, specifically, and in reverse order, from acute to chronic to transplant, some general issues about their overall significance deserve mention.

Those who desire more information on all issues relating to kidney disease should peruse the KDOQI Clinical Practice Guidelines published in the American Journal of Kidney Diseases. The guidelines on diabetes and chronic kidney disease (CKD) (KDOQI, 2007) cover areas that go beyond the focus of this chapter on hypertension in both acute and CKD. The web site of U.S. Renal Data System provides yearly statistics on CKD and end-stage renal disease (ESRD). The British National Institute for Clinical Excellence (NICE) has also recently published guidelines for the identification and management of CKD (Crowe et al., 2008).

CKD is one of the many factors that can lead to resistant hypertension. The approach that should be taken to elucidate the causes and improve the management of resistant hypertension is covered in Chapter 7. Additional information directed to CKD and resistant hypertension is provided in the Core Curriculum in Nephrology (Parker, 2008).

THE SCOPE OF THE PROBLEM

One of the major crises facing health care in the United States and all developed societies is the need to provide renal replacement therapy (RRT) to the rapidly growing number of people with kidney damage that progresses into ESRD. Hypertension is responsible for much of this progressive damage, playing a major role as well in the other major risk factor, obesity-induced diabetes. Between them, they represent by far the most common risk factors across the entire spectrum of renal disease (Whaley-Connell et al., 2008) (Fig. 9-1). In addition, low hemoglobin, higher serum uric acid, history of nocturia, and finally the history of kidney disease are independent risk factors for ESRD (Hsu et al., 2009).

As the incidence of both hypertension and obesity-induced diabetes is growing rapidly, the burden of CKD promises to expand even beyond its currently bloated share of health care resources. Moreover, as RRT keeps many ESRD patients alive longer, they end up as major contributors to cardiovascular disease, both heart attacks and stroke (McCullough et al., 2008). Some specific data about the overall situation:

• As noted in early 2008 (MMWR, 2008a):

Thirteen percent of U.S. adults (i.e., 26 million adults) were estimated to have chronic kidney disease in 2000, and most of these adults were not aware of their condition (Coresh et al., 2007).... In 2005, approximately 100,000 persons began treatment for ESRD in the United States, nearly half a million persons were living on chronic dialysis or with a kidney transplant, and total Medicare expenditures for ESRD reached approximately $20 billion, accounting for 6.4% of the total Medicare budget (U.S. Renal Data System, 2007). Of the new cases of ESRD in 2005, 71% had diabetes or hypertension listed as the primary cause.

By 2020, with the aging of the population and the increasing prevalence of diabetes, nearly 150,000 persons in the U.S. are projected to begin therapy for ESRD, nearly 800,000 will be living on chronic dialysis or with a kidney transplant, and costs for ESRD are projected to reach $54 billion.

• The overall prevalence of CKD has risen from 10% of the adult population in 1988 to 13% in 2004 and has reached 38% of people over the age of 70 years (Coresh et al., 2008). The definition and clarification of CKD used in these surveys include both microalbuminuria

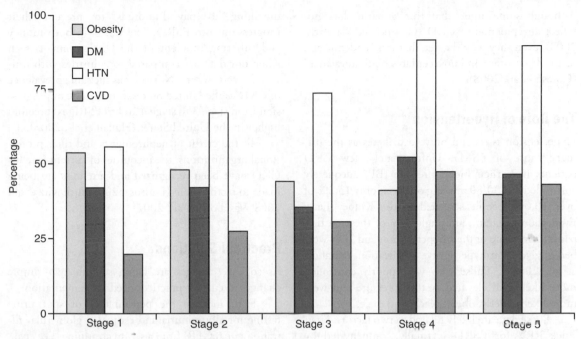

FIGURE 9-1   The prevalence of four risk factors (obesity, diabetes, hypertension, and cardiovascular disease) in patients screened in the Kidney Early Evaluation Program, grouped by the stage of chronic renal disease. (Reproduced from Whaley-Connell AI, Sowers JR, Stevens LA, et al. CKD in the United States: Kidney Early Evaluation Program (KEEP) and National Health and Nutrition Examination Survey (NHANES) 1999–2004. *Am J Kidney Dis* 2008;51:S13–S20.)

(more than 30 mg/g creatinine) and an estimated glomerular filtration rate (eGFR) below 60 mL per minute per 1.73 m² (Table 9-1). These increases from 1988 to 2004 pertain to both the milder stages, i.e., 1 and 2, and the more serious stages, 3 and 4, of CKD. Similar, or even higher, prevalences have been found in other developed societies (Tsukamoto, 2008; Wen et al., 2008). As developing countries become more developed, their burden will also grow: by 2030, it is estimated that 70% of ESRD will be among their residents, while they possess only 15% of the world economy (Barsoum, 2006).

• At least in the United States and Japan, the increasing incidence of new ESRD has slowed, but the number of patients receiving RRT continues to rise rapidly (U.S. Renal Data System, 2008). This likely reflects two opposing forces: the adequate treatment of more (though still only a fraction) of susceptible patients before they progress into ESRD versus the continually expanding population whom nephrologists are willing to enter into chronic dialysis.

• Most patients in the United States with CKD are not aware of their condition: only 6% of those with

stage 3, 38% with stage 4, and 47% with stage 5 (Saab et al., 2008).

• Most major trials on treatment of either hypertension or cardiovascular disease either exclude patients with CKD or provide little data on their course (Coca et al., 2006).

TABLE 9.1	Classification of Chronic Kidney Disease

	GFR (estimated from MDRD equation in mL/min/1.73 m²)	Albuminuria (calculated from urine albumin/creatinine rate in mg/g)	Percent of CKD
Stage 1	>90	>30	20
Stage 2	60–89	>30	27
Stage 3	30–59	—	50
Stage 4	25–29	—	(4 and 5) 3
Stage 5	<15	—	

Although some argue that this scenario does not reflect an epidemic of CKD (Glassock & Winearls, 2008), even they would agree that it is "endemic at a relatively constant and unacceptably high prevalence" (Coresh et al., 2008).

The Role of Hypertension

Hypertension is second only to diabetes as the primary cause of ESRD. Unfortunately, few CKD patients have their blood pressure (BP) adequately controlled to 130/80 mm Hg or lower: only 13.2% of over 10,000 people screened in the Kidney Early Evaluation Program, although 80% of these participants were aware of their hypertension and 70% were being given antihypertensive medication (Sarafidis et al., 2008a). Those who were poorly controlled more likely had elevated systolic pressure and were more likely elderly, obese, black, and male.

These data are likely related to two factors. First, since RRT for ESRD is totally compensated by Medicare, black men have unrestricted access to RRT (Duru et al., 2008) and actually do better than Caucasian men when they start dialysis (Norris et al., 2008). On the other hand, black men are much less likely to receive medical care that could prevent their progressing into ESRD (Duru et al., 2008). This obviously reflects the absence of a rational health care system in the United States (Wesson, 2008). Unfortunately, black men in particular, and poor people in general, will continue to suffer the consequences of a skewed health care delivery system willing to pay millions to keep ESRD patients alive but unwilling to pay hundreds to prevent their progression into ESRD. The waste, in both money and suffering inherent in the U.S. system, is seen when our data are compared to countries with universal access to care: Norway has the same prevalence of CKD as the United States, but the rate of progression from stage 3 to stage 4 and to ESRD is threefold higher in the United States (Hallan et al., 2006).

To the credit of nephrologists and their professional organizations, the inequities of current care for CKD have been recognized and attempts are being made to rectify them (DuBose, 2007; Jurkovitz et al., 2008; Vassalotti et al., 2007).

Practical Solutions

As societal changes are being sought, two simple changes in current practices need implementation:

First, increase the performance of spot urine testing for albuminuria and estimated glomerular filtration rate (eGFR) from a serum creatinine (Lee et al., 2009). Now fewer than 20% of primary care practitioners obtain these tests, even on elderly patients with diabetes (Minutolo et al., 2008) and only 38% of U.S. clinical labs report eGFR when they measure serum creatinine (Accetta et al., 2008).

Second, encourage primary caregivers to treat those with stage 1 or 2 disease more intensely. There are not enough nephrologists to care even for those with stage 3 disease, which is the level of CKD that is now the criterion for referral to a nephrologist. Table 9-2 provides a nine-item list for prevention of the progression of kidney damage (Graves, 2008).

TABLE 9.2	**Measures to Prevent Progression of Kidney Disease**

1. Control hypertension to a level < 130/80 mm Hg
2. Control diabetes to a hemoglobin A1c level < 7.0
3. Control lipid levels to an LDL-C level < 100 mg/dL
4. Use antiproteinuric antihypertensive agents: Angiotensin-converting enzyme inhibitors, angiotensin receptor blockers, aldosterone inhibitors, diltiazem
5. Avoid NSAIDs
6. Recommend dietary modification: Low fat, low salt, fewer calories if overweight
7. Avoid radio-contrast radiographic tests and premedicate the patient if required
8. Advise patients to discuss their condition with any physician who intends to prescribe a new medication
9. Encourage regular visits to a nephrologist (every 6–12 months)

SI conversion factor: To convert LDL-C values to mmol/L, multiply by 0.0259.
LDL-C, low-density lipoprotein cholesterol; NSAIDs, nonsteroidal anti-inflammatory drug. Modified from Graves JW. Diagnosis and management of chronic kidney disease. *Mayo Clin Proc* 2008;83:1064–1069.

We will now examine the specific varieties of renal disease and how they relate to hypertension, starting from acute renal insults and progressing eventually to posttransplantation. Renovascular hypertension is covered in the next chapter. It should always be kept in mind as a potentially curable form of CKD.

ACUTE KIDNEY DISEASE

A rapid decline in renal function may appear from various causes: prerenal (e.g., volume depletion), intrinsic (e.g., glomerulonephritis), or postrenal (e.g., obstructive uropathy). Nonsteroidal anti-inflammatory drugs (NSAIDs) are among the most common causes of acute renal failure, particularly in patients whose already reduced renal perfusion depends on prostaglandin-mediated vasodilation. Hypertension is rarely a problem because most of these patients are also volume contracted from prior therapy with diuretics and ACEI or ARB therapy (Braden et al., 2004). However, hypertension is frequent in most intrinsic and postrenal conditions.

Acute Kidney Injury

A striking increase in hospitalizations for acute kidney injury (AKI) has been recorded in the U.S. National Hospital Discharge Survey (MMWR, 2008b). In 2004, there were 221,000 hospitalizations for AKI versus 19,000 for CKD, a reversal from 1980 when there was a fivefold greater rate for CKD than for AKI.

AKI is defined differently in different studies (Zappitelli et al., 2008). Perhaps the best is the RIFLE classification, which provides a gradation of severity, starting with stage 1 or "risk" as oliguria for more than 6 hours or an increase in serum creatinine of more than 50% and proceeding to stage 2 as "injury" and stage 3 as "failure" with greater disease severity (Kellum et al., 2008).

Waikar et al. (2008), in their review of AKI, list these as the most common precipitations, all more common in the elderly, the diabetic, and those with preexisting CKD (Hsu et al., 2008):

• Sepsis
• Coronary interventions: catheterization, angioplasty, and bypass surgery
• Aortic aneurysm repair
• Intravenous contrast for radiologic examinations
• Nephrotoxic antibiotics

The reported mortality rate for those who develop AKI varies from 36% to 71%. Among survivors, those over age 65 have less recovery of kidney function (Schmitt et al., 2008),

Gadolinium and Nephrogenic Systemic Fibrosis

Contrast agents have long been known to reduce renal function (Weisbord et al., 2008), but a more specific syndrome—nephrogenic systemic fibrosis—has recently been identified as a serious consequence of the use of gadolinium as contrast for magnetic resonance imaging (MRI) in patients with preexisting ESRD (Kallen et al., 2008).

Recognition of AKI

The need for an early recognition of AKI is obvious, since immediate correction of causative factors is critical for survival. Among many markers that have been proposed, the plasma and urine measurements of neutrophil gelatinase-associated lipocalin (NGAL) are the most promising. NGAL is one of the most rapidly induced proteins in the kidney after acute injury (Mishra et al., 2003) and it can easily be measured in one drop of blood or 0.2 mL of urine (Devarajan, 2008). In a prospective cohort study of 635 patients with suspected AKI, the urinary NGAL provided a 90% sensitivity and a 99.5% specificity, superior to other markers and highly predictive of clinical outcomes (Nickolas et al., 2008).

Hypotension, rather than hypertension, is frequent in many AKI patients because vasodilation and volume depletion may occur at the onset of the injury. If hypertension supervenes, it often reflects iatrogenic volume overload in an attempt to increase renal perfusion. Renin released from hypoperfused kidneys may also be involved.

Acute Glomerulonephritis

The classic presentation of acute glomerulonephritis is a child with recent streptococcal pharyngitis or impetigo who suddenly passes dark urine and develops facial edema. The renal injury represents the trapping of antibody-antigen complexes within the glomerular capillaries. Although the syndrome has become less common, it still occurs, sometimes in adults past middle age. Typically, in the acute phase, patients are hypertensive, and there is a close temporal relation between oliguria, edema, and hypertension. On occasion, hypertension of a severe, even malignant, nature may be the overriding feature.

The hypertension should be treated by salt and water restriction and, in mild cases, diuretics and other oral antihypertensives. In keeping with an apparent role of renin, ACEI and ARB therapies have been effective (Catapano et al., 2008). In the classic disease, the patient is free of edema and hypertension within days, of proteinuria within weeks, and of hematuria within months. Hypertension was found in only three of 88 children followed up for 10 to 17 years (Popovic-Rolovic et al., 1991).

More common than poststreptococcal glomerulonephritis are a variety of primary renal diseases (e.g., IgA nephropathy) and systemic diseases (e.g., systemic lupus erythematosus), which may present with acute renal crises marked by hypertension (Haas et al., 2008). The hypertension may be effectively treated with an ACEI, with or without an ARB (Catapano et al., 2008).

Various viral infections may precipitate renal damage, more likely chronic than acute (Berns & Bloom, 2008). HIV-infected patients may have only microalbuminuria (Baekken et al., 2008) or severe antiglomerular basement membrane disease (Wechsler et al., 2008), manifested by heavy proteinuria (Rhee et al., 2008) or malignant hypertension (Morales et al., 2008).

Urinary Tract Obstruction and Reflux

Vesicoureteric reflux is seen in 1% to 2% of otherwise normal children and can lead to hypertension, renal scarring, and ESRD (Gargollo & Diamond, 2007). Among 157 hypertensives in India over the age of 18 years, vesicoureteral reflux was found in 30 (19.1%) without overt evidence of renal parenchymal damage (Barai et al., 2004).

Hypertension may develop after unilateral (Shin et al., 2008) or bilateral (Kiryluk et al., 2008) obstruction to the urinary tract. Unilateral hydronephrotic mice have enhanced reactivity of afferent arterioles in both kidneys accompanied by reduced NO availability (Carlstrom et al., 2008). In most patients, the hypertension is fairly mild, but significant hypertension and severe renal insufficiency may occur with hydronephrosis from prostatic obstruction (Sacks et al., 1989). Catheter drainage of the residual urine may lead to rapid resolution of the hypertension and circulatory overload (Ghose & Harindra, 1989).

Other Causes of Acute Renal Disease

Other causes of acute renal disease with hypertension include:

- Bilateral renal artery occlusion, either by emboli or thromboses (Svarstad et al., 2005).
- Removal of angiotensin II support of blood flow with ACEI or ARB therapy in the presence of bilateral renal artery disease (Safian & Textor, 2001).
- Trauma to the kidney (Watts & Hoffbrand, 1987).
- Cholesterol emboli, which may shower the kidney after radiologic or surgical procedures, producing rapidly worsening renal function and hypertension (Vidt, 1997).
- Extracorporeal shock wave lithotripsy for kidney stones is only rarely followed by rises in BP (Eassa et al., 2008).

Renal Donors

Removal of half of a living donor's renal mass could be looked upon as an acute injury, but in normal humans, the removal of a kidney does not usually result in hypertension, likely because of downward adjustments in glomerular hemodynamics to maintain normal fluid volume (Guidi et al., 2001). However, the possibility of subsequent damage to the remaining kidney has been raised, since the removal of one kidney could lead to hyperperfusion and progressive glomerulosclerosis in the other.

In a meta-analysis of 48 studies with 5,145 donors whose average age at donation was 41 years and whose BP averaged 121/77, follow-up for at least 5 years revealed a 6/4 mm Hg increase in BP (Boudville et al., 2006). However, at a mean follow-up of 12.2 years, the survival and incidence of ESRD were similar in 255 donors compared to those in the general population (Ibrahim et al., 2009).

CHRONIC KIDNEY DISEASE

Of the various discernable primary causes of ESRD among patients starting dialysis in the United States, diabetic nephropathy is the most common, comprising about 40%, followed by vascular diseases, including hypertensive nephrosclerosis (20%), primary glomerular disease (18%), tubulointerstitial diseases (7%), and cystic diseases (5%) (Whaley-Connell et al., 2008).

There are some differences in the prevalence of hypertension and the responses to antihypertensive therapy among these various causes of kidney disease: chronic pyelonephritis may be less commonly associated with hypertension (Goodship et al., 2000); polycystic diseases may be more commonly associated (Grantham, 2008), even before significant renal dysfunction develops (Reed et al., 2008). Patients with these various causes of CKD may start at either end of the spectrum: hypertension without overt renal damage on the one end and severe renal insufficiency without hypertension on the other. Eventually, however, both groups move toward the middle— renal insufficiency with hypertension—so that hypertension is found in approximately 85% of patients with CKD of diverse causes (Sarafidis et al., 2008a) and is closely related to the progression of nephropathy. Renal insufficiency as a consequence of primary hypertension is described in Chapter 4 with coverage of the recently published data incriminating genetic polymorphism, at least in Blacks and nondiabetics, and not preexisting hypertension as the cause of the focal segmental glomerulosclerosis underlying what has been called "hypertensive nephrosclerosis" (Freedman & Sedor, 2008).

This section examines the development of hypertension as a secondary process in the presence of primary renal disease or diabetes. The special features of diabetic nephropathy are covered separately, but most cases of CKD are similar in their course and treatment. Moreover, almost half of patients clinically defined as having diabetic nephropathy have been shown to actually have nondiabetic renal disease by kidney biopsy (Zhou J et al., 2008).

Patients whose underlying problem is bilateral renovascular disease may present with refractory hypertension and renal insufficiency (Guo et al., 2007). The recognition of the renovascular etiology of these patients' condition is critical because revascularization may relieve their hypertension and improve their renal function. More about this important group of patients with ischemic nephropathy is provided in the next chapter, as well as hypertension associated with renal tumors.

The Role of Hypertension

Hypertension accelerates the progression of renal damage, regardless of the cause. Perhaps the best evidence for this tight relationship is the repeatedly observed slowing of the progression of established CKD as initially elevated BPs are lowered. This was demonstrated first for patients with diabetic nephropathy (Mogensen, 1976) and subsequently for those with other causes of CKD, as in the Modification of Diet in Renal Disease Study (MDRD) (Lazarus et al., 1997). In the MDRD trial, 585 patients with a GFR between 25 and 55 mL per minute and 255 patients with a GFR between 13 and 24 mL per minute were studied. Among those with proteinuria of more than 1 g per day at baseline, the rate of decline in GFR was significantly less over a mean follow-up of 2.2 years in both the groups whose BPs remained an average of 5 mm Hg lower as a result of more intensive therapy.

Along with their higher prevalence of hypertension, African Americans have an increased susceptibility to CKD and ESRD. Non-diabetic CKD in African Americans has been attributed to "hypertensive neprosclerosis," i.e. hypertension causing CKD. The diagnosis is usually made by exclusion with non-specific focal segmental glomerulosclerosis (FSGS) on biopsy.

Two studies in the October 2008 issue of Nature Genetics report a genetic locus, MYH9, that explains much of the increased risk of FSGS in African Americans (Kao et al., 2008; Kopp et al., 2009).

In patients with CKD, ambulatory BP monitoring, which often identifies a loss of nocturnal dipping, is better than office readings in predicting progression of renal damage and mortality (Pogue et al., 2009). Nondipping in CKD has been attributed to a compensation for diminished natriuresis during the daytime and to enhanced pressure-natriuresis during the night (Kimura, 2008). Out-of-office BP measurements in patients with CKD are also critical to identify the considerable proportion with white-coat hypertension, 32% in one series (Minutolo et al., 2007a), to avoid unnecessary and potentially harmful overtreatment.

Mechanisms

Hypertension develops and progresses in patients with renal diseases for multiple reasons (Table 9-3). Most of these funnel into a common path: Impaired renal autoregulation that normally attenuates the transmission of elevated systemic pressure to the glomeruli, resulting in high perfusion pressure (Mori et al., 2008). The resultant glomerular

TABLE 9.3   Features Associated with High Blood Pressure in Chronic Kidney Disease

Preexisting primary (essential) hypertension
Extracellular fluid volume expansion
Arterial stiffness
Renin-angiotensin-aldosterone system stimulation
Increased sympathetic activity
Endothelin
Low birth weight with reduced nephron number
Decrease in vasodilatory prostaglandins
Obesity and insulin resistance
Sleep apnea
Smoking
Hyperuricemia
Erythropoietin administration
Parathyroid hormone secretion/increased intracellular calcium/hypercalcemia
Renal vascular disease and renal arterial stenosis
Aldosterone-induced fibrosis and sodium retention
Asymmetric dimethylarginine
Advanced glycation end products
Chronic allograft dysfunction
Cadaver allografts, especially from a donor with a family history of hypertension
Immunosuppressive and corticosteroid therapy
Heritable factors

hypertension damages the glomerular cells and leads to progressive sclerosis, setting off a vicious cycle (Anderson & Brenner, 1989) (Fig. 9-2).

As the extent of renal damage increases, arteries within the kidneys and throughout the body become sclerotic and stiff. As a consequence, systolic pressure rises, diastolic falls, and pulse pressure widens (Cheng et al., 2008). The stiffness that is responsible for the rising systolic pressure makes it increasingly difficult to lower this pressure. As more and more antihypertensive drugs are added, the systolic barely moves, but the diastolic falls, exposing the CKD patient to potential harm from too low a diastolic pressure to maintain perfusion to the brain, heart, and kidneys (Peralta et al., 2007).

Of the contributing or aggravating factors listed in Table 9-3, volume expansion from impaired natriuresis has traditionally been given primacy. However, in view of the increased peripheral vascular resistance typically seen in these patients, both an activated renin-angiotensin-aldosterone mechanism (Hollenberg, 2004) and an overactive sympathetic

nervous system (Neumann et al., 2004) have received increasing attention. Obesity, particularly abdominal, accelerates the progression of CKD and the attendant hypertension (Ritz, 2008; Wang et al., 2008).

Proteinuria

The degree of proteinuria serves as a strong predictor of the rate of progression of CKD. Increased protein trafficking through the glomerular capillaries directly damages the podocytes and tubular interstitium (Schieppati & Remuzzi, 2003). The role of heavy proteinuria in progression of renal damage was documented in a meta-analysis of data from 11 randomized controlled trials involving 1,860 patients (Jafar et al., 2003). As seen in Figure 9-3, proteinuria above 1 g per day was associated with a higher relative risk for progression at all levels of systolic BP above 120 mm Hg. The greater the proteinuria, the more the progression. Beyond its inherent toxicity, proteinuria is a useful marker of the type and extent of CKD (Table 9-4).

Measures of Glomerular Filtration Rate

In addition to proteinuria, the presence and degree of CKD is based on the rate of glomerular filtration (GFR) (see Table 9-1). Increasingly, the GFR has been estimated from equations measuring creatinine clearance, the Cockcroft-Gault equation, or, more accurately, the eGFR by the MDRD equation using the serum creatinine level, age, gender, and race (Ruilope et al., 2007).

These equations have been shown to be less accurate when the GFR is above 60 mL per minute per 1.73 m^2 and the eGFR to underestimate measured decreases in renal function over time (Xie et al., 2008). Therefore, attention has turned to the measurement of serum cystatin C, an endogenous protein filtered by glomeruli and reabsorbed and catabolized by tubular epithelial cells with only small amounts excreted in the urine. Unlike equations using serum creatinine, cystatin C levels are not affected by muscle mass and they are closely correlated to outcomes in patients with CKD (Menon et al., 2007) and the incidence of hypertension in people without CKD (Kestenbaum et al., 2008). The most accurate estimate of GFR appears to be the combination of serum cystatin C levels with the MDRD equation (Stevens et al., 2008b).

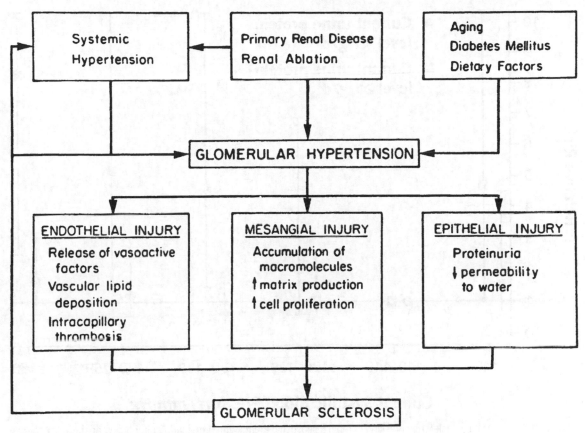

FIGURE 9 2 Pivotal role in glomerular hypertension in the initiation and progression of structural injury. (Modified from Anderson S, Brenner BM. Progressive renal disease: A disorder of adaptation. *QJM* 1989;70:185–189.)

Management

Intensity of Therapy

Reduction of BP and proteinuria has been clearly shown to slow the rate of progression of CKD (Jafar et al., 2003; Lewis, 2007). However, as seen in Figure 9-3, only those with proteinuria above 1 g per day have been shown to benefit from more intensive lowering of BP. This was found in the MDRD study (Lazarus et al., 1997) and reconfirmed in the African American Kidney Disease and Hypertension (AASK) study (Wright et al., 2002). In the AASK study, no additional slowing of the progression of hypertensive nephrosclerosis was found in those given more therapy to provide an average BP of 128/78 compared to those given less therapy who ended up with an average BP of 141/85. Moreover, 759 of the original 1,094 enrollees in the AASK were followed for another 5 years while receiving an ACEI (Appel et al., 2008).

Despite achieving a mean BP of 133/78, most of the patients continued to suffer a decline in renal function.

The reason why there is no benefit of lowered BP on renal function in those with lesser degrees of proteinuria remains unknown. The reason why those with heavy proteinuria benefit likely reflects the damage induced by heavy loads of protein traversing the nephron and the slowing of this damage as proteinuria is reduced, either by any drug that lowers renal perfusion pressure or by drugs that have a special ability to lower intraglomerular pressure, i.e., renin-angiotensin suppressants.

Hazards of More Intensive Therapy

In multiple trials of patients with CKD, an *increased* incidence of cardiovascular morbidity and mortality has been noted when systolic pressures are lowered to below 120 mm Hg or diastolic pressure below 85 mm Hg

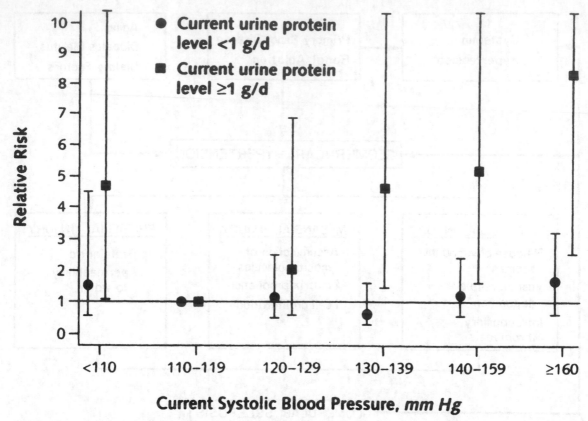

FIGURE 9-3 The relative risk for progression of renal disease in patients with proteinuria either below or above 1 g per day by levels of systolic BP. The reference group (RR = 1) is a systolic pressure of 110 to 119 mm Hg. (Modified from Jafar TH, Stark PC, Schmid CH, et al. Progression of chronic kidney disease; The role of blood pressure control, proteinuria, and angiotensin-converting enzyme inhibition: A patient-level meta-analysis. *Ann Intern Med* 2003;139:244–252.)

TABLE 9.4	Importance of Proteinuria in Chronic Kidney Disease (CKD)
Interpretation	**Explanation**
1. Marker of CKD	Urine albumin-creatinine ratio > 30 mg/g for 3 months diagnostic
2. Clue to the type of CKD	Higher proteinuria suggests diabetic or glomerular diseases
3. Risk factor	Higher proteinuria predicts faster progression
4. Predictor of response to therapy	Higher proteinuria predicts better response
5. Hypothesized surrogate for outcome	Reducing proteinuria may be a goal of the therapy

Adapted from Vassalotti JA, Stevens LA, Levey AS. Testing for chronic kidney disease: A position statement from the National Kidney Foundation. *Am J Kidney Dis* 2007;50:169–180.

(Berl et al., 2005; Kovesdy et al., 2006; Pohl et al., 2005; Weiner et al., 2007). As seen in Figure 9-4, in the Irbesartan Diabetic Nephropathy Trial (IDNT), a progressive decrease in renal endpoints occurred with achieved systolic BP between 121 and 130 mm Hg, but all-cause mortality strikingly increased in those few who achieved systolic BP below 121 (Pohl et al., 2005).

However, one other large trial did *not* find an increase in stroke among 1,757 patients with stage 3 or more CKD, who had a significant fall in BP (Ninomiya et al., 2008). In the Perindopril Protection Against Recurrent Stroke Study (PROGRESS, 2001), all 6,105 participants had known cerebrovascular disease, and half were treated with an ACEI plus a diuretic, if needed, to lower the BP. The 1,757 patients with CKD had a progressively lower rate of recurrent stroke with reductions of BP even to below 120/70 mm Hg though the number of patients at each achieved level of BP has not been provided to enable a close examination of the data.

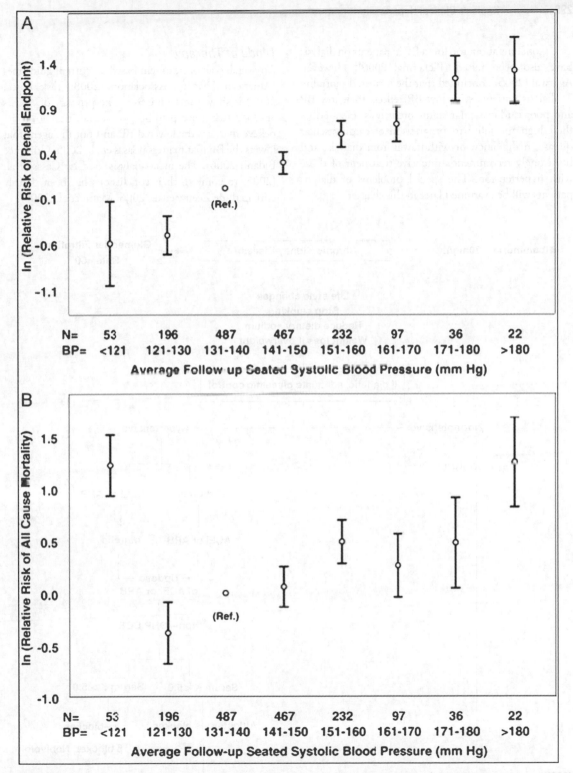

FIGURE 9-4   A: The relative risk for reaching a renal end point by level of achieved follow-up systolic blood pressure (SBP). **B:** The relative risk for all-cause mortality by level of achieved SBP. The number of patients who were at risk is shown above each level of achieved SBP. (Reproduced from Pohl MA, Blumenthal S, Cordonnier DJ, et al. Independent and additive impact of BP control and angiotensin II receptor blockade on renal outcomes in the Irbesartan Diabetic Nephropathy Trial: Clinical implications and limitations. *J Am Soc Nephrol* 2005;16:3027–3037, with permission.)

Concerns about too low a BP in patients on dialysis have also been raised (Pickering, 2006). However, Agarwal (2005) concluded that the increased mortality in dialysis patients with low BP reflects their low BP and poor cardiovascular status predialysis. He ascribes their high mortality to progression of cardiovascular disease, malignancy, or withdrawal from dialysis, and he strongly recommends intensive treatment of those with hypertension. The special problems of dialysis patients will be examined later in this chapter.

Mode of Therapy

An overall plan of treatment based on current guidelines (American Diabetes Association, 2008; Task Force, 2007) is shown in Figure 9-5. The primacy of ACEIs and/or ARBs is accepted by most authorities, but some believe that it is the lowered BP and not the agent that lowers the BP that matters (Casas et al., 2005; Griffin & Bidani, 2006). The meta-analysis used by Casas et al. (2005) to come to their conclusions has been sharply criticized (de Zeeuw et al., 2006; Mann et al., 2006).

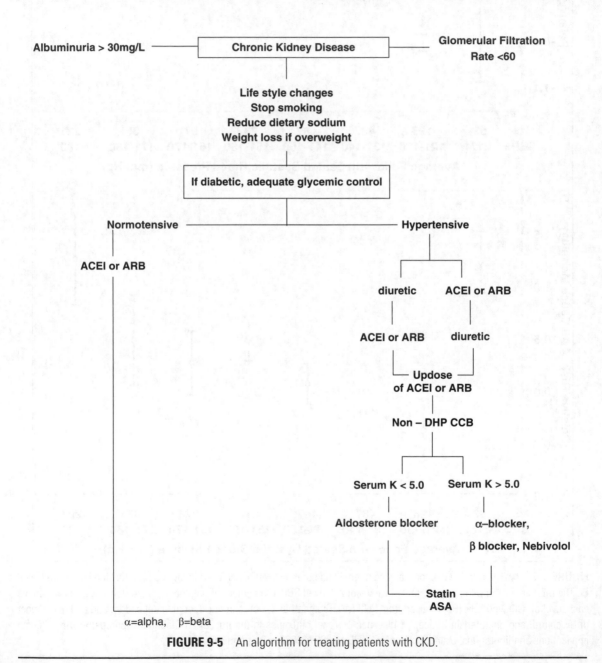

FIGURE 9-5   An algorithm for treating patients with CKD.

Lifestyle Changes

All hypertensives with or without CKD, with or without diabetes, should be intensively encouraged to change their unhealthy lifestyles and given as much help as possible to achieve these changes.

Cessation of smoking is paramount, since smoking is a major risk for progression of CKD (Orth & Hallan, 2008).

Reduction in dietary sodium becomes increasingly more critical as CKD progresses and renal sodium excretory capacity becomes weaker (Mimran & du Cailar, 2008). As will be noted, dialysis patients need to limit their interdialytic weight gain, almost all attributable to excessive sodium and water intake (Inrig et al., 2007).

Sodium reduction to the range of 1 to 2 g per day (sodium, 44 to 88 mEq per day) is both feasible and often necessary to control the hypertension in CKD patients (De Nicola et al., 2004). The importance of dietary sodium restriction in proteinuric patients goes beyond the ability to enhance the antihypertensive effect of all drugs (save calcium channel blockers [CCBs]). In a study of 38 patients with CKD and an average of 3.8 g per day proteinuria, reduction of dietary sodium from 196 to 92 mmol per day provided a 22% reduction in proteinuria (Vogt et al., 2008). Losartan alone reduced the level by 30%, and when the low sodium diet was combined with losartan, the proteinuria level fell by 70%.

Weight reduction: Obese hypertensive people are now likely to develop CKD (Gomez et al., 2006). Abdominal obesity rather than weight per se is the culprit (Elsayed et al., 2008). An increased likelihood of sleep apnea adds to the risk of obesity (Tsioufis et al., 2008).

Glycemic control: If only they could lose their excess weight, most type 2 diabetics would likely avoid their subsequent risk of CKD.

Renin-Angiotensin System (RAS) Inhibitors

Both ACEIs and ARBs reduce proteinuria and slow the progression of CKD equally (Kunz et al., 2008; Sarafidis et al., 2008b). The renoprotective effect has been shown in CKD caused by diabetes (Sarafidis et al., 2008b), nondiabetic disease (Jafar et al., 2003), and in patients with polycystic disease (Jafar et al., 2005). The place of direct renin inhibitors (DRIs) remains uncertain since the only one now available has not been adequately tested.

Despite their benefits, neither ACEIs nor ARBs have been found to reduce all-cause mortality, in patients with CKD. Presumably, nonrenal events, which may become increasingly common, the longer the CKD is held in check, are responsible.

ACEIs

ACEIs are recommended for initial antihypertensive drug therapy by most authorities. The evidence favoring the special benefits of ACEIs in patients with nondiabetic CKD is impressive: in the 11 RCTs analyzed by Jafar et al. (2003), the use of an ACEI was associated with a 33% decrease in risk of progression after adjustments for the reduction of

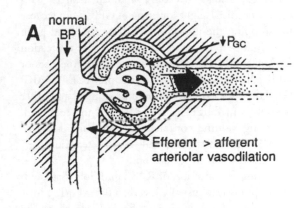

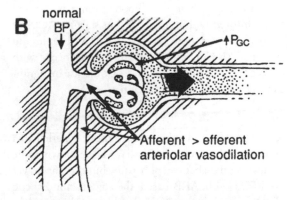

FIGURE 9-6   Effect of antihypertensive treatment on glomerular hemodynamics as determined by micropuncture studies in rats. **A:** Angiotensin-converting enzyme inhibition results in normalization of BP associated with vasodilatation, predominantly of the efferent arteriole, resulting in the normalization of intraglomerular capillary pressure (P_{GC}). **B:** With CCBs, reduction of BP is offset by afferent arteriolar vasodilatation, and, therefore, P_{GC} remains elevated. (Modified from Tolins JP, Raij L. Antihypertensive therapy and the progression of chronic renal disease: Are there renoprotective drugs? *Semin Nephrol* 1991;11:538–548.)

both BP and proteinuria. In eight RCTs including 142 patients with advanced polycystic kidney disease, ACEIs were effective in reducing proteinuria (Jafar et al., 2005).

These better effects of renin-angiotensin system (RAS) inhibitors likely reflect their greater ability to reduce intraglomerular pressure by their preferential dilation of efferent arterioles (Fig. 9-6) (Tolins & Raij, 1991). The reduction in intraglomerular pressure protects the glomeruli from progressive sclerosis and reduces the escape of protein into the tubule. At the same time, GFR is reduced and serum creatinine increased, usually to only a small degree. This expected, initial slight lowering of GFR is not a cause for stopping the use of an ACEI or ARB and is, in fact, followed by an even greater renal protection (Bakris et al., 2000). If the serum creatinine rises or GFR falls more than 30% of the pre-ACEI or ARB level, the ACEI or ARB should be stopped and other possible contributing causes identified and corrected, including volume contraction, concomitant use of NSAIDs, or most dramatically, the presence of bilateral renovascular hypertension.

Another reflection of RAS inhibition is a rise in serum potassium, usually less than 0.5 mEq/L. However, if hyperkalemia above 5.5 mEq/L develops, the dose of ACEI or ARB should be reduced or the drug discontinued. Obviously, blood chemistries should be monitored within a few days of starting ACEI or ARB therapy in patients with CKD as a rapid and sustained rise in serum creatinine may occur with unrecognized bilateral renovascular disease or significant hyperkalemia may develop.

ARBs

An ARB may be added in those without hyperkalemia (Saruta et al., 2009). ARBs have been shown to be protective in diabetic nephropathy but there are as yet no RCTs with ARB-based therapy in nondiabetic CKD. Certainly, an ARB should be substituted in those who develop an ACEI-induced cough. However, as noted in the next section, ARBs have not been shown to reduce mortality in diabetic nephropathy whereas ACEIs have, so preference should be given to an ACEI.

Combination of ACEI and ARB

Kunz et al. (2008) showed that the combination of an ACEI and an ARB reduced proteinuria an additional 20% over that seen with either drug alone. As they collected their data, they noted serious discrepancies in the data from the one trial which first appeared to document the benefit of combination therapy, the COOPERATE trial (Nakao et al., 2003).

Two more serious blocks to the rapidly expanding rush to use ACEI + ARB in CKD have risen. First, patients with microalbuminuria, i.e., stage 1, or 2, CKD, were found to lower their albuminuria as well with the ACEI ramipril alone as with ramipril plus the ARB irbesartan (Bakris et al., 2007).

Even more seriously, the massive (25,620 participants) ONgoing Telmisartan Alone and in combination with Ramipril Global Endpoint Trial (ONTARGET) found that the combination of the ACEI and the ARB in the same doses as were used alone did not reduce proteinuria more than either drug alone but *worsened* major renal outcomes (Mann et al., 2008). The worsening was reflected in more hypotension, more doubling of serum creatinine, and more entering dialysis. Messerli (2009) concludes that "dual RAS blockade should no longer be used in clinical practice."

ARB plus Direct Renin Inhibitor

Another dual RAS blockade has been tested. The DRI aliskerin, starting at 150 mg per day and advancing to 300 mg per day, was added to 100 mg of the ARB losartan in half of 599 patients with type 2 diabetic nephropathy (Parving et al., 2008). The patients were receiving, in addition to the losartan, a number of other antihypertensive drugs, 60% on three or more, so they were normotensive (mean BP = 135/79) when aliskerin was added. After 6 months on aliskerin, the BP had fallen only 2/1 mm Hg, but the mean urinary albumin-to-creatinine ratio in an early morning urine sample fell by 20%. There were equal numbers of adverse events in the aliskerin add-on group and the placebo group.

The investigators conclude that "aliskerin may have renoprotective effects that are independent of its BP-lowering effect." The potential for such an independent effect of the DRI on renal function could reflect the presence of high levels of prorenin, the precursor of renin, in diabetics and the inhibition of some of the deleterious renal actions of prorenin by the DRI (Schmieder, 2007). The question remains, however, if the still patented and expensive DRI is needed to further reduce proteinuria when other less expensive ways are available.

Other Combinations

The combination of an ACEI, benazepril, with a diuretic, hydrochlorothiazide, provided a greater decrease in albuminuria than did the combination of the ACEI with a CCB, amlodipine, despite a greater BP fall with the CCB + ACEI (Bakris et al., 2008).

In the BENEDICT study, the ACEI trandolapril alone was as effective as its combination with the non-DHP-CCB, verapamil, in preventing the onset of microalbuminuria in 1,204 hypertensives with diabetes but normal urinary albumin excretion (Remuzzi et al., 2006b).

Higher Dose ACEI/ARB Therapy

Doses of either ACEIs or ARBs in excess of those approved by the U.S. F.D.A. have been tested in a few hundred patients to determine if further reductions in proteinuria could be obtained beyond that achieved by the usual doses. In a summary of four trials with ACEIs and eight with ARBs, Berl (2008) concludes that the use of high doses has shown an overall further decrement in proteinuria, but the benefit likely reflects a significant effect in only a minority of patients. Since these responders are not identifiable, Berl states: "a temporary trial at higher doses seems cogent to provide more robust antiproteinuric benefit to such patients. The cost of doing so in terms of side effects is low and warrants the approach" (Berl, 2008).

Putative Danger of Prolonged RAS Inhibition

However, a warning about the potential for exacerbation of renal failure by prolonged use of high doses has been published by two Mayo Clinic nephrologists (Onuigbo & Onuigbo, 2005; 2006). They described five patients whose renal function had deteriorated while on an ACEI but had improved when the ACEI was discontinued. Soon after their report, Suissa et al. (2006) reported a nested case-control analysis of 102 diabetic patients who developed ESRD. Relative to the use of thiazides diuretics, the ratio of ESRD was 2.5 higher in those who used an ACEI, compared to 0.8 for β-blockers and 0.7 for CCBs. This increase was observed only after 3 years of ACEI use, with a risk ration of only 0.8 for the first 3 years, but 4.2 thereafter. These reports are observational, but it should be noted that none of the many trials that have shown renoprotection by RAS inhibitors have followed patients as long as 3 years.

Without doubt, there is an epidemic of ESRD in diabetic patients. In their analysis of possible causes, Jones et al. (2005) discount the possibility that the increasing use of ACEIs could be responsible, because the incidence of ESRD attributable to hypertensive nephrosclerosis has not increased despite the similar increase in the use of ACEIs among hypertensives as among the diabetics. However, Jones et al. (2005) offer no other explanation for the almost threefold increase in ESRD caused by diabetic nephropathy from 1990 to 2000. Perhaps the diabetic kidney is in some way more susceptible to injury from ACEIs than the nondiabetic kidney. As counterintuitive and well-nigh heretical as this seems, rats given ACEIs develop renal fibrosis in spite of reductions in BP and proteinuria (Hamming et al., 2006a). Hamming et al. (2006b) state in their comment on the study by Suissa:

> The incidence of end-stage renal disease is increasing worldwide, despite extensive use of renin-angiotensin system blockers. It would be prudent not to take their long-term renoprotective effect for granted, scrutinize their effects on renal structural damage in experimental studies, and critically evaluate their outcome in humans during long-term follow-up.

Anemia with RAS Inhibitors

Both ACEIs and ARBs have been found to reduce hemoglobin levels in CKD patients, an effect attributed to the blockade of erythropoietic effects of angiotensin II on RBC precursors and to the improved oxygenation from increased renal blood flow (Mohanram et al., 2008). In the patients enrolled in the RENAAL trial given the ARB losartan, the greatest effect on hemoglobin was seen at 1 year, but there was no impact on the renoprotective effect of the ARB.

Trials of Prevention

Despite all these real and putative problems with long-term use of RAS inhibition to treat CKD, the practice has become virtually routine in any patient with proteinuria on low eGFR (Sarafidis & Bakris, 2008). The practice has been applied to prevention as well.

The previously noted BENEDICT trial is only one of many that have shown that an ACEI or ARB can delay the appearance of microalbuminuria in hypertensive diabetics (Strippoli et al., 2006). Estacio et al. (2006) showed that in 129 diabetics with normal BP (126/84 mm Hg), higher doses of the ARB valsartan to lower the BP to 118/75 mm Hg reduced microalbuminuria more than with lower doses of the ARB that lowered the BP to 124/80 mm Hg (However, two large and long RCTs, failed to find renoprotection in the absence of macroalbuminuria (Bilous et al., 2009; Mann et al., 2009). The ACE genotype may predict the response to ACEI or ARB therapy. However, in three large trials performed in France, the ACE insertion/deletion polymorphism did not predict the response to ACEI therapy (Hadjadj et al., 2008).

Palmer et al. (2008) addressed the question of whether screening all hypertensive type 2 diabetics for urinary microalbuminuria and treating all with a positive test with an ARB would be cost-effective. They estimated a cost of $20,011 per quality-adjusted life year with a 77% probability that this approach is cost-effective.

Diuretics

Either before or after RAS inhibitors, a diuretic will likely be needed to bring the hypertension to near the 130/80 mm Hg goal that current guidelines recommend for CKD patients. A therapeutic cross fire is often encountered: On the one hand, the need for a diuretic becomes progressively greater as renal function deteriorates and sodium cannot be excreted, so the intravascular volume is expanded and the BP rises (Sica, 2008). On the other hand, as renal function deteriorates, diuretics may not work. All diuretics must gain entry to the tubular fluid and have access to the luminal side of the nephron to work. They reach the tubular fluid by secretion across the proximal tubule by way of organic acid secretory pathways. Patients with CKD are thus resistant to acidic diuretics such as thiazides and the loop diuretics because of the accumulation of organic acid end products of metabolism that compete for the secretory pump.

In practice, thiazides diuretics in usual doses (12.5 to 50 mg) are usually not adequate when eGFR falls to below 50 mL per minute per 1.73 m². Fortunately, loop diuretics can be safely given at high enough doses to cross the secretory barrier and exert a diuresis, even with much lower eGFR. To do so, enough must be given by the process of "sequential doubling of single doses until a ceiling dose is reached" (Brater, 1988). Once the ceiling dose is reached, that dose should be given as often as needed as a maintenance dose. In those with stage 4 or 5 CKD, that dose may be as high as 360 mg or more of furosemide or the equivalent of other loop diuretics.

If volume control is still not achieved, metolazone alone, or, even better, with a loop diuretic will usually achieve a diuresis even in ESRD, if some residual renal function is present (Sica & Gehr, 2003).

Caution is needed not to overdiurese by carefully monitoring the body weight.

Aldosterone Blockers

Aldosterone is now recognized to be an accelerator of renal damage by stimulating inflammation and fibrosis (Remuzzi et al., 2008). Since its secretion is largely controlled by angiotensin, the suppression of aldosterone synthesis by RAS inhibitors is considered to be responsible for at least part of the overall benefits of RAS inhibitors. However, a breakthrough of aldosterone secretion in the face of continued RAS inhibition has been recognized, first in the treatment of heart failure (Lee et al., 1999), then in the treatment of hypertension (Sato & Saruta, 2001), and then in patients with CKD (Sato et al., 2003). Bomback and Klemmer (2007) identified eight well-performed studies, with a range of incidence of breakthrough varying from 10% over 6 months to 53% over 1 year.

When an aldosterone blocker is added to an ACEI or ARB in CKD patients, proteinuria decreases from the level achieved by the RAS inhibitor by 15% to 54% and a significant fall in BP occurs in 40% of the patients (Bomback et al., 2008). Whether these impressive benefits occur only, or usually, in the presence of aldosterone breakthrough is not known, but aldosterone blockers are being increasingly used in CKD patients not adequately managed by RAS inhibition. In the algorithm shown in Figure 9-5, the use of an aldosterone blocker is relegated to the fourth line of therapy and only in those with a normal serum potassium because of the potential for hyperkalemia from the inhibition of potassium excretion by the aldosterone blocker. However, with the increasing recognition of their remarkable ability to bring resistant hypertension into control (Chapman et al., 2007), the cautious use of aldosterone blockers even earlier in the treatment of CKD may become more acceptable.

Calcium Channel Blockers

In Figure 9-5, nondihydropyridine calcium channel blockers (non-DHP-CCBs) are recommended as third choices. The advocacy of non-DHP-CCBs is based on their greater antiproteinuric effect than seen with DHP-CCBs in a review of 28 randomized trials (Bakris et al., 2004). This difference is attributed by Bakris et al. to a greater effect of non-DHP-CCBs on efferent arteriolar vasodilation than seen with DHP-CCBs in experimental models (Griffin et al., 1999). In addition, non-DHP-CCBs have been found to reduce glomerular permeability (Russo et al., 2002).

These differences in antiproteinuric effects, though in themselves a cause for concern, have *not* been shown to eventuate in differences in renal protection between DHP-CCBs and non-DHP-CCBs. However, additional concern arose from the AASK trial of patients with CKD from hypertensive nephrosclerosis, wherein those with proteinuria greater than 300 mg per day had a faster decline in GFR if started on the DHP-CCB amlodipine than if started on the ACEI ramipril (Agodoa et al., 2001). It should be noted, however, that the majority of the patients in the AASK trial had proteinuria less than 300 mg per day and among them, GFR was better preserved in those on amlodipine. Moreover, in the Ramipril Efficacy in Nephropathy (REIN) trial, the use of DHP-CCBs improved renoprotection when added to an ACEI and when BP was reduced effectively (Ruggenenti et al., 1998).

In conclusion, non-DHP-CCBs may be preferable to DHP-CCBs but either type of CCB can safely and effectively be used *when added to an ACEI or ARB* in patients with CKD.

α-Blockers

Peripheral α-blockers, e.g., doxazosin, may be used without dose adjustment. The central α-blocker clonidine is often used as a bridge to lower BP on the days between dialysis, but its side effects and propensity to rebound makes it a poor substitute for adequate control of fluid volume.

β-Blockers

Now that their use has been shown to be less effective for primary prevention (see Chapter 7), β-blockers should be used only for secondary prevention of cardiac problems, e.g., post-MI, CHF, or tachyarrhythmias. If one is to be used, the choice should logically be one that is not cleared through the kidney, e.g., propanolol or timolol. The α/β agents carvedilol and labetalol will cause less metabolic mischief than a β-blocker, and carvedilol has been shown to reduce proteinuria in CKD patients (Bakris et al., 2006). The vasodilating β-blocker nebivolol likely would do as well.

Minoxidil

In the past, those with refractory hypertension and CKD were successfully treated with minoxidil (Toto et al., 1995). However, when added to a regimen that included maximal doses of an ACEI or ARB, proteinuria increases, despite the lower BP (Diskin et al., 2006).

Timing of Therapy

The potential for additional adverse effects of the persistently elevated nocturnal BP, i.e., nondipping, that is frequently present in patients with CKD has prompted studies comparing a shift in the timing of antihypertensive drug intake from morning to evening. Hermida et al. (2005) found a decrease in the level of microalbuminuria among 200 hypertensives when the ARB valsartan was given at bedtime, compared to when it was given in the morning. A similar benefit was reported among 32 CKD patients whose proteinuria was decreased from 235 to 167 mg per day, when they took any one of their average daily intake of 2.4 medications in the evening (Minutolo et al., 2007b).

The addition of a diuretic (Uzu et al., 2005) or the use of a long-acting antihypertensive taken in the morning may reduce the nocturnal pressure, at least in one study, by increasing the daytime natriuresis, so the residual vascular volume is reduced (Fukuda et al., 2008). Similar benefit should be provided by a lower dietary sodium intake since, by the nature of CKD, renal sodium excretion is impaired (Bankir et al., 2008).

Restriction of Dietary Protein

A protein-restricted diet has been recommended for predialysis patients (Walser et al., 1999), and an analysis of multiple randomized trials has shown a delay in ESRD or death (Fouque et al., 2000), but individualized decisions seem appropriate in view of the malnutrition often seen with CKD (Levey, 2002).

Correction of Anemia

Anemia is a risk factor for progression of CKD and left ventricular hypertrophy (Rossing et al., 2004). However, treatment with erythropoietin to achieve a hemoglobin level above 12 g/L has been found to increase serious adverse events, so the current recommendations are to maintain a level of 11 g/L (Moist et al., 2008).

Lipid-Lowering Agents

In view of the common presence of dyslipidemia in CKD patients and the high rate of atherosclerotic vascular disease they suffer, the use of lipid-lowering agents seems appropriate. In a review of 50 trials involving 30,144 patients with CKD, statin therapy was found to reduce the risk of cardiovascular morbidity and mortality but had no effect on all-cause mortality and had uncertain renoprotective effects (Strippoli et al., 2008). The protection against cardiovascular disease is enough to make statin therapy to lower LDL-cholesterol to below 100 mg per day part of the current standard of care for CKD patients (Bogaert & Chonchol, 2008).

Dose Modification of Other Drugs

The presence of CKD can influence the dosing of a variety of drugs, in particular those with considerable renal clearance (Table 9-5) (Kappel & Calissi, 2002). In stage 4 and 5 CKD, the metabolism and transport of nonrenally cleared drugs may also be altered (Nolin et al., 2008).

Beyond the impact of CKD on the handling of various drugs, used either for its own treatment or for the treatment of concomitant diseases, it is important to recognize the potential for renal damage from both commonly used drugs, e.g., analgesics (Chang et al., 2008), and over-the-counter herbal remedies (Laliberte et al., 2007), as well as newer chemotherapeutic agents (Jain & Townsend, 2007).

Attention should also be given to the potential for metabolic mischief, particularly the worsening of insulin sensitivity, by high doses of diuretics and β-blockers (Gupta et al., 2008) as described in Chapter 7.

CKD in the Elderly

As the fastest growing part of our population, those over age 65 are becoming the largest burden of CKD: the medium age of new dialysis patients in the United States is now 65 years of age, and the fastest growing group of new dialysis patients is of those older than

TABLE 9.5	Dose Modification for Patients with Renal Insufficiency	
Drugs requiring dose modification	**Drugs not requiring dose modification**	
All antibiotics	EXCEPT	Cloxacillin, clindamycin, metronidazole, macrolides
Antihypertensives Atenolol, nadolol, angiotensin-converting enzyme inhibitors	*Antihypertensives* CCBs, minoxidil, angiotensin receptor blockers, clonidine, α- blockers	
Other cardiac medications Digoxin, sotalol	*Other cardiac medications* Amiodarone, nitrates	
Diuretics AVOID potassium-sparing diuretics in patients with creatinine clearance < 30 mL/min	*Narcotics* Fentanyl hydromorphone, morphine	
Lipid-lowering agents HMG-CoA reductase inhibitors, benafibrate, clofibrate, fenofibrate	*Psychotropics* Tricyclic antidepressants, nefazodone, other selective serotonin reuptake inhibitors	
Narcotics Codeine, meperidine	*Antidiabetic agents* Repaglinide, rosiglitazone	
Psychotropics Lithium, chloral hydrate, gabapentin, trazodone, paroxetine, primidone, topiramate, vigabatrin	*Miscellaneous* Proton pump inhibitors	
Antidiabetic agents Acarbose, chlorpropamide, glyburide, gliclazide, metformin, insulin		
Miscellaneous Allopurinol, colchicine, histamine$_2$ receptor antagonists, diclofenac, ketorolac, terbutaline		

Modified from Kappel J, Calissi P. Nephrology: 3. Safe drug prescrbing for patients with renal insufficiency. *CMAJ* 2002;166:473–477.

75 years of age (Stevens et al., 2008a) (Fig. 9-7). Although the diminution of renal structure and function with age may largely reflect the impact of nonrenal diseases, e.g., hypertension or diabetes (Fliser, 2005), the kidney ages even in their absence (Zhou et al., 2008). Moreover, with the same level of eGFR, the elderly have higher mortality rates than the younger (O'Hare et al., 2007).

The loss of renal function with age is often heralded by increasing nocturia, as sodium ingested during the day is more slowly excreted into the night (Kujubu & Aboseif, 2008). More seriously, cognitive impairment closely accompanies progressive CKD (Kurella et al., 2008).

Moreover, among a group of elderly Japanese patients (mean age = 63 ± 14) with varying degrees of CKD of various etiologies, 56% were found to have a silent brain infarction by MRI (Kobayashi et al., 2009). The prevalence increased with the severity of CKD and was twofold higher in those with CKD caused by hypertensive nephrosclerosis than seen in those with other etiologies. In keeping with the evidence described in Chapter 7 for better stroke protection with drugs that raise circulating levels of angiotensin II (ARBs, diuretics, and CCBs), compared to those that lower the A-II levels (ACEIs and β-blockers), the prevalence of stroke was 1.75 higher in those who took the A-II lowering drugs.

More in the United States than elsewhere, older patients with advanced CKD are increasingly started on RRT, including dialysis and transplantation. However, the societal costs and the individual discomforts of such intensive treatment are well recognized. Calls for more limited management are being made,

particularly for those afflicted with other life-threatening conditions (Abaterusso et al., 2008).

Even as currently available therapies may be less vigorously used in some elderly patients, the inability to prevent or overcome the progression of CKD in most people has spurred the research into more protective therapies.

Therapy in the Future

Though the intensive application of currently available therapies will slow and occasionally reverse the progression of renal disease (Ruggenenti et al., 2008), the growing impact of obesity-induced diabetes is overwhelming the wider use of traditional therapies (Fox & Munter, 2008).

As the scope of causative and aggravating factors for CKD widens (Schlondorff, 2008), more varied therapies are being considered to counter them. A partial list includes:

- Stem-cell infusion (LeBleu & Kalluri, 2008)
- Vitamin D receptor activation (Alborzi et al., 2008)
- Pentoxifulline (McCormick et al., 2008)
- Antioxidants (Paravicini & Touyz, 2008)
- Endothelin receptor antagonists (Barton, 2008)
- Activation of hypoxia-inducible transcription factors (Fine & Norman, 2008)
- A number of inhibitors of transforming growth factor—β-1 and other inflammatory cytokines, proliferative mitogens, cell-cycle inhibitors, and other targets of renal damage (Khwaja et al., 2007).

DIABETIC NEPHROPATHY

Most of the preceding coverage of CKD applies to the most common of its causes—diabetic nephropathy. However, diabetes provokes additional pathology and requires additional therapy (Table 9-6) (KDOQI, 2007).

Pathology and Clinical Features

As delineated by Kimmelstiel and Wilson (1936), renal disease occurs among diabetics with a high incidence and with a particular glomerular pathology—nodular intercapillary glomerulosclerosis. The clinical description has been improved very little since their original paper (Kimmelstiel & Wilson, 1936):

> The clinical picture appears... to be almost as characteristic as the histological one: the patients are relatively

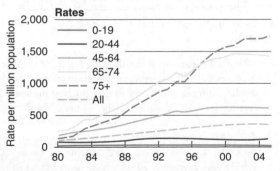

FIGURE 9-7 Rates of new cases of ESRD in patients at various ages treated by dialysis or transplantation in the United States, by years from 1980 to 2004. (Modified from U.S. Renal data systems. Chronic kidney disease. *USRDS 2007*, Bethesda NIH, NIDDKD 2008.)

TABLE 9.6	Goals for Risk Factor Management in Diabetic Patients
Risk Factor	**Goal of Therapy**
Cigarette smoking	Complete cessation
BP	<130/80 mm Hg
LDL-C	<100 mg/dL
Triglycerides > 200 mg/dL; HDL-C < 40 mg/dL	Increase HDL-C
Prothrombotic state	Aspirin
Glucose	HbA$_{1c}$ <7%
Overweight and obesity (BMI ≥ 25 kg/m^2)	Significant weight loss
Physical inactivity	Regular exercise

LDL-C, low-density lipoprotein cholesterol; HDL-C, high-density lipoprotein cholesterol; HbA$_{1c}$, hemoglobin A$_{1c}$.

old; hypertension is present, usually of the benign type, and the kidneys frequently show signs of decompensation; there is a history of diabetes, usually of long standing; the presenting symptoms may be those of edema of the nephrotic type, renal decompensation or heart failure; the urine contains large amounts of albumin and there is usually impairment of concentrating power with or without nitrogen retention.

The clinical description should be altered to include younger patients who have been diabetic for more than 15 years, to involve hypertension in approximately 50% to 60% of patients, and to almost always be accompanied by retinal capillary microaneurysms.

Course

Persistent microalbuminuria, as the first manifestation of diabetic nephropathy, has been observed in about one third of newly diagnosed type 1 diabetics within 20 years (Hovind et al., 2004) and in about one quarter of newly diagnosed type 2 diabetics within 10 years (Adler et al., 2003). The difference in time of onset may largely reflect the long asymptomatic background of type 2 compared to the usual abrupt onset of type 1. Rather surprisingly, regression of microalbuminuria has been observed in a significant percentage of type 1 diabetics, generally associated with lower levels of BP and glycemia (Hovind et al., 2004; Perkins et al., 2003).

Nelson et al. (1996) studied renal function every 6 to 12 months over 4 years in 194 Pima Indians who were selected as the representatives of different stages

in the development of diabetic nephropathy: from normal glucose tolerance to overt diabetes; from normal albumin excretion to macroalbuminuria. As shown in Figure 9-8, the major findings generally were as follows: Glomerular hyperfiltration is present from the onset until macroalbuminuria appears. Thereafter, GFR declines rapidly because of a progressive loss of intrinsic ultrafiltration capacity. Although the rather abrupt fall in GFR that occurs after approximately 15 years was not prevented by the control of BP, higher baseline pressures predicted an increasing urinary albumin excretion, which in turn mediated a fall in GFR.

Mechanisms

A great amount of research has delineated the mechanisms of diabetic nephropathy (Jefferson et al., 2008; Qian et al., 2008; Remuzzi et al., 2006a). Figure 9-9 portrays current evidence of the interplay of multiple factors that eventuate in diabetic nephropathy (Jefferson et al., 2008).

The critical role of glomerular hypertension as reflected by the hyperfiltration seen in Figure 9-8 has been strongly supported by the ability of antihypertensive therapy to prevent the progression of nephropathy. In addition to multiple clinical studies, the role is supported by the observation that nodular glomerulosclerosis developed in only the nonobstructed kidney of a diabetic patient with unilateral renal artery stenosis (Berkman & Rifkin, 1973). Moreover, normal kidneys transplanted into diabetic patients develop typical diabetic lesions (Mauer et al., 1983), denying an essential role for genetic factors.

The progression from glomerular hypertension to overt nephropathy has been portrayed by Adler (2004):

Mesangial expansion is the defining lesion in diabetic nephropathy.... The mesangial expansion encroaches on capillary lumena and results in slow progression toward end-stage renal disease. But the diabetic lesion also involves podocyte injury mediated by signal transduction change, cytoskeletal change, alterations in the podocyte slit pore membrane, detachment from the GBM, and apoptosis, all of which contribute to the development of proteinuria. In turn, proteinuria accelerates progression by its effects on tubulointerstitial fibrosis and atrophy, the final common pathway of progressive renal insufficiency. Adding insult to injury are the arterial and arteriolar sclerotic lesions, which superimpose ischemia on each of the other three renal regions.

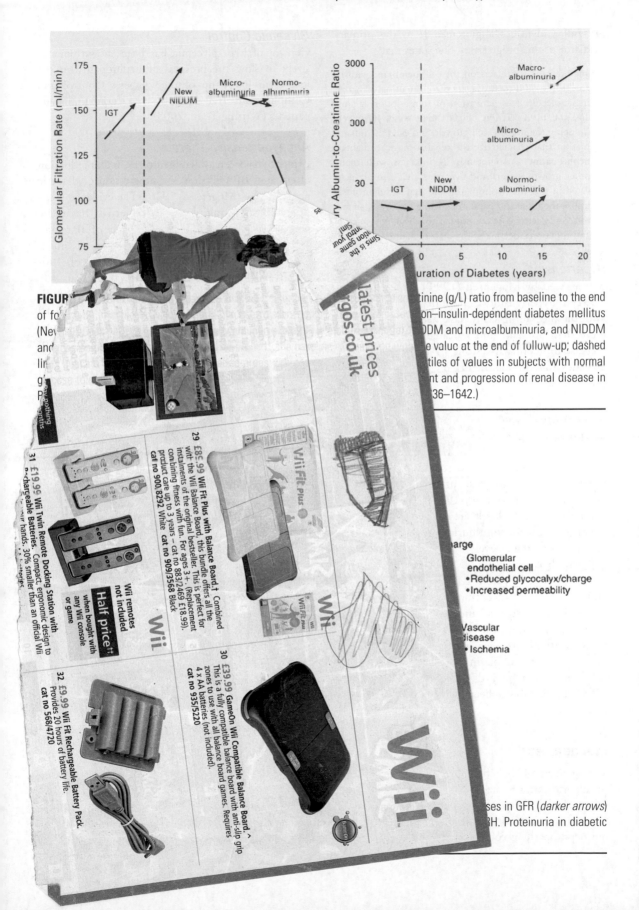

FIGUR... ...tinine (g/L) ratio from baseline to the end
of fo... ...on–insulin-dependent diabetes mellitus
(New... ...DDM and microalbuminuria, and NIDDM
and... ...e value at the end of follow-up; dashed
li... ...tiles of values in subjects with normal
g... ...nt and progression of renal disease in
P... ...36–1642.)

...ses in GFR (*darker arrows*)
...H. Proteinuria in diabetic

...arge
  Glomerular
  endothelial cell
  •Reduced glycocalyx/charge
  •Increased permeability

...Vascular
...disease
  • Ischemia

Dr. Adler identifies angiotensin II as the primary mediator of this progression. She states that:

> angiotensin II interacts on the cell membrane with its receptor(s), and then triggers the elaboration of signaling molecules, the activation of transcription factors, and the up-regulation of gene expression, ultimately inducing the fibrosis, cell growth, and even the inflammation that characterize the renal damage in diabetic nephropathy.... Angiotensin II interacts with many other growth factors and cytokines that also are activated in diabetic nephropathy and that simultaneously utilize the same and parallel signaling pathways, all factors or systems contributing to the histologic picture and functional decline of the diabetic kidney.

Hypertension

As reviewed by Mogensen (1999), the associations between hypertension and both increasing albuminuria and falling GFR have been recognized for more than 30 years and repeatedly confirmed. An increase in nocturnal systolic BP has been found to precede the development of microalbuminuria (Lurbe et al., 2003).

Renin-Angiotensin

The progressive glomerulosclerosis would be expected to knock out the juxtaglomerular cells that secrete renin and, in some diabetics, a state of *hyporeninemic hypoaldosteronism* appears, usually manifested by hyperkalemia (Perez et al., 1977). However, serum renin and prorenin levels are often increased before the onset of microalbuminuria, serving as a potential marker for the development of nephropathy (Dronavalli et al., 2009). Moreover, the intrarenal RAS is activated in both type 1 (Hollenberg et al., 2003) and type 2 (Mezzano et al., 2003) diabetics. These findings suggest autonomy of the intrarenal renin system and set the stage for the major benefits of RAS inhibitors seen in diabetic nephropathy. Moreover, elevated plasma aldosterone levels have been noted in type 1 diabetics (Hollenberg et al., 2004), presumably reflecting an activated systemic RAS.

Management

Management of diabetic nephropathy is similar to the algorithm for management of hypertension in all CKDs shown in Figure 9-5, but there are differences. The management of hypertension in diabetics without nephropathy is covered in Chapter 7.

Glycemic Control

Control of hyperglycemia has been shown conclusively to slow the progress of nephropathy in the long-term follow-up of the Diabetes Control and Complications Trial study of 1,349 type 1 diabetic patients (Writing Team, 2003).

Antihypertensive Therapy

Evidence has been available since 1976 that reduction of elevated BP will slow the progression of diabetic nephropathy (Mogensen, 1976). The evidence accumulated from multiple subsequent trials has made two certain conclusions: First, the degree of BP reduction needed to protect against progression is much lower than the previously accepted goal of 140/90 mm Hg and, second, multiple drugs will usually be needed to achieve the necessary goal (KDOQI, 2007). The evidence is nicely portrayed in Figure 9-10 (Bakris et al., 2000) showing that the rate of progression of nephropathy was directly related to the level of BP achieved in these six trials of patients with diabetic nephropathy and the three trials in nondiabetic renal disease. It required on average more than two, sometimes four or more, drugs to achieve the lower targets of therapy. More so than with nondiabetic CKD, considerable evidence supports a goal of therapy to below 130/80 in diabetic CKD (KDOQI, 2007). However, overly aggressive therapy that lowers systolic pressure below 120 mm Hg or diastolic below 70 may increase all-cause mortality (Pohl et al., 2005).

Choices of Drugs
ACEIs, ARBs, and DRIs

Although the renoprotection provided in the original trials by Mogensen (1976) and Parving et al. (1983) used diuretics, β-blockers, and direct vasodilators—the major drugs available in the 1970s—more recent trials have almost all used ACEIs or ARBs as the primary drug. As reviewed earlier in this chapter, ACEIs and ARBs (and DRIs) theoretically should reduce intraglomerular pressure better than do other drugs and, practically, they do. The evidence, starting with overt nephropathy in hypertensive type 1 diabetics, has now progressed to encompass normotensive diabetics with, or without, microalbuminuria (Estacio et al., 2006).

As with nondiabetic CKD, the wisest course would be to start with an ACEI or an ARB. The combination of an ACEI and an ARB may be appropriate for some proteinuric patients, but with the knowledge that the combination may lower BP too

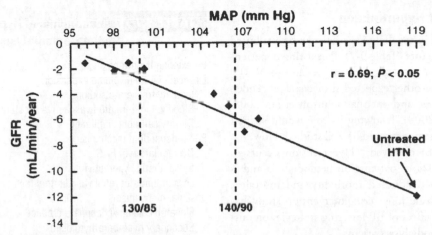

FIGURE 9-10   Relationship between the achieved BP control and declines in GFR in six clinical trials of diabetic and three trials of nondiabetic renal disease. HTN, hypertension; MAP, mean arterial pressure. (Modified from Bakris GL, Williams M, Dworkin L, et al. Preserving renal function in adults with hypertension and diabetes: A consensus approach. *Am J Kidney Dis* 2000;36:646–661.)

much or induce hyperkalemia (ONTARGET Investigators, 2008).

Additional Drugs

More than one drug will usually be needed and the second one should almost always be a diuretic (Mogensen et al., 2003), as volume expansion is usual with any degree of renal insufficiency. A CCB may be needed to achieve BP control. As noted previously in this chapter, evidence of lesser decreases in proteinuria with DHP-CCBs than seen with non–DHP-CCBs (Bakris et al., 2004) has prompted the recommendation that non-DHP-CCBs be used as add-on therapy in patients with diabetic nephropathy. It should be noted that over half of the ARB-based group in the RENAAL trial received a DHP-CCB with no apparent loss of renal protection (Brenner et al., 2001). Therefore, while a non–DHP-CCB may be theoretically preferable, a DHP-CCB will likely do as well when added to maximal ACEI or ARB (Contreras et al., 2005).

Other choices for third or fourth add-ons include α-blockers or vasodilating β-blockers. Although aldosterone antagonists were usually avoided in CKD patients because of the threat of hyperkalemia, particularly on top of an ACEI or ARB, aldosterone escape has been noted in 40% of ACEI-treated patients with diabetic nephropathy (Sato et al., 2003). Therefore, cautious use of an aldosterone antagonist is appropriate, and perhaps earlier, in the algorithm.

Other Therapies

As with nondiabetic CKD, a *low-protein diet* should be helpful. *Moderate sodium restriction* is clearly necessary (Vogt et al., 2008). *Control of dyslipidemia* may also lower the BP, reduce proteinuria, slow the decline in GFR, and reduce cardiovascular events (Strippoli et al., 2008). As an aid to achieve control of hyperglycemia, a *thiazolidinedione* may also lower the BP (Parulkar et al., 2001).

Gaede et al. (2008) have provided a striking demonstration of the ability of a multifaceted approach involving tight control of hypertension, hyperglycemia, and dyslipidemia, along with aspirin and an ACEI, to reduce the progression of nephropathy as well as retinopathy and autonomic neuropathy in patients with type 2 diabetes and microalbuminuria. Despite the costs and problems of such intensive therapy, the benefits are surely worth the expense and effort.

CHRONIC DIALYSIS

Although only a small proportion of CKD patients progress to ESRD and start dialysis, they constitute an inordinate personal and societal burden. They represent 1.7% of U.S. Medicare patients but consume 6.4% of Medicare's budget and, as noted at the beginning of this chapter, their numbers are projected to continue to climb rapidly.

The Role of Hypertension

Hypertension in the dialysis patient can be attributed to a host of factors (Table 9-7). Preexisting hypertension is a major risk factor for progression to ESRD, along with the other expected suspects: age, gender, eGFR, diabetes, and anemia (Johnson et al., 2008; Levin et al., 2008). Knowing its role would suggest that its management would be well studied. However, as Toto (2008) observed: "Hypertension occurs in more than 80% of patients on hemodialysis and is associated with increased morbidity and mortality, yet no large-scale long-term intervention study has examined the effect of BP lowering strategies on outcomes in hemodialysis patients."

The little that is known supports the continuation of diuretics if there is any residual renal function (Bragg-Gresham et al., 2007) and the use of ACEIs or ARBs (Fang et al., 2008; Suzuki et al., 2008).

However, there are even more fundamental unanswered issues in regard to dialysis and hypertension including:

- How to ascertain the presence of hypertension? The best way seems to be an average of the readings taken before, during, and after dialysis (Agarwal et al., 2008).
- What is the role of BP variability? It seems to be detrimental (Brunelli et al., 2008).
- What is the best BP for dialysis patients? As Luther and Golper (2008) note, the upper and lower limits have never been established, and few dialysis centers achieve the arbitrarily set standards of less than 140/90 mm Hg predialysis and less than 130/80 mm Hg postdialysis.
- How to avoid intradialytic hypotension, much less its cause and treatment? Davenport et al. (2008) found that the incidence of this serious problem was significantly greater in centers that achieved the highest rate of meeting the postdialysis BP target. As reviewed by Palmer and Henrich (2008), there are many factors responsible and many ways to avoid, or treat, this hemodynamic instability (Table 9-8).

Management in the Future

Intradialytic hypotension is only one of the many problems facing the dialysis patient, with early mortality, usually from a cardiovascular event, being the most obvious.

TABLE 9.7	Mechanisms of Hypertension in the Hemodialysis Patient

Preexisting hypertension
Extracellular fluid volume expansion
   Inability to excrete sodium
   Blood volume–related vasoactive substances
   Dietary salt noncompliance
Renal-dependent mechanisms
   Dysregulation of RAS
   Sympathetic hyperactivity
   Loss of inherent renal vasodilatory factors
Vascular mechanisms
   Elevated calcium/phosphate product
   Secondary hyperparathyroidism
   Vascular calcification and stiffening
Medications and toxins
   Sympathomimetics
   Erythropoietin
   Cigarette smoking
   Lead exposure
Circulating factors
   Endogenous inhibitors of nitric oxide system
   Endogenous inhibitors of vascular Na^+, K^+-ATPase
   Parathyroid hormone
   "Uremic toxins"
Hemodialysis prescription
   Dialysate Na^+ and K^+ concentrations
   Shorter dialysis sessions
   Overestimation of dry weight
   Impaired sleep; sleep apnea

Modified from Khosla and Johnson, *Am J Kidney Dis*, 2004;43(4): 739–751.

TABLE 9.8	Causes of Dialysis-Related Hypotension

Excessive ultrafiltration
Decrease of plasma osmolality
Dialysate problems: temperature, bioincompatibility
Hyperinsulinemia from dialysate-induced hyperglycemia
Reflex sympathetic inhibition
Autonomic neuropathy
Bleeding
Electrolyte abnormalities (hypokalemia, hyperkalemia, hypocalcemia)
Sepsis
Heart disease (ischemia, arrhythmias, pericardial effusion with cardiac tamponade)
Restoration of nitric oxide by the removal of endogenous inhibitors

As to hypertension, the simplest, but perhaps the most difficult to obtain, is rigid reduction of dietary sodium intake to maintain the "dry weight" and limit the fluid volume expansion between dialysis, as long preached by the late Belding Scribner (1999) and repeatedly shown to be helpful (Agarwal et al., 2009; Ozkahya et al., 2006). More antihypertensive drugs will almost certainly not play a prominent role.

The best solution to almost all of the problems faced by dialysis patients, including their hypertension and hypotension, has been described in over 300 papers over the past 40 years—daily hemodialysis. As described by Kjellstrand et al. (2008):

> The first study of daily dialysis in patients with end-stage renal disease (ESRD) began four decades ago in 1967 (DePalma et al., 1969). Since then many have studied daily haemodialysis and reported improvements in biochemistry, cardiovascular physiology, clinical symptoms and quality of life.

Reimbursement problems, the virtual disappearance of home haemodialysis training programs in the USA and other countries, difficult logistics, physician and patient reluctance and conservatism have limited adoption of daily dialysis.

Support for the use of daily home hemodialysis is growing. Data on large number of patients successfully managed have been published (Culleton et al., 2007; Kjellstrand et al., 2008).

The survival data on 415 patients treated by short daily hemodialysis, either at home or in centers, are striking: much better than with thrice-a-week dialysis and similar to what is achieved by renal transplantation (Kjellstrand et al., 2008) (Fig. 9-11).

A rational proposal to increase the adoption of home hemodialysis while minimizing any additional costs to Medicare has been presented (Hodge, 2008). Hodge's proposal involves a one-time subsidy for each patient converted from conventional clinic hemodialysis to frequent dialysis at home.

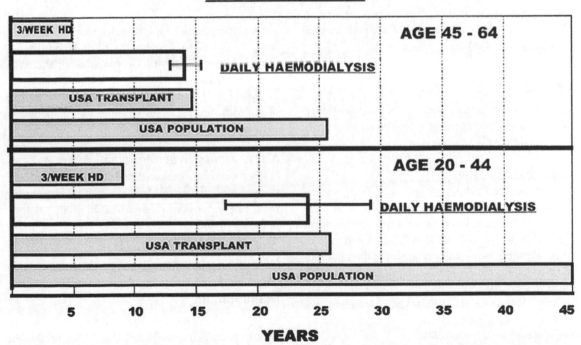

FIGURE 9-11 Life expectancy by age group for three times per week hemodialysis (HD), daily hemodialysis, deceased donor renal transplant recipients and the U.S. population. The life expectancy of both the younger and older daily hemodialysis patients is three times that of patients treated by conventional three times per week hemodialysis and equal to that of recipients of deceased donor renal transplants. The life expectancies are 9 to 15 years longer than those of the age-matched US hemodialysis patients. (Reproduced from Kjellstrand *LM*, et al., *Nephrol Dial Transplant* 2008;23(10):3283, with permission).

As Hodge writes:

> This will accelerate conversion of patients to frequent dialysis and brighten their presently grim outlook and poor quality of life, lessen the revenue-cost strain for dialysis organizations, and stimulate research and private investment in new renal replacement technologies. Costs to Medicare are modest, controllable, and easily discontinued without affecting already converted patients.

This proposal is likely only one of many that could eventuate in the maintenance of a longer and better life for patients with ESRD.

HYPERTENSION AFTER KIDNEY TRANSPLANTATION

As more patients are receiving renal transplants and living longer thereafter, hypertension has been recognized as a major complication, one that may, if uncontrolled, quickly destroy the transplant or add to the risk of cardiovascular disease (Gill, 2008). The majority of transplant recipients are hypertensive, and the higher the level of BP at 1 year after transplantation, the lower is the rate of allograft survival (Mange et al., 2004).

Causes

Table 9-9 lists a number of causes of posttransplantation hypertension beyond the persistence of primary hypertension.

Immunosuppression
Cyclosporine and tacrolimus can cause both nephrotoxicity and hypertension, and the two are often interrelated. Tacrolimus, when compared to cyclosporine, provides better survival and lower acute rejection rates, while allowing most patients to discontinue steroids (Kramer et al., 2008). Sirolimus, which is not a calcineurin inhibitor, causes less hypertension and nephrotoxicity (Morath et al., 2007). Other regimens that avoid calcineurin inhibitors are based on mycophenolate mofetil (Guba et al., 2008).

Posttransplantation Renal Artery Stenosis
Renal artery stenosis, often at the suture line, is found in approximately 1% to 5% of patients with posttransplantation hypertension (Bruno et al., 2004) and should be suspected by appearance of a bruit. The diagnosis should be suspected if hypertension

TABLE 9.9	Causes of Posttransplantation Hypertension

Immunosuppressive therapy
  Steroids
  Cyclosporine, tacrolimus
Allograft failure
  Chronic rejection
  Recurrent disease
Potentially surgically remediable causes
  Allograft renal artery stenosis
  Native kidneys
Volume expansion
  Erythrocytosis
  Sodium retention
Speculative cause
  Recurrent essential hypertension
    As a primary cause of ESRD
    From a hypertensive or prehypertensive donor
Other pressor mechanisms including:
  Endothelin
  Transforming growth factor β
  Decreased nitric oxide

suddenly appears or rapidly progresses or if allograft function deteriorates after an ACEI or ARB is begun. Duplex sonography with measurement of the resistive index is the preferred way to begin evaluation; if a stenosis is seen, arteriography followed by angioplasty with stenting is the usual corrective maneuver (Bruno et al., 2004).

Native Kidney Hypertension
If graft stenosis is excluded and the allograft is functioning well, the native kidneys may be responsible for the hypertension. If hypertension persists despite intensive medical therapy including ACEIs or ARBs, the native kidneys may have to be removed (Fricke et al., 1998).

Management
CCBs have been most widely used to treat hypertension in transplant recipients, but RAS inhibitors, ACEIs, and ARBs are being used increasingly. Their use, as reviewed by Cruzado et al. (2008), has both pros and cons. The pros include a decrease in transforming growth factor—β-1 and other markers of fibrosis—greater reduction in proteinuria, better control of hypertension, and prevention of posttransplant erythrocytosis. They also are effective in regress-

ing left ventricular hypertrophy which further protects against cardiac events (Paoletti et al., 2007). The cons of RAS inhibition include hyperkalemia, anemia, and a possible decline in renal function (Cruzado et al., 2008).

Most posttransplant hypertension will require at least two drugs for control. An ACEI or ARB and a CCB are the most likely combination.

Other drugs including diuretics, α-blockers, and β-blockers may be needed to control posttransplant hypertension that is not related to discernable and correctable causes. However it's done, the intensive control of hypertension to below 130/80 is necessary to protect the kidney while close attention is directed toward all other treatable cardiovascular risk factors, including new-onset diabetes (Bloom & Crutchlow, 2008).

Now that normal parenchymal diseases have been covered, hypertension caused by renovascular diseases will be examined.

REFERENCES

Abaterusso C, Lupo A, Ortalda V, et al. Treating elderly people with diabetes and stages 3 and 4 chronic kidney disease. *Clin J Am Soc Nephrol* 2008;3:1185–1194.

Accetta NA, Gladstone EH, DiSogra C, et al. Prevalence of estimated GFR reporting among US clinical laboratories. *Am J Kidney Dis* 2008;52:778–787.

Adler S. Diabetic nephropathy: Linking histology, cell biology, and genetics. *Kidney Int* 2004;66:2095–2106.

Adler AL, Stevens RJ, Manley SE, et al. Development and progression of nephropathy in type 2 diabetes: The United Kingdom Prospective Diabetes Study (UKPDS 64). *Kidney Int* 2003;63:225–232.

Agarwal R. Hypertension and survival in chronic hemodialysis patients–past lessons and future opportunities. *Kidney Int* 2005;67:1–13.

Agarwal R, Alborzi P, Satyan S, et al. Dry-weight reduction in hypertensive hemodialysis patients (DRIP): A randomized, controlled trial. *Hypertension* 2009;53:500–507.

Agarwal R, Metiku T, Tegegne GG, et al. Diagnosing hypertension by intradialytic blood pressure recordings. *Clin J Am Soc Nephrol* 2008;3:1364–1372.

Agodoa LY, Appel L, Bakris GL, et al. Effect of ramipril vs amlodipine on renal outcomes in hypertensive nephrosclerosis. *JAMA* 2001;285:2719–2728.

Alborzi P, Patel NA, Peterson C, et al. Paricalcitol reduces albuminuria and inflammation in chronic kidney disease: A randomized double-blind pilot trial. *Hypertension* 2008;52:249–255.

American Diabetes Association. Standards of medical care in diabetes-2008. *Diabetes Care* 2008;31:524–526.

Anderson S, Brenner BM. Progressive renal disease: a disorder of adaptation. *QJM* 1989;70:185–189.

Appel LJ, Wright JT Jr, Greene T, et al. Long-term effects of renin-angiotensin system-blocking therapy and a low blood pressure goal on progression of hypertensive chronic kidney disease in African Americans. *Arch Intern Med* 2008;168:832–839.

Baekken M, Os I, Sandvik L, et al. Microalbuminuria associated with indicators of inflammatory activity in an HIV-positive population. *Nephrol Dial Transplant* 2008;23:3130–3137.

Bakris GL, Ritz E. The message for World Kidney Day 2009: Hypertension and kidney disease: A marriage that should be prevented. *Kidney Int* 2009;75:449–452.

Bakris GL, Hart P, Ritz E. Beta blockers in the management of chronic kidney disease. *Kidney Int* 2006;70:1905–1913.

Bakris GL, Ruilope L, Locatelli F, et al. Treatment of microalbuminuria in hypertensive subjects with elevated cardiovascular risk: Results of the IMPROVE trial. *Kidney Int* 2007;72:879–885.

Bakris GL, Toto RD, McCullough PA, et al. Effects of different ACE inhibitor combinations on albuminuria: Results of the GUARD study. *Kidney Int* 2008;73:1303–1309.

Bakris GL, Weir MR, Secic M, et al. Differential effects of calcium antagonist subclasses on markers of nephropathy progression. *Kidney Int* 2004;65:1991–2002.

Bakris GL, Williams M, Dworkin L, et al. Preserving renal function in adults with hypertension and diabetes: A consensus approach. *Am J Kidney Dis* 2000;36:646–661.

Bankir L, Bochud M, Maillard M, et al. Nighttime blood pressure and nocturnal dipping are associated with daytime urinary sodium excretion in African subjects. *Hypertension* 2008;51:891–898.

Barai S, Bandopadhayaya GP, Bhowmik D, et al. Prevalence of vesicoureteral reflux in patients with incidentally diagnosed adult hypertension. *Urology* 2004;63:1045–1049.

Barsoum RS. Chronic kidney disease in the developing world. *N Engl J Med* 2006;354:997–999.

Barton M. Reversal of proteinuric renal disease and the emerging role of endothelin. *Nat Clin Pract Nephrol* 2008;4:490–501.

Berkman J, Rifkin H. Unilateral nodular diabetic glomerulosclerosis (Kimmelstiel-Wilson): Report of a case. *Metabolism* 1973;22:715–722.

Berl T. Maximizing inhibition of the renin-angiotensin system with high doses of converting enzyme inhibitors or angiotensin receptor blockers. *Nephrol Dial Transplant* 2008;23:2443–2447.

Berl T, Hunsicker LG, Lewis JB, et al. Impact of achieved blood pressure on cardiovascular outcomes in the Irbesartan Diabetic Nephropathy Trial. *J Am Soc Nephrol* 2005;16:2170–2179.

Berns JS, Bloom RD. Viral nephropathies: Core curriculum 2008. *Am J Kidney Dis* 2008;52:370–381.

Bilous R, Chaturvedi N, Sjolie AK, et al. Effect of candesartan on microalbuminuria and albumin excretion rate in diabetes: Three randomized trials. *Ann Inter Med* 2009;151:11–14.

Bloom RD, Crutchlow MF. New-onset diabetes mellitus in the kidney recipient: Diagnosis and management strategies. *Clin J Am Soc Nephrol* 2008;3 (Suppl 2):S38–S48.

Bogaert YE, Chonchol M. Assessing the benefits and harms of statin treatment in patients with chronic kidney disease. *Nat Clin Pract Nephrol* 2008;4:470–471.

Bomback AS, Klemmer PJ. The incidence and implications of aldosterone breakthrough. *Nat Clin Pract Nephrol* 2007;3:486–492.

Bomback AS, Kshirsagar AV, Amamoo MA, et al. Change in proteinuria after adding aldosterone blockers to ACE inhibitors or angiotensin receptor blockers in CKD: A systematic review. *Am J Kidney Dis* 2008;51:199–211.

Boudville N, Prasad GV, Knoll G, et al. Meta-analysis: Risk for hypertension in living kidney donors. *Ann Intern Med* 2006;145:185–196.

Braden GL, O'Shea MH, Mulhern JG, et al. Acute renal failure and hyperkalemia associated with cyclooxygenase-2 inhibitors. *Nephrol Dial Transplant* 2004;19:1149–1153.

Bragg-Gresham JL, Fissell RB, Mason NA, et al. Diuretic use, residual renal function, and mortality among hemodialysis patients in the Dialysis Outcomes and Practice Pattern Study (DOPPS). *Am J Kidney Dis* 2007;49:426–431.

Brater DC. Use of diuretics in chronic renal insufficiency and nephrotic syndrome. *Semin Nephrol* 1988;8:333–341.

Brenner BM, Cooper ME, de Zeeuw D, et al. Effects of losartan on renal and cardiovascular outcomes in patients with type 2 diabetes and nephropathy. *N Engl J Med* 2001;345:861–869.

Brunelli SM, Thadhani RI, Lynch KE, et al. Association between long-term blood pressure variability and mortality among incident hemodialysis patients. *Am J Kidney Dis* 2008;52:716–726.

Bruno S, Rumuzzi G, Ruggenenti P. Transplant renal artery stenosis. *J Am Soc Nephrol* 2004;15:134–141.

Carlstrom M, Lai EY, Steege A, et al. Nitric oxide deficiency and increased adenosine response of afferent arterioles in hydronephrotic mice with hypertension. *Hypertension* 2008;51:1386–1392.

Casas JP, Chua W, Loukogeorgakis S, et al. Effect of inhibitors of the renin-angiotensin system and other antihypertensive drugs on renal outcomes: Systematic review and meta-analysis. *Lancet* 2005;366:2026–2033.

Catapano F, Chiodini P, De NL, et al. Antiproteinuric response to dual blockade of the renin-angiotensin system in primary glomerulonephritis: Meta-analysis and metaregression. *Am J Kidney Dis* 2008;52:475–485.

Chang SH, Mathew TH, McDonald SP. Analgesic nephropathy and renal replacement therapy in Australia: Trends, comorbidities and outcomes. *Clin J Am Soc Nephrol* 2008;3:768–776.

Chapman N, Dobson J, Wilson S, et al. Effect of spironolactone on blood pressure in subjects with resistant hypertension. *Hypertension* 2007;49:839–845.

Cheng LT, Gao YL, Gu Y, et al. Stepwise increase in the prevalence of isolated systolic hypertension with the stages of chronic kidney disease. *Nephrol Dial Transplant* 2008;23(12):3895–3900.

Coca SG, Krumholz HM, Garg AX, et al. Underrepresentation of renal disease in randomized controlled trials of cardiovascular disease. *JAMA* 2006;296:1377–1384.

Contreras G, Greene T, Agodoa LY, et al. Blood pressure control, drug therapy, and kidney disease. *Hypertension* 2005;46(1):44–50.

Coresh J, Selvin E, Stevens LA, et al. Prevalence of chronic kidney disease in the United States. *JAMA* 2007;298:2038–2047.

Coresh J, Stevens LA, Levey AS. Chronic kidney disease is common: What do we do next? *Nephrol Dial Transplant* 2008;23:1122–1125.

Crowe E, Halpin D, Stevens P. Early identification and management of chronic kidney disease: Summary of NICE guidance. *Br Med J* 2008;337:a1530.

Cruzado JM, Rico J, Grinyo JM. The renin angiotensin system blockade in kidney transplantation: pros and cons. *Transplant Int* 2008;21:304–313.

Culleton BF, Walsh M, Klarenbach SW, et al. Effect of frequent nocturnal hemodialysis vs conventional hemodialysis on left ventricular mass and quality of life: A randomized controlled trial. *JAMA* 2007;298:1291–1299.

Davenport A, Cox C, Thuraisingham R. Achieving blood pressure targets during dialysis improves control but increases intradialytic hypotension. *Kidney Int* 2008;73:759–764.

De Nicola L, Minutolo R, Bellizzi V, et al. Achievement of target blood pressure levels in chronic kidney disease: A salty question? *Am J Kidney Dis* 2004;43:782–795.

De Zeeuw, Lewis EJ, Remuzzi G, et al. Renoprotective effects of renin-angiotensin-system inhibitors. *Lancet* 2006;367:899–900.

Devarajan P. NGAL in acute kidney injury: From serendipity to utility. *Am J Kidney Dis* 2008;52:395–399.

Diskin CJ, Stokes TJ, Dansby LM, et al. Does the hyperfiltration of minoxidil result in increased proteinuria and loss of renoprotection conferred by angiotensin inhibition? *Kidney Blood Press Res* 2006;29:54–59.

Dronavelli S, Duka I, Bakris GL. The pathogenesis of diabetic nephropathy *Nat Clin Pract Endocrinol Metab* 2008;4:444–452.

DuBose TD Jr. American Society of Nephrology Presidential Address 2006: Chronic kidney disease as a public health threat–new strategy for a growing problem. *J Am Soc Nephrol.* 2007;18:1038–1045.

Duru OK, Li S, Jurkovitz C, et al. Race and sex differences in hypertension control in CKD: Results from the Kidney Early Evaluation Program (KEEP). *Am J Kidney Dis* 2008;51:192–198.

Eassa WA, Sheir KZ, Gad HM, et al. Prospective study of the long-term effects of shock wave lithotripsy on renal function and blood pressure. *J Urol* 2008;179:964–968.

Elsayed EF, Sarnak MJ, Tighiouart H, et al. Waist-to-hip ratio, body mass index, and subsequent kidney disease and death. *Am J Kidney Dis* 2008;52:29–38.

Estacio RO, Coll JR, Tran ZV, et al. Effect of intensive blood pressure control with valsartan on urinary albumin excretion in normotensive patients with type 2 diabetes. *Am J Hypertens* 2006;19:1241–1248.

Fang W, Oreopoulos DG, Bargman JM. Use of ACE inhibitors or angiotensin receptor blockers and survival in patients on peritoneal dialysis. *Nephrol Dial Transplant* 2008;23:3704–3710.

Fine LG, Norman JT. Chronic hypoxia as a mechanism of progression of chronic kidney diseases: From hypothesis to novel therapeutics. *Kidney Int* 2008;74:867–872.

Fliser D. Ren sanus in corpore sano: The myth of the inexorable decline of renal function with senescence. *Nephrol Dial Transplant* 2005;20:482–485.

Fougue D, Wang P, Laville M et al. Low protein diets delay end-stage renal disease in non-diabetic adults with chronic renal failure. *Nephrol Dial Transplant* 2000;15:1986–1992.

Fox CS, Muntner P. Trends in diabetes, high cholesterol, and hypertension in chronic kidney disease among U.S. adults: 1988–1994 to 1999–2004. *Diabetes Care* 2008;31:1337–1342.

Freedman BI, Sedor JR. Hypertension-associated kidney disease: Perhaps no more. *J Am Soc Nephrol* 2008;19:2047–2051.

Fricke L, Doehn C, Steinhoff J, et al. Treatment of posttransplant hypertension by laparoscopic bilateral nephrectomy? *Transplantation* 1998;65:1182–1187.

Fukuda M, Yamanaka T, Mizuno M, et al. Angiotensin II type 1 receptor blocker, olmesartan, restores nocturnal blood pressure decline by enhancing daytime natriuresis. *J Hypertens* 2008;26:583–588.

Gaede P, Lund-Andersen H, Parving HH, et al. Effect of a multifactorial intervention on mortality in type 2 diabetes. *N Engl J Med* 2008;358:580–591.

Gargollo PC, Diamond DA. Therapy insight: What nephrologists need to know about primary vesicoureteral reflux. *Nat Clin Pract Nephrol* 2007;3:551–563.

Ghose RR, Harindra V. Unrecognised high pressure chronic retention of urine presenting with systemic arterial hypertension. *Br Med J* 1989;298:1626–1628.

Gill JS. Cardiovascular disease in transplant recipients: Current and future treatment strategies. *Clin J Am Soc Nephrol* 2008;3 (Suppl 2):S29–S37.

Glassock RJ, Winearls C. An epidemic of chronic kidney disease: Fact or fiction? *Nephrol Dial Transplant* 2008;23:1117–1121.

Gomez P, Ruilope LM, Barrios V, et al. Prevalence of renal insufficiency in individuals with hypertension and obesity/overweight: The FATH study. *J Am Soc Nephrol* 2006;17:S194–S200.

Goodship THJ, Stoddart JT, Martinek V, et al. Long-term follow-up of patients presenting to adult nephrologists with chronic pyelonephritis and "normal" renal function. *Q JM* 2000;93:799–803.

Grantham JJ. Clinical practice: Autosomal dominant polycystic kidney disease. *N Engl J Med* 2008;359:1477–1485.

Graves JW. Diagnosis and management of chronic kidney disease. *Mayo Clin Proc* 2008;83:1064–1069.

Griffin KA, Bidani AK. Progression of renal disease: Renoprotective specificity of renin-angiotensin system blockade. *Clin J Am Soc Nephrol* 2006;1:1054–1065.

Griffin KA, Picken MM, Bakris GL, et al. Class differences in the effects of calcium channel blockers in the rat remnant kidney model. *Kidney Int* 1999;44:1849–1860.

Guba M, Rentsch M, Wimmer CD, et al. Calcineurin-inhibitor avoidance in elderly renal allograft recipients using ATG and basiliximab combined with mycophenolate mofetil. *Transplant Int* 2008;21:637–645.

Guidi E, Cozzi MG, Minetti E, et al. Effect of familial hypertension on glomerular hemodynamics and tubuloglomerular feedback after uninephrectomy. *Am J Hypertens* 2001;14:121–128.

Guo H, Karla PA, Gilbertson DT, et al. Artherosclerotic renovascular disease in older US patients starting dialysis, 1996 to 2001. *Circulation* 2007;115:50–58.

Gupta AK, Dahlof B, Dobson J, et al. Determinants of new-onset diabetes among 19,257 hypertensive patients randomized in the Anglo-Scandinavian Cardiac Outcomes Trial–Blood Pressure Lowering Arm and the relative influence of antihypertensive medication. *Diabetes Care* 2008;31:982–988.

Haas M, Rahman MH, Cohn RA, et al. IgA nephropathy in children and adults: Comparison of histologic features and clinical outcomes. *Nephrol Dial Transplant* 2008;23:2537–2545.

Hallan SI, Coresh J, Astor BC, et al. International comparison of the relationship of chronic kidney disease prevalence and ESRD risk. *J Am Soc Nephrol* 2006;17:2275–2284.

Hamming I, Goor H, Navis GJ. ACE inhibitor use and the increased long-term risk of renal failure in diabetes. *Kidney Int* 2006a;70:1377–1378.

Hamming I, Navis G, Kocks MJ, et al. ACE inhibition has adverse renal effects during dietary sodium restriction in proteinuric and healthy rats. *J Pathol* 2006b;209:129–139.

Hermida RC, Calvo C, Ayala DE, et al. Decrease in urinary albumin excretion associated with the normalization of nocturnal blood pressure in hypertensive subjects. *Hypertension* 2005;46:960–968.

Hodge MH. Practicable frequent hemodialysis: A proposal to meet the needs of patients and the requirements of Medicare. *Am J Kidney Dis* 2008;52:387–390.

Hollenberg NK, Price DA, Fisher NDL, et al. Glomerular hemodynamics and the renin-angiotensin system in patients with type 2 diabetes mellitus. *Kidney Int* 2003;63:172–178.

Hollenberg NK, Stevanovic R, Agarwal A, et al. Plasma aldosterone concentration in the patient with diabetes mellitus. *Kidney Int* 2004;65:1435–1439.

Hovind P, Tarnow L, Rossing P, et al. Predictors for the development of microalbuminuria and macroalbuminuria in patients with type 1 diabetes: Inception cohort study. *Br Med J* 2004;328:1105–1109.

Hsu CY, Iribarren C, McCulloch CE, et al. Risk factors for end-stage renal disease: 25-year follow-up. *Arch Intern Med* 2009;169:342–350.

Hsu CY, Ordonez JD, Chertow GM, et al. The risk of acute renal failure in patients with chronic kidney disease. *Kidney Int* 2008;74:101–107.

Ibrahim HN, Foley R, Tan L, et al. Long-term consequences of kidney donation. *N Engl J Med* 2009;360:459–469.

Inrig JK, Patel UD, Gillespie BS, et al. Relationship between interdialytic weight gain and blood pressure among prevalent hemodialysis patients. *Am J Kidney Dis* 2007;50:108–18, 118.

Jafar TH, Stark PC, Schmid CH, et al. Progression of chronic kidney disease; the role of blood pressure control, proteinuria, and angiotensin-converting enzyme inhibition: A patient-level meta-analysis. *Ann Intern Med* 2003;139:244–252.

Jafar TH, Stark PC, Schmid CH, et al. The effect of angiotensin-converting-enzyme inhibitors on progression of advanced polycystic kidney disease. *Kidney Int* 2005;67:265–271.

Jain M, Townsend RR. Chemotherapy agents and hypertension: A focus on angiogenesis blockade. *Curr Hypertens Rep* 2007;9: 320–328.

Jefferson JA, Shankland SJ, Pichler RH. Proteinuria in diabetic kidney disease: A mechanistic viewpoint. *Kidney Int* 2008;74: 22–36.

Johnson ES, Thorp ML, Platt RW, et al. Predicting the risk of dialysis and transplant among patients with CKD: A retrospective cohort study. *Am J Kidney Dis* 2008;52:653–660.

Jones CA, Krolewski AS, Rogus J, et al. Epidemic of end-stage renal disease in people with diabetes in the United States population: Do we know the cause? *Kidney Int* 2005;67:1684–1691.

Jurkovitz CT, Qiu Y, Wang C, et al. The Kidney Early Evaluation Program (KEEP): Program design and demographic characteristics of the population. *Am J Kidney Dis* 2008;51:S3–S12.

Kallen AJ, Jhung MA, Cheng S, et al. Gadolinium-containing magnetic resonance imaging contrast and nephrogenic systemic fibrosis: A case-control study. *Am J Kidney Dis* 2008;51: 966–975.

Kao WH, Klag MJ, Meoni LA et al. MYH9 is associated with non-diabetic end-stage renal disease in African Americans. *Nat Genet* 2008;40:1185–1192.

Kappel J, Calissi P. Nephrology: 3. Safe drug prescribing for patients with renal insufficiency. *CMAJ* 2002; 166: 473–477.

KDOQI clinical practice guidelines and clinical practice recommendations for diabetes and chronic kidney disease. *Am J Kidney Dis* 2007;49:S12–S154.

Kellum JA, Bellomo R, Ronco C. Definition and classification of acute kidney injury. *Nephron Clin Pract* 2008;109:c182–187.

Kestenbaum B, Rudser KD, de Boer, IH, et al. Differences in kidney function and incident hypertension: the multi-ethnic study of atherosclerosis. *Ann Intern Med* 2008;148: 501–508.

Khwaja A, El KM, Floege J, et al. The management of CKD: a look into the future. *Kidney Int* 2007;72:1316–1323.

Kimmelstiel P, Wilson C. Intercapillary lesions in the glomeruli of the kidney. *Am J Pathol* 1936;12:83–97.

Kimura G. Kidney and circadian blood pressure rhythm. *Hypertension* 2008;51:827–828.

Kiryluk K, Rabenou RA, Goldberg ER, et al. The Case: Thirty-one-year old woman with hypertension and abnormal renal imaging. *Kidney Int* 2008;73:659–660.

Kjellstrand CM, Buoncristiani U, Ting G et al. Short daily haemodialysis: Survival in 415 patients treated for 1006 patient-years. *Nephrol Dial Transplant* 2008;23:3283–3289.

Kobayashi M, Hirawa N, Yatsu K, et al. Relationship between silent brain infarction and chronic kidney disease. *Nephrol Dial Transplant* 2009;24(1):201–209.

Kopp JB, Smith MW, Nelson GW et al . MYH9 is a major-effect risk gene for focal segmental glomerulosclerosis. *Nat Genet* 2008;40:1175–1184.

Kovesdy CP, Trivedi BK, Kalantar-Zadeh K, et al. Association of low blood pressure with increased mortality in patients with moderate to severe chronic kidney disease. *Nephrol Dial Transplant* 2006;21:1257–1262.

Kramer BK, Del CD, Margreiter R, et al. Efficacy and safety of tacrolimus compared with ciclosporin A in renal transplantation: three-year observational results. *Nephrol Dial Transplant* 2008;23:2386–2392.

Kujubu DA, Aboseif SR. An overview of nocturia and the syndrome of nocturnal polyuria in the elderly. *Nat Clin Pract Nephrol* 2008;4:426–435.

Kunz R, Friedrich C, Wolbers M, et al. Meta-analysis: Effect of monotherapy and combination therapy with inhibitors of the renin-angiotensin system on proteinuria in renal disease. *Ann Intern Med* 2008;148:30–48.

Kurella TM, Wadley V, Yaffe K, et al. Kidney function and cognitive impairment in US adults: The Reasons for Geographic and Racial Differences in Stroke (REGARDS) Study. *Am J Kidney Dis* 2008;52:227–234.

Laliberte MC, Normandeau M, Lord A, et al. Use of over-the-counter medications and natural products in patients with moderate and severe chronic renal insufficiency. *Am J Kidney Dis* 2007;49:245–256.

Lazarus JM, Bourgoignie JJ, Buckalew VM, et al. Achievement and safety of a low blood pressure goal in chronic renal disease. The modification of diet in renal disease study group. *Hypertension* 1997;29:641–650.

LeBleu VS, Kalluri R. Stem cell-based therapy for glomerular diseases: An evolving concept. *J Am Soc Nephrol* 2008;19: 1621–1623.

Lee AF, MacFadyen RJ, Struthers AD. Neurohormonal reactivation in heart failure patients on chronic ACE inhibitor therapy: A longitudinal study. *Eur J Heart Fail* 1999;1:401–406.

Lee D, Levin A, Simon DR, et al. Longitudinal analysis of performance of estimated glomerular filtration rate as renal function declines in chronic kidney disease. *Nephrol Dial Transplant* 2009;24;109–116.

Levey AS. Nondiabetic kidney disease. *N Engl J Med* 2002;347: 1505–1511.

Levin A, Djurdjev O, Beaulieu M, et al. Variability and risk factors for kidney disease progression and death following attainment of stage 4 CKD in a referred cohort. *Am J Kidney Dis* 2008; 52:661–671.

Lewis EJ. Treating hypertension in the patient with overt diabetic nephropathy. *Semin Nephrol* 2007;27:182–194.

Lurbe E, Redon J, Kesani A, et al. Increase in nocturnal blood pressure and progression to microalbuminuria in type 1 diabetes. *N Engl J Med* 2002;347:797–805.

Luther JM, Golper TA. Blood pressure targets in hemodialysis patients. *Kidney Int* 2008;73:667–668.

Mange KC, Feldman HI, Joffe MM, et al. Blood pressure and the survival of renal allografts from living donors. *J Am Soc Nephrol* 2004;15:187–193.

Mann JF, Ritz E, Kunz R. Renoprotective effects of renin-angiotensin-system inhibitors. *Lancet* 2006;367:900–902.

Mann JF, Schmieder RE, Dyal L et al. Effect of telmisartan on renal outcomes: A randomized trial. *Ann Intern Med* 2009;151: 1–2.

Mann JF, Schmieder RE, McQueen M, et al. Renal outcomes with telmisartan, ramipril, or both, in people at high vascular risk (the ONTARGET study): A multicentre, randomised, double-blind, controlled trial. *Lancet* 2008;372:547–553.

Mauer SM, Steffes MW, Connett J, et al. The development of lesions in the glomerular basement membrane and mesangium after transplantation of normal kidneys to diabetic patients. *Diabetes* 1983;32:948–952.

McCormick BB, Sydor A, Akbari A, et al. The effect of pentoxifylline on proteinuria in diabetic kidney disease: A meta-analysis. *Am J Kidney Dis* 2008;52:454–463.

McCullough PA, Li S, Jurkovitz CT, et al. CKD and cardiovascular disease in screened high-risk volunteer and general populations: The Kidney Early Evaluation Program (KEEP) and National Health and Nutrition Examination Survey (NHANES) 1999–2004. *Am J Kidney Dis* 2008;51:S38–S45.

Menon V, Shlipak MG, Wang X, et al. Cystatin C as a risk factor for outcomes in chronic kidney disease. *Ann Intern Med* 2007;147:19–27.

Messerli FH. The sudden demise of dual renin-angiotensin system blockade or the soft science of the surrogate end point. *J Am Coll Cardiol* 2009;53:468–470.

Mezzano S, Droguett A, Burgos E, et al. Renin-angiotensin system activation and interstitial inflammation in human diabetic nephropathy. *Kidney Int* 2003;64:S64–S70.

Mimran A, du Cailar G. Dietary sodium: The dark horse amongst cardiovascular and renal risk factors. *Nephrol Dial Transplant* 2008;23:2138–2141.

Minutolo R, Borrelli S, Scigliano R, et al. Prevalence and clinical correlates of white coat hypertension in chronic kidney disease. *Nephrol Dial Transplant* 2007a;22:2217–2223.

Minutolo R, De NL, Mazzaglia G, et al. Detection and awareness of moderate to advanced CKD by primary care practitioners: A cross-sectional study from Italy. *Am J Kidney Dis* 2008;52: 444–453.

Minutolo R, Gabbai FB, Borrelli S, et al. Changing the timing of antihypertensive therapy to reduce nocturnal blood pressure in CKD: An 8-week uncontrolled trial. *Am J Kidney Dis* 2007b;50: 908–917.

Mishra J, Ma Q, Prada A, et al. Identification of neutrophil gelatinase-associated lipocalin as a novel early urinary biomarker for ischemic renal injury. *J Am Soc Nephrol* 2003;14: 2534–2543.

Mogensen CE. Progression of nephropathy in long-term diabetes with proteinuria and effect of initial hypertensive treatment. *Scand J Clin Lab Invest* 1976;36:383–388.

Mogensen CE. Microalbuminuria, blood pressure and diabetic renal disease: Origin and development of ideas. *Diabetologia* 1999;42:263–285.

Mogensen CE, Viberti G, Halimi S, et al. Effect of low-dose perindopril/indapamide on albuminuria in diabetes: Preterax in Albuminuria Regression: PREMIER. *Hypertension* 2003;41: 1063–1071.

Mohanram A, Zhang Z, Shahinfar S, et al. The effect of losartan on hemoglobin concentration and renal outcome in diabetic nephropathy of type 2 diabetes. *Kidney Int* 2008;73:630–636.

Moist LM, Foley RN, Barrett BJ, et al. Clinical practice guidelines for evidence-based use of erythropoietic-simulating agents. *Kidney Int* 2008;74:S12–S18.

Morales E, Gutierrez-Solis E, Gutierrez E, et al. Malignant hypertension in HIV-associated glomerulonephritis. *Nephrol Dial Transplant* 2008.

Morath C, Arns W, Schwenger V, et al. Sirolimus in renal transplantation. *Nephrol Dial Transplant* 2007;22 (Suppl 8): viii61–viii65.

MMWR. Morbidity and mortality weekly report. *www cdc gov/ mmwr* 2008a;57:8.

MMWR. Morbidity and mortality weekly report. *www cdc gov/ mmwr* 2008b;57:12.

Mori T, Polichnowski A, Glocka P, et al. High perfusion pressure accelerates renal injury in salt-sensitive hypertension. *J Am Soc Nephrol* 2008;19:1472–1482.

Nakao N, Yoshimura A, Morita H, et al. Combination treatment of angiotensin-II receptor blocker and angiotensin-converting-enzyme inhibitor in non-diabetic renal disease (COOPERATE): A randomised controlled trial. *Lancet* 2003;361:117–124.

Nelson RG, Bennett PH, Beck GJ, et al. Development and progression of renal disease in Pima Indians with non-insulin-dependent diabetes mellitus. *N Engl J Med* 1996;334:1636–1642.

Nickolas TL, O'Rourke MJ, Yang J, et al. Sensitivity and specificity of a single emergency department measurement of urinary neutrophil gelatinase-associated lipocalin for diagnosing acute kidney injury. *Ann Intern Med* 2008;148:810–819.

Ninomiya T, Perkovic V, Gallagher M, et al. Lower blood pressure and risk of recurrent stroke in patients with chronic kidney disease: PROGRESS trial. *Kidney Int* 2008;73:963–970.

Nolin TD, Naud J, Leblond FA, et al. Emerging evidence of the impact of kidney disease on drug metabolism and transport. *Clin Pharmacol Ther* 2008;83:898–903.

Norris K, Mehrotra R, Nissenson AR. Racial differences in mortality and ESRD. *Am J Kidney Dis* 2008;52:205–208.

O'Hare AM, Choi AI, Bertenthal D, et al. Age affects outcomes in chronic kidney disease. *J Am Soc Nephrol* 2007;18:2758–2765.

ONTARGET Investigators. Telmisartan, ramipril, or both in patients at high risk for vascular events. *N Engl J Med* 2008;358:1547–1559.

Onuigbo MA, Onuigbo NT. Late onset renal failure from angiotensin blockade (LORFFAB): A prospective thirty-month Mayo Health System clinic experience. *Med Sci Monit* 2005;11: CR462–CR469.

Onuigbo MA, Onuigbo NT. Use of ultrahigh RAAS blockade: Implications for exacerbation of renal failure. *Kidney Int* 2006;69:194–195.

Orth SR, Hallan SI. Smoking: A risk factor for progression of chronic kidney disease and for cardiovascular morbidity and mortality in renal patients–absence of evidence or evidence of absence? *Clin J Am Soc Nephrol* 2008;3:226–236.

Ozkahya M, Ok E, Toz H, et al. Long-term survival rates in haemodialysis patients treated with strict volume control. *Nephrol Dial Transplant* 2006;21:3506–3513.

Palmer BF, Henrich WL. Recent advances in the prevention and management of intradialytic hypotension. *J Am Soc Nephrol* 2008;19:8–11.

Paoletti E, Cassottana P, Amidone M, et al. ACE inhibitors and persistent left ventricular hypertrophy after renal transplantation: A randomised clinical trial. *Am J Kidney Dis* 2007;50:133–142.

Paravicini TM, Touyz RM. NADPH oxidases, reactive oxygen species, and hypertension: Clinical implications and therapeutic possibilities. *Diabetes Care* 2008;31 (Suppl 2):S170–S180.

Parker MG. Resistant hypertension: Core Curriculum 2008. *Am J Kidney Dis* 2008;52:796–802.

Parulkar AA, Pendergrass ML, Granda-Ayala R, et al. Nonhypoglycemic effects of thiazolidinediones. *Ann Intern Med* 2001;134:61–71.

Parving HH, Persson F, Lewis JB, et al. Aliskiren combined with losartan in type 2 diabetes and nephropathy. *N Engl J Med* 2008;358:2433–2446.

Parving HH, Smidt UM, Andersen AR, et al. Early aggressive antihypertensive treatment reduces rate of decline in kidney function in diabetic nephropathy. *Lancet* 1983;1:1175–1179.

Peralta CA, Shlipak MG, Wassel-Fyr C, et al. Association of antihypertensive therapy and diastolic hypotension in chronic kidney disease. *Hypertension* 2007;50:474–480.

Perez GO, Lespier L, Knowles R, et al. Potassium homeostasis in chronic diabetes mellitus. *Arch Intern Med* 1977;137: 1018–1022.

Perkins BA, Ficociello LH, Silva KH, et al. Regression of microalbuminuria in type 1 diabetes. *N Engl J Med* 2003;348:2285–2293.

Pickering TG. Target blood pressure in patients with end-stage renal disease: Evidence-based medicine or the emperor's new clothes? *J Clin Hypertens (Greenwich)* 2006;8:369–375.

Pogue V, Rahman M, Lipkowitz M, et al. Disparate estimates of hypertension control from ambulatory and clinic blood pressure measurements in hypertensive kidney disease. *Hypertension* 2009;53:20–27.

Pohl MA, Blumenthal S, Cordonnier DJ, et al. Independent and additive impact of blood pressure control and angiotensin II receptor blockade on renal outcomes in the Irbesartan Diabetic Nephropathy Trial: Clinical implications and limitations. *J Am Soc Nephrol* 2005;16:3027–3037.

Popovic-Rolovic M, Kostic M, Antic-Peco A, et al. Medium- and long-term prognosis of patients with acute poststreptococcal glomerulonephritis. *Nephron* 1991;58:393–399.

PROGRESS Collaborative Group. Randomised trial of a perindopril-based blood-pressure-lowering regimen among 6,105 individuals with previous stroke or transient ischaemic attack. *Lancet* 2001; 358:1033–1041.

Qian Y, Feldman E, Pennathur S, et al. From fibrosis to sclerosis: Mechanisms of glomerulosclerosis in diabetic nephropathy. *Diabetes* 2008;57:1439–1445.

Reed B, McFann K, Kimberling WJ, et al. Presence of De Novo Mutations in autosomal dominant polycystic kidney disease patients without family history. *Am J Kidney Dis* 2008.

Remuzzi G, Benigni A, Remuzzi A. Mechanisms of progression and regression of renal lesions of chronic nephropathies and diabetes. *J Clin Invest* 2006a;116:288–296.

Remuzzi G, Cattaneo D, Perico N. The aggravating mechanisms of aldosterone on kidney fibrosis. *J Am Soc Nephrol* 2008;19:1459–1462.

Remuzzi G, Macia M, Ruggenenti P. Prevention and treatment of diabetic renal disease in type 2 diabetes: The BENEDICT study. *J Am Soc Nephrol* 2006b;17:S90–S97.

Rhee MS, Schmid CH, Stevens LA, et al. Risk factors for proteinuria in HIV-infected and -uninfected Hispanic drug users. *Am J Kidney Dis* 2008;52:683–690.

Ritz E. Obesity and CKD: How to assess the risk? *Am J Kidney Dis* 2008;52:1–6.

Rossing K, Christensen PK, Hovind P, et al. Progression of nephropathy in type 2 diabetic patients. *Kidney Int* 2004; 66: 1596.

Ruggenenti P, Perna A, Benini R, et al. Effects of dihydropyridine calcium channel blockers, angiotensin-converting enzyme inhibition, and blood pressure control on chronic, nondiabetic nephropathies. *J Am Soc Nephrol* 1998;9:2096–2101.

Ruggenenti P, Perticucci E, Cravedi P, et al. Role of remission clinics in the longitudinal treatment of CKD. *J Am Soc Nephrol* 2008;19:1213–1224.

Ruilope LM, Zanchetti A, Julius S, et al. Prediction of cardiovascular outcome by estimated glomerular filtration rate and estimated creatinine clearance in the high-risk hypertension population of the VALUE trial. *J Hypertens* 2007;25:1473–1479.

Russo LM, Bakris GL, Comper WD. Renal handling of albumin: A critical review of basic concepts and perspective. *Am J Kidney Dis* 2002;39:899–919.

Saab G, Whaley-Connell AT, McCullough PA, et al. CKD awareness in the United States: The Kidney Early Evaluation Program (KEEP). *Am J Kidney Dis* 2008;52:382–383.

Sacks SH, Aparicio SAJR, Bevan A, et al. Late renal failure due to prostatic outflow obstruction: A preventable disease. *Br Med J* 1989;298:156–159.

Safian RD, Textor SC. Renal-artery stenosis. *N Engl J Med* 2001;344:431–442.

Sarafidis PA, Bakris GL. Renin-angiotensin blockade and kidney disease. *Lancet* 2008;372:511–512.

Sarafidis PA, Li S, Chen SC, et al. Hypertension awareness, treatment, and control in chronic kidney disease. *Am J Med* 2008a;121:332–340.

Sarafidis PA, Stafylas PC, Kanaki AI, et al. Effects of renin-angiotensin system blockers on renal outcomes and all-cause mortality in patients with diabetic nephropathy: An updated meta-analysis. *Am J Hypertens* 2008b;21:922–929.

Saruta T, Hayashi K, Ogihara T et al. Effects of candesartan and amlodipine on cardiovascular events in hypertensive patients with chronic kidney disease: Subanalysis of the CASE-J Study. *Hypertens Res* 2009;32:505–512.

Sato A, Saruta T. Aldosterone escape during angiotensin-converting enzyme inhibitor therapy in essential hypertensive patients with left ventricular hypertrophy. *J Int Med Res* 2001;29: 13–21.

Sato A, Hayashi K, Naruse M, et al. Effectiveness of aldosterone blockade in patients with diabetic nephropathy. *Hypertension* 2003;41:64–68.

Schieppati A, Remuzzi G. The future of renoprotection: Frustration and promises. *Kidney Int* 2003;64:1947–1955.

Schlondorff DO. Overview of factors contributing to the pathophysiology of progressive renal disease. *Kidney Int* 2008;74:860–866.

Schmieder RE. The potential role of prorenin in diabetic nephropathy. *J Hypertens* 2007;25:1323–1326.

Schmitt R, Coca S, Kanbay M, et al. Recovery of kidney function after acute kidney injury in the elderly: A systematic review and meta-analysis. *Am J Kidney Dis* 2008;52:262–271.

Scribner BH. Can antihypertensive medications control BP in haemodialysis patients: Yes or no? *Nephrol Dial Transplant* 1999;14:2599–2601.

Shin GT, Kim DR, Lim JE, et al. Upregulation and function of GADD45gamma in unilateral ureteral obstruction. *Kidney Int* 2008;73:1251–1265.

Sica DA. The kidney and hypertension: Causes and treatment. *J Clin Hypertens (Greenwich)* 2008;10:541–548.

Sica DA, Gehr TW. Diuretic use in stage 5 chronic kidney disease and end-stage renal disease. *Curr Opin Nephrol Hypertens* 2003;12:483–490.

Stevens LA, Coresh J, Levey AS. CKD in the elderly–old questions and new challenges: World Kidney Day 2008. *Am J Kidney Dis* 2008a;51:353–357.

Stevens LA, Coresh J, Schmid CH, et al. Estimating GFR using serum cystatin C alone and in combination with serum creatinine: A pooled analysis of 3,418 individuals with CKD. *Am J Kidney Dis* 2008b;51:395–406.

Strippoli GF, Craig MC, Schena FP, et al. Role of blood pressure targets and specific antihypertensive agents used to prevent diabetic nephropathy and delay its progression. *J Am Soc Nephrol* 2006;17:S153–S155.

Strippoli GF, Navaneethan SD, Johnson DW, et al. Effects of statins in patients with chronic kidney disease: Meta-analysis and meta-regression of randomised controlled trials. *Br Med J* 2008;336:645–651.

Suissa S, Hutchinson T, Brophy JM, et al. ACE-inhibitor use and the long-term risk of renal failure in diabetes. *Kidney Int* 2006;69:913–919.

Suzuki H, Kanno Y, Sugahara S, et al. Effect of angiotensin receptor blockers on cardiovascular events in patients undergoing hemodialysis: An open-label randomized controlled trial. *Am J Kidney Dis* 2008;52:501–506.

Svarstad E, Ureheim L, Iversen BM. Critical renal artery stenoses may cause spectrum of cardiorenal failure and associated thromboembolic events. *Clin Nephrol* 2005;63:487–492.

Task Force. The Task Force for the Management of Arterial Hypertension of the European Society of Hypertension (ESH) and of the European Society of Cardiology (ESC). *J Hypertens* 2007;25:1105–1187.

Tolins JP, Raij L. Antihypertensive therapy and the progression of chronic renal disease. Are there renoprotective drugs? *Semin Nephrol* 1991;11:538–548.

Toto RD. Improving outcomes in hemodialysis patients: The need for well-designed clinical trials. *Am J Kidney Dis* 2008;52:400–402.

Toto RD, Mitchell HC, Smith RD, et al. "Strict" blood pressure control and progression of renal disease in hypertensive nephrosclerosis. *Kidney Int* 1995;48:851–859.

Tsioufis C, Thomopoulos C, Dimitriadis K, et al. Association of obstructive sleep apnea with urinary albumin excretion in essential hypertension: A cross-sectional study. *Am J Kidney Dis* 2008;52:285–293.

Tsukamoto Y. End-stage renal disease (ESRD) and its treatment in Japan. *Nephrol Dial Transplant* 2008;23:2447–2450.

U.S. Renal data systems. Chronic kidney disease. *USRDS 2007*, Bethesda NIH, NIDDKD 2008.

Uzu T, Harada T, Namba T, et al. Thiazide diuretics enhance nocturnal blood pressure fall and reduce proteinuria in immunoglobulin A nephropathy treated with angiotensin II modulators. *J Hypertens* 2005;23:861–865.

Vassalotti JA, Stevens LA, Levey AS. Testing for chronic kidney disease: A position statement from the National Kidney Foundation. *Am J Kidney Dis* 2007;50:169–180.

Vidt DG. Cholesterol emboli: A common cause of renal failure. *Annu Rev Med* 1997;48:375–385.

Vogt L, Waanders F, Boomsma F, et al. Effects of dietary sodium and hydrochlorothiazide on the antiproteinuric efficacy of losartan. *J Am Soc Nephrol* 2008;19:999–1007.

Waikar SS, Liu KD, Chertow GM. Diagnosis, epidemiology and outcomes of acute kidney injury. *Clin J Am Soc Nephrol* 2008;3:844–861.

Walser M, Mitch WE, Maroni BJ, et al. Should protein intake be restricted in predialysis patients? *Kidney Int* 1999;55:771–777.

Wang Y, Chen X, Song Y, et al. Association between obesity and kidney disease: A systematic review and meta-analysis. *Kidney Int* 2008;73:19–33.

Watts RA, Hoffbrand BI. Hypertension following renal trauma. *J Hum Hypertens* 1987;1:65–71.

Wechsler E, Yang T, Jordan SC, et al. Anti-glomerular basement membrane disease in an HIV-infected patient. *Nat Clin Pract Nephrol* 2008;4:167–171.

Weiner DE, Tighiouart H, Levey AS, et al. Lowest systolic blood pressure is associated with stroke in stages 3 to 4 chronic kidney disease. *J Am Soc Nephrol* 2007;18:960–966.

Weisbord SD, Mor MK, Resnick AL, et al. Prevention, incidence, and outcomes of contrast-induced acute kidney injury. *Arch Intern Med* 2008;168:1325–1332.

Wen CP, Cheng TY, Tsai MK, et al. All-cause mortality attributable to chronic kidney disease: A prospective cohort study based on 462 293 adults in Taiwan. *Lancet* 2008;371:2173–2182.

Wesson DE. Is the ethnic disparity in CKD a symptom of dysfunctional primary care in the US? *J Am Soc Nephrol* 2008;19:1249–1251.

Whaley-Connell AT, Sowers JR, Stevens LA, et al. CKD in the United States: Kidney Early Evaluation Program (KEEP) and National Health and Nutrition Examination Survey (NHANES) 1999–2004. *Am J Kidney Dis* 2008;51:S13–S20.

Wright JT Jr., Bakris G, Greene T, et al. Effect of blood pressure lowering and antihypertensive drug class on progression of hypertensive kidney disease: Results of the AASK trial. *JAMA* 2002;288:2421–2431.

Writing Team for the Diabetes Control and Complications Trial/ Epidemiology of Diabetes Interventions and Complications Research Group. Sustained effect of intensive treatment of type 1 diabetes mellitus on development and progression of diabetic nephropathy: The Epidemiology of Diabetes Interventions and Complications (EDIC) study. *JAMA* 2003;290:2159–2167.

Xie D, Joffe MM, Brunelli SM, et al. A comparison of change in measured and estimated glomerular filtration rate in patients with nondiabetic kidney disease. *Clin J Am Soc Nephrol* 2008;3:1332–1338.

Young CJ, Gaston RS. Renal transplantation in black Americans. *N Engl J Med* 2000;343:1545–1552.

Zappitelli M, Parikh CR, kcan-Arikan A, et al. Ascertainment and epidemiology of acute kidney injury varies with definition interpretation. *Clin J Am Soc Nephrol* 2008;3:948–954.

Zhou J, Chen X, Xie Y, et al. A differential diagnostic model of diabetic nephropathy and non-diabetic renal diseases. *Nephrol Dial Transplant* 2008;23:1940–1945.

Zhou XJ, Rakheja D, Yu X, et al. The aging kidney. *Kidney Int* 2008;74:710–720.

Renovascular Hypertension

O f all of the fairly common identifiable causes of hypertension, renovascular hypertension (RVHT) remains the most puzzling: Although its pathophysiology seems clear, uncertainty remains as to its prevalence, natural history, diagnosis, and treatment (Levin et al., 2007).

These uncertainties reflect a confluence of factors:

• Structural renovascular disease (RVD) is becoming more prevalent as the population becomes older, hypertensive, and atherosclerotic (Kuczera et al., 2009).

• The presence of structural renovascular disease is being more frequently recognized, particularly by "drive by" renal arteriography done in patients having coronary angiography (de Mast and Buetler, 2009).

• Revascularization by percutaneous angioplasty/ stenting of structural renovascular disease that has not been documented to be the cause of functional RVHT, though technically easy and financially rewarding, has not been found to be helpful in most patients (Bax et al., 2009).

• With increasing scrutiny, tests to document functional RVHT (such as renal vein sampling) have been found to have poor predictability (Aparico et al., 2009).

• Data are currently not available to prove the superiority of medical therapy, balloon angioplasty and/ or stenting, or surgical repair of those with functional RVHT (Leeser et al., 2009).

The dilemma is obvious: more patients have structural renovascular disease that can induce hypertension and renal ischemia but uncertainty remains as to how to diagnose and treat them (Textor, 2008).

In this chapter, a more conservative approach is recommended than the increasingly common practice of immediate angioplasty/stenting whenever a "significant" renal artery stenosis is identified, a practice being performed, even in patients with easily controlled hypertension and normal renal function. This has led

to more than a twofold increase in renal artery stenting from 1996 to 2000 as a consequence of the 3.9-fold increase in the procedure by cardiologists (Murphy et al., 2007). Long-term cost-benefit advantages may follow such "prophylactic" revascularization (van Helvoort-Postulart et al., 2007) but, in view of complications seen even under the best of circumstances and the absence of evidence that it improves outcomes (Hackam et al., 2008), caution seems advisable.

On the other hand, patients with refractory hypertension and/or worsening renal function should be evaluated for RVHT and appropriately treated. In such patients, it is important to consider this disease because, if identified, it can be relieved; if left untreated, it may destroy the kidneys. The presence of bilateral renal artery stenosis should be considered in all patients with unexplained progressive renal insufficiency leading to dialysis, because ischemic nephropathy may be involved in as many as 11% of such patients (Guo et al., 2007). Even in patients with end-stage renal disease (ESRD), relief of renal artery stenosis may prevent, delay, or overcome, the need for dialysis (Thatipelli et al., 2008).

RENOVASCULAR DISEASE VERSUS RENOVASCULAR HYPERTENSION

RVHT refers to hypertension caused by renal ischemia. It is important to realize that renovascular *disease* (RVD) may or may not cause sufficient hypoperfusion to set off the processes that lead to hypertension. The problem is simply that renovascular disease is much more common than is RVHT. For example, arteriography revealed some degree of renal artery stenosis in 32% of 303 normotensive patients and in 67% of 193 hypertensives with an increasing prevalence with advancing age (Eyler et al., 1962) (Table 10-1). Note that in Table 10-1,

TABLE 10.1	Prevalence of Renal Arterial Lesions in Normotensive and Hypertensive Patients			
Age	Normotensive		Hypertensive	
Years	Normal	Lesion	Normal	Lesion
31–40	7	3	6	10
41–50	26	8	14	22
51–60	99	35	28	50
60+	69	56	15	48

Data from Eyler WR, Clark MD, Garman JE, et al. Angiography of the renal areas including a comparative study of renal arterial stenosis in patients with and without hypertension. *Radiology* 1962;78:879–892.

almost half of *normotensive* patients older than 60 had atherosclerotic lesions in their renal vessels.

More recent studies show similar data. Among patients having coronary angiograms whose average blood pressure (BP) was 143/80 and serum creatinine was 1.1 mL/dL, 47% had renovascular disease by renal angiography (Rihal et al., 2002).

Before procedures were available to prove the functional significance of stenotic lesions, surgery was frequently performed on hypertensive patients with a unilateral small kidney who did not have reversible RVHT. Smith (1956) recognized this as early as 1948 as a misguided application of Goldblatt's experimental model of hypertension induced by clamping the renal artery. Smith reported that only 25% of patients were relieved of their hypertension by nephrectomy and warned that only about 2% of all hypertensives probably could be helped by surgery.

PREVALENCE OF RENOVASCULAR HYPERTENSION

Smith's (1956) estimate of the true prevalence of RVHT may be right. The prevalence varies with the nature of the hypertensive population:

• In nonreferred hypertensive patient populations, the prevalence is likely less than 1% (Kalra et al., 2005).
• In patients with suggestive clinical features, the prevalence is higher, 7.3% of 837 patients with suggestive clinical features had at least a 70% stenosis of one or both renal arteries by renal angiography (Buller et al., 2004). Since most RVHT is atherosclerotic in origin,

the prevalence, not surprisingly, increases with age (Guo et al., 2007).

• Among patients with accelerated-malignant hypertension, the prevalence is even higher: of 123 adults with diastolic BP greater than 125 mm Hg and grade III or IV retinopathy, 4% of blacks and 32% of whites had RVHT (Davis et al., 1979).
• High-grade renal artery stenosis also is seen more frequently in hypertensive patients with atherosclerotic disease in peripheral (Leertouwer et al., 2001), carotid, or coronary arteries (Buller et al., 2004); in elderly patients with heart failure (Missouris et al., 2000); and in patients with severe hypertension and rapidly progressing renal insufficiency, particularly if it develops after institution of angiotensin-converting enzyme inhibitor (ACEI), angiotensin II receptor blocker (ARB), or direct renin inhibitor (DRI) therapy (Krijnen et al., 2004).
• On the other hand, RVHT is less common in blacks; in one series, it was found in 12% of blacks versus 28% of whites (Hansen et al., 1998).
• Diabetics, even though they have a higher prevalence of renal artery disease (Freedman et al., 2004), have less RVHT (Valabhji et al., 2000).
• RVHT has been recognized in neonates (Tapper et al., 1987), children (Tullus et al., 2008), and pregnant women (Thorsteinsdottir et al., 2006).

MECHANISMS OF HYPERTENSION

Animal Models

The pathophysiology of RVHT was first identified by Goldblatt et al. (1934) who, looking not for RVHT, but for a renal cause for primary hypertension, put clamps on both renal arteries of dogs. The clamps were inserted on separate occasions so that they could observe the effect of unilateral obstruction (Fig. 10-1). However, with the modest degree of constriction that they used, unilateral clamping caused only transient hypertension. For permanent hypertension, both renal arteries had to be clamped, or one clamped and the contralateral kidney removed (Goldblatt, 1975).

After significant renal ischemia and the initial marked rise in renin secretion, renin levels fall but remain inappropriately high and are largely responsible for the hemodynamic changes (Welch, 2000). Figure 10-2 shows a stepwise scheme for the hemodynamic and hormonal changes that underlie RVHT.

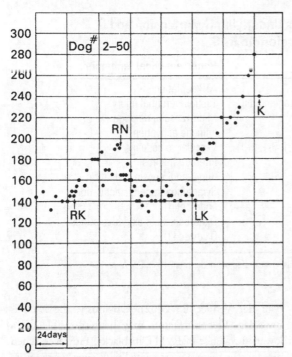

FIGURE 10-1 Results from one of Goldblatt's original experiments. The graph shows the mean BP of a dog whose right kidney was first moderately constricted (RK), with subsequent hypertension that was relieved after right nephrectomy (RN). After severe constriction of the left renal artery (LK), more severe hypertension occurred, and the animal was sacrificed (K). (Reprinted from Hoobler SW. History of experimental renovascular hypertension. In: Stanley JC, Ernst CB, Fry WJ, eds. *Renovascular Hypertension*. Philadelphia, PA: Saunders, 1984:12–19, with permission.)

Other factors may be involved that interrelate to these primary mechanisms, including those listed by Textor (2008) (Table 10-2):

Studies in Humans

As in the animal models, RVHT in humans is caused by increased renin release from the ischemic kidney (Welch, 2000). Simon (2000) suggests that the stenosis must obstruct at least 80% of the arterial lumen to set off the process. The resultant high level of angiotensin II increases renal vascular resistance, causing a shift in the pressure-natriuresis curve; thus, fluid volume is maintained despite markedly elevated BP (Granger & Schnackenberg, 2000). Chronically, the ischemic kidney continues to secrete excess renin and BP falls when angiotensin inhibitors are given. When the stenosis is relieved, hypertension recedes by a fall in peripheral resistance and fluid volume (Valvo et al., 1987).

As in animal models, humans may enter into a third phase, wherein removal of the stenosis or the entire affected kidney will not relieve the hypertension because of widespread arteriolar damage and glomerulosclerosis, i.e., ischemic nephropathy (Garovic & Textor, 2005). This phenomenon is clinically relevant: The sooner an arterial lesion that is causing RVHT is removed, the greater the chance of relieving the hypertension. Among 110 patients, corrective surgery for unilateral RVHT was successful in 78% of those with hypertension of less than 5 years' duration but in only 25% of those with hypertension of longer duration (Hughes et al., 1981).

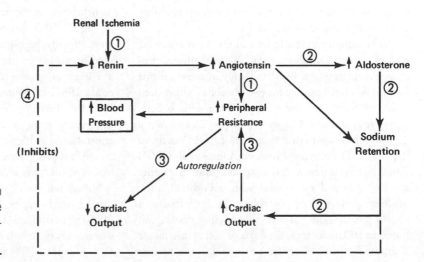

FIGURE 10-2 Hypertension with renovascular disease. Stepwise hemodynamic changes in the development of RVHT.

TABLE 10.2	Interactive Mechanisms Underlying Hypertension and Kidney Injury in Atherosclerotic RAS	
Tissue Underperfusion	**Recurrent Local Ischemia**
Activation of renin-angiotensin system	ATP depletion
Altered endothelial function (endothelin, NO, prostaglandins)	Tubulointerstitial injury
Sympathoadrenergic activation	Microvascular damage
Increased reactive oxygen species	Immune activation
Cytokine release/inflammation (NF-κB, TNF, TGF-β, PAI-1, IL-1)	Vascular remodeling
Impaired tubular transport functions	Interstitial fibrosis
Apoptosis/necrosis	Renin-angiotensin activation
	Sympathoadrenergic activation
	Endothelin
	Disturbances of oxidative stress
	Oxidized LDL

Modified from Textor SC. Atherosclerotic renal artery stenosis: Overtreated but underrated? *J Am Soc Nephrol* 2008;19:656–659.

CLASSIFICATION AND COURSE

The most common cause of RVHT is atherosclerotic stenosis of the main renal artery; most of the remaining cases are fibroplastic, but a number of both intrinsic and extrinsic lesions can induce RVHT (Table 10-3). The general features of the most common types of renal artery stenosis are listed in Table 10-4.

Atherosclerotic Lesions

As compared to patients with primary hypertension, patients with atherosclerotic RVHT are older and have higher systolic pressure, more extensive renal damage, and vascular disease elsewhere (Buller et al., 2004); more extensive left ventricular hypertrophy; ischemic heart disease; renal insufficiency (Zoccali et al., 2002), and, not surprisingly, lower probability of survival (Conlon et al., 2000).

The atherosclerotic lesions in the renal artery are part of systemic atherosclerosis. Why the process progresses enough to set off RVHT only in some patients is unknown but evidence for two possibilities have been provided: infectious and genetic. The genetic associations are uncertain: Olivieri et al. (2002) reported a 2.25-fold increased odds ratio with the DD variant of the ACE I/D polymorphism; van Onna et al. (2004) found no association with the polymorphism but rather a 44% increased odds ratio with endothelial nitric oxide synthase gene polymorphism. As for infection, a sixfold greater odds ratio of renovascular disease was found in 100 patients clinically suspected of this disease if antibodies to Chlamydia pneumonia were present

(van der Ven et al., 2002). Obviously, the issue is unsettled. Genetic factors may be responsible for a lower prevalence of RVHT in blacks. However, when present, the disease is associated with even more severe hypertension and extrarenal vascular disease than are seen in nonblacks with RVHT (Novick et al., 1994).

Natural History

As noted by Levin et al. (2007): "Large cohort studies systematically evaluating specific populations to characterize the natural history of renal artery stenosis have not been done."

The natural history of atherosclerotic renal artery stenosis has been examined by repeated renal artery duplex scans in a total of 295 kidneys in 170 patients over a mean of 33 months (Caps et al., 1998a). These patients had been referred because of progressive renal insufficiency in the presence of hypertension. As seen in Figure 10-3, progression was common in those with initially high-grade (≥60%) stenosis accompanied by a 21% incidence of renal atrophy, defined as a 1.0 cm or greater decrease in renal length (Caps et al., 1998b). Progression was associated with a systolic BP above 160 mm Hg, diabetes mellitus, and high-grade stenosis in either the ipsilateral or the contralateral kidney.

A less progressive loss of renal function has been observed in two studies of patients with at least a 50% renal artery stenosis, recognized incidentally during angiography for coronary (Conlon et al., 2000) or peripheral (Leertouwer et al., 2001) vascular disease. Even though the degree of renal artery stenosis was at least 70% in a significant portion of these

TABLE 10.3	Types of Lesions Associated with RVHT

Intrinsic lesions
  Atherosclerosis
  Fibromuscular dysplasia
    Intimal
    Medial
      Dissection (Edwards et al., 1982)
      Segmental infarction (Salifu et al., 2000)
    Adventitial
  Aneurysm (English et al., 2004)
  Emboli (Scolari et al., 2007)
  Arteritis
    Large artery vasculitis (Slovut & Olin, 2004)
    Takayasu's (Cakar et al., 2008)
  Arteriovenous malformation or fistula (Lekuona et al., 2001)
  Renal artery (Kolhe et al., 2004) or aortic dissection (Rackson et al., 1990)
  Angioma (Farreras-Valenti et al., 1965)
  Neurofibromatosis[a] (Watano et al., 1996)
  Tumor thrombus (Jennings et al., 1964)
  Thrombosis with the antiphospholipid syndrome (Riccialdelli et al., 2001)
  Thrombosis after antihypertensive therapy (Dussol et al., 1994)
  Rejection of renal transplant (Kasiske et al., 2004)
  Injury to the renal artery
    Stenosis after transplantation (Tedla et al., 2007)
    Trauma (Myrianthefs et al., 2007)
    Radiation (Shapiro et al., 1977)
    Lithotripsy (Smith et al., 1991)
  Intrarenal cysts (Torres et al., 1991)
  Congenital unilateral renal hypoplasia[a] (Ask-Upmark kidney) (Steffens et al., 1991)
  Unilateral renal infection (Siamopoulos et al., 1983)
Extrinsic lesions
  Pheochromocytoma or paraganglioma (Nakano et al., 1996)
  Congenital fibrous band[a] (Silver & Clements, 1976)
  Pressure from diaphragmatic crus[a] (Deglise et al., 2007)
  Tumors (Restrick et al., 1992)
  Subcapsular or perirenal hematoma (Nomura et al., 1996)
  Retroperitoneal fibrosis (Castle, 1973)
  Perirenal pseudocyst (Kato et al., 1985)
  Stenosis of celiac axis with steal of renal blood flow (Alfidi et al., 1972)

[a]More common in children.

patients, end- stage renal failure developed in only 1 of the 188 with coronary disease over 4 years and in none of the 126 with peripheral vascular disease over 10 years (Leertouwer et al., 2001). All three of the studies examined patients with known renal vascular disease. Perhaps a better reflection of the natural history of RVHT comes from an 8-year follow-up of 119 "free living" subjects who had renal duplex sonography at an average age of 82 years (Pearce et al., 2006). Renal artery stenoses were identified in 6.8% initially. After 8 years, none of these had progressed to occlusion. In the entire group, renal artery stenoses were now seen in 14%, with 4% of the lesions considered significant. The average BP of the group had changed from 136/80 to 145/72 mm Hg, serum creatinine from 1.0 to 1.3 mg/dL, and renal size decreased by a mean of 0.4 cm.

These prospective studies give additional meaning to Textor's statement in 2008 that "The published literature cannot support the observed, massive expansion of endovascular intervention." At the least, a clear distinction should be made between the likelihood of progression of renal artery disease identified in patients with clinically suggestive features of RVHT and evidence of renal ischemia, on the one hand, and patients with no clinical or functional evidence of RVHT, on the other. Even in the presence of high-grade bilateral disease, the progress of renal damage can be slowed without revascularization if the hypertension is intensively treated: 85% of 68 such patients treated medically had stable renal function through 3 years of follow-up (Chábová et al., 2000).

Since atherosclerotic RVD is a local manifestation of a systemic disease, the relatively slow rate of progression of the renal lesion is countered by the more common cause of death by cardiovascular disease (Kalra et al., 2005).

Fibromuscular Dysplasia

Figure 10-4 shows the two most common types of fibromuscular stenoses (Lüscher et al., 1987). Of these, fibromuscular dysplasia is the most common, whereas focal fibroplastic lesions are more common in children (Tullus et al., 2008).

Medial fibromuscular dysplasia is usually noted in young women but has been found in older patients, often incidentally (Plouin et al., 2007). The process often involves multiple other arteries, most frequently the carotid and vertebral vessels. Intracranial aneurysms are not infrequent but most cerebrovascular

TABLE 10.4	Features of the Two Major Forms of Renal Artery Stenosis

Renal Artery Disease History	Incidence, %	Age, years	Location of Lesion in Renal Artery	Natural History
Atherosclerosis	90	>50	Ostia and proximal 2 cm	Progression is common, sometimes to occlusion
Fibromuscular dysplasias Intimal	1–2	Children, young adults	Middle main renal artery	Progression in most
Medial	10	15–50	Distal main renal artery and branches	Progression in 33%
Adventitial	<1	15–30	Mid to distal main renal artery	Progression in most

involvement is asymptomatic (Slovut & Olin, 2004). With high-resolution echograms, Boutouyrie et al. (2003) found abnormal patterns of the carotid artery and thickness of the radial artery in most of 70 patients with renal fibromuscular dysplasia.

The cause of fibromuscular dysplasia remains unknown, though cigarette smoking and hypertension are associated with an increased risk, as in the presence of the disease in first-degree relatives (Slovut & Olin, 2004). Other vascular diseases, in particular large-artery

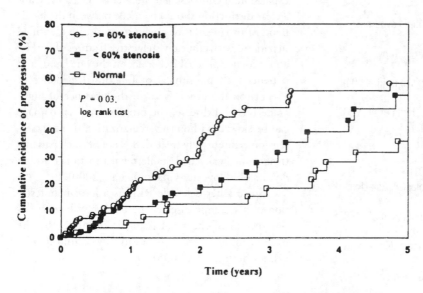

FIGURE 10-3 Cumulative incidence of renal disease progression stratified according to baseline degree of renal artery narrowing. Standard errors were less than 10% for all plots through 5 years. (Reprinted from Caps MT, Perissinotto C, Zierler E, et al. Prospective study of atherosclerotic disease progression in the renal artery. *Circulation* 1998a;98:2866–2872, with permission.)

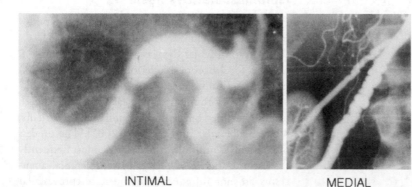

INTIMAL   MEDIAL

FIGURE 10-4 Representative radiographs of the two major types of fibromuscular dysplasia. (Reprinted from Lüscher TF, Lie JT, Stanson AW, et al. Arterial fibromuscular dysplasia. *Mayo Clin Proc* 1987;62:931–952, with permission.)

vasculitis, may require angiography to be distinguished from fibromuscular dysplasia (Plouin et al., 2007).

Patients with the less common but more sharply localized fibroplastic lesions intimal and adventitial—usually show rapid progression, so severe stenosis and hypertension are frequently observed (Sperati et al., 2009).

Other Causes

Of the myriad causes of RVHT listed in Table 10-2, a few deserve additional comment.

Aneurysm

Aneurysms are common with medial fibroplasia. Saccular aneurysms, usually at the bifurcation of the renal artery, may induce hypertension by various mechanisms. They rarely rupture and need not be ablated if less than 2.0 cm in diameter in the absence of symptoms or severe hypertension (English et al., 2004).

Emboli

Most commonly seen as a complication of angiography or vascular surgery, renal cholesterol emboli can induce renal failure or RVHT (Scolari et al., 2007). Cutaneous, ocular, and other visceral lesions are usually seen, and the diagnosis may be documented by biopsy of skin lesions.

Arteritis

Progressive aortic arteritis (Takayasu arteritis or pulseless disease) is seen infrequently in North America and Europe but is a common cause of RVHT in China, India, Japan, Mexico, and Brazil (Weaver et al., 2004). It is seen mainly in children and young adults and is often associated with signs of chronic inflammation (Cakar et al., 2008).

RVHT is common in various vasculitic syndromes with renal involvement, including Wegener granulomatosis (Woodrow et al., 1990), systemic lupus erythematosus (Ward & Studenski, 1992), and the antiphospholipid syndrome (Riccialdelli et al., 2001). These patients may enter into an acute, severe hypertensive phase, usually associated with markedly elevated plasma renin levels, likely reflecting intrarenal stenosis from multiple arteriolar lesions. The hypertension can sometimes be rather remarkably reversed by ACEI therapy (Coruzzi & Novarini, 1992).

Aortic Dissection

RVHT was found in nearly 20% of patients with aortic dissection (Rackson et al., 1990).

CLINICAL FEATURES

General

Clinical features suggestive of renovascular disease as the cause of hypertension are presented in Table 10-5 (White et al., 2006). Some of these features were identified in a cooperative study involving 2,442 hypertensive patients, 880 with renovascular disease (Maxwell et al., 1972). Of the 880, 502 had surgery; of these, 60% had atherosclerotic lesions, and 35% had fibromuscular disease. The clinical characteristics of 131 patients with surgically cured renovascular disease were compared to those in a carefully matched group with essential hypertension (Simon et al., 1972). Of the clinical features more common in patients with RVHT, only an abdominal bruit was of clear discriminatory value, heard in 46% of those with RVHT but in only 9% of those with essential hypertension. The bruit was heard over the flank in 12% of those with RVHT and in only 1% of those with essential hypertension. As nicely reviewed by Turnbull (1995), most systolic bruits are innocent, but systolic-diastolic bruits in hypertensives are suggestive of RVHT.

TABLE 10.5	Clinical Clues for RVHT

History
  Onset of hypertension before age 30 in women with no
    family history (fibromuscular dysplasia)
  Abrupt onset or worsening of hypertension
  Severe or resistant hypertension
  Symptoms of atherosclerotic disease elsewhere
  Smoker
  Worsening renal function with ACE inhibition or AII
    receptor blockade
  Recurrent flash pulmonary edema
Examination
  Abdominal bruits
  Other bruits
  Advanced hypertensive retinopathy
Laboratory
  Secondary aldosteronism
    Higher plasma renin
    Low serum potassium
    Low serum sodium
  Proteinuria, usually moderate
  Elevated serum creatinine
  >1.5 cm difference in kidney size on sonography
  Cortical atrophy on CT angiography

Additional Features
Hyperaldosteronism

Patients with RVHT occasionally have profound secondary aldosteronism with hypokalemia due to urinary potassium wasting but low serum sodium unlike the high serum sodium seen in primary aldosteronism. (Agarwal et al., 1999)—all reversed with relief of RVHT.

Nephrotic Syndrome

Proteinuria is common, and a few patients with RVHT have nephrotic-range proteinuria, usually with more severe renal damage and, often, renal artery thrombosis (Halimi et al., 2000).

Polycythemia

Polycythemia has been seen occasionally in patients with RVHT but elevated peripheral and renal venous erythropoietin levels without polycythemia are much more common (Grützmacher et al., 1989).

Dyslipidemia

Not surprisingly, those with atherosclerotic RVHT may have dyslipidemia, in particular low apolipoprotein A_1 levels (Scoble et al., 1999). Correction of dyslipidemia may reverse RVHT (Khong et al., 2001), and statin therapy may improve the outcome (Silva et al., 2008).

Cortical Atrophy

Cortical atrophy demonstrable by computed tomography (CT) angiography may be an even earlier morphological marker of ischemic damage than overall renal length (Mounier-Vehier et al., 2002).

Ischemic Nephropathy

Beyond hypertension, the second most common clinical presentation of renal artery stenosis is ischemic nephropathy, which is estimated to be the cause of ESRD in at least 5% of patients entering chronic dialysis (Levin et al., 2007). The usual definition of ischemic nephropathy is "impairment of renal function beyond occlusive disease of the main renal arteries" (Garovic & Textor, 2005). However, as these authors note:

> deterioration of renal function does not necessarily reflect true "ischemia." Because a major function of the kidney is filtration, blood flow to the kidney provides a vast oversupply of oxygenated blood per se. Less than 10% of the blood flow is needed for metabolic requirements of the

> kidney.... To materially affect renal function on a vascular basis alone, the entire renal mass must be affected. Thus, a reduction in glomerular filtration rate (GFR) for patients with unilateral renovascular disease implies some other parenchymal disease in the contralateral kidney and rarely improves after renal revascularization.

Assuming this scenario is correct, the use of the two therapies directed toward relief of the occlusive disease need reconsideration. First, the use of antihypertensive drugs reduces perfusion pressure to the kidney, activating pressor mechanisms to restore perfusion, including some, or all, of those listed in Table 10-2. As Garovic and Textor state:

> In clinical settings, antihypertensive therapy is directed at lowering systemic pressures to achieve proven benefits in reducing cardiovascular morbidity. The price of lowering pressure for patients with renovascular disease may be underperfusion of the poststenotic kidney(s). This can develop during therapy with any antihypertensive agent and can produce a loss of GFR when perfusion pressures fall below those needed for autoregulation. Revascularization of the kidney can remove the pressure dependence of GFR in such patients.

This leads to the second reconsideration of therapy, that directed at mechanical relief of the stenosis by angioplasty and stents. As observed by Levin et al. (2007):

> One could hypothesize that less severe lesions allow transmission of high pressures to compromised renal vasculature, thereby exacerbating the sclerotic process by activating local tissue factors associated with endothelial shear stress. If so, then aggressive treatment of less severe lesions may be important to prevent progressive parenchymal injury.... Prevailing opinion holds that intervention in lesions <70% is not helpful. However, if relatively less severe lesions affected downstream events, it would seem reasonable to intervene earlier in the course of RAS.

Patients with ischemic nephropathy may be difficult to distinguish from the larger number with primary hypertension or primary renal parenchymal disease which progresses into renal failure. The possibility of bilateral renovascular disease should be considered in the following groups (Chonchol & Linas, 2006):

- Young women with severe hypertension, in whom fibroplastic disease is common.
- Older patients with extensive atherosclerotic disease who suddenly have a worsening of renal function.
- Azotemic hypertensives who develop multiple episodes of acute pulmonary edema.

- Any hypertensive who develops rapidly progressive renal failure without evidence of obstructive uropathy.
- Patients in whom renal function quickly deteriorates after treatment with an ACEI, ARB, or DRI.

Such patients, if they are candidates for intervention, should have an appropriate workup to determine the presence of occlusive disease, but no controlled trials in such patients have been performed to determine the best strategy. However, among 59 patients who had angioplasty, better improvement in renal function was seen in those whose serum creatinine levels had rapidly increased before the procedure (Muray et al., 2002).

Variants

Hypertension After Renal Transplantation

As described in Chapter 9, patients who develop severe hypertension after renal transplantation should be evaluated for stenosis of the renal artery. Posttransplant stenoses have been reported in from 1% to 23% of all renal allografts (Bruno et al., 2004).

Hypertension and the Hypoplastic Kidney

As described in Chapter 9, those patients with a small kidney but without a stenotic lesion who respond to nephrectomy usually have increased levels of plasma renin activity (PRA) from the venous blood draining the diseased kidney, suggesting a renovascular etiology (Mizuiri et al., 1992). Similarly, in patients with a small kidney and totally occluded renal artery, the presence of increased levels of renin from the occluded kidney is highly predictive of relief of hypertension by nephrectomy (Rossi et al., 2002).

DIAGNOSTIC TESTS

Before any tests are performed for the diagnosis of RVHT, the clinician should consider whether, if renovascular disease is present, revascularization would be indicated to provide likely benefit despite the possible complications (Textor, 2003). As listed on the right side of Table 10-6, for those patients with stable renal function and longstanding, stable hypertension that is responsive to easily tolerated antihypertensive drugs, revascularization would likely provide no benefit; therefore, no tests should be performed in them. On the other hand, in those with one or more factors that make a favorable response to revascularization more likely, listed on the left side of Table 10-6, testing should be performed to define the extent of renovascular disease and its functional significance. In those with a high likelihood of RVHT, catheter-directed angiography and, if significant stenosis are seen, immediate revascularization are appropriate.

| TABLE 10.6 | Factors Indicative of Response to Revascularization for Atherosclerotic RVHT |

Favorable	Nonfavorable
BP response likely	BP response less likely
Treatment-resistant hypertension	Longstanding stable hypertension
Recent onset/progression of hypertension	Acceptable BPs/tolerable medication regimen
Hypertension aggravating acute coronary syndromes	
Impaired cardiac function/"flash" pulmonary edema	
Renal functional response likely	Renal function less likely to benefit
Entire renal mass affected: solitary functioning kidney/ bilateral RAS	Unilateral RAS with normal contralateral circulation
Recent fall in GFR	Bilateral parenchymal disease (elevated resistance index in contralateral kidney)
Viable kidneys: blood flow preserved on nephrogram/ favorable resistance index by Doppler ultrasound	Stable kidney function
Acute renal failure during antihypertensive therapy, especially with angiotensin-converting enzyme inhibitors/angiotensin receptor blockers	
Patient considered viable with reasonable life expectancy	Patient with limited viability
	Severe comorbid disease likely to limit life expectancy

Clinical Prediction Rule

Beyond the listing in Table 10-6, more formal protocols have been proposed to grade the clinical features into degrees of likelihood to guide the decision for additional workup for RVHT. Mann and Pickering (1992) provided an Index of Clinical Suspicion, dividing patients into *low* (who should *not* be further tested), *moderate* (who should have noninvasive testing), or *high* (who may be considered for proceeding directly to renal arteriography (Table 10-7).

Krijnen et al. (1998) performed logistic regression analysis of data from 477 hypertensive patients who underwent renal angiography because of suspicion of RVHT on the basis of drug-resistant hypertension or increases in serum creatinine after ACE inhibition. Their scoring model included age, gender, presence of atherosclerotic vascular disease, recent onset of hypertension, body mass index, presence of abdominal bruit, serum creatinine and cholesterol levels, and smoking. The probability of renal artery stenosis sharply increased as total score rose above 10, reaching almost 100% with sum scores of 25. In these patients, the diagnostic accuracy of their model was similar to that of renal scintigraphy.

Although the predictive power of these clinical indices has not been validated by the results of revascularization, their application would sharply reduce the number of workups that might otherwise be performed in patients with little likelihood of having RVHT. Only those patients with clinical features indicating the presence of RVHT that would likely respond favorably to revascularization would undergo diagnostic testing. The algorithm shown in Figure 10-5 starts with noninvasive tests that can confirm the clinical likelihood of the presence of RVHT that would likely respond favorably to revascularization and then proceeds to an imaging study.

As noted in Table 10-7, those patients with a high index of clinical suspicion, in whom it is essential to identify RVHT if it is present, should start with catheter-directed contrast angiography and, if a significant stenosis is found, have immediate angioplasty/stenting.

Tests to Predict the Response to Revascularization

Renin Measurements

According to the pathophysiology described earlier, RVHT should be associated with hypersecretion of renin from a kidney that is significantly hypoperfused.

TABLE 10.7 **Testing for RVHT: Clinical Index of Suspicion as a Guide to Selecting Patients for Workup**

Index of Clinical Suspicion

Low (should not be tested)
  Borderline, mild to moderate hypertension, in the absence of clinical clues
Moderate (noninvasive tests recommended)
  Severe hypertension (DBP > 120 mm Hg)
  Hypertension refractory to standard therapy excluding ACEIs and AII-blockers
  Abrupt onset of sustained, moderate to severe hypertension at age <20 or >50
  Hypertension with a suggestive abdominal or flank bruit
  Moderate hypertension (DBP > 105 mm Hg) in a smoker, a patient with evidence of occlusive vascular disease (cerebro-vascular, coronary, peripheral vascular), or a patient with unexplained but stable elevation of serum creatinine
  Normalization of BP by an ACEI in a patient with moderate to severe hypertension (particularly a smoker or a patient with recent onset of hypertension)
High (may consider proceeding directly to arteriography)
  Severe hypertension (DBP > 120 mm Hg) with either progressive renal insufficiency or refractoriness to aggressive treatment, particularly in a patient who has been a smoker or has other evidence of occlusive arterial disease
  Accelerated or malignant hypertension (grade III or IV retinopathy)
  Hypertension with recent elevation of serum creatinine, either unexplained or reversibly induced by an ACEI, AII receptor blocker, or direct renin inhibitor
  Moderate to severe hypertension with incidentally detected asymmetry of renal size

---

Modified from Mann SJ, Pickering TG. Detection of renovascular hypertension. State of the art: 1992. *Ann Intern Med* 1992;117:845–853.

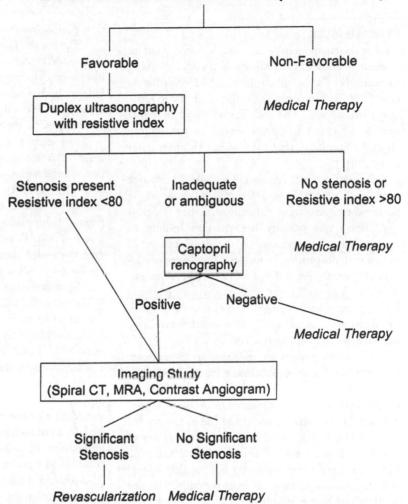

FACTORS INDICATIVE OF RESPONSE TO REVASCULARIZATION (Table 10.6)

FIGURE 10-5 An algorithm for evaluation and therapy of RVHT based on the presence of factors indicative of a response to revascularization (shown in Table 10-6).

Peripheral Blood

Although increased levels of PRA are found in some patients with RVHT, they are not elevated in many (Rudnick & Maxwell, 1984), in keeping with the experimental evidence that secretion of renin from the clipped kidney falls to "normal" soon after RVHT is induced, whereas renin release from the contralateral kidney is suppressed.

Various maneuvers have been used to augment renin release in the hope that patients with curable disease would show a hyperresponsiveness, thereby improving the discriminatory value of PRA levels (Wilcox, 2000). The most widely used maneuver, response of PRA to captopril, has been found to

have limited value as a screening study (Vasbinder et al., 2001).

Comparison of Renal Vein Renins

The comparison of renin levels in blood from each renal vein, obtained by percutaneous catheterization, has been used to establish both the diagnosis and reversibility of RVHT with a ratio greater than 1.5:1.0 between the two renal veins considered abnormal or lateralizing. In initial reports, an abnormal ratio was 92% predictive of curability; however, 65% of those whose renal vein PRA level ratio did not lateralize also were improved by surgery (Rudnick & Maxwell, 1984). More recently, the procedure has been found to have poor predictive value (Hasbak et al., 2002).

Duplex Ultrasonography with Resistive Index

Duplex ultrasonography is a moderately accurate screening test with the peak systolic velocity having a sensitivity of 85% and sensitivity of 92% (Williams et al., 2007). Moreover, the estimation of the resistance index from the end-diastolic and maximal systolic velocities has been shown to predict the clinical response to revascularization (Radermacher et al., 2001).

Patients may not respond to technically effective revascularization because of structural damage to the poststenotic vasculature, either because their underlying disease was primary hypertension leading to nephrosclerosis or because of the development of ischemic nephropathy. To measure the degree of vascular resistance beyond the stenosis, the velocities of blood flow within the renal artery are estimated by Doppler ultrasonography and the resistive index calculated by the equation: $[1 - (\text{end-diastolic velocity} \div \text{maximal systolic velocity})] \times 100$.

The resistive index was measured in 138 patients with renovascular disease before revascularization by angioplasty or surgery (Radermacher et al., 2001). In the 35 who had a resistive index value of 80 or higher, only one had a subsequent 10 mm Hg or greater fall in BP. In the 96 patients with a resistive index value of less than 80, the mean BP fell by at least 10 mm Hg in 90. In other series, the index has predicted postrevascularization changes in renal function, but not in BP (Crutchley et al., 2009).

The RI has been shown to correlate with renal pathology in tissue obtained by biopsy (Ikee et al., 2005), but has had less predictive accuracy in others' experience (Drieghe et al., 2008; Krumme & Hollenbeck, 2007). As seen in Figure 10-5, duplex ultrasonography with RI is given as the first study in those with favorable indications for revascularization.

Renal Scans

It seems logical that hypoperfusion of the affected kidney would be seen with RVHT. However, at least two factors may be involved in reducing the discriminatory power of renal perfusion studies. First, for reasons that are not apparent, considerable asymmetry of renal blood flow is present in the absence of RVHT. Asymmetry, defined as a 25% or greater difference

between the two kidneys, was found in 51% of 148 hypertensive patients whose renal arteries were patent by angiography (van Onna et al., 2003). Not surprisingly, the presence of asymmetry increased the rate of false-positive results of renal scintigraphy.

The second factor that may play a role is the frequent development of either bilateral renovascular disease or ischemic nephropathy in the contralateral kidney, both leading to a decreased differential of blood flow. Nonetheless, renal perfusion scans may serve to predict the response to revascularization.

Renography may be done with radiolabeled agents that are excreted either by glomerular filtration—technetium-99 diethylenetriamine pentaacetic acid (^{99}Tc-DTPA)—or partially by filtration but mainly by tubular secretion to measure renal blood flow—^{131}I-hippurate, or ^{99}Tc-mercaptoacetyltriglycine (^{99}Tc-MAG$_3$). When used alone, isotopic renograms provided about 75% sensitivity and specificity for the diagnosis of RVHT (Pickering, 1991).

Soon after the observation that renal function in an ischemic kidney could abruptly be reduced further after a single dose of the ACEI captopril (Hricik et al., 1983), the effect of captopril on renal uptake of ^{99}Tc-DTPA was reported (Wenting et al., 1984). Either a reduction of the uptake of ^{99}Tc-DTPA or a slowing of the excretion of ^{131}I-hippurate or ^{99}Tc-MAG$_3$ can be used to identify the effect of the ACEI in removing the protective actions of the high levels of angiotensin II on the autoregulation of glomerular filtration and on the maintenance of renal blood flow, respectively (Fig. 10-6).

To reduce the cost and time of the workup, the postcaptopril renal scan should be done first. If the result is negative (as it will be most of the time), there is no need for a precaptopril renogram. If the test is positive, the procedure should be repeated the next day without captopril to ensure that the differences are related to reversible vascular disease and not parenchymal damage.

As reviewed by Taylor (2000), ACEI renography is highly accurate in patients with a moderate likelihood of RVHT and normal renal function, wherein sensitivity and specificity are approximately 90%. By combining data from ten studies which evaluated the effects of revascularization in 291 patients, the mean positive predictive value of ACEI renography was 92%. Less impressive results have been reported more recently in patients who had angioplasty (Soulez et al., 2003; van Jaarsveld & Deinum, 2001). As expected, the test is less sensitive

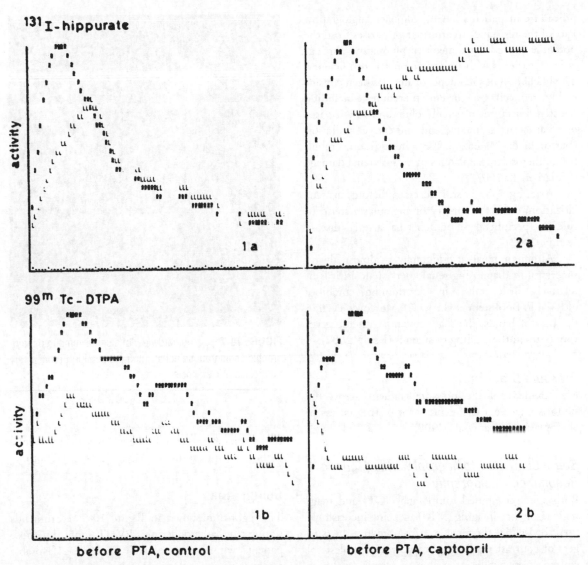

FIGURE 10-6 Renography in a 42-year-old man with hypertension and stenosis of the left renal artery. L, left kidney; R, right kidney. After percutaneous transluminal angioplasty (PTA), his hypertension was cured. The upper half of the figure shows ^{131}I-hippurate (a) and the lower half shows ^{99m}Tc-diethylenetriamine pentaacetic acid (DTPA) (b) time-activity curves in two different circumstances: (1) before PTA without any medication (control) and (2) before PTA but with 25 mg captopril taken orally 1 hour before the investigation. Captopril slowed down the excretion of ^{131}I-hippurate and reduced the uptake of ^{99m}Tc-DTPA in only the left kidney. (Reprinted from Geyskes GG, Oei HY, Puylaert BAJ, et al. Renovascular hypertension identified by captopril-induced changes in the renogram. *Hypertension* 1987;9:451–458, with permission.)

in patients with renal insufficiency; as many as half will have an "indeterminate" test. The test can be done in patients taking various antihypertensive drugs although sensitivity is reduced in patients who are on ACEI or ARB therapy (Pedersen, 2000) which should be discontinued at least 3 days before renography.

Tests Imaging the Renal Arteries

Catheter-Directed Renal Arteriography

For many years, catheter-directed arteriography was the only procedure available to visualize the renal vessels. As noninvasive imaging became available, arteriography has been utilized less except as a "drive-by" procedure in patients having coronary angiography. Part of the resistance to arteriography arises from the potential for contrast media nephropathy, particularly in patients with underlying renal insufficiency. The likelihood of such nephropathy has been considerably reduced by current procedures, including selective injections of small volumes of low- or iso-osmolar contrast media and preventive hydration (Bartorelli & Marenzi, 2008). In addition, emboli from atherosclerotic plaques may cause renal damage (Scolari et al., 2007).

Arteriography is still necessary before revascularization, either by surgery or angioplasty/stent, to rule out peripheral or branch renal arterial disease (Reidy, 2002).

Although renal arteriography is almost always successful in diagnosing renal artery stenosis, it is of relatively little value in determining curability of RVHT (Bookstein et al., 1972). Moreover, even in the best of hands, there is substantial interobserver variability in the grading of stenosis (Reidy, 2002).

Pressure Gradient

Measurement of the pressure gradient across the stenosis may be a useful predictor of the success of angioplasty (Leesar et al., 2009).

Spiral Computed Tomography and Magnetic Resonance Angiography

Both spiral computed tomography (CT) and magnetic resonance imaging (MRI) are being increasingly used to visualize the renal arteries, to reduce the dangers of contrast media nephropathy and cholesterol embolization while providing excellent sensitivity (Textor, 2009). The most important advantages of spiral computed tomographic angiography are the injection of contrast medium intravenously rather than directly into the renal arteries, the ability to visualize both the arterial lumen and wall in three dimensions, and the ability to visualize accessory and distal vessels (Fig. 10-7).

MRA with gadolinium enhancement involves no ionizing radiation. The serious complication of nephrogenic systemic fibrosis likely occurs only in patients with ESRD (Marckmann, 2008). In addition to imaging the renal arteries, MRA can provide useful data on total renal length and volume. In the future, newer procedures such as the use of MR to evaluate renal tissue oxygenation may improve recognition of intrarenal ischemia (Textor et al., 2008).

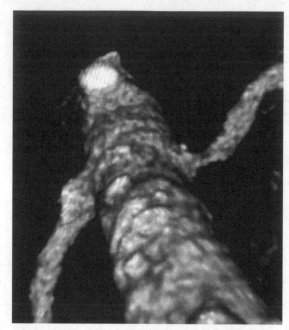

FIGURE 10-7 An upward view of a spiral computed tomographic angiogram demonstrating proximal left renal artery atherosclerotic stenosis.

Moreover, newer technology enables MRA to be done without a contrast media (Miyazaki & Lee, 2008).

Conclusion

The algorithm shown in Figure 10-5 recommends testing for atherosclerotic RVHT only in those patients who are more likely to have a favorable response to revascularization. No accurate estimates of the numbers of such patients are available, but they likely make up less than 5% of the total hypertensive population. The algorithm can be applied to patients with fibromuscular dysplasia. Being younger, they are usually easier to identify on clinical grounds, less likely to have renal insufficiency or extensive atherosclerosis, and more likely to have a favorable response to medical therapy or revascularization.

Except in those relatively few patients with such high likelihood of RVHT in whom immediate direct angiography is indicated, the algorithm starts with a study to confirm the clinical evidence for a favorable response to revascularization. Only those likely to respond would then have an imaging study to visualize the extent of renovascular disease, thereby pointing to the appropriate mode of revascularization.

Since Doppler ultrasonography with measurement of the resistive index can both identify renovascular disease and, according to still limited experience, ascertain the likelihood of a respond to revascularization, this procedure is a logical way to begin. If duplex sonography is unavailable or technically inadequate, captopril renography is recommended.

THERAPY

Even if renal artery stenosis is incidentally detected, its presence indicates that the patient is at increased risk for future cardiovascular and renal events (Hackam et al., 2007). Therefore, regardless of the clinical scenario, all patients with recognized renal artery disease should be given intensive medical therapy. If the disease is found to be functionally significant, renal artery revascularization may be indicated.

The smaller number of patients with functionally significant fibromuscular dysplasia are usually helped by angioplasty, and surgery is needed only in those with disease in segmental arteries (Plouin et al., 2007).

Once an atherosclerotic lesion is found and proved to be functionally significant, three choices are available for treatment: medical therapy, angioplasty, and surgical revascularization. In addition, intensive control of all concomitant cardiovascular risk factors is mandatory.

Over the past few years, angioplasty with stenting has far surpassed surgery when revascularization is deemed necessary (Murphy et al., 2004). At the same time, as the limitations of revascularization have become obvious, more patients are being treated medically, at least until they show evidence of progression of renal damage or resistant hypertension.

Medical Therapy

The largest experience has been with renin-angiotensin inhibition, in particular ACEIs. The largest published experience is a population-based cohort study of 3,570 patients in whom the diagnosis of renovascular disease had been made by various techniques (Hackam et al., 2008). All patients were 65 years of age or older with a mean age of 74.5. Hypertension was diagnosed in over 85% and 64% had CKD. The mean follow-up was 2 years.

The primary end point of death, myocardial infarction or stroke, occurred in 10 per 100 patient years in the 53% who were prescribed an ACEI and 13 per 100 patient years in the 47% who were not prescribed an ACEI, a difference that was highly significant after adjustment for a number of possible confounding factors. In addition, the number of hospitalizations for heart failure and institutionalization of long-term dialysis were reduced by over 30%.

The major problem, as expected in patients whose renal perfusion is based on high level of angiotensin, was acute renal failure. This developed in 1.2 per 100 patient years in those on ACEI versus 0.6 per 100 patient years in those not on ACEI. Again as expected, most acute renal failure occurred in those with CKD, diabetes, or those taking loop diuretics.

These data are keeping with the results of more controlled but far smaller studies (Baxter et al., 2009; Hackam et al., 2007).

As these data reconfirm, careful monitoring of renal function is mandatory in patients who are either known to have renovascular disease or who are more likely to have renovascular, i.e., patients in the "Moderate" and "High" categories in Table 10-7, when an ACEI, an ARB, or a DRI is started. If the serum creatinine rises beyond 30% of baseline, the renin-angiotensin inhibitor should be stopped and revascularization considered (Cohen & Townsend, 2008).

Angioplasty

After the first report of successful treatment of RVHT by percutaneous transluminal renal angioplasty (Grüntzig et al., 1978), the technical aspects have continually improved, including the use of filtering devices to recapture debris which could otherwise induce atheroembolization (Corriere et al., 2007). The high rate of restenosis with balloon angioplasty has led to increasing use of stents, particularly in those with atherosclerotic ostial lesions (Corriere et al., 2008) or posttransplant RVHT (Bruno et al., 2003).

After many thousands of patients with renovascular disease, with or without proof of its functional significance, have had angioplasty ± stenting, a proper trial has been completed and another is in progress to determine if the procedure is better than medical therapy. The two trials are summarized in Table 10-8.

Results of the Angioplasty and Stenting for Renal Artery Lesion (ASTRAL) trial were presented on April 1, 2008 but as of early 2009 not published. Press releases from the presentation, available on the web, indicate that angioplasty and stenting offer no

TABLE 10.8 Clinical Trials of Medical Therapy ± Angioplasty Factors Stent in Patients with Atherosclerotic Renal Artery Stenosis

	Astral	Coral
No. of patients	806	1,080
Inclusion criteria	Renal artery suitable for angioplasty ± stent placement; no prior revascularization procedure for atherosclerotic renovascular disease	80%–99% renal artery stenosis, or 60%–80% stenosis with ≥20 mm Hg transstenotic gradient; systolic BP ≥ 155 mm Hg on ≥2 BP meds
Interventions	Angioplasty ± stent vs. medical R_x alone	Angioplasty ± stent vs. medical Rx alone
Primary end point	Mean slope of 1/Scr vs. time	Composite of CV death, stroke, MI, HF hospitalization, or ESRD
Secondary end points	BP, urinary protein excretion, serious vascular events, ESRD, angiography patency at 12 months	Mortality, subgroup analyses, 1/Scr vs. time, BP, renal artery patency, renal resistive index, quality of life, cost-effectiveness
Recruitment period	6 years	≈4 years
Planned mean follow-up	1 year	2+ years

ACE, angiotensin converting enzyme; ARBs, angiotensin II receptor blockers; ASTRAL, Angioplasty and Stent for Renal Artery Lesions; BP, blood pressure; CORAL, Cardiovascular Outcomes in Renal Atherosclerotic Lesions; CV, cardiovascular; ESRD, end-stage renal disease; HF, heart failure; MI, myocardial infarction; R_x, therapy; Scr, serum creatinine.

benefit over medical therapy. The trial enrolled 806 patients with atherosclerotic renovascular disease, all with some degree of renal failure (average serum creatinine 2.0 mg/dL), an average BP of 151/76 mm Hg, and an average 76% stenosis of one renal artery. The angioplasty and stent procedure was considered technically successful in 88%. After at least 1-year follow-up, there were no differences in BP, changes in serum creatinine, rates of acute renal failure, or cardiovascular events between the revascularized or the medically treated halves.

Another large trial, the Cardiovascular Outcomes with Renal Atherosclerotic Lesions (CORAL), is in progress (Cooper et al., 2006).

Surgery

There are many uncontrolled observational studies showing benefits for both BP and renal function by surgery (Cherr et al., 2002; Marone et al., 2004). Despite the increasing likelihood that patients who are referred for surgical repair will either have failed to respond to angioplasty or have extensive atherosclerotic disease in the aorta or mesenteric vessels that also needs repair, the overall results with surgery seem generally comparable to those seen with technically successful angioplasty (Galaria et al., 2005). Not surprisingly, mortality is higher, averaging 10% in the immediate postoperative period (Modrall et al., 2008).

Surgery may be the only choice for patients with major renal artery involvement by arteritis (Weaver et al., 2004). In addition, nephrectomy may be appropriate for patients with refractory hypertension and an atrophic, nonfunctioning kidney (Canzanello, 2004).

The Choice of Therapy

In reviewing the recent literature, a number of points become obvious:

• Patients with fibroplastic disease do better than do those with atherosclerotic disease when treated medically or by revascularization (Slovut & Olin, 2004). Their better response likely reflects their younger age, less prolonged hypertension, and less atherosclerosis in other organs. Those who do not respond well to medical therapy should have percutaneous transluminal angioplasty (PTA), usually without a stent. Angioplasty cures or improves 70% to 90% (Slovut & Olin, 2004).
• For atherosclerotic RVHT, *medical therapy*, usually with an ACEI or ARB and often with a calcium channel blocker, may be effective over many years (Hackam et al., 2007).
• *Angioplasty* with a stent should be performed in patients who do not tolerate or respond to medical therapy or who have progressive renal impairment (Textor, 2008).

- *Surgical revascularization* is much less commonly indicated, except when angioplasty with stenting is not feasible or is unsuccessful or when abdominal vascular surgery is required.
- Revascularization or angioplasty may be indicated for ischemic nephropathy, more to preserve renal function than to control hypertension (Levin et al., 2007).

Obviously, uncertainties remain about both the diagnosis and treatment of RVHT. The separation of patients with atherosclerotic renovascular disease, who comprise about 90% of those with RVHT, into those who are either likely or unlikely to have a favorable response to revascularization (shown in Table 10-6), should be of considerable help. However, the uncertainties that remain seem so formidable that clinicians experienced with the management of RVHT should almost always be involved in the evaluation and treatment of these patients.

RENIN-SECRETING TUMORS

Renin-secreting tumors are not common. Since the recognition of the first case in 1967 (Robertson et al., 1967), only about 90 have been reported (Wong et al., 2008). Since it has been so well described, fewer will be deemed worthy of publication. Most such tumors are relatively small and are composed of renin-secreting juxtaglomerular cells (i.e., hemangiopericytomas). Other causes of hypertension and high renin levels include

- Wilms tumor in children, usually associated with high levels of prorenin (Leckie et al., 1994).
- Renal cell carcinoma (Moein & Dehghani, 2000); tumors of various extrarenal sites, including lung, ovary, liver, pancreas, sarcomas, and teratomas (Pursell & Quinlan, 2003), and adrenal paraganglionoma (Arver et al., 1999).
- Large intrarenal tumors that compress renal vessels.
- Unilateral juxtaglomerular cell hyperplasia (Kuchel et al., 1993).

Most of the renin-secreting tumors of renal origin fit a rather typical pattern:

- Severe hypertension in relatively young patients: The mean age of the reported cases is 27 years (Wong et al., 2008).
- Secondary aldosteronism, usually manifested by hypokalemia.

- Very high prorenin and renin levels in the peripheral blood: Even higher levels from the kidney harboring the tumor.
- Tumor recognizable by computed tomographic scan.
- Morphologically, a hemangiopericytoma arising from the juxtaglomerular apparatus.

Now that the renal causes of hypertension have been covered, we turn to those associated with hormonal excesses that are usually adrenal in origin.

REFERENCES

Agarwal M, Lynn KL, Richards AM, et al. Hyponatremic-hypertensive syndrome with renal ischemia. *Hypertension* 1999;33: 1020–1024.

Alfidi RJ, Tarar R, Fosmoe RJ, et al. Renal splanchnic steal and hypertension. *Radiology* 1972;102:545–549.

Aparicio L, Boggio G, Waisman G et al. Advances in noninvasive methods for functional evaluation of renovascular disease. *J Am Soc Hypertens* 2009;3:42–51.

Arver S, Jacobsson H, Cedermark B, et al. Malignant human renin producing paraganglionoma—localization with ^{123}I-MIBG and treatment with ^{131}I-MIBG. *Clin Endocrinol* 1999;51:631–635.

Bartorelli AL, Marenzi G. Contrast-induced nephropathy. *J Interven Cardiol* 2008;21:74–85.

Bax L, Woittiez AJ, Kouwenberg HJ et al. Stent placement in patients with atherosclerotic renal artery stenosis and impaired renal function: A randomized trial. *Ann Intern Med* 2009;150:840–841.

Bookstein JJ, Abrams HL, Buenger RE, et al. Radiologic aspects of renovascular hypertension. Part 3. Appraisal of arteriography. *JAMA* 1972;221:368–374.

Boutouyrie P, Gimenez-Roqueplo A-P, Fine E, et al. Evidence for carotid and radial artery wall subclinical lesions in renal fibromuscular dysplasia. *J Hypertens* 2003;21:2287–2295.

Bruno S, Remuzzi G, Ruggenenti P. Transplant renal artery stenosis. *J Am Soc Nephrol* 2004;15:134–141.

Buller CE, Norareda JG, Ramanathan K, et al. The profile of cardiac patients with renal artery stenosis. *J Am Coll Cardiol* 2004;43:1606–1613.

Cakar N, Yalcinkaya F, Duzova A, et al. Takayasu arteritis in children. *J Rheumatol* 2008;35:913–919.

Canzanello VJ. Medical management of renovascular hypertension. In: Mansoor GA, ed. *Secondary Hypertension: Clinical Presentation, Diagnosis, and Treatment.* Totowa, NJ: Humana Press Inc.; 2004:91–107.

Caps MT, Perissinotto C, Zierler RE, et al. Prospective study of atherosclerotic disease progression in the renal artery. *Circulation* 1998a;98:2866–2872.

Caps MT, Zierler RE, Polissar NL, et al. Risk of atrophy in kidneys with atherosclerotic renal artery stenosis. *Kidney Int* 1998b; 53:735–742.

Castle CH. Iatrogenic renal hypertension: Two unusual complication of surgery for familial pheochromocytoma. *JAMA* 1973; 225:1085–1088.

Chábová V, Schirger A, Stanson AW, et al. Outcomes of atherosclerotic renal artery stenosis managed without revascularization. *Mayo Clin Proc* 2000;75:437–444.

Cherr GS, Hansen KJ, Craven TE, et al. Surgical management of atherosclerotic renovascular disease. *J Vasc Surg* 2002;35: 236–245.

Chonchol M, Linas S. Diagnosis and management of ischemic nephropathy. *Clin J Am Soc Nephrol* 2006;1:172–181.

Cohen DL, Townsend RR. What should the physician do when creatinine increases after starting an angiotensin-converting enzyme inhibitor or an angiotensin receptor blocker? *J Clin Hypertens (Greenwich)* 2008;10:803.

Conlon PJ, O'Riordan E, Kalra PA. New insights into the epidemiologic and clinical manifestations of atherosclerotic renovascular disease. *Am J Kidney Dis* 2000;35:573–587.

Cooper CJ, Murphy TP, Matsumoto A, et al. Stent revascularization for the prevention of cardiovascular and renal events among patients with renal artery stenosis and systolic hypertension: Rationale and design of the CORAL trial. *Am Heart J* 2006;152:59–66.

Corriere MA, Crutchley TA, Edwards MS. Is embolic protection during renal artery intervention really necessary? *J Cardiovasc Surg (Torino)* 2007;48:443–453.

Corriere MA, Pearce JD, Edwards MS et al. Endovascular management of atherosclerotic renovascular disease: Early results following primary intervention. *J Vasc Surg* 2008;48:580–587.

Coruzzi P, Novarini A. Which antihypertensive treatment in renal vasculitis? *Nephron* 1992;62:372.

Crutchley TA, Pearce JD, Craven TE, et al. Clinical utility of the resistive index in atherosclerotic renovascular disease. *J Vasc Surg* 2009;49:148–155.

Davis BA, Crook JE, Vestal RE, et al. Prevalence of renovascular hypertension in patients with grade III or IV hypertensive retinopathy. *N Engl J Med* 1979;301:1273–1276.

Deglise S, Corpataux JM, Haller C, et al. Bilateral renal artery entrapment by diaphragmatic crura: A rare cause of renovascular hypertension with a specific management. *J Comput Assist Tomogr* 2007;31:481–484.

de Mast Q, Beutler J. The prevalence of artherosclerotic renal artery stenosis in risk groups: A systemic literature review. *J Hypertens* 2009;27:1333–1340.

Drieghe B, Madaric J, Sarno G, et al. Assessment of renal artery stenosis: Side-by-side comparison of angiography and duplex ultrasound with pressure gradient measurements. *Eur Heart J* 2008;29:517–524.

Dussol B, Nicolino F, Brunet P, et al. Acute transplant artery thrombosis induced by angiotensin-converting inhibitor in a patient with renovascular hypertension. *Nephron* 1994;66:102–104.

Edwards BS, Stanson AW, Holley KE, et al. Isolated renal artery dissection. Presentation, evaluation, management, and pathology. *Mayo Clin Proc* 1982;57:564–571.

English WP, Pearce JD, Craven TE, et al. Surgical management of renal artery aneurysms. *J Vasc Surg* 2004;40:53–60.

Eyler WR, Clark MD, Garman JE, et al. Angiography of the renal areas including a comparative study of renal arterial stenosis in patients with and without hypertension. *Radiology* 1962;78:879–892.

Farreras-Valenti P, Rozman C, Jurado-Grau J, et al. Gröblad-Strandberg-Touraine syndrome with systemic hypertension due to unilateral renal angioma. *Am J Med* 1965;39:355–360.

Freedman BI, Hsu FC, Langefeld CD et al. Renal artery calcified plaque associations with subclinical renal and cardiovascular disease. *Kidney Int.* 2004;65:2262–2267.

Galaria II, Surowiec SM, Rhodes JM, et al. Percutaneous and open renal revascularizations have equivalent long-term functional outcomes. *Ann Vasc Surg* 2005;19:218–228.

Garovic VD, Textor SC. Renovascular hypertension and ischemic nephropathy. *Circulation* 2005;112:1362–1374.

Goldblatt H. Reflections. *Urol Clin North Am* 1975;2:219–221.

Goldblatt H, Lynch J, Hanzal RF, et al. Studies on experimental hypertension. I. The production of persistent elevation of systolic blood pressure by means of renal ischemia. *J Exp Med* 1934;59:347–378.

Granger JP, Schnackenberg CG. Renal mechanisms of angiotensin II-induced hypertension. *Semin Nephrol* 2000;20:417–425.

Grüntzig A, Kuhlmann U, Vetter W, et al. Treatment of renovascular hypertension with percutaneous transluminal dilatation of a renal-artery stenosis. *Lancet* 1978;1:801–802.

Grützmacher P, Radtke HW, Stahl RA, et al. Renal artery stenosis and erythropoietin [Abstract]. *Kidney Int* 1989;35:326.

Guo H, Karla PA, Gilbertson DT, et al. Artherosclerotic renovascular disease in older US patients starting dialysis, 1996 to 2001. *Circulation* 2007;115:50–58.

Hackam DG, Duong-Hua ML, Mamdani M, et al. Angiotensin inhibition in renovascular disease: A population-based cohort study. *Am Heart J* 2008;156:549–555.

Hackam DG, Spence JD, Garg AX, et al. Role of renin-angiotensin system blockade in atherosclerotic renal artery stenosis and renovascular hypertension. *Hypertension* 2007;50:998–1003.

Halimi J-M, Ribstein J, Du Cailar G, et al. Nephrotic-range proteinuria in patients with renovascular disease. *Am J Med* 2000;108:120–126.

Hansen KJ, Deitch JS, Dean RH. Renovascular disease in blacks: Prevalence and result of operative management. *Am J Med Sci* 1998;315:337–342.

Hasbak P, Jensen LT, Ibsen H, et al. Hypertension and renovascular disease: Follow-up of 100 renal vein renin samplings. *J Hum Hypertens* 2002;16:275–280.

Hricik DE, Browning PJ, Kopelman R, et al. Captopril-induced functional renal insufficiency in patients with bilateral renal-artery stenosis or renal-artery stenosis in a solitary kidney. *N Engl J Med* 1983;308:373–376.

Hughes JS, Dove HG, Gifford RW Jr, et al. Duration of blood pressure elevation in accurately predicting surgical cure of renovascular hypertension. *Am Heart J* 1981;101:408–413.

Ikee R, Kobayashi S, Hemmi N, et al. Correlation between the resistive index by Doppler ultrasound and kidney function and histology. *Am J Kidney Dis* 2005;46:603–609.

Jennings RC, Shaikh VAR, Allen WMC. Renal ischaemia due to thrombosis of renal artery resulting in metastases from primary carcinoma of bronchus. *Br Med J* 1964;2:1053–1054.

Kalra PA, Guo H, Kausz AT, et al. Artherosclerotic renovascular disease in United States patients aged 67 years and older: Risk factors, revascularization, and prognosis. *Kidney Int* 2005;68:293–301.

Kasiske BL, Anjum S, Shah R, et al. Hypertension after kidney transplantation. *Am J Kidney Dis* 2004;43:1071–1081.

Kato K, Takashi M, Narita H, et al. Renal hypertension secondary to perirenal pseudocyst: Resolution by percutaneous drainage. *J Urol* 1985;134:942–943.

Khong TK, Mossouris CG, Belli AM, et al. Regression of atherosclerotic renal artery stenosis with aggressive lipid lowering therapy. *J Hum Hypertens* 2001;15:431–433.

Kolhe N, Downes M, O'Donnell P, et al. Renal artery dissection secondary to medial hyperplasia presenting as loin pain haematuria syndrome. *Nephrol Dial Transplant* 2004;19:495–497.

Krijnen P, van Jaarsveld BC, Deinum J, et al. Which patients with hypertension and atherosclerotic renal artery stenosis benefit from immediate intervention? *J Hum Hypertens* 2004;18:91–96.

Krijnen P, van Jaarsveld BC, Steyerberg EW, et al. A clinical prediction rule for renal artery stenosis. *Ann Intern Med* 1998;129:705–711.

Krumme B, Hollenbeck M. Doppler sonography in renal artery stenosis—does the Resistive Index predict the success of intervention? *Nephrol Dial Transplant* 2007;22:692–696.

Kuchel O, Horky K, Cantin M, et al. Unilateral juxtaglomerular hyperplasia, hyperreninism and hypokalaemia relieved by nephrectomy. *J Hum Hypertens* 1993;7:71–78.

Kuczera P, Wloszczynska E, Adamczak M et al. Frequancy of renal artery stenosis and variants of renal vascularization in hypertensive patients: Analysis of 1550 angiographies in one centre. *J Human Hypertens* 2009;23:396–401.

Leckie BJ, Birnie G, Carachi R. Renin in Wilms' tumor: Prorenin as an indicator. *J Clin Endocrinol Metab* 1994;79:1742–1746.

Leertouwer TC, Pattynama PMT, van den Berg-Huysmans A. Incidental renal artery stenosis in peripheral vascular disease. *Kidney Int* 2001;59:1480–1483.

Leesar MA, Varma J, Shapira A et al. Prediction of hypertension improvement after stenting of renal artery stenosis: comparative accuracy of translesional pressure gradients, intravascular ultrasound, and angiography. *J Am Coll Cardiol* 2009;53:2363–2371.

Lekuona I, Laraudogoitia E, Salcedo A, et al. Congestive heart failure in a hypertensive patient. *Lancet* 2001;357:358.

Levin A, Linas S, Luft FC, et al. Controversies in renal artery stenosis: A review by the American Society of Nephrology Advisory Group on Hypertension. *Am J Nephrol* 2007;27:212–220.

Lüscher TF, Lie JT, Stanson AW, et al. Arterial fibromuscular dysplasia. *Mayo Clin Proc* 1987;62:931–952.

Mann SJ, Pickering TG. Detection of renovascular hypertension. State of the art: 1992. *Ann Intern Med* 1992; 117:845–853.

Marckmann P. Nephrogenic systemic fibrosis: Epidemiology update. *Curr Opin Nephrol Hypertens* 2008;17:315–319.

Marone LK, Clouse WD, Dorer DJ, et al. Preservation of renal function with surgical revascularization in patients with atherosclerotic renovascular disease. *J Vasc Surg* 2004;39:322–329.

Maxwell MH, Bleifer KH, Franklin SS, et al. Demographic analysis of the study. *JAMA* 1972;220:1195–1204.

Missouris CG, Belli A-M, MacGregor GA. "Apparent" heart failure: A syndrome caused by renal artery stenosis. *Heart* 2000;83:152–155.

Miyazaki M, Lee VS. Nonenhanced MR angiography. *Radiology* 2008;248:20–43.

Mizuiri S, Amagasaki Y, Hosaka H, et al. Hypertension in unilateral atrophic kidney secondary to ureteropelvic junction obstruction. *Nephron* 1992;61:217–219.

Modrall JG, Rosero EB, Smith ST, et al. Operative mortality for renal artery bypass in the United States: Results from the National Inpatient Sample. *J Vasc Surg* 2008;48:317–322.

Moein MR, Dehghani VO. Hypertension: A rare presentation of renal cell carcinoma. *J Urol* 2000;164:2019.

Mounier-Vehier C, Lions C, Devos P, et al. Cortical thickness: An early morphological marker of atherosclerotic renal disease. *Kidney Int* 2002;61:591–598.

Muray S, Martín M, Amoedo ML, et al. Rapid decline in renal function reflects reversibility and predicts the outcome after angioplasty in renal artery stenosis. *Am J Kidney Dis* 2002;39:60–66.

Murphy TP, Soares G, Kim M. Increase in utilization of percutaneous renal artery interventions by Medicare beneficiaries, 1996–2000. *Am J Radiol* 2004;183:561–568.

Myrianthefs P, Aravosita P, Tokta R, et al. Resolution of Page kidney-related hypertension with medical therapy: A case report. *Heart Lung* 2007;36:377–379.

Nakano S, Kigoshi T, Uchida K, et al. Hypertension and unilateral renal ischemia (Page kidney) due to compression of a retroperitoneal paraganglioma. *Am J Nephrol* 1996;16:91–94.

Nomura S, Hashimoto A, Shutou K, et al. Page kidney in a hemodialyzed patient. *Nephron* 1996;72:106–107.

Novick AC, Zaki S, Goldfarb D, et al. Epidemiologic and clinical comparison of renal artery stenosis in black patients and white patients. *J Vasc Surg* 1994;20:1–5.

Olivieri O, Grazioli S, Pizzolo F, et al. Different impact of deletion polymorphism of gene on the risk of renal and coronary artery disease. *J Hypertens* 2002;20:37–43.

Pearce JD, Craven BL, Craven TE, et al. Progression of atherosclerotic renovascular disease: A prospective population-based study. *J Vasc Surg* 2006;44:955–962.

Pedersen EB. New tools in diagnosing renal artery stenosis. *Kidney Int* 2000;57:2657–2677.

Pickering TG. The role of laboratory testing in the diagnosis of renovascular hypertension. *Clin Chem* 1991;37:1831–1837.

Plouin PF, Perdu J, La Batide-Alanore A, et al. Fibromuscular dysplasia. *Orphanet J Rare Dis* 2007;2:28.

Pursell RN, Quinlan PM. Secondary hypertension due to a renin-producing teratoma. *Am J Hypertens* 2003;16:592–595.

Rackson ME, Lossef SV, Sos TA. Renal artery stenosis in patients with aortic dissection: Increased prevalence. *Radiology* 1990;177:555–558.

Radermacher J, Chavan A, Bleck A, et al. Use of Doppler ultrasonography to predict the outcome of therapy for renal-artery stenosis. *N Engl J Med* 2001;344:410–417.

Reidy JF. New diagnostic techniques for imaging the renal arteries. *Curr Opin Nephrol Hypertens* 2002;11:635–639.

Restrick LJ, Ledermann JA, Hoffbrand BI. Primary malignant retroperitoneal germ cell tumour presenting with accelerated hypertension. *J Hum Hypertens* 1992;6:243–244.

Riccialdelli L, Arnaldi G, Giacchetti G, et al. Hypertension due to renal artery occlusion in a patient with antiphospholipid syndrome. *Am J Hypertens* 2001;14:62–65.

Rihal CS, Textor SC, Breen JF, et al. Incidental renal artery stenosis among a prospective cohort of hypertensive patients undergoing coronary angiography. *Mayo Clin Proc* 2002;77:309–316.

Robertson PW, Klidjian A, Harding LK, et al. Hypertension due to a renin-secreting renal tumour. *Am J Med* 1967;43:963–976.

Rossi GP, Cesari M, Chiesura-Corona M, et al. Renal vein renin measurements accurately identify renovascular hypertension caused by total occlusion of the renal artery. *J Hypertens* 2002;20:975–984.

Rudnick MR, Maxwell MH. Limitations of renin assays. In: Narins RG, ed. *Controversies in Nephrology and Hypertension*. New York: Churchill Livingstone; 1984:123–160.

Salifu MO, Gordon DH, Friedman EA, et al. Bilateral renal infarction in a black man with medial fibromuscular dysplasia. *Am J Kidney Dis* 2000;36:184–189.

Scoble JE, de Takats D, Ostermann ME, et al. Lipid profiles in patients with atherosclerotic renal artery stenosis. *Nephron* 1999;83:117–121.

Scolari F, Ravani P, Gaggi R, et al. The challenge of diagnosing atheroembolic renal disease: Clinical features and prognostic factors. *Circulation* 2007;116:298–304.

Shapiro AL, Cavallo T, Cooper W, et al. Hypertension in radiation nephritis. Report of a patient with unilateral disease, elevated renin activity levels, and reversal after unilateral nephrectomy. *Arch Intern Med* 1977;137:848–851.

Siamopoulos K, Sellars L, Mishra SC, et al. Experience in the management of hypertension with unilateral chronic pyelonephritis: Results of nephrectomy in selected patients. *QJM* 1983;52:349–362.

Silva VS, Martin LC, Franco RJ, et al. Pleiotropic effects of statins may improve outcomes in atherosclerotic renovascular disease. *Am J Hypertens* 2008;21:1163–1168.

Silver D, Clements JB. Renovascular hypertension from renal artery compression by congenital bands. *Ann Surg* 1976;183:161–166.

Simon G. What is critical renal artery stenosis? *Am J Hypertens* 2000;13:1189–1193.

Simon N, Franklin SS, Bleifer KH, et al. Clinical characteristics of renovascular hypertension. *JAMA* 1972;220:1209–1218.

Slovut DP, Olin JW. Fibromuscular dysplasia. *N Engl J Med* 2004;350:1862–1871.

Smith HW. Unilateral nephrectomy in hypertensive disease. *J Urol* 1956;76:685–701.

Smith LH, Drach G, Hall P, et al. National High Blood Pressure Education Program (NHBPEP) review paper on complications of shock wave lithotripsy for urinary calculi. *Am J Med* 1991;91:635–641.

Soulez G, Therasse E, Qanadli SD, et al. Prediction of clinical response after renal angioplasty: Respective value of renal Doppler sonography and scintigraphy. *AJR* 2003;181:1029–1035.

Sperati CJ, Aggarwal N, Arepally A, et al. Fibromuscular dysplasia. *Kidney Int* 2009; 75:333–336.

Steffens J, Mast GJ, Braedel HU, et al. Segmental renal hypoplasia of vascular origin causing renal hypertension in a 3-year-old girl. *J Urol* 1991;146:826–829.

Tapper D, Brand T, Hickman R. Early diagnosis and management of renovascular hypertension. *Am J Surg* 1987;153:495–500.

Taylor A. Functional testing: ACEI renography. *Semin Nephrol* 2000;20:437–444.

Tedla F, Hayashi R, McFarlane SI, et al. Hypertension after renal transplant. *J Clin Hypertens (Greenwich)* 2007;9:538–545.

Textor SC. Stable patients with atherosclerotic renal artery stenosis should be treated first with medical management. *Am J Kidney Dis* 2003;42:858–863.

Textor S. Current approaches to renovascular hypertension. *Med Clin North Am* 2009;3:717–732.

Textor SC. Atherosclerotic renal artery stenosis: Overtreated but underrated? *J Am Soc Nephrol* 2008;19:656–659.

Textor SC, Glockner JF, Lerman LO, et al. The use of magnetic resonance to evaluate tissue oxygenation in renal artery stenosis. *J Am Soc Nephrol* 2008;19:780–788.

Thatipelli M, Misra S, Johnson CM, et al. Renal artery stent placement for restoration of renal function in hemodialysis recipients with renal artery stenosis. *J Vasc Interv Radiol* 2008;19:1563–1568.

Thorsteinsdottir B, Kane GC, Hogan MJ, et al. Adverse outcomes of renovascular hypertension during pregnancy. *Nat Clin Pract Nephrol* 2006;2:651–656.

Torres VE, Wilson DM, Burnett JC Jr, et al. Effect of inhibition of converting enzyme on renal hemodynamics and sodium management in polycystic kidney disease. *Mayo Clin Proc* 1991; 66:1010–1017.

Tullus K, Brennan E, Hamilton G, et al. Renovascular hypertension in children. *Lancet* 2008;371:1453–1463.

Turnbull JM. Is listening for abdominal bruits useful in the evaluation of hypertension? *JAMA* 1995;274:1299–1301.

Valabhji J, Robinson S, Poulter C, et al. Prevalence of renal artery stenosis in subjects with type 2 diabetes and coexistent hypertension. *Diabetes Care* 2000;23:539–543.

Valvo E, Bedogna V, Gammaro L, et al. Systemic haemodynamics in renovascular hypertension: Changes after revascularization with percutaneous transluminal angioplasty. *J Hypertens* 1987; 5:629–632.

van der Ven AJAM, Hommels MJ, Kroon AA, et al. *Clamydia pneumoniae* seropositivity and systemic and renovascular atherosclerotic disease. *Arch Intern Med* 2002;162:786–790.

van Helvoort-Postulart D, Dirksen CD, Nelemans PJ, et al. Renal artery stenosis: Cost-effectiveness of diagnosis and treatment. *Radiology* 2007;244:505–513.

van Jaarsveld BC, Deinum J. Evaluation and treatment of renal artery stenosis: Impact on blood pressure and renal function. *Curr Opin Nephrol Hypertens* 2001;10:399–404.

van Onna M, Houben JHM, Kroon AA, et al. Asymmetry of renal blood flow in patients with moderate to severe hypertension. *Hypertension* 2003;41:108–113.

van Onna M, Kroon AA, Houben AJHM, et al. Genetic risk of atherosclerotic renal artery disease: The Candidate Gene Approach in a Renal Angiography cohort. *Hypertension* 2004;44:448–453.

Vasbinder GBC, Nelemans PJ, Kessels AGH, et al. Diagnostic tests for renal artery stenosis in patients suspected of having renovascular hypertension. *Ann Intern Med* 2001; 135:401–411.

Ward MM, Studenski S. Clinical prognostic factors in lupus nephritis. The importance of hypertension and smoking. *Arch Intern Med* 1992;152:2082–2088.

Watano K, Okamoto H, Takagi C, et al. Neurofibromatosis complicated with XXX syndrome and renovascular hypertension. *J Intern Med* 1996;239:531–535.

Weaver FA, Kumar SR, Yellin AE, et al. Renal revascularization in Takayasu arteritis-induced renal artery stenosis. *J Vasc Surg* 2004;39:749–757.

Welch WJ. The pathophysiology of renin release in renovascular hypertension. *Semin Nephrol* 2000;20:394–401.

Wenting GJ, Tan-Tjiong H, Derkx FHM, et al. Split renal function after captopril in unilateral renal artery stenosis. *Br Med J* 1984;288:886–890.

White CJ, Jaff MR, Haskal ZJ, et al. Indications for renal arteriography at the time of coronary arteriography: A science advisory from the American Heart Association Committee on Diagnostic and Interventional Cardiac Catheterization, Council on Clinical Cardiology, and the Councils on Cardiovascular Radiology and Intervention and on Kidney in Cardiovascular Disease. *Circulation* 2006;114:1892–1895.

Wilcox CS. Functional testing: Renin studies. *Semin Nephrol* 2000;20:432–436.

Williams GJ, Macaskill P, Chan SF, et al. Comparative accuracy of renal duplex sonographic parameters in the diagnosis of renal artery stenosis: Paired and unpaired analysis. *Am J Roentgenol* 2007;188:798–811.

Wong L, Hsu TH, Perlroth MG, et al. Reninoma: Case report and literature review. *J Hypertens* 2008;26:368–373.

Woodrow G, Cook JA, Brownjohn AM, et al. Is renal vasculitis increasing in incidence? *Lancet* 1990;336:1583.

Zoccali C, Mallamaci F, Finocchiaro P. Atherosclerotic renal artery stenosis: Epidemiology, cardiovascular outcomes, and clinical prediction rules. *J Am Soc Nephrol* 2002;13:S179–S183.

Primary Aldosteronism

F or over 40 years after Jerome Conn characterized the syndrome, primary aldosteronism (PA) was generally held to be a relatively rare cause of hypertension, present in fewer than 1% of all patients. However, over the past few years, the prevalence of this condition has been reported to be much higher, reaching 40% in highly selected groups and around 10% in referred patients (Rossi et al., 2006a), so it is now referred to as "the most common cause of secondary hypertension" (Young, 2007b). These figures may be inflated by the confounding effect of referral and selection (Kaplan, 2007) but the availability of a simple screening test has led to an increased recognition of the milder forms of this condition, particularly those related to bilateral adrenal hyperplasia (BAH) (Funder et al., 2008).

This chapter will cover those syndromes listed in Table 11-1 in which secretion of the physiologic mineralocorticoid aldosterone is primarily increased. Chapter 13 will cover syndromes caused by increased secretion of other mineralocorticoids, e.g., deoxycorticosterone in congenital adrenal hyperplasias, or by cortisol acting on mineralocorticoid receptors, e.g., apparent mineralocorticoid excess.

As milder degrees of PA have been recognized by the wider application of the plasma aldosterone to renin ratio (ARR) as a screening or case-finding test, it has become increasingly clear that the majority of patients with an elevated ARR do not have a solitary adrenal adenoma that can be recognized by computed tomography (CT) or MRI (Mulatero et al., 2008). Therefore, bilateral adrenal venous sampling (AVS), a procedure that requires considerable expertise in performance and adds considerable expense to the workup is now recognized to be necessary for confirmation of the type of pathology (Young & Stanson 2009).

The need to establish the type of pathology is critical: Adenomas usually should be surgically removed; bilateral hyperplasia should never be surgically attacked but will almost always respond to medical therapy (Catena et al., 2007; Sukor et al., 2009).

The clinician is left in a dilemma: As the diagnosis of PA has become easier, the recognition of the type of pathology has become more difficult. Since CT imaging and MRI are often misleading and AVS requires considerable expertise, patients increasingly need referral to a center for definitive testing which is often difficult and always expensive.

To avoid this dilemma, this text will present the view that the ARR screening study should not be done except in hypertensive patients with unexplained hypokalemia, resistance to three-drug therapy, after the finding of an adrenal incidentaloma (as described in Chapter 12), or in the relatives of patients with a familial syndrome. This view does not take in all of the patients recommended for screening in the Clinical Practice Guidelines of the Endocrine Society (Funder et al., 2008) although the major categories are similar. Even if PA is sometimes missed, medical therapy—in particular the aldosterone receptor blockers spironolactone or eplerenone—will almost always control the hypertension and, if present, the hypokalemia and all of the additional harmful effects of aldosterone excess since they are mediated through the mineralocorticoid receptor. Thereby, the patients who have PA will likely be identified while expensive laboratory procedures, invasive diagnostic tests, and unnecessary surgery will be avoided in the majority of patients who do not.

This view, which will be detailed in the remainder of this chapter, may be too conservative. However, as of now, it seems to be the best balance between the multiple costs of diagnosis and the infrequency of the syndrome.

TABLE 11.1	Syndromes of Mineralocorticoid Excess

Aldosterone-producing adenoma
Bilateral hyperplasia
Primary unilateral adrenal hyperplasia
GRA Familial hyperaldosteronism, type I Familial
  hyperaldosteronism, type II
Adrenal carcinoma

DEFINITIONS

Primary aldosteronism is the syndrome resulting from the autonomous hypersecretion of aldosterone, almost always from the adrenal cortex, usually by a solitary adenoma or by bilateral hyperplasia, rarely by the variants of these two (Table 11-1).

Most aldosteronism seen in clinical practice is secondary to an increase in renin-angiotensin activity in response to a reduced renal profusion as seen with renal artery stenosis or chronic edematous states. The ability to measure plasma renin activity (PRA) has made the differentiation much easier, since renin is elevated in secondary aldosteronism and suppressed in PA.

INCIDENCE

After recognition of the multiple features of aldosterone excess in a single patient who was found at surgery to have a solitary adrenal adenoma, Conn (1955) went on to characterize the syndrome. Over the next decade, Conn et al. (1965) reported a high frequency of PA, found in almost 20% of the hypertensive patients at the University of Michigan. This high prevalence was subsequently thought to reflect the nature of the patients referred to that center, highly selected and suspected of having the disease. In most series of unselected patients reported in the 1970s and 1980s, classic PA was found in fewer than 0.5% of hypertensives (Kaplan, 1967; Gifford, 1969; Sinclair et al., 1987).

However, in the early 1990s, by the use of a simple screening test—the plasma ARR—one group of investigators in Brisbane, Australia, reported the finding of PA in 8.5% of 199 patients (Gordon et al., 1993). Subsequently, an abnormal ARR has been reported in 4% to 39% of hypertensives (Kaplan, 2007) but, as will be indicated later, that alone does not establish the diagnosis. Though the incidence of

PA is higher than previously thought, it is likely not to be as common as some now believe.

CLINICAL FEATURES

The disease is usually seen in patients between the ages of 30 and 50 years (though cases have been found in patients from the age of 3 to 75 years), and in women more frequently than in men. The syndrome has been recognized during pregnancy in hypokalemic patients with even higher aldosterone levels than expected and, most important, suppressed PRA (Al-Ali et al., 2007).

The classic clinical features of PA are hypertension, hypokalemia, excessive urinary potassium excretion, hypernatremia, and metabolic alkalosis (Fig. 11-1). The usual presence of these features reflects the pathophysiology of aldosterone excess.

Hypertension

Patients with PA are hypertensive, with very few exceptions (Medeau et al., 2008). The blood pressure (BP) may be quite high—the mean in one series of 136 patients was 205/123 (Ferriss et al., 1978b). In another series of 140 patients, 28 had severe, resistant hypertension (Bravo et al., 1988). More than a dozen cases have had malignant hypertension (Kaplan, 1963; Zarifis et al., 1996). The BP decline

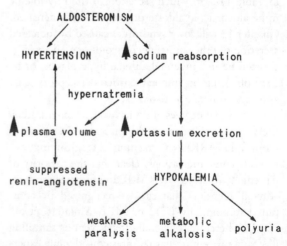

FIGURE 11-1 Pathophysiology of primary aldosteronism (Reprinted from Kaplan NM. Primary aldosteronism. In: Astwood EB, Cassidy CE, eds. *Clinical Endocrinology.* Vol. 2. New York: Grune & Stratton; 1968:468–472, with permission.)

(dip) during the night is usually attenuated (Zelinka et al., 2004).

Looked at in another way, increased levels of aldosterone and lower levels of renin may be seen before hypertension becomes manifest. Among 3,326 normotensive participants in the Framingham Heart Study, there was a continuous gradient of increased risk of BP progression with increasing ARR levels (Newton-Cheh et al., 2007). Similar findings were noted in a 5-year follow-up of 1,984 normotensives in France (Meneton et al., 2008).

Complications

Aldosterone levels inappropriate to sodium status exert deleterious effects on various tissues by rapid, nongenomic effects through their interaction with mineralocorticoid receptors (Rocha & Funder, 2002). Thereby vascular damage (Holaj et al., 2007) and fibrosis in the heart (Diez, 2008) and kidney (Reinke et al., 2009) occur so that cardiovascular complications reflect more than the accompanying hypertension (Milliez et al., 2005). In particular, left ventricular hypertrophy is usually disproportionate to the level and duration of hypertension (Muiesan et al., 2008).

Hemodynamics

Aldosterone infusions in conscious sheep induce hypertension by effects on the kidney (Sosa León et al., 2002) and, in humans, the hypertension is hemodynamically characterized by a slightly expanded plasma volume, an increased total body and exchangeable sodium content, and an increased peripheral resistance (Bravo, 1994; Williams et al., 1984). When ten patients with PA, previously well controlled on spironolactone, were studied 2 weeks after the drug was stopped and the hypertension reappeared, cardiac output and sodium content (both plasma volume and total exchangeable sodium) rose initially (Wenting et al., 1982) (Fig. 11-2). Between weeks 2 and 6, the hemodynamic patterns separated into two types: In five patients, the hypertension was maintained through increased cardiac output; in the other five, cardiac output and blood volume returned to their initial values, but total peripheral resistance rose markedly. Total body sodium space remained expanded in both groups, though more so in those with increased cardiac output (Man in't Veld et al., 1984). After surgery, the cardiac output fell in the high-flow patients, and the peripheral resistance fell in the high-resistance patients.

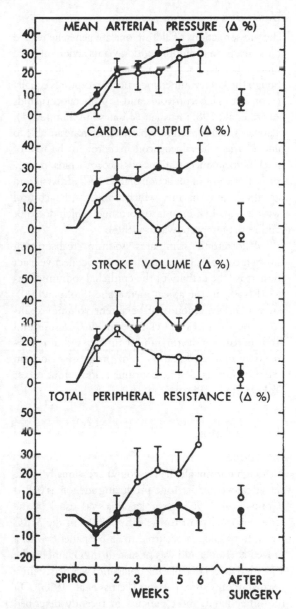

FIGURE 11-2 Changes (mean ± SEM) in systemic hemodynamics after discontinuation of spironolactone treatment (SPIRO) and after surgery in ten patients with primary aldosteronism. Note the fall in stroke volume and cardiac output after 2 weeks in the five patients with high-resistance hypertension (*open circles*) compared to the five with high-flow hypertension (*closed circles*). (Reprinted from Wenting GJ, Man in't Veld AJ, Derkx FHM, et al. Recurrence of hypertension in primary aldosteronism after discontinuation of spironolactone. Time course of changes in cardiac output and body fluid volumes. *Clin Exp Hypertens* 1982;4:1727–1748, with permission.)

Mechanism of Sodium Retention

The pressor actions of aldosterone are generally related to its effects on sodium retention via its action on renal mineralocorticoid receptors (Baxter et al., 2004). Even though the kidney mineralocorticoid receptor is equally receptive to glucocorticoids and to mineralocorticoids (Arriza et al., 1987; Farman & Rafestin-Oblin, 2001), relatively small concentrations of aldosterone are able to bind to the mineralocorticoid receptor in the face of much higher concentrations of glucocorticoids (mainly cortisol) because of the action of the 11β-hydroxysteroid dehydrogenase enzyme, which converts the cortisol (with its equal affinity) into cortisone, which does not bind to the receptor (Walker, 1993).

Aldosterone stimulates sodium reabsorption through complex genomic effects that collectively act to increase the activity of the epithelial sodium channel (ENaC) in the apical membrane (Stokes, 2000). After a certain amount of persistent volume expansion, the increases in renal perfusion pressure and atrial natriuretic factor inhibit further sodium reabsorption so that "escape" from progressive sodium retention occurs, despite continued aldosterone excess (Yokota et al., 1994).

Hypokalemia

Incidence

Although normokalemia was found occasionally in the classic cases of aldosterone-producing adenomas (APA) (Conn et al., 1965), hypokalemia was usual in the series reported prior to the early 1990s. In the MRC series, hypokalemia occurred in all 62 patients with a proved adenoma and was persistent in 53; among the 17 with hyperplasia, plasma potassium was persistently normal in only three patients (Ferriss et al., 1983). On the other hand, most patients in recently described series are normokalemic (Funder et al., 2008). There are a number of possible reasons why hypokalemia is now less common. These include:

- Most cases now being recognized are caused by BAH whose manifestations are usually milder than seen with APA. This includes the degree of potassium wastage.
- With more extensive screening, most cases are being recognized much earlier, before significant hypokalemia develops.
- Patients may experience considerable potassium loss without having the serum K^+ fall to the level as defined as hypokalemia. Whereas a patient's usual K^+ level

may be 4.8 mmol/L, a fall to 3.6 mmol/L may reflect significant K^+ loss but not be so recognized.
- There may be a disconnect between hypertension and hypokalemia. Hypertension may develop by other nongenomic effects of aldosterone in addition to the genomic mediation of increased renal sodium reabsorption. Thereby, hypertension may develop before significant K^+ wastage.
- If patients reduce the sodium intake for relief of hypertension, K^+ wastage will decrease.
- Caution should be used to ensure that hypokalemia is not inadvertently missed. A number of factors may cause a temporary and spurious rise in plasma potassium, including: A difficult and painful venipuncture may cause plasma potassium to rise for multiple reasons: If the patient hyperventilates, the respiratory alkalosis causes potassium to leave cells; repeated fist clenching causes potassium to leave the exercising muscles; if the tourniquet is left on, plasma potassium rises from venous stasis. In a series of 152 patients with PA, serum potassium was above 3.6 mmol/L in only 10.5% in samples obtained without fist clenching but in 69.1% after fist clenching with a tourniquet in place (Abdelhamid et al., 2003).
- Any degree of hemolysis.
- Efflux of potassium from blood cells if separation of plasma by centrifugation is delayed or if the sample is placed on ice.

With significant falls in serum and body K^+, aldosterone secretion may fall, even from otherwise autonomous adenomas (Kaplan, 1967). Therefore, potassium levels should be restored before aldosterone levels are measured.

Suppression of Renin Release

As a consequence of the initial expansion of vascular volume and the elevated BP, the baroreceptor mechanism in the walls of the renal afferent arterioles suppresses the secretion of renin to the point that renin mRNA may be undetectable in the kidney (Shionoiri et al., 1992). Almost all patients with PA have low levels of PRA that respond poorly to upright posture and diuretics, two maneuvers that usually raise PRA (Montori et al., 2001). Rarely, concomitant renal damage may stimulate renin release (Oelkers et al., 2000) but renin levels are almost always suppressed, even in those with malignant hypertension (Wu et al., 2000). The presence of a low renin in patients with therapy-resistant hypertension is a clue to the presence of PA (Eide et al., 2004).

Other Effects

- Hypernatremia is usual, unlike most forms of edematous secondary aldosteronism in which the sodium concentration is often quite low or with diuretic-induced hypokalemia in which slightly low serum sodium is usually found. Thus, the serum sodium concentration may provide a useful clinical separation between primary and secondary aldosteronism.
- Hypomagnesemia from excessive renal excretion of magnesium may produce tetany.
- Sodium retention and potassium wastage may be demonstrable wherever such exchange is affected by aldosterone: sweat, saliva, and stool.
- Atrial natriuretic peptide (ANP) levels are appropriately elevated for a state of volume expansion (Opocher et al., 1992).
- An increased prevalence of the "metabolic syndrome" has been noted in patients with PA (Pimenta & Calhoun, 2009). However, no such relationship was seen in a retrospective case-control study of 460 patients with PA beyond that seen in patients with primary (essential) hypertension (Matrozova et al., 2009). Moreover, plasma aldosterone levels were correlated with body mass index in patients with primary hypertension but not in patients with PA (Rossi et al., 2008a).

Familial Hyperaldosteronism Type II

Familial occurrence of PA was first reported in 1991 (Gordon et al., 1991) and now has been recognized in multiple families, involving over 100 patients (Sukor et al., 2008). No specific genetic mutation has been identified but studies have been consistent with linkage to a locus at chromosome 7p22.

The syndrome is referred to as FH type II because Gordon and associates have chosen to refer to glucocorticoid-remediable aldosteronism (GRA) as familial hyperaldosteronism type I.

Resistant Hypertension

Resistant hypertension refers to the persistence of BP above 140/90 mm Hg despite therapy with three antihypertensive drugs, including a diuretic, in full doses. Primary aldosteronism has been reported to be present in 20% to 40% of patients with resistant hypertension (Calhoun, 2007) based on the findings in small groups of patients. In a larger study of 251 patients with resistant hypertension, Pimenta

et al. (2007) made the diagnosis of PA in 59 patients (24%) on the basis of hormonal studies. These patients were subsequently reported to have higher aldosterone levels and indirect evidence of intravascular volume expansion (Gaddam et al., 2008). As in other reports of a high prevalence of PA among resistant hypertensives, the patients were studied while taking a variety of drugs that can variably alter both renin and aldosterone levels. The average number of such drugs was 4.2 per patient and 71% were on a β-blocker which is known to lower renin more than aldosterone, giving rise to falsely positive tests for PA.

In a much more convincing study of 1,616 patients with resistant hypertension, a number far larger than the total in all previous reports, the patients were studied after all antihypertensive drugs that could alter renin and aldosterone levels were discontinued (Douma et al., 2008). PA was diagnosed in 11.3% of these patients, using multiple tests to confirm the diagnosis. The authors conclude that since resistant hypertension is found in about 10% of hypertensive patients and since PA is present in about 10% of them, the overall prevalence of PA "in the general unselected hypertensive population is much lower than currently reported."

DIAGNOSIS

The diagnosis of PA is easy to make in patients with unprovoked hypokalemia and other manifestations of the fully expressed syndrome. The fact that hypokalemia was present in most patients in series published before 1990 likely reflects the failure to look for the syndrome in normokalemic hypertensives. Over the past decade, many more hypertensive patients have been found to have PA, the majority without hypokalemia. This higher frequency is largely the consequence of broader use of the ARR for case detection. The Clinical Practice Guideline (Funder et al., 2008) lists these groups as having a high prevalence of PA and therefore in need of testing:

- Moderate or severe hypertension, i.e., patients with systolic BP greater than 160 or diastolic BP greater than 100 mm Hg
- Resistant hypertension defined as BP above 140/90 despite treatment with three antihypertensive medications (This definition does not require the inclusion of a diuretic)
- Hypertensives with spontaneous or *diuretic-induced hypokalemia*
- Hypertension with adrenal incidentaloma

The adoption of these guidelines would call for testing of a large segment of the hypertensive population and, before their adoption, the warning by Grimes and Schulz (2002) should be noted:

> Screening has a darker side that is often overlooked. It can be inconvenient, unpleasant, and expensive... A second wave of injury can arise after the initial screening insult: false-positive results and true-positive results leading to dangerous interventions.

It therefore seems prudent to restrict testing to only portions of the four groups listed in the Guideline (Funder et al., 2008) for the following reasons:

- "Moderate" hypertension, from 160 to 180 systolic or 100 to 110 diastolic would subsume about 25% of all hypertensives.
- Hypertension should not be considered "resistant" unless therapy includes a diuretic. The prevalence of apparent resistance may subsume 30% of all hypertensives although far fewer, about 10%, are truly resistant.
- Hypokalemia induced by a diuretic may reflect nothing more than an effective diuretic that induces secondary aldosteronism. If such hypokalemia is resistant to the replacement of potassium, the likelihood of PA is likely greater.
- Only about 1% of adrenal incidentalomas have been found to have PA (Young, 2007a).

Urine Potassium

Although the ARR has largely replaced other case detection testing, if hypokalemia is present, a 24-hour urine sample should be collected for sodium and potassium levels before starting potassium-replacement therapy but 3 to 4 days after diuretics have been stopped. If the urine sodium is above 100 mmol/24 hours (to ensure that enough sodium is present to allow potassium wastage to express itself), the presence of a potassium level above 30 mmol/24 hours indicates a driven renal wastage of potassium. In addition to the action of excess mineralocorticoid in the syndromes of PA, a number of other conditions may require consideration, conditions in which hypokalemia is coupled with renal potassium wastage (Table 11-2).

Once the renal origin of hypokalemia is recognized, it may be preferable to correct the hypokalemia with potassium supplements, 40 to 80 mmol per day, after the discontinuation of diuretics before performing additional workup. To restore total body potassium

TABLE 11.2	Causes of Hypokalemia Due to Renal Loss of Potassium

I. High flow rate of potassium in the cortical collecting duct (CCD)
   A. Increased sodium excretion, e.g., diuretics
   B. Increased organic osmoles
      1. Glucose
      2. Urea
      3. Mannitol
II. High potassium concentration in the CCD
   A. With expanded intravascular volume (low plasma renin)
      1. Primary mineralocorticoid excess (Table 11-1)
      2. Liddle syndrome
      3. Amphotericin B
   B. With contracted intravascular volume (high plasma renin)
      1. Bartter syndrome
      2. Giletman syndrome
      3. Magnesium depletion
      4. Increased bicarbonate excretion
      5. Secondary aldosteronism, e.g., nephrotic syndrome

deficits after a prolonged diuretic use, a minimum of 3 weeks is needed, and it may take months. After a suitable interval, the supplemental potassium should be stopped for at least 3 days and the plasma potassium level should be rechecked. If plasma potassium is normal, plasma renin and aldosterone levels should bemeasured. Recall that if the plasma aldosterone is not definitely elevated in the presence of hypokalemia, it should be rechecked after potassium replenishment.

Plasma Aldosterone:Renin Ratio

The ARR is derived by dividing the plasma aldosterone (normal = 5 to 20 ng/dL) by the PRA (normal = 1 to 3 ng/mL/hour). If plasma aldosterone is measured in picomoles per liter and PRA in nanograms per liter, the values should be 27.7-fold higher, i.e., a ratio of 20 equals a ratio of 555 in SI units.

If plasma renin concentration (PRC)—also called "direct" or "active" renin assay—is obtained, ARR results will likely be reported as plasma aldosterone in pmol/L divided by PRC in mU/L (PA/PRC). The PRC values are approximately seven times the PRA values. In view of the limited experience with the direct renin assay, Mattsson and Young (2006) advise that it should not replace the PRA in testing.

The ARR should be performed with attention to a number of factors that can interfere with its validity as described in the Clinical Practice Guideline (Funder et al., 2008) (Table 11-3).

The first evidence that the ARR identified far more patients with PA than the small percentage previously recognized came from Gordon et al. (1993) from the Greenslopes Hospital in Brisbane, Australia. The Brisbane group's findings of a high prevalence of an elevated ARR have been replicated by a number of investigators in various countries throughout the world, mostly on patients referred to study centers (Table 11-4).

As noted in Table 11-4, there are considerable differences in the definition of an elevated ARR, with most of the ARR threshold levels representing the upper values obtained in patients presumed to have essential hypertension. The reported prevalence of an elevated ARR in hypertensive patients varies from 6% to as high as 39% in those referred because of resistant hypertension (Calhoun, 2007).

Despite the widespread use of the ARR to make important diagnostic and therapeutic decisions, very little study has been made of its test characteristics, i.e., sensitivity, specificity, and likelihood ratios at different cutoff values. At the conclusion of a systematic review of all of the literature on the ARR published from January 1966 to October 2001, Montori and Young (2002) state: "There are no published valid estimates of the test characteristics of the aldosterone-renin ratio when used as a screening test for primary aldosteronism in patients with presumed essential hypertension."

In an attempt to better characterize the ARR, Montori et al. (2001) studied 497 patients under varying circumstances. They made two conclusions: First, the ratio varied considerably in the same

---

TABLE 11.3   Measurement of the ARR

A. Preparation
 1. Correct hypokalemia if present
 2. Encourage patient to liberalize sodium intake
 3. Withdraw agents for at least 4 weeks that raise renin but may lower aldosterone causing false negatives
    a. Spironolactone, eplerenone, amiloride, and triamterene
    b. Potassium-wasting diuretics
    c. Products derived from licorice root
 4. Withdraw other medications that may affect the ARR for at least 2 weeks
    a. β-Adrenergic blockers, central α-2 agonist (e.g., clonidine), nonsteroidal antiinflammatory drugs which lower renin more than aldosterone causing false positives
    b. Angiotensin-converting enzyme inhibitors, angiotensin receptor blockers, direct renin inhibitors, dihydropyridine calcium channel blockers which raise renin and lower aldosterone causing false positives
 5. If necessary to maintain hypertension control, use other antihypertensive medications that have lesser effects on the ARR (e.g., verapamil slow-release, doxazosin)
 6. Estrogen-containing medications may cause false-positive ARR when PRC (rather than PRA) is measured
B. Conditions for collection of blood
 1. Collect blood midmorning, after the patient has been out of bed for at least 2 h and seated for 5–15 min
 2. Collect blood carefully, avoiding stasis and hemolysis
 3. Maintain the sample at room temperature (and not on ice, because this will promote conversion of inactive to active renin) before centrifugation and rapid freezing of plasma components pending assay
C. Factors to take into account when interpreting results
 1. Age: in patients aged >65 year, renin can be lowered more than aldosterone by age alone, leading to a raised ARR
 2. Time of the day, recent diet, posture, and the length of time in that posture
 3. Medications
 4. Method of blood collection, including any difficulty doing so
 5. Potassium levels
 6. Renal disease may raise aldosterone through hyperkalemia while lowering the secretion of renin, causing false positives

---

ARR, aldosterone to renin ratio; PRC, plasma renin concentration; PRA, plasma renin activity.
Modified from Funder JW, Carey RM, Fardella C, et al. Case detection, diagnosis, and treatment of patients with primary aldosteronism: An Endocrine Society clinical practice guideline. *J Clin Endocrinol Metab* 2008;93:3266–3281.

TABLE 11.4	The Prevalence of Autonomous Hyperaldosteronism and Aldosterone-Producing Adenomas (APA) in Patients Tested by Plasma Aldosterone to Plasma Renin Activity Ratio (ARR)[a]				
Reference	No. of Patients	ARR Threshold[a]	Raised ARR	Abnormal Suppression by Salt Loads	Proven APA
Hiramatsu (1981)	348	40	7.4%	NA[b]	2.6%
Gordon et al. (1993)	199	30	20.0%	8.5%	2.5%
Lim (1999)	125	27	14.0%	NA	NA
Lim (2000)	495	27	16.6%	9.2%	0.4%
Nishikawa (2000)	1020	20	6.4%	NA	4.2%
Loh (2000)	350	20 + PA > 15	18.0%	4.6%	1.7%
Rayner (2000)	216	36 + PA > 18	32.0%	NA	2.3%
Fardella (2000)	305	25	9.5%	4.9%	0.3%
Douma (2001)	978	30 + PA[c,d]	21.2%	13.8%	NA
Rossi (2002)	1046	35	12.8%	6.3%	1.5%
Hood (2002)	835	40	12.3%	NA	0.7%
Mulatero (2002)	2160	50	10.6%	7.0%	1.6%
Calhoun (2002)	88	20	NA	20.4%	NA
Girerd (2003)	143	NA	39%	NA	6%
Fogari (2003)	750	25	12%	6%	2%
Strauch (2003)	403	50	21.6%	19%	6.5%
Stowasser (2003)	~300	30	18.6%	17.7%	5%
Mosso (2003)	609	25	10.2%	6.1%	0%
Olivieri (2004)	287	50	32.4%	NA	NA
Giacchetti (2006)	157	40 + PA > 7 after IV saline	38.8%	100	16.6%
Williams (2006)	347	25 + PA > 8	7.5%	3.2	NA
Rossi (2006a,b)	1,125	40	11.2%	NA	4.8%
Douma (2008)	1,616	65 + PA > 15	20.9%	11.3	NA

[a]ARR expressed as plasma aldosterone in ng/dL, divided by PRA in ng/Ml/h.
[b]NA, not available.
[c,d]increased.

patients whose posture changed from supine to standing and even more so after diuretic therapy (25 mg of hydrochlorothiazide daily) for 4 weeks; second, the ratio was "strongly and inversely dependent on the PRA level," leading to the conclusion that "the aldosterone:renin ratio does not provide a renin-independent measure of circulating aldosterone that is suitable for determining whether plasma aldosterone concentration is elevated relative to PRA...Elevation of the ARR is predominantly an indicator of low PRA" (Montori et al., 2001).

Further concern over the sensitivity of the ARR has been raised by the data on repeated studies in 71 patients with a proven unilateral APA (Tanabe et al., 2003). The ARR was normal (below 35) in 31% of these patients on at least one occasion and only 37% had an abnormal ARR on all occasions.

The confounding effect of diuretic therapy noted by Montori et al. (2001) also applies to other antihypertensive medications. β-Blockers, by reducing PRA more than plasma aldosterone, can increase the number of false-positive ARRs and an ACE inhibitor or angiotensin receptor blocker may cause false-negative results (Mulatero et al., 2002). As seen in Table 11-3, the effect of these and other drugs must be considered in the preparation of the patient before performance of the ARR test.

Another probable source of inaccuracy with the ARR is the potential errors introduced by the increasing use of commercial renin activity and aldosterone assay kits in nonresearch labs (Stowasser & Gordon, 2006a).

As noted by Montori et al. (2001), the most common reason for false-positive ARRs is the presence of a low level of PRA as often found in the elderly, blacks, and hypertensives. With a not-unusual low PRA level of 0.3 ng/mL/hour, the presence of a normal plasma aldosterone level of 12 ng/dL would provide an ARR of 40 which by most investigators' current criteria (Table 11-4) would be abnormal.

To reduce this source of false-positive tests, some require an absolutely elevated plasma aldosterone level of 16 ng/dL or higher to call the ARR abnormal (Young, 2002). However, the Brisbane group does not, since in a description of 54 patients with documented PA, 20 had plasma aldosterone levels of 15 ng/dL or lower (Stowasser et al., 2003). Nonetheless, the wisdom of requiring an elevated plasma aldosterone has been documented in recent series, reducing false-positives from 30% to 3% in one (Seiler et al., 2004).

There is a need for establishing the "correct" cut-off of the ARR, so as to miss very few with PA, i.e., high sensitivity, and not to require additional workup in those without PA, i.e., high specificity. Many attempts have been made including a study by Bernini et al. (2008) which concluded that an ARR of 69 provided the best balance of sensitivity, 98%, and specificity, 85%. However, their high ARR could reflect their patient population who had severe degrees of aldosteronism and who were on a sodium-restricted diet.

The continued confusion over the performance and interpretation of the ARR has led the authors of the Clinical Practice Guideline to this conclusion:

> Although it would clearly be desirable to provide firm recommendations for ARR and plasma aldosterone cut-offs, the variability of assays between laboratories and the divided literature to date make it more prudent to point out relative advantages and disadvantages, leaving clinicians the flexibility to judge for themselves (Funder et al., 2008)

This position is clearly not suitable for the guidance of practitioners who must manage most patients. The best advice is to carefully follow all of the steps listed in Table 11-3, ensuring that patients are properly prepared and the blood sample is obtained under appropriate conditions. Then the levels of plasma aldosterone and renin activity should be examined without calculating a ratio. If the PRA is definitely low (below 0.5 ng/mL/hour) and the plasma aldosterone is definitely high (above 15 mg/dL), the same measurement of aldosterone and renin activity should be obtained on another occasion as recommended by Gordon and Stowasser (2007). If both low PRA and

high aldosterone levels are found again, a confirmatory test should be performed.

All of this, of course, assumes that the patient is willing and able to undergo a laparoscopic adrenalectomy if the remainder of the workup confirms the presence of an APA.

Confirmatory Tests

Elevated and Nonsuppressible Aldosterone

If the PRA is low and the aldosterone is high, the presence of an inappropriately elevated and nonsuppressible aldosterone level should be documented. This was first demonstrated with the saline suppression test of plasma aldosterone (Kem et al., 1971). Plasma aldosterone is measured before and after the infusion of 2 L of normal saline over 4 hours. Patients with PA have higher basal levels but, more importantly, fail to suppress these levels after saline to below 5 ng/dL (Mulatero et al., 2006). Some patients with adrenal hyperplasia may suppress to a level between 5 and 10 ng/dL after saline (Holland et al., 1984), but the level was not found to discriminate between an APA and a bilateral hyperplasia (Rossi et al., 2007).

Some prefer to measure urine aldosterone levels after 3 days of oral sodium loading, with an abnormal level being above 12 (Young, 2002) or 14 μg/24 hours (Bravo, 1994). However, the Brisbane group has found that both the intravenous and oral salt loading tests are often inaccurate and they utilize a high salt diet plus large doses of the mineralocorticoid Florinef over a 4-day hospitalization, the FST test (Stowasser et al., 2003).

Captopril Suppression

Whereas plasma aldosterone levels were markedly suppressed 3 hours after oral intake of 1 mg captopril per kilogram of the body weight in patients with essential hypertension or renovascular hypertension, they remained elevated in patients with primary hyperaldosteronism (Thibonnier et al., 1982). The normal response is a full in plasma aldosterone of 30% or more (Funder et al., 2008).

Rule Out Glucocorticoid-Remediable Aldosteronism

GRA should be considered in a young patient, particularly if other family members have aldosteronism or hemorrhagic stroke. This is most easily confirmed by demonstrating the hybrid gene in a blood sample (see below).

Excluding Other Diseases

Various causes of secondary aldosteronism are easily excluded by the presence of edema and high levels of peripheral blood PRA. In addition, there are a number of monogenic forms of hypertension, most involving renal tubular disorders, some associated with hypertension and hypokalemia, that should not be confused with PA (Stowasser & Gordon, 2006b) (Table 11-5).

Those listed under Hypertension and Hypokalemia also have suppressed, low PRA but all have low aldosterone levels, either because of the secretion of other mineralocorticoids (glucocorticoid-remediable hyperaldosteronism and congenital adrenal hyperplasia caused by either 11β-hydroxylase or 17-α-hydroxylase deficiency) or because of increased cortisol acting as a mineralocorticoid (apparent mineralocorticoid excess, to be covered in Chapter 14), increased sodium reabsorption from activated sodium channels (Liddle syndrome), or increased activity of mineralocorticoid receptors (Geller et al., 2000).

Glucocorticoid-Remediable Aldosteronism (Familial hyperaldosteronism, Type I)

Sutherland et al. (1966) described a father and son with classic features of PA whose entire syndrome was completely relieved by dexamethasone, 0.5 mg four times a day (i.e., glucocorticoid remediable). Subsequently, the syndrome was shown to follow an autosomal dominant mode of inheritance and to be associated with increased levels of 18-hydroxylated cortisol. Ulick et al. (1990) postulated that the syndrome was the result of the acquisition of aldosterone

synthase activity by cells of the zona fasciculata. This would explain the high levels of 18-hydroxylated steroids which can be suppressed by exogenous glucocorticoid which in turn suppresses ACTH, the normal stimulus to synthetic activity within the zona fasciculata.

Genetic Confirmation

The correctness of Ulick et al.'s postulate was proven by Lifton et al. (1992) who found "complete linkage of glucocorticoid-remediable aldosteronism to a gene duplication arising from unequal crossing over, fusing the 5 regulatory region of 11-beta-hydroxylase to the 3' coding sequences of aldosterone synthase" (Fig. 11-3). The two genes lie next to one another on human chromosome 8 and are 94% identical, likely explaining the propensity to cross over (Dluhy & Lifton, 1999).

Clinical and Laboratory Features

As more patients with GRA have been identified, variations in both genotype and phenotype have been identified (Holloway et al., 2009). Different sites of gene crossover do not seem to influence the phenotype, and considerably different phenotypes have been seen within a single family that are not accounted for by different genotypes (Fallo et al., 2004).

The hyperaldosteronism is usually evident at birth with inheritance as an autosomal dominant trait, occurring equally among men and women. The hypertension is often severe, poorly responsive to usual antihypertensive therapy, but some affected subjects in pedigrees are normotensive. An increased prevalence of strokes, particularly cerebral hemorrhage from intracranial aneurysm, has been reported

---

TABLE 11.5   Monogenic Forms of Hypertension

Disorder	Inheritance	Consequence of Mutant Gene
Hypertension and Hypokalemia		
Glucocorticoid-remediable aldosteronism (familial hyperaldosteronism, type I)	Dominant	Increased mineralocorticoids from chimeric 11-β-hydroxylase and aldosterone synthase genes
Apparent mineralocorticoid excess	Recessive	Reduced inactivation of cortisol due to 11-β-HSD deficiency
Mutation of mineralocorticoid receptor	Dominant	Increased activity of mineralocorticoid receptor
Liddle syndrome	Dominant	Increased activity of epithelial sodium channel
Hypertension and Hyperkalemia		
Pseudohypoaldosteronism, type II (Gordon syndrome)	Dominant	Increased chloride reabsorption in distal tubule

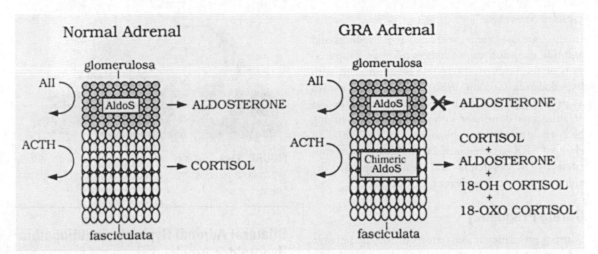

FIGURE 11-3 Regulation of aldosterone production in the zona glomerulosa and cortisol production in the zona fasciculate in the normal adrenal, and model of the physiologic abnormalities in the adrenal cortex in GRA. Ectopic expression of aldosterone synthase enzymatic activity in the adrenal fasciculate results in GRA. (Reprinted from Lifton RP, Dluhy RG, Powers M, et al. Hereditary hypertension caused by chimaeric gene duplications and ectopic expression of aldosterone synthase. *Nature Genet* 1992;2:66–74, with permission.)

(Dluhy & Lifton, 1999). About half of affected patients are normokalemic, explained by a number of factors, including a lesser mineralocorticoid activity of the 18-hydroxylated steroids and the inability of dietary potassium to stimulate aldosterone secretion when it arises from the zona fasciculata (Litchfield et al., 1997).

Diagnosis

Initially, the definitive diagnosis was based on dexamethasone suppression of aldosterone but now that genetic testing is so readily available, this is the preferred procedure. The genetic test can be arranged by sending an e-mail to Richard.lifton@yale.edu.

Treatment

Suppressive doses of exogenous glucocorticoid will usually control the hypertension even if all the hormonal perturbations are not normalized (Stowasser et al., 2000). Spironolactone with or without a thiazide diuretic has been used without glucocorticoid suppression (Dluhy & Lifton, 1999).

Nonglucocorticoid-remediable aldosteronism

Geller et al. (2008) have reported another familial form of aldosteronism with severe hypertension appearing by age 7 with very high levels of 18-hydroxylated steroids which were not suppressed by dexamethasone.

Bilateral adrenalectomy was performed because of unrelenting hypertension and massive hyperplasia was found.

Liddle Syndrome

Liddle et al. (1963) described members of a family with hypertension, hypokalemic alkalosis, and negligible aldosterone secretion, apparently resulting from an unusual tendency of the kidneys to conserve sodium and excrete potassium even in the virtual absence of mineralocorticoids. Such patients have a mutation of the β or γ subunits of the renal epithelial sodium channel which causes increased sodium reabsorption in the distal nephron (Furuhashi et al., 2005). As will be noted in Chapter 13, these clinical features are also seen in apparent mineralocorticoid excess caused by mutations in 11β-hydroxysteroid dehydrogenase, preventing conversion of cortisol to cortisone.

Activation of Mineralocorticoid Receptor

Geller et al. (2000) identified a mutation in the mineralocorticoid receptor that causes early-onset hypertension that is markedly exacerbated in pregnancy. The exacerbation is a consequence of an altered receptor specificity so that the high levels of progesterone and other steroids lacking 21-hydroxyl groups become potent agonists.

Gordon Syndrome

In this rare syndrome, increased renal sodium and chloride retention causes hypertension and suppression of the renin-aldosterone mechanism, but with hyperkalemia (Gordon, 1986). The syndrome, known as pseudohypoaldosteronism type II, is inherited as an autosomal dominant with at least three loci having been recognized (Disse-Nicodème et al., 2000). An elevated ARR has been noted with aldosterone stimulated by hyperkalemia and renin suppressed by volume expansion (Stowasser, 2000).

During Pregnancy

Normal pregnancy is associated with elevated plasma aldosterone but also elevated renin activity. In 31 reported cases of PA diagnosed during pregnancy, usually presenting with marked hypokalemia, renin levels were reduced (Lindsay & Nieman, 2006). Moreover, preexisting hypertension due to PA may be ameliorated during pregnancy, perhaps by antagonism of the effects of elevated aldosterone by the high progesterone levels (Murakami et al., 2000). Management is complicated by the inability to use most medical therapies and laparoscopic adrenalectomy may be the preferred treatment.

TYPES OF ADRENAL PATHOLOGY

Once the diagnosis of PA is made, the type of adrenal pathology must be ascertained since the choice of therapy is different: surgical for an adenoma, medical for hyperplasia. This need is even greater today than in the past as recognition of patients with milder manifestations of aldosteronism is so much easier and more frequently performed.

Aldosterone-Producing Adenomas

Solitary benign adenomas (Fig. 11-4) are almost always unilateral and most are small, weighing less than 6 g and measuring less than 3 cm in diameter. In various series, from 20% to 85% are smaller than 1 cm (Rossi et al., 2001). Histologically, most adenomas are composed of lipid-laden cells arranged in small acini or cords, similar in appearance and arrangement to the normal zona fasciculata, the middle zone of the adrenal cortex. Moreover, focal or diffuse hyperplasia, as seen in Figure 11-4, is usually present in both the remainder of the adrenal with the adenoma and the contralateral gland (Lack et al., 1990).

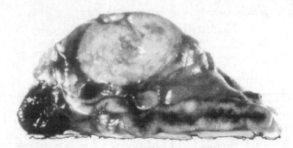

FIGURE 11-4 Solitary adrenal adenoma with diffuse hyperplasia removed from a patient with primary aldosteronism.

Bilateral Adrenal Hyperplasia (Idiopathic Hyperaldosteronism)

In the late 1960s, reports of hyperaldosteronism with no adenoma but rather with BAH began to appear (Davis et al., 1967) and it was referred to as idiopathic hyperaldosteronism (IHA) (Biglieri et al., 1970). As more patients have been screened, the proportion of PA related to BAH has steadily increased from less than one third in the 1970s to more than two thirds in the 2000s (Young, 2007b).

The better detail provided by newer imaging procedures may lead to confusion: Because the hyperplasia that often accompanies an adenoma can now be recognized, bilateral hyperplasia may be mistakenly diagnosed on the one hand; because nodularity is often seen with hyperplasia, an adenoma may be mistakenly diagnosed on the other (Young, 2007b). The presence of bilateral hyperplasia suggests a secondary response to some stimulatory mechanism rather than a primary neoplastic growth but none has been identified. Lim et al. (2002) postulate that in susceptible hypertensives, an increased sensitivity to angiotensin II may gradually induce adrenal hyperplasia that becomes autonomous, i.e., "tertiary aldosteronism."

It should be recalled that, soon after the description of hyperaldosteronism associated with BAH, members of the MRC BP Unit at the Western Infirmary in Glasgow published a series of papers with convincing evidence that this condition was totally different from Conn syndrome of aldosterone-producing adenoma (Table 11-6) (Ferriss et al., 1970). They referred to BAH as simply a form of "low-renin essential hypertension" (McAreavey et al., 1983).

Moreover, there is a progressive increase in adrenal nodular hyperplasia with age having no relationship to hypertension (Tracy & White, 2002). Therefore, the increased frequency of cases with hyperplasia may simply reflect the natural changes with age: increased adrenal nodular hyperplasia, progressively lower renin but maintained aldosterone levels (Guthrie et al., 1976), giving rise to an elevated aldosterone:renin ratio without hyperaldosteronism. This scenario is in keeping with the MRC investigators' belief that these patients have "low-renin essential hypertension" (McAreavey et al., 1983).

Unilateral Hyperplasia

Even more difficult to explain than the presence of bilateral hyperplasia are the 30 reported cases of hyperaldosteronism that apparently are caused by hyperplasia of only one adrenal gland (Goh et al., 2007).

Other Pathologies
Carcinoma

Aldosterone-producing carcinomas are rare, with only 58 having been reported from 1955 to 2003 (Seccia et al., 2005). Most are associated with concomitant hypersecretion of other adrenal hormones,

but a few may hypersecrete only aldosterone (Touitou et al., 1992).

Associated conditions

Patients have been reported with PA caused by an adrenal adenoma in association with acromegaly (Dluhy & Williams, 1969), primary hyperparathyroidism, the multiple endocrine neoplasia I syndrome (Gordon et al., 1995), neurofibromatosis (Biagi et al., 1999), familial adenomatous polyposis (Alexander et al., 2000), renal artery stenosis (Mansoor et al., 2002), and end-stage renal disease (Kazory & Weiner, 2007).

Extra-adrenal tumors

Single ectopic aldosterone-producing tumors have been found in the kidney (Abdelhamid et al., 1996) and ovary (Kulkarni et al., 1990).

DIAGNOSING THE TYPE OF ADRENAL PATHOLOGY

Various procedures have been used to diagnose the type of adrenal pathology but AVS is now recommended even when there is no apparent ambiguity by CT scans because of the vagaries of adrenal pathology

TABLE 11.6 Differences Between Aldosterone-Producing Adenoma, Bilateral Adrenal Hyperplasia, and Low-Renin Hypertension[a]

	Aldosterone-Producing Adenoma	Bilateral Adrenal Hyperplasia	Low-Renin Essential Hypertension
Clinical Features			
Age	Middle-aged	Older	Older
Hypokalemia	Frequent	Less common	Uncommon
Hemodynamics			
Body sodium content	Increased	Normal	Normal
Plasma aldosterone in response to standing	Fall	Rise	Rise
Hormonal			
Plasma renin levels	Very low	Low	Low
Plasma aldosterone levels	Very high	High-normal	Normal
Aldosterone secretion	Autonomous	Responsive to AII[b]	Responsive to AII[b]
Aldosterone suppressibility to volume loads	Minimal	Partial	Complete
Aldosterone to angiotensin relation	Inverse	Direct	Direct
Hybrid steroids	Present	Absent	Absent
Relief by surgical removal	Usual	Extremely rare	Never

[a]Based on data included in Ferris et al. (1970) and McAreavey et al. (1983).
[b]AII, angiotensin II.

(Funder et al., 2008). Erros still occur: BAH is operated upon, with limited success (Sukor et al., 2009).

Ancillary Procedures

In general, autonomous lesions that can be cured by surgery (adenomas and the rare primary adrenal hyperplasia) display their autonomy from the normal control of aldosterone production by the renin-angiotensin mechanism by having (a) high levels of aldosterone and its precursor 18-OH-corticosterone (Auchus et al., 2007), (b) little or no response to stimulation of renin-angiotensin such as during an upright posture test, and (c) the production of hybrid steroids such as 18-OH-cortisol. None of these are now recommended for measurement.

Adrenal Computed Tomography

The Clinical Practice Guideline recommends an adrenal CT scan "as the initial study in subtype testing" (Funder et al., 2008). Other investigators also recommend routine CT scans (Mattsson & Young, 2006; Mulatero et al., 2008; Schirpenbach & Reincke, 2007). However, as stated by Rossi et al. (2008b), "adrenal imaging is insufficient to achieve discrimination between APA and IHA" and they did not include CT scanning in their algorithm for the diagnostic workup of PA.

The inaccuracy of CT scans (which are preferable to MRI) was clearly demonstrated in the Mayo Clinic series of 194 patients with PA who had both CT scan and AVS, the most accurate discriminator (Young et al., 2004). The CT scan correctly identified only 53% with either unilateral or bilateral lesions. CT scans showed an APA in 24% who had bilateral lesions and who would thereby be subjected to inappropriate adrenalectomy. CT scans showed bilateral disease in 21% who had an APA and would thereby be denied an indicated adrenalectomy. CT scans showed an APA in the wrong adrenal in 12 patients. Similar data showing the fallibility of CT scans when compared to AVS have been published by other investigators (Magill et al., 2001; Nwariaku et al., 2006).

The Mayo Clinic investigators (Mattsson & Young, 2006) continue to rely on the presence by CT scan of a solitary unilateral macroadenoma, larger than 1 cm, with normal contralateral adrenal morphology in patients with PA below age 40 (who are much more likely to have an adenoma than BAH) to recommend surgery without AVS. However, they too recognize the frequent need for AVS in most patients whose CT findings are less certain.

Adrenal Venous Sampling

AVS is now recognized as the definitive procedure to differentiate unilateral from bilateral disease in patients with confirmed PA. One of the first reports of the value of AVS was that of Rossi et al. (2001) who reported their findings in 104 patients with PA and equivocal CT or MRI findings. AVS was feasible in 97.1% of attempts and, in 80.6% of cases, bilateral samples were obtained almost simultaneously. With bilateral selective AVS, a value of aldosterone/cortisol of one side over the contralateral side of 2 or greater identified a unilateral source of excess aldosterone in 80% of the patients. However, at least 10 ways to perform and interpret AVS have been published (Kline et al., 2008). These investigators conclude that the greatest accuracy is obtained when hormonal levels are used to confirm the catheter positioning before samples are obtained to calculate the lateralization. They also note that the true specificity and sensitivity of AVS have not been validated since only those with lateralization undergo surgery.

AVS should only be performed in centers with experience with the procedure. Even in the hands of such experienced investigators, 20% of patients cannot be correctly characterized by AVS, although better results have been reported in more recent series (Nwariaku et al., 2006; Young et al., 2004).

All who perform AVS or who wish to interpret data from the procedure should read the Clinical Practice Guideline (Funder et al., 2008).

Adrenal Scintigraphy

Adrenal scintiscans with the isotope 6-β-[^{131}I]-iodomethyl-19-norcholesterol (NP-59) have been used to identify the site of aldosterone hypersecretion (Rossi et al., 2008b). Since small adenomas with relatively low uptake of the tracer may give false-negative results (Nakahama et al., 2003), this procedure will rarely need to be utilized.

Overall Plan

As seen in Figure 11-5, the diagnosis of PA should be looked for in patients considered to have an increased prevalence. Only 10% to 20% of these patients will have the combination of a low PRA and high aldosterone level. Those should then have a test to confirm autonomous hyperaldosteronism. Approximately half of these will be confirmed and they should have AVS. As noted earlier, there seems to be no value and a potential for serious mistakes by CT scanning so this is not part of the algorithm.

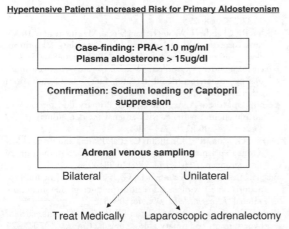

Hypertensive Patient at Increased Risk for Primary Aldosteronism

Case-finding: PRA< 1.0 mg/ml
Plasma aldosterone > 15ug/dl

Confirmation: Sodium loading or Captopril suppression

Adrenal venous sampling

Bilateral   Unilateral

Treat Medically   Laparoscopic adrenalectomy

FIGURE 11-5 A diagnosis flow chart for evaluating and treating patients with primary aldosteronism. PA, primary aldosteronism; PRA, plasma renin activity.

Remember that young patients and particularly those with a family history of aldosteronism should be evaluated for GRA, as described earlier in this chapter. The problem of excluding adrenal hyperfunction in patients with an adrenal incidentaloma is addressed in the first portion of Chapter 12.

THERAPY

Once the type of adrenal pathology has been ascertained, surgery should be done if the diagnosis is *adenoma*, and medical therapy is indicated if the diagnosis is *bilateral hyperplasia*. There are reports of relief of aldosteronism by removal of a unilaterally hyperplastic gland (Goh et al., 2007), so surgery should only be performed if AVS clearly defines a unilateral source of the aldosterone hypersecretion.

Surgical Treatment

Preoperative Management
Once the diagnosis of adenoma is made, a 3- to 5-week course of spironolactone therapy may be given to normalize the various disturbances of electrolyte composition and fluid volume, easing anesthetic, surgical, and postoperative management.

Surgical Technique
With improved preoperative diagnosis of an adenoma, laparoscopic adrenalectomy has become the procedure of choice (Funder et al., 2008). If hyperplasia is found at surgery despite the preoperative diagnosis of an adenoma, only a unilateral adrenalectomy should be done. In view of the poor overall results with bilateral adrenalectomy and its complications, one gland should be left intact.

Postoperative Course
Hypertension is relieved without the need for antihypertensive drugs in 35% to 60% and improved in most of the remainder (Letavernier et al., 2008; Pang et al., 2007; Zarnegar et al., 2008). The likelihood of complete resolution of hypertension is greater in those patients who required only two or fewer antihypertensive drugs pre-operatively, who are not obese, who are female, and who have had hypertension for less than 6 years (Zarnegar et al., 2008).

Postoperative Complications
Hypoaldosteronism
The patient, even if given spironolactone preoperatively, may develop hypoaldosteronism with an inability to conserve sodium and excrete potassium. This may persist for some time after renin levels return to normal, analogous to the slowness of the return of cortisol production after prolonged ACTH suppression by exogenous glucocorticoids.

The aldosterone deficiency is usually not severe or prolonged and can be handled simply by providing adequate salt without the need for exogenous glucocorticoid or mineralocorticoid therapy.

Sustained Hypertension
The hypertension may persist for some time; a few patients require years for the return of normal BP. If the BP fails to respond, hyperfunctioning adrenal tissue may have been left. More likely is the presence of coincidental primary hypertension, as would be expected in at least 20% of cases, or the occurrence of significant renal damage from the prolonged hypertension (Reincke et al., 2009). In 99 patients who had bilateral hyperplasia, relief of hypertension after unilateral or bilateral adrenalectomy occurred in only 19% (Funder et al., 2008).

Medical Treatment
Chronic medical therapy with spironolactone or eplerenone or, if those are not tolerated, amiloride with or without a thiazide diuretic is the treatment of choice for patients with hyperplasia, patients with an adenoma who are unable or unwilling to have surgery, patients who remain hypertensive after

surgery, and patients with equivocal findings (Funder et al., 2008).

Spironolactone usually lowers the BP and keeps it down (Ferriss et al., 1978a). PA patients treated with spironolactone had a slower but eventually equal regression of left ventricular hypertrophy as those who had unilateral adrenalectomy (Catena et al., 2007). Although higher doses may initially be needed, a satisfactory response may then be maintained with as little as 25 to 50 mg a day. The combination of spironolactone with a thiazide diuretic may provide even better control and allow for smaller doses of spironolactone. With these lower doses, the various side effects are generally minor, and in only three of 95 cases were they severe enough to lead to withdrawal of the drug (Ferriss et al., 1978a). A more selective aldosterone receptor antagonist, eplerenone, is now available, providing somewhat less receptor blockade but fewer side effects than spironolactone (McManus et al., 2008), and it will likely be the medical therapy of choice. If additional antihypertensive therapy is needed, CCBs may be preferable since, in high doses, they have some aldosterone receptor antagonist activity (Dietz et al., 2008).

In patients with adrenal cancer, various inhibitors of steroidogenesis are useful. These are described in the next chapter in the section "Treatment of Cushing Syndrome."

CONCLUSIONS

Primary aldosteronism remains a fascinating disease that is more common than previously thought but less common than some now claim. Other mineralocorticoid-induced forms of hypertension are covered in the next chapter.

REFERENCES

Abdelhamid S, Blomer R, Hommel G, et al. Urinary tetrahydroaldosterone as a screening method for primary aldosteronism: A comparative study. *Am J Hypertens* 2003;16:522–530.

Abdelhamid S, Müller-Lobeck, Pahl S, et al. Prevalence of adrenal and extra-adrenal Conn syndrome in hypertensive patients. *Arch Intern Med* 1996;156:1190–1195.

Al-Ali NA, El-Sandabesee D, Steel SA, et al. Conn's syndrome in pregnancy successfully treated with amiloride. *J Obstet Gynaecol* 2007;27:730–731.

Alexander GL, Thompson GB, Schwartz DA. Primary aldosteronism in a patient with familial adenomatous polyposis. *Mayo Clin Proc* 2000;75:636–637.

Arriza JL, Weinberger C, Cerelli G, et al. Cloning of human mineralocorticoid receptor complementary DNA: Structural and functional kinship with the glucocorticoid receptor. *Science* 1987;237:268–275.

Auchus RJ, Chandler DW, Singeetham S, et al. Measurement of 18-hydroxycorticosterone during adrenal vein sampling for primary aldosteronism. *J Clin Endocrinol Metab* 2007;92:2648–2651.

Baxter JD, Funder JW, Apriletti JW, et al. Towards selectively modulating mineralocorticoid receptor function: Lessons from other systems. *Mol Cell Endocrinol* 2004;217:151–165.

Bernini G, Moretti A, Argenio G, et al. Primary aldosteronism in normokalemic patients with adrenal incidentalomas. *Eur J Endocrinol* 2002;146:523–529.

Bernini G, Moretti A, Orlandini C, et al. Plasma and urine aldosterone to plasma renin activity ratio in the diagnosis of primary aldosteronism. *J Hypertens* 2008;26:981–988.

Biagi P, Alessandri M, Campanella G, et al. A case of neurofibromatosis type 1 with an aldosterone-producing adenoma of the adrenal. *J Intern Med* 1999;246:509–512.

Biglieri EG, Schambelan M, Slaton PE Jr, et al. The intercurrent hypertension of primary aldosteronism. *Circ Res* 1970;26/27 (Suppl I): I195–I202.

Bravo EL. Primary aldosteronism: Issues in diagnosis and management. *Endocrinol Metab Clin* 1994;23:271–283.

Bravo EL, Fouad-Tarazi FM, Tarazi RC, et al. Clinical implications of primary aldosteronism with resistant hypertension. *Hypertension* 1988;11(Suppl 1):207–211.

Calhoun DA. Is there an unrecognized epidemic of primary aldosteronism? *Pro. Hypertension* 2007;50:447–453.

Calhoun DA, Nishizaka MK, Zaman MA, et al. Hyperaldosteronism among black and white subjects with resistant hypertension. *Hypertension* 2002;40:892–896.

Catena C, Colussi G, Lapenna R, et al. Long-term cardiac effects of adrenalectomy or mineralocorticoid antagonists in patients with primary aldosteronism. *Hypertension* 2007;50:911–917.

Conn JW. Part I. Painting background. Part II. Primary aldosteronism, a new clinical syndrome. *J Lab Clin Med* 1955;43:317.

Conn JW, Cohen ED, Rovner DR, et al. Normokalemic primary aldosteronism: A detectable cause of curable "essential" hypertension. *JAMA* 1965;193:200–206.

Davis WW, Newsome HH Jr, Wright LD Jr, et al. Bilateral adrenal hyperplasia as a cause of primary aldosteronism with hypertension, hypokalemia and suppressed renin activity. *Am J Med* 1967;42:642–647.

Dietz JD, Du S, Bolten CW, et al. A number of marketed dihydropyridine calcium channel blockers have mineralocorticoid receptor antagonist activity. *Hypertension* 2008;51:742–748.

Diez J. Effects of aldosterone on the heart: Beyond systemic hemodynamics? *Hypertension* 2008;52:462–464.

Disse-Nicodème S, Achard JM, Desitter I, et al. A new locus on chromosome 12p13.3 for pseudohypoaldosteronism type II, an autosomal dominant form of hypertension. *Am J Hum Genet* 2000;67:302–310.

Dluhy RG, Lifton RP. Glucocorticoid-remediable aldosteronism. *J Clin Endocrinol Metab* 1999;84:4341–4344.

Dluhy RG, Williams GH. Primary aldosteronism in a hypertensive acromegalic patient. *J Clin Endocrinol* 1969;29:1319–1324.

Douma S, Petidis K, Vogiatzis K, et al. The aldosterone/PRA ratio (ARR) application in the diagnosis of primary aldosteronism [Abstract]. *J Hypertens* 2001;19(Suppl 2):S12.

Douma S, Petidis K, Doumas M, et al. Prevalence of primary hyperaldosteronism in resistant hypertension: a retrospective observational study. *Lancet* 2008;371:1921–1926.

Eide IK, Torjesen PA, Drolsum A, et al. Low-renin status in therapy-resistant hypertension: A clue to efficient treatment. *J Hypertens* 2004;22:2217–2226.

Fallo F, Pilon C, Williams TA, et al. Coexistence of different phenotypes in a family with glucocorticoid-remediable aldosteronism. *J Hum Hypertens* 2004;18:47–51.

Fardella CE, Mosso L, Gomez-Sanchez C, et al. Primary aldosteronism in essential hypertensives: prevalence, biochemical profile, and molecular biology. *J Clin Endocrinol Metab* 2000;85: 1863–1867.

Farman N, Rafestin-Oblin M-E. Multiple aspects of mineralocorticoid sensitivity. *Am J Physiol Renal Physiol* 2001;280:F181–F192.

Ferriss JB, Beevers DG, Boddy K, et al. The treatment of low-renin ("primary") hyperaldosteronism. *Am Heart J* 1978a;96: 97–109.

Ferriss JB, Beevers DG, Brown JJ, et al. Clinical, biochemical and pathological features of low-renin ("primary") hyperaldosteronism. *Am Heart J* 1978b;95:375–388.

Ferriss JB, Brown JJ, Fraser R, et al. Hypertension with aldosterone excess and low plasma-renin: Preoperative distinction between patients with and without adrenocortical tumour. *Lancet* 1970;2:995–1000.

Ferriss JB, Brown JJ, Fraser R, et al. Primary aldosterone excess: Conn's syndrome and similar disorders. In: Robertson JIS, ed. *Handbook of Hypertension*. Vol. 2, Clinical Aspects of Secondary Hypertension, New York: Elsevier; 1983.

Fogari R, Preti P, Mugellini A, et al. Prevalence of primary aldosteronism among hypertensive pateints [Abstract]. *J Hypertens* 2003; 21(Suppl 4): S142.

Freedman BI, Hsu FC, Langefeld CD et al. Renal artery calcified plaque associations with subclinical renal and cardiovascular disease. *Kidney Int* 2004;65:2262–2267.

Funder JW, Carey RM, Fardella C, et al. Case detection, diagnosis, and treatment of patients with primary aldosteronism: An Endocrine Society clinical practice guideline. *J Clin Endocrinol Metab* 2008;93:3266–3281.

Furuhashi M, Kitamura K, Adachi M, et al. Liddle's syndrome caused by a novel mutation in the proline-rich PY motif of the epithelial sodium channel β-subunit. *J Clin Endocrinol Metab* 2005;90:340–344.

Gaddam KK, Nishizaka MK, Pratt-Ubunama MN, et al. Characterization of resistant hypertension: Association between resistant hypertension, aldosterone, and persistent intravascular volume expansion. *Arch Intern Med* 2008;168: 1159–1164.

Geller DS, Farhl A, Pinkerton N, et al. Activating mineralocorticoid receptor mutation in hypertension exacerbated by pregnancy. *Science* 2000;289:119–123.

Geller DS, Zhang J, Wisgerhof MV, et al. A novel form of human mendelian hypertension featuring nonglucocorticoid-remediable aldosteronism. *J Clin Endocrinol Metab* 2008;93:3117–3123.

Giacchetti G, Ronconi V, Lucarelli G, et al. Analysis of screening and confirmatory tests in the diagnosis of primary aldosteronism: Need for a standardized protocol. *J Hypertens* 2006; 24:737–745.

Gifford RW Jr. Evaluation of the hypertensive patient with emphasis on detecting curable causes. *Milbank Mem Fund Q* 1969;47:170–186.

Girerd X, Villeveuve F, Lemaire A, et al. A clinical prediction rule for primary aldosteronism in drug-resistant hypertensive patients referred to an hypertension clinic [Abstract]. *J Hypertens* 2003;21(Suppl 4):S145.

Goh BK, Tan YH, Chang KT, et al. Primary hyperaldosteronism secondary to unilateral adrenal hyperplasia: An unusual cause of surgically correctable hypertension. A review of 30 case. *World J Surg* 2007;31:72–79.

Gordon RD. Syndrome of hypertension and hyperkalemia with normal glomerular filtration rate. *Hypertension* 1986;8:93–102.

Gordon RD, Stowasser M. Primary aldosteronism: The case for screening. *Nat Clin Pract Nephrol* 2007;3:582–583.

Gordon RD, Klemm SA, Stowasser M, et al. How common is primary aldosteronism? Is it the most frequent cause of curable hypertension? *Curr Sci* 1993;11(Suppl 5):S310–S311.

Gordon RD, Stowasser M, Klemm SA, et al. Primary aldosteronismsome genetic, morphological, and biochemical aspects of subtypes. *Steroids*. 1995;60:35–41.

Gordon RD, Stowasser M, Tunny TJ, et al. Clinical and pathological diversity of primary aldosteronism, including a new familial variety. *Clin Exp Pharmacol Physiol* 1991;18:283–286.

Grimes DA, Schulz KF. Uses and abuses of screening tests. *Lancet* 2002;359:881–884.

Guthrie GP Jr, Genest J, Nowaczynski W, et al. Dissociation of plasma renin activity and aldosterone in essential hypertension. *J Clin Endocrinol Metab* 1976;43:446–448.

Hiramatsu K, Yamada T, Yukimura Y, et al. A screening test to identify aldosterone-producing adenoma by measuring plasma renin activity. Results in hypertensive patients. *Arch Intern Med* 1981;141:1589–1593.

Holaj R, Zelinka T, Wichterle D, et al. Increased intima-media thickness of the common carotid artery in primary aldosteronism in comparison with essential hypertension. *J Hypertens* 2007;25:1451–1457.

Holland OB, Brown H, Kuhnert L, et al. Further evaluation of saline infusion for the diagnosis of primary aldosteronism. *Hypertension* 1984;6:717–723.

Holloway CD, MacKenzie R, Fraser S. Effects of genetic variation in the aldosterone synthase (CYO11B2) gene on enzyme function. *Clinical Endocrinology* 2009;70:363–371.

Hood S, Cannon J, Scanlon M, Brown MJ. Prevalence of primary hyperaldosteronism measured by aldosterone to renin ratio and spironolactone testing: Pharst study [Abstract]. *J Hypertens* 2002;20(Suppl 4):S119.

Kaplan NM. Primary aldosteronism with malignant hypertension. *N Engl J Med* 1963;269:1282–1286.

Kaplan NM. Hypokalemia in the hypertensive patient: With observation on the incidence of primary aldosteronism. *Ann Intern Med* 1967;66:1079–1090.

Kaplan NM. Is there an unrecognized epidemic of primary aldosteronism?(Con). *Hypertens* 2007;50:454–458.

Kazory A, Weiner ID. Primary hyperaldosteronism in a ptient with end-stage renal disease. *Nephrol Dial Transplant* 2007;22: 917–919.

Kem DC, Weinberger MH, Mayes DM, et al. Saline suppression of plasma aldosterone in hypertension. *Arch Intern Med* 1971;128:380–386.

Kline GA, Harvey A, Jones C, et al. Adrenal vein sampling may not be a gold-standard diagnostic test in primary aldosteronism: Final diagnosis depends upon which interpretation rule is used. Variable interpretation of adrenal vein sampling. *Int Urol Nephrol* 2008;40:1035–1043.

Kulkarni JN, Mistry RC, Jamat MR, et al. Autonomous aldosterone-secreting ovarian tumor. *Gynecol Oncol* 1990;37: 284–289.

Lack EE, Travis WD, Oertel JE. Adrenal cortical nodules, hyperplasia, and hyperfunction. In: Lack EE, ed. *Contemporary Issues in Surgical Pathology*. Vol. 14, Pathology of the Adrenal Glands. New York: Churchill Livingstone; 1990:75–113.

Letavernier E, Peyrard S, Amar L, et al. Blood pressure outcome of adrenalectomy in patients with primary hyperaldosteronism with or without unilateral adenoma. *J Hypertens* 2008;26: 1816–1823.

Liddle GW, Bledsoe T, Coppage WS Jr. A familial renal disorder simulating primary aldosteronism but with negligible aldosterone secretion. *Trans Assoc Am Phys* 1963;76:199–213.

Lifton RP, Dluhy RG, Powers M, et al. Hereditary hypertension caused by chimaeric gene duplications and ectopic expression of aldosterone synthase. *Nature Genet* 1992;2:66–74.

Lim PO, Rodgers P, Cardale K, et al. Potentially high prevalence of primary aldosteronism in a primary-care population. *Lancet* 1999;353:40.

Lim PO, Brennan G, Jung RT, et al. High prevalence of primary aldosteronism in the Tayside hypertension clinic population. *J Hum Hypertens* 2000;14:311–315.

Lim PO, Struthers AD, MacDonald TM. The neurohormonal natural history of essential hypertension: Towards primary or tertiary aldosteronism? *J Hypertens* 2002;20:11–15.

Lindsay JR, Nieman LK. Adrenal disorders in pregnancy. *Endocrinol Metab Clin N Am* 2006;30:1–20.

Litchfield WR, Coolidge C, Silva P, et al. Impaired potassium-stimulated aldosterone production: A possible explanation for normokalemia in glucocorticoid-remediable aldosteronism. *J Clin Endocrinol Metab* 1997;82:1507–1510.

Loh K-C, Koay ES, Khaw M-C, et al. Prevalence of primary aldosteronism among Asian hypertensive patients in Singapore. *J Clin Endocrinol Metab* 2000;85:2854–2859.

Magill SB, Raff H, Shaker JL, et al. Comparison of adrenal vein sampling and computed tomography in the differentiation of primary aldosteronism. *J Clin Endocrinol Metab* 2001;86:1066–1071.

Man in't Veld AJ, Wenting GJ, Schalekamp MADH. Distribution of extracellular fluid over the intra- and extravascular space in hypertensive patients. *J Cardiovasc Pharmacol* 1984;6:S143–S150.

Mansoor GA, Malchoff CD, Arici MH, et al. Unilateral adrenal hyperplasia causing primary aldosteronism: Limitations of I-131 norcholesterol scanning. *Am J Hypertens* 2002;15:459–464.

Matrozova J, Steichen O, Amar L, et al. Carbohydrate and lipid metabolism disorders in patients with primary aldosteronism: A controlled cross-sectional study. *Hypertension* 2009;53:506–510.

Mattsson C, Young WF Jr. Primary aldosteronism: diagnostic and treatment strategies. *Nat Clin Pract Nephrol* 2006;2:198–208.

McAreavey D, Murray GD, Lever AF, et al. Similarity of idiopathic aldosteronism and essential hypertension. *Hypertension* 1983;5:116–121.

McManus F, McInnes G, McConnell J. Drug insight: Eplerenone, a mineralcorticoid-receptor antagonist. *Nat Clin Pract Endocrinol Metab* 2008;4:44.

Medeau V, Moreau F, Trinquart L, et al. Clinical and biochemical characteristics of normotensive patients with primary aldosteronism: A comparison with hypertensive cases. *Clin Endocrinol (Oxf)* 2008;69:20–28.

Meneton P, Galan P, Bertrais S, et al. High plasma aldosterone and low renin predict blood pressure increase and hypertension in middle-aged Caucasian populations. *J Hum Hypertens* 2008;22:550–558.

Milliez P, Girerd X, Plouin PF, et al. Evidence for an increased rate of cardiovascular events in patients with primary aldosteronism. *J Am Coll Cardiol* 2005;45:1243–1248.

Montori VM, Young WF Jr. Use of plasma aldosterone concentration-to-plasma renin activity ratio as a screening test for primary aldosteronism: A systematic review of the literature. *Endocrinol Metab Clin NA* 2002;31:619–632.

Montori VM, Schwartz GL, Chapman AB, et al. Validity of the aldosterone-renin ratio used to screen for primary aldosteronism. *Mayo Clin Proc* 2001;76:877–882.

Mosso L, Carvajal C, Gonzalez A, et al. Primary aldosteronism and hypertensive disease. *Hypertension* 2003;42:161–165.

Muiesan ML, Salvetti M, Paini A, et al. Inappropriate left ventricular mass in patients with primary aldosteronism. *Hypertension* 2008;52:529–534.

Mulatero P, Bertello C, Rossato D, et al. Roles of clinical criteria, computed tomography scan, and adrenal vein sampling in differential diagnosis of primary aldosteronism subtypes. *J Clin Endocrinol Metab* 2008;93:1366–1371.

Mulatero P, Milan A, Fallo F, et al. Comparison of confirmatory tests for the diagnosis of primary aldosteronism. *J Clin Endocrinol Metab* 2006;91:2618–2623.

Mulatero P, Rabbia F, Milan A, et al. Drug effects on aldosterone/plasma renin activity ratio in primary aldosteronism. *Hypertension* 2002;40:897–902.

Murakami T, Ogura EW, Tanaka Y, et al. High blood pressure lowered by pregnancy. *Lancet* 2000;356:1980.

Nakahama H, Fukuchi K, Yoshihara F, et al. Efficacy of screening for primary aldosteronism by adrenocortical scintigraphy without discontinuing antihypertensive medication. *Am J Hypertens* 2003;16:725–728.

Newton-Cheh C, Guo CY, Gona P, et al. Clinical and genetic correlates of aldosterone-to-renin ratio and relations to blood pressure in a community sample. *Hypertension* 2007;49:846–856.

Nishikawa T, Omura T. Clinical characteristics of primary aldosteronism: Its prevalence and comparative studies on various causes of primary aldosteronism in Yokohama Rosai Hospital. *Biomed Pharmacother* 2000;54(Suppl 1):83–85.

Nwariaku FE, Miller BS, Auchus R, et al. Primary hyperaldosteronism: Effect of adrenal vein sampling on surgical outcome. *Arch Surg* 2006;141:497–502.

Oelkers W, Diederich S, Bähr V. Primary hyperaldosteronism without suppressed renin due to secondary hypertensive kidney damage. *J Clin Endocrinol Metab* 2000;85:3266–3270.

Olivieri O, Ciacciarelli A, Signorelli D et al. Aldosterone to Renin ratio in a primary care setting: the Bussolengo study. *J Clin Endocrinol Metab* 2004;89:4221–4226.

Opocher G, Rocco S, Carpenéa G, et al. Usefulness of atrial natriuretic peptide assay in primary aldosteronism. *Am J Hypertens* 1992;5:811–816.

Pang TC, Bambach C, Monaghan JC, et al. Outcomes of laparoscopic adrenalectomy for hyperaldosteronism. *ANZ J Surg* 2007;77:768–773.

Pimenta E, Calhoun DA. Aldosterone and metabolic dysfunction. An unresolved issue. *Hypertens* 2009;53:585–586.

Pimenta E, Gaddam KK, Pratt-Ubunama MN, et al. Aldosterone excess and resistance to 24-h blood pressure control. *J Hypertens* 2007;25:2131–2137.

Rayner BL, Opie LH, Davidson JS. The aldosterone/renin ratio as a screening test for primary aldosteronism. *S Afr Med J* 2000;90:394–400.

Reincke M, Rump LC, Quinkler M, et al. Risk factors associated with low glomerular filtration rate in primary aldosteronism. *J Clin Endocrinol Metab* 2009; 94:869–875.

Rocha R, Funder JW. The pathophysiology of aldosterone in the cardiovascular system. *Ann NY Acad Sci* 2002;970:89–100.

Rossi GP, Belfiore A, Bernini G, et al. Prospective evaluation of the saline infusion test for excluding primary aldosteronism due to aldosterone-producing adenoma. *J Hypertens* 2007;25:1433–1442.

Rossi GP, Belfiore A, Bernini G, et al. Body mass index predicts plasma aldosterone concentrations in overweight-obese primary hypertensive patients. *J Clin Endocrinol Metab* 2008a;93:2566–2571.

Rossi GP, Bernini G, Caliumi C, et al. A prospective study of the prevalence of primary aldosteronism in 1,125 hypertensive patients. *J Am Coll Cardiol* 2006a;48:2293–2300.

Rossi GP, Bernini G, Desideri G, et al. Renal damage in primary aldosteronism: Results of the PAPY Study. *Hypertension* 2006b;48:232–238.

Rossi GP, Pessina AC, Heagerty AM. Primary aldosteronism: An update on screening, diagnosis and treatment. *J Hypertens* 2008b;26:613–621.

Rossi E, Regolisti G, Negro A, et al. High prevalence of primary aldosteronism using postcaptopril plasma aldosterone to renin ratio as a screening test among Italian hypertensives. *Am J Hypertens* 2002;15:896–902.

Rossi GP, Sacchetto A, Chiesura-Corona M, et al. Identification of the etiology of primary aldosteronism with adrenal vein sampling in patients with equivocal computed tomography and magnetic resonance findings. *J Clin Endocrinol Metab* 2001;86:1083–1090.

Schirpenbach C, Reincke M. Primary aldosteronism: Current knowledge and controversies in Conn's syndrome. *Nat Clin Pract Endocrinol Metab* 2007;3:220–227.

Seccia TM, Fassina A, Nussdorfer GG, et al. Aldosterone-producing adrenocortical carcinoma: an unusal cause of Conn's syndrome with an ominous clinical course. *Endocrinol Relat Cancer* 2005;12:149–159.

Seiler L, Rump LC, Schulte-Mönting J, et al. Diagnosis of primary aldosteronism: Value of different screening parameters and influence of antihypertensive medication. *Eur J Endocrinol* 2004;150:329–337.

Shionoiri H, Hirawa N, Ueda S-I, et al. Renin gene expression in the adrenal and kidney of patients with primary aldosteronism. *J Clin Endocrinol Metab* 1992;74:103–107.

Sinclair AM, Isles CG, Brown I, et al. Secondary hypertension in a blood pressure clinic. *Arch Intern Med* 1987;147:1289–1293.

Sosa León LA, McKinley MJ, McAllen RM, et al. Aldosterone acts on the kidney, not the brain, to cause mineralocorticoid hypertension in sheep. *J Hypertens* 2002;20:1203–1208.

Stokes JB. Understanding how aldosterone increases sodium transport. *Am J Kidney Dis* 2000;36:866–870.

Stowasser M. How common is adrenal-based mineralocorticoid hypertension? *Curr Opin Endocrinol Diabetes* 2000;7:143–150.

Stowasser M, Gordon RD. Monogenic mineralocorticoid hypertension. *Best Pract Res Clin Endocrinol Metab* 2006b;20:401–420.

Stowasser M, Gordon RD. Aldosterone assays: An urgent need for improvement. *Clin Chem* 2006a;52:1640–1642.

Stowasser M, Bachmann, AW, Huggard PR, et al. Treatment of familial hyperaldosteronism type I: Only partial suppression of adrenocorticotropin required to correct hypertension. *J Clin Endocrinol Metab* 2000;85:3313–3318.

Stowasser M, Gordon RD, Gunasekera TG, et al. High rate of detection of primary aldosteronism, including surgically treatable forms, after 'non-selective' screening of hypertensive patients. *J Hypertens* 2003;21;2149–2157.

Strauch B, Zelinka T, Hampf M, et al. Prevalence of primary hyperaldosteronism in moderate to severe hypertension in the Central Europe region. *J Human Hypertens* 2003;17:349–352.

Sukor N, Mulatero P, Gordon RD, et al. Further evidence for linkage of familial hyperaldosteronism type II at chromosome 7p22 in Italian as well as Australian and South American families. *J Hypertens* 2008;26:1577–1582.

Sukor N, Gordon RD, Ku YK et al. Role of unilateral adrenalectomy in bilateral primary aldosteronism: A 22 year single center experience. *J Clin Endocrinol Metab* 2009;94:2437–2445.

Sutherland DJA, Ruse JL, Laidlaw JC. Hypertension, increased aldosterone secretion and low plasma renin activity relieved by dexamethasone. *Can Med Assoc J* 1966;95:1109–1119.

Tanabe A, Naruse M, Takagi S, et al. Variability in the renin/aldosterone profile under random and standardized sampling conditions in primary aldosteronism. *J Clin Endocrinol Metab* 2003;88:2489–2494.

Thibonnier M, Sassano P, Joseph A, et al. Diagnostic value of a single dose of captopril in renin- and aldosterone-dependent,

surgically curable hypertension. *Cardiovasc Rev Rep* 1982;3:1659–1667.

Touitou Y, Boissonnas A, Bogdan A, et al. Concurrent adrenocortical carcinoma and Conn's adenoma in a man with primary hyperaldosteronism: In vivo and in vitro studies. *Acta Endocrinol* 1992;127:189–192.

Tracy RE, White S. A method of quantifying adrenocortical nodular hyperplasia at autopsy: Some use of the method in illuminating hypertension and atherosclerosis. *Ann Diagn Pathol* 2002;6:20–29.

Ulick S, Chan CK, Gill JR Jr, et al. Defective fasciculata zone function as the mechanism of glucocorticoid-remediable aldosteronism. *J Clin Endocrinol Metab* 1990;71:1151–1157.

Walker BR. Defective enzyme-mediated receptor protection: Novel mechanisms in the pathophysiology of hypertension. *Clin Sci* 1993;85:257–263.

Wenting GJ, Man in't Veld AJ, Derkx FHM, et al. Recurrence of hypertension in primary aldosteronism after discontinuation of spironolactone: Time course of changes in cardiac output and body fluid volumes. *Clin Exp Hypertens* 1982;A4:1727–1748.

Williams ED, Boddy K, Brown JJ, et al. Body elemental composition, with particular reference to total and exchangeable sodium and potassium and total chlorine, in untreated and treated primary hyperaldosteronism. *J Hypertens* 1984;2:171–176.

Williams JS, Williams GH, Raji A. Prevalence of primary hyperaldosteronism in mild to moderate hypertension without hypokalemia. *J Hum Hypertens* 2006;20:129–136.

Wu F, Bagg W, Drury PL. Progression of accelerated hypertension in untreated primary aldosteronism. *Aust NZ J Med* 2000;30:91.

Yokota N, Bruneau BG, Kuroski de Bold ML, et al. Atrial natriuretic factor significantly contributes to the mineralocorticoid escape phenomenon: Evidence of a guanylate cyclase-mediated pathway. *J Clin Invest* 1994;94:1938–1946.

Young WF Jr. Primary aldosteronism: Management issues. *Ann NY Acad Sci* 2002;970:61–76.

Young WF, Jr. Clinical practice: The incidentally discovered adrenal mass. *N Engl J Med* 2007a;356:601–610.

Young WF. Primary aldosteronism: Renaissance of a syndrome. *Clin Endocrinol (Oxf)* 2007b;66:607–618.

Young WF, Stanson AW. What are the keys to successful adrenal venous sampling (AVS) in patients with primary aldosteronism? *Clin Endocrinol* 2009;70:14–17.

Young WF Jr, Stanson AW, Thompson GB, et al. Role for adrenal venous sampling in primary aldosteronism. *Surgery* 2004;136:1227–1235.

Zarifis J, Lip GY, Leatherdale B, et al. Malignant hypertension in association with primary aldosteronism. *Blood Press* 1996;5:250–254.

Zarnegar R, Young WF Jr, Lee J, et al. The aldosteronoma resolution score: Predicting complete resolution of hypertension after adrenalectomy for aldosteronoma. *Ann Surg* 2008;247:511–518.

Zelinka T, Štrauch B, Pecen L, et al. Diurnal blood pressure variation in pheochromocytoma, primary aldosteronism and Cushing's syndrome. *J Hum Hypertens* 2004;18:107–111.

Pheochromocytoma (with a Preface about Incidental Adrenal Masses)

THE INCIDENTAL ADRENAL MASS

In considering the adrenal causes of hypertension in this and the next two chapters, we will start with an increasingly common clinical problem—the incidentally discovered adrenal mass. An *adrenal incidentaloma* is an adrenal mass, generally 1 cm or more in diameter, discovered serendipitously on an abdominal CT or MRI scan performed for a nonadrenal indication (Young, 2007b). While most are benign and most are nonfunctional, an adrenal incidentaloma must never be ignored because 10% to 15% will be either malignant or functionally active. Early resection can be lifesaving. A missed diagnosis can have life-threatening consequences, including extra-adrenal metastasis and hypertensive crisis.

Prevalence

Whether estimated from autopsy studies or CT scans, the prevalence of adrenal incidentaloma is 4% to 6% (Barzon et al., 2003; Bovio et al., 2006). The prevalence increases sharply with age—from 0.2% of CT scans performed on patients 20 to 29 years of age to 7% on patients over the age of 70 years (Young, 2007b).

Differential Diagnosis

Every adrenal incidentaloma must be evaluated for malignancy and functional activity (Young, 2007b). As shown in Table 12-1, the differential diagnosis includes adrenal adenocarcinoma, adrenal metastases, subclinical Cushing syndrome, pheochromocytoma, and aldosterone-producing adenoma.

Evaluation for Malignancy

Potential malignancy is an overriding concern. Among 2,005 patients with adrenal incidentaloma, adrenocortical carcinoma was detected in 4.7% and metastatic cancer in 2.5% (Young, 2007b).

As shown in Table 12-2, the size of the mass and its appearance on CT or MRI—the *imaging phenotype*—are the two key indicators of malignancy (Young, 2007b).

Size

Adrenocortical carcinomas typically are large; 90% are at least 4 cm in diameter. Among the patients with adrenal incidentaloma greater than 4 cm in diameter, one in four will have adrenocortical carcinoma (Young, 2007b). The smaller the carcinoma at the time of resection, the lower will be the tumor stage and the better the prognosis (Libe et al., 2007).

Imaging Phenotype

In adenomas, the cytosol typically is laden with fat, yielding characteristic features on MRI and CT (Young, 2007b). On T_2-weighted MRI, adenomas are isointense to the liver. On chemical shift MRI, signal loss occurs on the out-of-phase images. On noncontrast CT, benign adenomas typically have a low attenuation value measured in Hounsefield units (HU). If the noncontrast CT attenuation value is less than 10 HU, the patient can be assured that the tumor is a benign lipid-rich adenoma (Hamrahian et al., 2005; Young, 2007b).

However, up to 30% of adenomas do not contain much fat and thus cannot be distinguished from malignancy or pheochromocytoma by MRI or non-contrast CT. In such cases, a contrast-enhanced CT is particularly helpful. If washout of the contrast material

TABLE 12.1	Clinical Evaluation of an Incidental Adrenal Mass

Disorder	Prevalence[a], %	Suggestive Clinical Features
Cushing syndrome	7.9	Weight gain and metabolic syndrome (glucose intolerance, dyslipidemia, central obesity) *plus* supraclavicular fat pads, facial plethora, easy bruising, purple striae, proximal muscle weakness, emotional and cognitive changes, opportunistic infections, altered reproductive function, acne, hirsuitism, osteoporosis, and leukocytosis with lymphopenia
Pheochromocytoma	5.6	Hypertension (paroxysmal or sustained) *plus* spells of sweating, headache, palpitations, and pallor
Primary aldosteronism	1.2	Refractory hypertension *with or without* hypokalemia
Adrenocortical carcinoma	4.7	Abdominal pain (mass effect), Cushing syndrome (cortisol effect), virilization (androgen effect), gynecomastia (estrogen effect), and hypokalemia (aldosterone effect)
Metastatic cancer	2.5	History of extra-adrenal cancer; cancer-specific signs

[a]Percentage of incidentally discovered adrenal masses with adrenal hyperfunction or cancer.
Modified from Young WF Jr. Clinical practice: The incidentally discovered adrenal mass. *N Engl J Med* 2007;356:601–610.

TABLE 12.2	Typical Imaging Features (Phenotype) of Incidental Adrenal Masses

Feature	Adrenal Adenoma	Adrenocortical Carcinoma	Pheo	Metastasis
Size	Small (<3 cm)	Large (>4 cm)	Large (>3 cm)	Variable
Shape	Round, smooth	Irregular	Round, clear margins	Irregular
Texture	Homogeneous	Heterogeneous	Heterogeneous, cystic areas (necrosis)	Heterogeneous
Laterality	Unilateral, solitary	Unilateral, solitary	Unilateral, solitary	Often bilateral
Unenhanced CT density (HU)	≤10	>10	>10	>10
Contrast-enhanced CT	Not vascular			
Vascularity	≥50%	Vascular	Vascular	Vascular
Washout @ 10 min		<50%	<50%	<50%
MRI[a]	Isointense	Hyperintense	Markedly hyperintense	Hyperintense
Growth rate	Stable or slow (<1 cm/year)	Rapid (>2 cm/year)	Slow (0.5–1.0 cm/year)	Variable

[a]Relative to liver on T_2-weighted imaging
Modified from Young WF JR. The incidentally discovered adrenal mass. *N Engl J Med* 2007;356:601–610.

is greater than 50% complete 10 minutes after injection, the patient can be reassured (with virtually 100% sensitivity and specificity) that this is a benign adenoma. Washout is slower with pheochromocytoma or adrenal malignancy (Szolar et al., 2005).

Metastases

Primary cancers that commonly metastasize to the adrenals are carcinomas of the lung, kidney, and GI track. Metastases tend to cause bilateral adrenal masses and the primary tumor almost always has been discovered before the adrenal incidentaloma(s) (Young, 2007b).

Evaluation for Hyperfunction

Table 12-3 lists the screening procedures and the confirmatory tests for adrenal hyperfunction,

TABLE 12.3	Laboratory Evaluation of an Incidental Adrenal Mass	
Adrenal Disorder	**Screening Tests**	**Confirmatory Tests**
Subclinical Cushing syndrome	Overnight dexamethasone (1 mg) suppression test	Serum corticotrophin, 24 h urine cortisol; mid-night salivary cortisol; 2-day high dose dexamethasone suppression test
Pheochromocytoma	Fractionated plasma or urine metanephrines	Contrast-enhanced CT, gadolinium-enhanced MRI, consider ^{123}I MIBG scan
Primary aldosteronism	Plasma renin and serum aldosterone; 24 h urine potassium excretion	Aldosterone-suppression testing with salt loading; adrenal vein sampling after proving nonsuppressible hyperaldosteronism; CT scan

Modified from Young WF Jr. Clinical practice: The incidentally discovered adrenal mass. *N Engl J Med* 2007;356:601–610.

i.e., autonomous production by an adrenal tumor of cortisol, catecholamines, or aldosterone. Among 3,868 patients with adrenal incidentaloma in 26 series, biochemical evidence of subclinical Cushing syndrome was found in 7.9%, pheo in 5.6%, and primary aldosteronism in 1.2% (Barzon et al., 2003).

It should be noted that one quarter to three quarters of adrenocortical carcinomas are hormonally active. Cosecretion of cortisol and androgens is the most common pattern and is highly suggestive of adrenocortical carcinoma (Libe et al., 2007).

Subclinical Cushing Syndrome

Subclinical Cushing syndrome needs to be considered when an adrenal incidentaloma is accompanied by subtle clinical signs of hypercortisolism. Patients can have hypertension, central obesity, diabetes, fatigue, and easy bruising; however, they do not have the wide nonblanching purple striae or other signs of full-blown Cushing syndrome (Barzon et al., 2003; Mitchell et al., 2007; Terzolo et al., 2007; Tsagarakis et al., 2006). Thus, the clinical picture is hard to distinguish from the garden-variety metabolic syndrome—except imaging studies have uncovered an adrenal mass. The standard screening tests for hypercortisolism—an elevated 24-hour urine-free cortisol excretion and the overnight 1-mg dexamethasone suppression test—are too insensitive, yielding normal or minimally elevated values in up to 25% of cases (Mitchell et al., 2007).

To improve the sensitivity of the 1-mg overnight dexamethasone suppression test, the Endocrinology and Endocrine Surgery groups at UT Southwestern recommend a lower-than-standard cutoff—1 mg/dL rather than 5 mg/dL—for an abnormally elevated 8 a.m. cortisol value (Mitchell et al., 2007). To avoid false positives, the minimally elevated value should be confirmed repeatedly and accompanied by additional biochemical evidence of excessive 24-hour cortisol production such as elevated unfractionated urinary cortisol (>2 times the reference value), feedback suppression of ACTH, and proximal steroidogenesis (plasma DHEA-S < 30 mg/dL) (Mitchell et al., 2007).

Clinically Silent Pheochromocytoma

In the Mayo Clinic series, approximately 5% of adrenal incidentalomas turned out to be pheochromocytomas (Young, 2007b). The likelihood of discovering a pheochromocytoma is approximately 25-fold higher when hypertension is accompanied by an adrenal incidentaloma than in the general hypertensive population. Currently, approximately one half of all pheochromocytomas are discovered incidentally; of these, one half are accompanied by neither hypertension nor other classical clinical features (Pacak et al., 2007b; Young, 2007b). The diagnosis is based on biochemistry, i.e., demonstration of catecholamine oversecretion by the adrenal chromaffin cells (see below).

Primary Aldosteronism

In the Mayo Clinic series, 1% of incidentalomas turned out to be aldosterone-producing adenomas (Young, 2007b). The best screening test is a blood sample looking for an elevated serum aldosterone level and suppressed plasma renin activity (Chapter 13).

Management

Figure 12-1 is an algorithm for evaluating the patient with an adrenal incidentaloma.

Initial hormonal evaluation should include the following three screening tests: (a) an overnight dexamethasone (1 mg) suppression test for subclinical Cushing syndrome, (b) measurement of plasma free metanephrines or of fractionated metanephrines and catecholamines in a 24-hour urine specimen for pheochromocytoma, and (c) measurement of serum aldosterone and plasma renin activity for primary aldosteronism.

Even clinically silent pheochromocytomas can trigger lethal hypertensive crisis and therefore should be resected after preoperative adrenergic blockade. Aldosterone-producing adenoma is an indication for laparoscopic adrenalectomy if accompanied by hypertension or hypokalemia.

The approach to subclinical Cushing syndrome is a work in progress. In an uncontrolled study of nine patients with this diagnosis, unilateral adrenalectomy ameliorated hypertension in six patients and reduced supraclavicular fat pads and other clinical features in all nine (Mitchell et al., 2007). Though preliminary, these provocative findings indicate the need for a large multicenter trial.

For now, adrenalectomy for subclinical Cushing syndrome should be considered in younger patients (under age 40) with recent onset or deterioration of hypertension, diabetes, and other clinical features of hypercortisolism. In middle age or older patients, a large adrenal mass favors resection. Most cortisol-producing adenomas are 2.5 cm or larger (Mitchell et al., 2007). If surgery is undertaken, glucocorticoid therapy should be administered to avoid perioperative adrenal crisis.

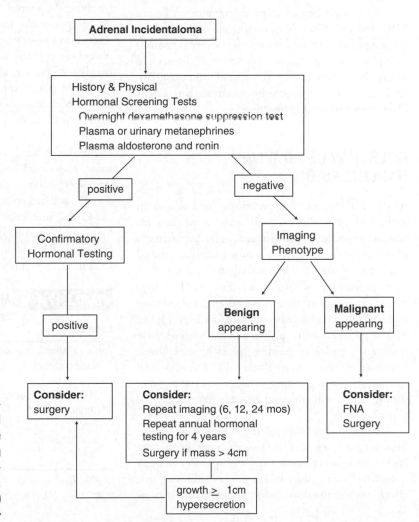

FIGURE 12-1 Algorithm for diagnostic evaluation of an incidental adrenal mass. FNA, fine needle aspiration. (Modified from Young WF Jr. Clinical practice: The incidentally discovered adrenal mass. *N Engl J Med* 2007b;356:601–610.)

Adrenalectomy is indicated when the radiologic appearance is suspicious for adrenal carcinoma, unless there are extenuating clinical circumstances related to advanced age and comorbidity. If an adrenal mass is ≥6 m in diameter, it needs to be resected. If an adrenal mass is 4 to 6 cm in diameter, the patient's age and imaging phenotype should be considered. Before age 30, adrenal incidentalomas are so rare that even a mass ≤4 cm merits consideration for resection, particularly if the imaging phenotype is suspicious (Young, 2007b).

Fine needle aspiration (FNA) biopsy is rarely needed to exclude malignancy because the imaging characteristics are so highly predictive (Young, 2007b). FNA is used mainly to exclude metastatic disease or infection (e.g., adrenal TB). A pheochromocytoma must be excluded first by biochemistry because FNA of a pheochromocytoma can trigger a hypertensive crisis.

If the mass has a benign appearance on CT or MRI and the initial hormonal studies are negative, imaging studies should be repeated every 6 months for up to 2 years and adrenal function studies should be repeated yearly for up to 4 years (Young, 2007b). Only then can the patient be reassured that there is little chance of further trouble.

OVERVIEW OF ADRENAL HYPERTENSION

As stated above, every hypertensive patient with an incidental adrenal mass will merit a workup for adrenal hypertension. Indeed, all hypertensive patients merit *consideration* of a potential adrenal cause but, without a known adrenal mass, only a small percentage will need an *evaluation*. The diagnostic challenge is that these adrenal diseases are rare and produce nonspecific signs and symptoms. Many patients with primary hypertension have recurrent spells suggesting pheochromocytoma, hypokalemia suggesting primary aldosteronism, and central obesity suggesting subclinical Cushing syndrome. Most will turn out to have normal adrenal function.

Although uncommon, the diagnosis of adrenal hypertension can lead to surgical cure or at least highly effective targeted drug therapy. Removing a hyperfunctioning adrenal tumor or blocking the effects of hormonal excess on target tissues may be

the only way to adequately control the hypertension and protect the patient from rampant target organ damage and premature death. This is particularly the case with pheochromocytoma.

PHEOCHROMOCYTOMA AND PARAGANGLIOMA

Pheochromocytomas are catecholamine-secreting tumors of adrenal chromaffin cells. *Paragangliomas* are extra-adrenal tumors of sympathetic or vagal ganglion cells. The odds that a paraganglioma will secrete catecholamines vary by location, as shown in Table 12-4. Catecholamine-secreting paragangliomas—often called "extra-adrenal pheos"—are located mainly in the abdomen or pelvis. Nonsecreting vagal paragangliomas are located mainly in the head and neck, most frequently involving the glomus cells of the carotid body. For clinical purposes, the term *pheo* generally refers to any catecholamine-secreting tumor, whether a true adrenal pheochromocytoma or a functional extra-adrenal paraganglioma (Pacak et al., 2007a; Young, 2007a).

Most pheochromocytomas and paragangliomas secrete both norepinephrine (NE) and epinephrine (EPI), with NE often predominating. Some primarily secrete EPI and an occasional tumor will secrete only dopamine. When correctly diagnosed and treated, most pheos are curable. When undiagnosed or improperly treated, they can be fatal.

Pheos often go unrecognized. In an autopsy series at Mayo Clinic, only 13 of 54 autopsy-proven pheos had been diagnosed during life (Young, 2007a). The remaining 41 undiagnosed pheos caused 30 deaths. In contrast, when pheo is diagnosed and managed by

TABLE 12.4	Location of Paraganglioma
Location	**Percentage**
Parasympathetic (non-secretory)	95
Head and neck	
Catecholamine-secreting	
Abdominal para-aortic	75
Urinary bladder	10
Thorax	10
Head and neck	3
Pelvis	2

Modified from Young WF Jr, Abboud AL. Editorial: Paraganglioma—all in the family. *J Clin Endocrinol Metab* 2006;91:790–792.

a highly experienced clinical team, the tumors can be successfully resected with minimal perioperative mortality (Pacak, 2007; Young, 2007a).

Prevalence

Pheos are rare. The estimated prevalence is less than 0.2% among unselected patients with hypertension but 5% among those with adrenal incidentaloma (Barzon et al., 2003; Young, 2007a). Because pheos are so rare and can cause lethal paroxysms, the clinician needs a high index of suspicion and a systematic approach to screening, localization, and surgery (Fig. 12-2).

Clinical Features

Table 12-5 lists the varied clinical features of pheo and Table 12-6 lists the long differential diagnosis.

Patients typically present with dramatic hyperadrenergic "spells." The classic clinical features are those of paroxysmal surges in catecholamine secretion. Excessive α- and β-adrenergic stimulation of the cardiovascular system produces the five "Ps" of the paroxysm (Young WF Jr, *Personal communication*, 2007c.):

• Paroxysmal hypertension
• Pounding headache

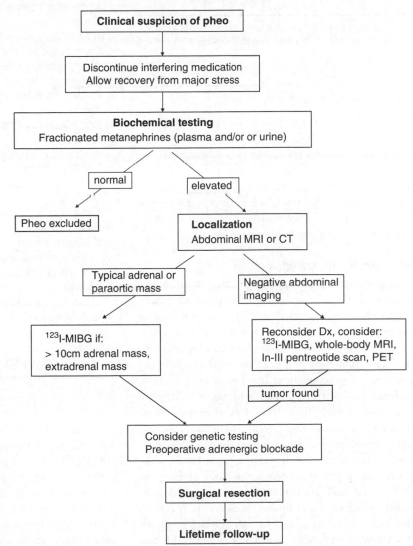

FIGURE 12-2 Algorithm for diagnostic evaluation of a suspected pheochromocytoma. Pheo, adrenal pheochromocytoma or extra-adrenal paraganglioma. In, indium. (Modified from Young WF Jr. Adrenal causes of hypertension: Pheochromocytoma and primary aldosteronism. *Rev Endocrinol Metab Disord* 2007a;8: 309–320.)

TABLE 12.5	Signs and Symptoms of Pheochromocytoma

More Common	Less Common
Hypertension (sustained or paroxysmal)	Postural hypotension
Excessive sweating	Flushing
Headaches	Weight loss
Palpitations	Decreased GI motility
Tachycardia	Increased respiratory rate
Anxiety/nervousness	Nausea/vomiting
Pallor	Pain in chest/abdomen
Tremulousness	Cardiomyopathy
Fasting hyperglycemia	Dizziness
Weakness, fatigue	Paresthesias
	Constipation (rarely diarrhea)
	Visual disturbances

Modified from Pacak K. Preoperative management of the pheochromocytoma patient. *J Clin Endocrinol Metab* 2007;92:4069–4079.

- Perspiration (often diffuse)
- Palpitations
- Pallor

Flushing is less common than pallor because NE—the dominant catecholamine—is a potent vasoconstrictor. Diabetes and weight loss are other signs of the hyperadrenergic state. Some patients are asymptomatic, some are normotensive, and others have symptoms due to concomitant conditions.

Paroxysmal Hypertension

The paroxysms represent the classic picture of the disease, but exclusively paroxysmal hypertension with intervening normotension is rare. Most patients have sustained hypertension with superimposed paroxysms. The paroxysms can be triggered by (a) mechanical compression of the tumor (by exercise, upright posture, bending over, urination, defecation, an enema, palpation of the abdomen, or a pregnant uterus), (b) injection of chemicals (anesthetic agents or radiology contrast material), (c) drugs that stimulate catecholamine synthesis (glucocorticoids) and secretion (histamine, opiates, or nicotine), (d) psychiatric drugs that inhibit biogenic amine reuptake transporters (tricyclic antidepressants, selective NE reuptake blockers, etc.), and (e) β-blockers, which leave α-adrenergic receptors relatively unopposed. A recent review of 11 case reports indicates that pheo crisis can be induced by

TABLE 12.6	Differential Diagnosis of Pheo-like Spells

Cardiovascular
  Labile primary hypertension
  Paroxysmal tachycardia
  Angina
  Acute pulmonary edema
  Eclampsia
  Hypertensive crisis during or after surgery
  Orthostatic hypotension
  Renovascular hypertension
Psychological
  Anxiety with hyperventilation
  Panic disorder
Neurological
  Autonomic neuropathy
  Migraine and cluster headaches
  Stroke
  Brain tumor
  Diencephalic seizures
  Autonomic hyperreflexia, as with quadriplegia
  Baroreceptor dysfunction
  Postural orthostatic tachycardia syndrome (POTS)
Endocrine
  Carbohydrate intolerance
  Thyrotoxicosis
  Insulinoma and hypoglycemia
  Medulllary thyroid carcinoma
  Menopausal syndrome
  Carcinoid
  Mastocytosis
Pharmacological
  Clonidine rebound
  Sympathomimetic drug ingestion (phenylephrine-containing cold remedies, cocaine, methamphetamines, Adderall
  Chlorpropamide-alcohol flush
  Monoamine oxidase inhibitor and decongestant
  Vancomycin "red man syndrome"
Factitious
  Ingestion of sympathomimetics

glucocorticoids, including ACTH, methylprednisolone, and high-dose (but not 1-mg low-dose) dexamethasone suppression testing (Rosas et al., 2008). The paroxysm does not occur immediately but rather 5 to 36 hours after the glucocorticoid administration and involves tumor necrosis (Rosas et al., 2008). Paroxysms also may occur without any clear provocation, sometimes from spontaneous tumor necrosis.

Among individual patients, paroxysms vary in frequency, duration, severity, and associated symptoms. They may occur many times per day or only every few months. Pheo paroxysms often are misdiagnosed as panic attacks. Patients may describe tightness in the abdomen rising into the chest or head, anxiety, tremors, sweating, palpitations, and weakness.

Pheo paroxysms, sometimes with BP greater than 250/150 mm Hg, can cause myocardial ischemia, catecholamine-induced cardiomyopathy with heart failure, and cardiac tachyarrhythmia (Brown et al., 2005; Kobal et al., 2008).

Hypotension

Predominantly EPI-secreting pheos can present as hypotension, as cyclic attacks of hypertension alternating with hypotension, and as acute coronary syndromes: diffuse ST-segment depression, chest pain, nausea/vomiting, and diaphoresis (Brown et al., 2005; Kobal et al., 2008). They can cause cardiogenic shock from catecholamine-induced cardiomyopathy. Profound hypotension may occur with spontaneous tumor necrosis or with α-blocker administration during the preoperative preparation for pheo surgery (Eisenhofer et al., 2008; Pacak, 2007; Young, 2007a). More commonly, patients have modest postural hypotension with tachycardia and dizziness. The postural hypotension indicates hypovolemia, which is a characteristic feature of pheo that has never been adequately explained (but we suspect that it is related to pressure natriuresis). In an untreated young hypertensive, postural hypotension and tachycardia may be a clue to the presence of a pheo.

Less-Common Presentations

Pheos also can present as an acute abdomen (from spontaneous tumor rupture), sudden death after minor abdominal trauma, lactic acidosis, or high fever and encephalopathy. Paragangliomas of the urinary bladder can cause painless hematuria and micturition syncope (Lenders et al., 2005).

The Revised Rule of 10s

Conventional teaching was that 10% of pheos are extra-adrenal (i.e., secretory paragangliomas), 10% occur in children, 10% are bilateral, 10% recur, 10% are malignant, 10% are discovered incidentally, and 10% are familial. Now, approximately 50% are discovered incidentally (Plouin & Gimenez-Roqueplo,

2006; Young, 2007a) and 15% to 25% are due to inherited germ line mutations (i.e., mutations occurring in all the cells of the body) (Gimenez-Roqueplo et al., 2006; Martin et al., 2007; Pacak et al., 2007a; Plouin & Gimenez-Roqueplo, 2006; Young, 2007a).

Familial Pheochromocytoma and Paraganglioma

Pheochromocytomas and paragangliomas can occur sporadically or they can be inherited as autosomal dominant traits alone or as part of one of several syndromes listed below. The known disease-causing genes are as follows:

- *VHL*, a tumor-suppressor gene associated with von Hippel-Lindau disease of pheochromocytomas (often bilateral), retinal and cerebellar angiomas, renal and pancreatic cysts, and renal cell carcinoma.
- *RET* (rearranged during transfection), a proto-oncogene associated with Multiple Endocrine Neoplasia (MEN) type 2A (pheochromocytoma, medullary carcinoma of the thyroid, hyperparathyroidism) or type 2B (pheochromocytoma, medullary carcinoma of the thyroid, mucosal neuromas, thickened corneal nerves, intestinal ganglioneuromatosis, slender facies).
- *NF-1*, associated with neurofibromatosis.
- *SDHD*, succinate dehydrogenase (mitochondrial complex II) gene subunit D which predisposes to familial paraganglioma.
- *SDHB*, succinate dehydrogenase gene subunit B which also predisposes to familial paraganglioma.
- *SDHC*, succinate dehydrogenase gene subunit C which mainly predisposes to nonsecretory vagal paragangliomas of the head and neck.

Differing Phenotypes of MEN2 and VHL Syndrome

The clinical and biochemical phenotypes of catecholamine-secreting tumors in the MEN2 and VHL syndromes were compared in a series of 49 patients (Pawlu et al., 2005). Patients with MEN2 are more likely to suffer from paroxysmal hypertension because MEN2 tumors mainly secrete NE whereas VHL tumors mainly secrete EPI. Compared with VHL tumors, MEN2 tumors have higher expression of both tyrosine hydroxylase, the rate-limiting enzyme in catecholamine synthesis, and phenylethanolamine *N*-methyltransferase (PNMT), the enzyme that converts NE to EPI.

With a clever use of contemporary human molecular genetics, Neumann et al. (2007) recently showed that the first description of pheochromocytoma from 1886 was, in fact, a case of MEN2 syndrome. The patient, an 18-year-old German girl named Mina Roll, presented with classic symptoms of pheo crisis and, at autopsy, was found to have vascular bilateral adrenal tumors that stained brown with chromate fixative (hence the name "pheo chrom" which means "chromate brown"). With a careful piece of detective work 120 years later, the geneticists searched the European-American Pheochromocytoma Registry to find four living family members with a germ line mutation in the *RET* gene, thus establishing the diagnosis of MEN2. These and other family members had pheochromocytomas and/or medullary carcinoma of the thyroid, the latter explaining the goiter in Mina Roll's original autopsy report (Neumann et al., 2007). Early clinical recognition of MEN2 syndrome is particularly important because medullary carcinoma of the thyroid—present in most of these patients—poses a major cause of death and thus merits immediate surgical removal.

Neurofibromatosis

Pheochromocytoma occurs in only 1% of patients with neurofibromatosis type 1. As of 2006, neurofibromatosis accounted for only 25 cases of the 565 total pheo cases in the European-American Pheochromocytoma Registry (Bausch et al., 2006). By comparison, von Hippel-Lindau syndrome accounted for 75 cases, paraganglioma syndromes for 54 cases, and sporadic pheochromocytoma for 380 cases. All 25 of 25 patients (100%) with neurofibromatosis had adrenal pheochromocytomas and, of these, three (12%) had metastatic disease.

Familial Paraganglioma

Discovered only in 2000, the familial paraganglioma syndromes are inherited as autosomal dominant traits (Martin et al., 2007; Pawlu et al., 2005; Plouin & Gimenez-Roqueplo, 2006; Young & Abboud, 2006). Of note, the *SDHD* mutation is characterized by *maternal imprinting*, meaning that the disease can only be inherited from one's father, emphasizing the importance of a detailed family history. The *SDHB* mutation is characterized by a high risk of malignancy including metastatic paraganglioma, renal cell carcinoma, and papillary carcinoma of the thyroid. The *SDHC* mutation is mainly associated with nonsecreting vagal paragangliomas (most often carotid body tumors) of the head and neck; however, the first two cases of pheochromocytoma with *SDHC* mutation have been reported (Peczkowska et al., 2008).

Tumorigenesis may involve (a) the failure of developmental apoptosis and/or (b) pseudohypoxic drive (Kaelin, 2007). Extra-adrenal chromaffin tissue normally plays an important role in catecholamine production in the developing fetus, but the tissue degenerates shortly after birth. Abnormal persistence of the fetal tissue may give rise to paraganglioma. The most common form of head and neck paraganglioma involves the hypoxia-sensing cells of the carotid body. Under hypoxic conditions, a hypoxia-inducible factor (HIF) normally translates from the cytosol to the nucleus, causing compensatory activation of the genes involved in angiogenesis, erythropoiesis, extracellular matrix turnover, and many other processes that defend against tissue hypoxia. In patients with familial paraganglioma, HIF remains activated—not by tissue hypoxia but rather by the abnormal accumulation of succinate. Such pseudohypoxic drive is also implicated in the molecular pathogenesis of tumorigenesis in VHL syndrome, as the VHL gene product normally is involved in the tonic restraint of HIF (Kaelin, 2007).

Other Associated Conditions

Catecholamine-secreting tumors also have been associated with the following nonfamilial conditions:

- *Carney's Triad* of secretory paraganglioma, GI stromal tumors, and pulmonary chondroma. Carney's triad does not appear to be inherited and the molecular basis for the association is unknown. In a recent study of 39 patients with Carney's Triad, the GI and pulmonary tumors were not caused by inactivating *SDH* mutations (Matyakhina et al., 2007).
- *Cholelithiasis*, seen in up to 30% of pheo patients (Gifford et al., 1994).
- *Diabetes*, with fasting glucose levels above 125 mg/dL in 14 of 60 patients (Stenstrom et al., 1984).
- *Hypercalcemia* in the absence of hyperparathyroidism (Kimura et al., 1990).
- *Polycythemia* due to increased erythropoietin production (Jacobs & Wood, 1994). More frequently, a high hematocrit is related to a contracted plasma volume.
- *Renovascular hypertension*, likely by external compression of a renal artery by the pheo (Gill et al., 2000).
- *Adrenocortical hyperfunction* may arise from ACTH secretion from the pheo, a coincidental

cortisol-secreting adenoma in the other adrenal, or bilateral adrenal hyperplasia (Pacak, 2007).

- *Rhabdomyolysis*, which has occurred with renal failure (Anaforoglu et al., 2008).
- *Megacolon*, reported in 17 cases (Sweeney et al., 2000).

Conditions Simulating Pheo

Most patients with hypertension and one or more of the manifestations of pheo turn out *not* to have that diagnosis. Table 12-6 lists the many conditions that can mimic a pheo. The most common are panic disorder and labile primary hypertension. Other common pheo mimics are rebound hypertension from clonidine withdrawal—especially with PRN dosing—obstructive sleep apnea (Chapter 3), and baroreflex failure (Chapter 2). The latter is suggested by a remote history of the head and neck surgery with mantle field radiation therapy, recent carotid endarterectomy, or surgical excision of bilateral carotid body tumors (i.e., vagal paragangliomas).

Pseudopheochromocytoma is a diagnosis of exclusion for patients with extremely labile hypertension and symptoms indistinguishable from a true pheo but negative biochemical testing (typically on multiple occasions) (Hunt & Lin, 2008; Mann, 2008; Sharabi et al., 2007). An emotional trigger may not be apparent and yet the paroxysms can become disabling. Excessive adrenomedullary secretion of EPI has been implicated but larger studies are needed (Hunt & Lin, 2008; Sharabi et al., 2007).

Death from Pheochromocytoma

Most deaths are related to failure to consider pheo in patients undergoing severe stress such as nonadrenal surgery or obstetric delivery. Many deaths are unexpected and sudden; this is likely related to catecholamine-induced effects on the cardiac muscle and conduction system. At least seven deaths have followed acute hemorrhagic necrosis of a pheo, most of them after β-blocker administration. Pheo should be considered before giving a β-blocker to control thyrotoxic symptoms (Ober, 1991), as this can precipitate a pheo crisis.

Evaluation

When and How to Screen?

The majority of hypertensive patients do *not* require screening for pheo. Screening indications are listed in Table 12-7. Many are derived from the patient's history.

TABLE 12.7	When to Screen for Pheo/paraganglioma?

Hyperadrenergic spells
Resistant hypertension
Family history of pheochromocytoma
Familial syndrome (e.g., MEN2, VHL)
Hypertensive response to anesthesia
Onset of hypertension before the age of 20 years
Hypertension with dilated cardiomyopathy
Adrenal incidentaloma

Screening is indicated in all patients with adrenal incidentalomas, even if the blood pressure is normal.

A systematic approach, such as outlined in Figure 12-2, will help to avoid missing the diagnosis and to avoid unnecessary—and expensive—laboratory testing (Yu et al., 2009). There are two steps to the diagnosis: (a) biochemical determination of autonomous catecholamine hypersecretion and (b) tumor localization.

Biochemical Diagnosis

In the past two decades, scientific breakthroughs in our understanding of the catecholamine metabolism and technical advances in the measurement of catecholamine metabolites have greatly improved the biochemical detection of pheo (Eisenhofer et al., 2008; Young, 2007a).

Scientific Rationale

Figure 12-3 depicts the clear view of catecholamine secretion, uptake, and metabolism provided by the work of Eisenhofer et al. at the NIH (Eisenhofer et al., 2004;2008; Goldstein et al., 2006).

Pheos contain large amounts of the enzyme catechol-*O*-methyl transferase (COMT), which converts NE and EPI to *O*-methylated derivatives, normetanephrine (NMN) and metanephrine (MN), which collectively are termed *metanephrines (mets)*. The metanephrines circulate free in the plasma and are sulfated as they pass through the GI circulation. The conjugated sulfates are filtered by the kidneys and excreted in the urine. Measurement of metanephrines either in a plasma sample or in a 24-hour urine sample is far superior to the measurement of the parent catecholamines and has revolutionized the diagnosis of pheo.

Elevated plasma or urine levels of metanephrines are highly sensitive diagnostic indicators of pheo for several reasons. Plasma levels of NMN and MN normally are very low. They are produced mainly within

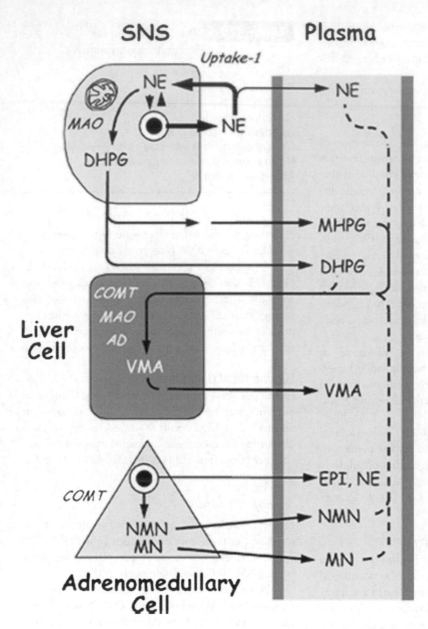

FIGURE 12-3 Catecholamine secretion, uptake, and metabolism. SNS, sympathetic nervous system; NE, norepinephrine; EPI, epinephrine; MAO, monoamine oxidase; DHPG, 3,4- dihydroxyphenylglycol; MHPG, 3-methoxy-4-hydroxyphenylglycol; COMT, catecholamine-*O*-methyl transferase; AD, aldehyde dehydrogenase; VMA, vanillylmandelic acid; NMN, normetanephrine; MN, metanephrine. (Modified from Goldstein DS, Eisenhofer G, Kopin IJ. Clinical catecholamine neurochemistry: A legacy of Julius Axelrod. *Cell Mol Neurobiol* 2006;26:695–702.

adrenal chromaffin cells and are not produced within the sympathetic nerves (as with the parent catecholamines) or within the liver (as with VMA). There is no COMT in peripheral sympathetic nerve terminals. As a result, most NMN and MN is generated within the adrenal chromaffin cells before being secreted into the circulation. In patients with pheo, metanephrines are continuously produced within the tumor and continuously secreted into the plasma by an autonomous process that is independent of vesicular catecholamine release, which is episodic (Goldstein et al., 2006). Whereas spikes in plasma NE and EPI may be missed

between the pheo spells, plasma metanephrines are continuously elevated and therefore provide a greater diagnostic sensitivity. A twofold elevation in plasma NE is associated with a sixfold elevation in plasma NMN (Eisenhofer et al., 2008). Metanephrines can be measured either in the plasma (as free metanephrines) or in a 24-hour urine specimen as the sulfate conjugates.

Which Test Is Best: Plasma or Urine Metanephrines?

Plasma and urine metanephrine measurements have their advantages, as well as disadvantages, and experts differ as to which test is best (Eisenhofer et al., 2008; Pacak, 2007; Young, 2007a). Plasma metanephrines are more convenient for the patient and have a high degree of sensitivity. Normal spot plasma metanephrine values virtually exclude the diagnosis of catecholamine-secreting tumor (except for the rare case of dopamine-secreting paraganglioma). However, the specificity is not ideal, with an overall false-positive rate of 15% in some series (Young, 2007a). The false-positive rate increases to approximately 25% in patients over age 60, because plasma catecholamine and metanephrine levels normally rise with age (Singh, 2004). Urinary measurements require an inconvenient 24-hour specimen collection but they have a lower false-positive rate of only 2% to 3% (Young, 2007a).

Participants in the First International Symposium on Pheochromocytoma debated this topic and concluded that either plasma or urinary metanephrines—or both—can be recommended as the initial screening test (Pacak et al., 2007a). The expert panel agreed on several other points and, of these, two merit special note. First, either test is far superior to the measurement of parent catecholamines alone. Second, the biochemical diagnosis should be compelling before ordering imaging tests to localize the tumor; thus, additional biochemical testing is needed when the initial biochemical results are equivocal.

In actuality, most clinicians are ordering plasma metanephrines because of the ease of specimen collection (Singh, 2004). If plasma metanephrines are normal, typically no further evaluation is needed. A fourfold or greater elevation in plasma-free NMN is approximately 100% diagnostic of a catecholamine-secreting tumor; imaging studies are indicated without further biochemical testing (Pacak, 2007; Pacak et al., 2007a).

However, gray zone results (e.g., twofold elevations above the reference values) are often encountered in clinical practice and necessitate additional biochemical testing (Pacak et al., 2007a). But again, which test is best? A retrospective study of 140 patients evaluated for pheo at the Mayo Clinic suggested that follow-up testing with either urine-fractionated metanephrines or plasma chromogranin A (another protein released by chromaffin cells) improves the diagnostic accuracy of plasma metanephrines (Algeciras-Schimnich et al., 2008). Whatever analytical method is used, careful attention to the technique can reduce false-positive testing, as discussed below.

Technique

To minimize acute stress reactions, the NIH laboratory recommends that blood samples be taken only after the patient has been supine for at least 20 minutes after the insertion of an indwelling venous cannula (Pacak, 2007). The Mayo Clinic laboratory obtains the sample from seated ambulatory patients by standard venipuncture and finds similar results (Kudva et al., 2003).

Urinary vanillylmandelic acid (VMA) assays are no longer routinely performed because of their poor sensitivity (Eisenhofer et al., 2004). About approximately 20% of VMA comes from the hepatic metabolism of the circulating catecholamines and metanephrines, with the remaining 80% from the metabolites of NE from sympathetic neurons (Fig. 12-2). Thus, large increases in adrenal catecholamine secretion by a pheo must occur before an increase in urinary VMA will be detected.

Increasingly, the measurement of total urinary metanephrines by spectrophotometry is being replaced by liquid chromatography-tandem mass spectrometry, which provides superior detection of total and fractionated metanephrines and avoids false-positive results from interference by sotalol, labetalol, acetaminophen, and other medications with structural similarity to metanephrines (Perry et al., 2007). Figure 12-4 shows that tandem mass spectrometry provides an excellent resolution of elevated urine total metanephrine values in pheo patients from normal values in nonpheo patients and normal volunteers (Perry et al., 2007). However, the ordering physician needs to know the expertise of his or her particular lab, as standards can vary (Singh et al., 2005). Except for α-blockers, most antihypertensives no longer need to be discontinued.

Table 12-8 lists the various tests and clinical cut-off values from the Mayo Clinic Laboratory.

Table 12-9 lists the common conditions that can elevate metanephrines, leading to a false-positive diagnosis of pheo. The most frequent are antidepressant medication, α-blockers, and sympathomimetics. Perioperative stress, acute myocardial infarction, and heart failure exacerbation can cause transient elevations in catecholamines, and biochemical testing for pheo should be delayed until the stress has subsided for 1 to 2 weeks (Fig. 12-2).

Patients with End-stage Renal Disease

Numerous case reports have described pheo in patients with renal failure (Saeki et al., 2003),

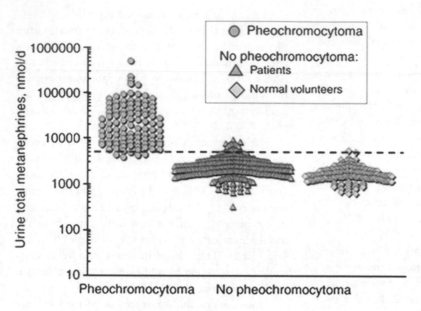

FIGURE 12-4 Comparison of 24-hour urinary excretion of total metanephrines (by tandem mass spectrometry in patients with histology-proven pheochromocytoma or paraganglioma (*circles, n =* 102), patients suspected of pheo but with a negative work up (*triangles, n =* 404), and normotensive healthy volunteers (*diamonds*, n = 221). The dashed line is the diagnostic cutoff value. (Modified from Perry CG, Sawka AM, Singh R, et al. The diagnostic efficacy of urinary fractionated metanephrines measured by tandem mass spectrometry in detection of pheochromocytoma. *Clin Endocrinol (Oxf)* 2007;66:703–708.)

including several cases of pheo and renal artery stenosis, the latter presumably due to an external compression by the tumor (rather than from atherosclerosis or FMD) (Kuzmanovska et al., 2001). Pheo presents a particular diagnostic challenge in patients with renal failure. Urinary metanephrines are invalid, even in patients who are not anuric, because of an impaired renal excretion. Plasma metanephrines are the only option but the false-positive rate is as high as 25% (Eisenhofer et al., 2005) because renal failure itself—either ESRD or moderate CKD—is characterized by sympathetic overactivity and impaired catecholamine clearance (Chapter 3). Thus, higher-than-usual cutoff values are recommended for biochemical evidence of pheo in the setting of CKD or ESRD (plasma NMN > 410 pg/mL, MN > 142 pg/mL) (Eisenhofer et al., 2005).

TABLE 12.8	Biochemical Diagnosis of Catecholamine-Secreting Tumor

Test	Cutoff Value[a]
Blood Test	
Plasma free normetanephrine	0.9 nmol/L
Plasma free metanephrine	0.5 nmol/L
Plasma norepineprine	750 pg/mL
Plasma epinephrine	110 pg/mL
Plasma dopamine	30 pg/mL
Urine Test	
Total metanephrines	1,300 µg/24 h
Normetanephrine	900 µg/24 h
Metanephrine	400 µg/24 h
Norepinephrine	170 µg/24 h
Epinephrine	300 µg/24 h
Dopamine	50 µg/24 h

[a]Supine values from the Mayo Clinic Laboratory.
Modified from Singh RJ. Advances in metanephrine testing for the diagnosis of pheochromocytoma. *Clin Lab Med* 2004;24:85–103.

TABLE 12.9	Causes of False-Positive Metanephrines

Medications that increase catecholamines
  Antidepressants
  Levodopa
  Clonidine withdrawal (PRN dosing)
  Antipsychotics
  α-Blockers
Conditions that increase catecholamines
  Major physical stress (surgery, stroke, MI, etc.)
  Obstructive sleep apnea

Modified from Young WF Jr, Pheochromocytoma. In: *ASH Clinical Hypertension Review Course Syllabus.* American Society of Hypertension, 481–494, 2007.

Dopamine-Secreting Paraganglioma

An occasional tumor will exclusively secrete dopamine because the tumor cells lack the enzyme dopamine-β-hydroxylase that converts dopamine to EPI and NE (Gangopadhyay et al., 2008). These tumors are extremely rare and are extra-adrenal paragangliomas rather than adrenal pheos. The diagnosis is easily missed because of the normal blood pressure and the normal plasma and urinary metanephrines. Rather than hyperadrenergic spells, the presenting symptoms are nausea, vomiting, or psychosis (due to excessive dopamine production) or an inflammatory syndrome of fever, weight loss, and an elevated sedimentation rate. Most are discovered incidentally on an abdominal CT or MRI for evaluation of abdominal pain. These paragangliomas are often large and metastatic by the time they are discovered, causing a poor prognosis. The diagnosis is made by an elevated 24-hour urinary dopamine level, which is usually dramatic (several fold the upper limit of normal of 3,300 nmol/24 hours).

Pharmacological Testing

With the improvement and widespread availability of metanephrine measurements, hazardous provocative tests (e.g., glucagon injection) have become obsolete. The clonidine suppression test, while safe, also is rarely needed to distinguish false-positive from true-positive elevations in metanephrines and may produce misleading results (Sartori et al., 2008). Plasma catecholamines and metanephrines are measured before and 3 hours after a single oral 0.3-mg dose of clonidine (Bravo & Tagle, 2003; Eisenhofer et al., 2008). The principle is that clonidine, a central sympatholytic, should cause a greater fall in plasma catecholamines and metanephrines when elevated plasma levels are due to the sympathetic neural overactivity than from an autonomously secreting tumor. However, false negatives can occur in patients with pheo and milder elevations in plasma catecholamines and metanephrines because much of the plasma NE and NMN is derived from sympathetic nerves which continue to function normally and remain responsive to clonidine (Sartori et al., 2008). The test cannot distinguish false-positive from true-positive elevations in MN and it is not needed to confirm the diagnosis of pheo when urine or plasma metanephrines are unequivocally elevated (Eisenhofer et al., 2008).

Localizing the Tumor
Abdominal CT and MRI

Once the biochemical diagnosis of autonomous catecholamine hypersecretion is certain, the next step is tumor localization in preparation for curative surgery (Fig. 12-2). Abdominal and pelvic MRI or CT is the initial imaging procedure, as 90% of catecholamine-secreting tumors are adrenal pheochromocytomas and 98% are located in the abdomen or pelvis (Young, 2007a).

Nevertheless, the diagnosis of pheo is not always straightforward. Figure 12-5 shows four different clinical scenarios to illustrate the importance of considering the imaging phenotype, the patient's symptoms, and the degree of biochemical abnormality (Young, 2007c). Patient 1 and Patient 3 had no symptoms and both presented with adrenal incidentalomas. In Patient 1, the imaging phenotype was suspicious for pheochromocytoma and the fivefold elevation in plasma NMN—in the absence of recent stress or confounding medication—confirmed the diagnosis. In Patient 3, the imaging phenotype was not suspicious for pheo and the normal plasma metanephrines excluded the diagnosis; no further evaluation was needed. Patient 2 presented with classic pheo symptoms and a classic imaging phenotype of a 3 to 10 cm cystic hyperintense adrenal mass with necrotic centers; the 20-fold elevation in plasma NMN confirmed the diagnosis. Patient 4 depicts a common clinical scenario of a gray-zone elevation in the plasma NMN ordered because of episodes of labile hypertension with flushing; subsequently, normal 24-hour urine metanephrine and catecholamine levels were sufficient to exclude the diagnosis without ordering the imaging studies.

In patients with suspected pheo, adrenergic blockade may not be necessary prior to contrast-enhanced imaging to prevent a hypertensive crisis during intravenous administration of the contrast material. No pheo paroxysms were observed in 17 patients with pheo who received nonionic contrast material (Bessell-Browne & O'Malley, 2007). According to Pacak (2007):

> Nonionic CT contrast does not have any appreciable effect on NE and EPI release in various types of pheochromocytoma patients; therefore, adrenergic blockade does not seem to be necessary as a specific precautionary measure before i.v. nonionic contrast.

While the results of this one small study await confirmation, gadolinium clearly does not stimulate pheos, thus eliminating the need for adrenergic blockade

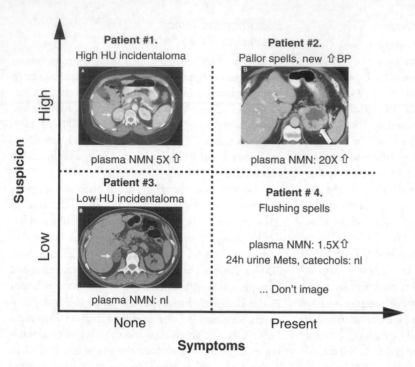

FIGURE 12-5 Examples of four patients in whom a pheo was suspected based on either symptoms or CT imaging studies. HU, Hounsefield units; NMN, normetanephrine; Mets, metanephrines. (Modified from Young WF Jr, Pheochromocytoma, ASH Clinical Hypertension Review Course Syllabus, American Society of Hypertension, 2007, pp. 481–494.)

prior to gadolinium-enhanced MRI. Both MRI and CT have similar sensitivities (90% to 100%) and specificities (70% to 80%) for adrenal pheo, whereas MRI may detect pelvic paragangliomas that are missed by CT or ^{131}I-metaiodobenzylguanidine (MIBG) (Garovic et al., 2004). Thus, gadolinium-enhanced MRI is the preferred technique if available.

Additional Imaging Studies

If abdominal imaging is negative, [^{123}I]-MIBG scintography can be used to localize the tumor (Fig. 12-2). The radiopharmaceutical is taken up selectively by the NE transporter in catecholamine-secreting tumors but has a false-negative rate of 15% (Young, 2007c). Some experts recommend confirmatory MIBG scanning before all pheo surgeries (Pacak, 2007); others believe that this is unnecessary as MIBG can produce both false-positive and false-negative results (Garovic et al., 2004). Additional localizing procedures include whole-body MRI, In-III pentreotide scanning, and PET scanning with ^{18}F-fluorodeoxyglucose is superior to MIBG scanning for detection of metastatic pheo (Timmers et al., 2009), ^{11}C-hydroxyephedrine, or 6-[^{18}F]fluorodopamine (Young, 2007a).

Genetic Testing

The goal of genetic testing is to identify individuals at high risk for developing new or recurrent catecholamine-secreting tumors. In such individuals, frequent biochemical screening and imaging may detect early tumors that have not yet metastasized, increasing the chance of surgical cure.

Some experts recommend genetic testing for all patients with catecholamine-secreting tumors and their first-degree relatives (Gimenez-Roqueplo et al., 2006; Pacak et al., 2007a), but others recommend a more selective, cost-effective approach (Eric & Neumann, 2009; Young, 2007a). The exact rate of familial inheritance is unknown due to missed diagnoses outside of academic centers and referral bias at academic centers conducting the research. Current estimates are that 20% to 30% of all pheos and paragangliomas are inherited, with germ line mutations being found in 7.5% to 27% of apparently sporadic tumors, i.e., those without the evidence of associated syndromes or family history after thorough evaluation (Gimenez-Roqueplo et al., 2006; Pacak et al., 2007a).

However, in the United States, the yield of routine genetic testing in patients with sporadic adrenal pheochromocytoma—defined by unilateral disease, a negative family history, and no syndromic signs or symptoms—is low (Young & Abboud, 2006). Nevertheless, all patients should be monitored for findings of one of the familial syndromes, some of which can be detected on physical examination. These include retinal angiomas in VHL syndrome, a thyroid mass in MEN2, cafe au lait spots in neurofibromatosis type 1, and a neck mass in paraganglioma syndromes. Evaluation and monitoring of first-degree relatives is also important since each of these disorders is transmitted as an autosomal dominant trait.

Who should be tested? Genetic testing has a higher yield and should be considered in patients with one or more of the following: (a) paraganglioma, (b) bilateral adrenal pheos, (c) unilateral adrenal pheo and a family history of pheo/paraganglioma, (d) unilateral adrenal pheo before the age of 40 years, and clinical findings suggestive of a syndromic disorder (Young & Abboud, 2006; Erlic & Neumann, 2009). Informed consent must be obtained and all family members should be offered genetic counseling. A list of clinically approved molecular genetic diagnostic laboratories is available at www.genetests.org.

Which genes should be tested? To eliminate the unneeded (and often non-reimbursable) expense of genetic testing for all known germ line mutations causing pheo or paraganglioma, genes should be tested sequentially with the order being driven by the clinical scenario (Young & Abboud, 2006; Erlic & Neumann, 2009). For example, a patient with a catecholamine-secreting abdominal paraganglioma is most likely to have a mutation in *SDHB*, *SDHD*, or *VHL*—in that order. Thus, the *SDHB* gene should be tested first and no further testing would be needed if a mutation were identified. A patient with bilateral adrenal pheos—but without medullary carcinoma of the thyroid—is most likely to have mutations in *VHL* followed by *RET*; if a *VHL* mutation is identified, *RET* does not need to be tested.

Management

Surgical resection is the treatment of choice. Most pheochromocytomas are benign and can be excised with high cure rates. Operative mortality is less than 3% when patients are managed by an experienced medical team (Pacak, 2007; Young, 2007a).

Preoperative Management

Both α- and β-adrenergic blockades are needed to prevent a pheo crisis in the operating room. Liberal salt intake is needed to prevent postoperative hypotension. Preoperative management should begin 10 days before surgery to ensure effective adrenergic blockade and volume expansion. In the absence of randomized controlled trials, the following approach is recommended by most experts (Pacak, 2007; Young, 2007a).

α-Blockade

Phenoxybenzamine is an irreversible α-blocker that produces more complete and more sustained α-adrenergic blockade than doxazosin or other α-blockers commonly used in general practice. Accordingly, side effects include orthostatic hypotension and reflex tachycardia, miosis, nasal congestion, ejaculation failure, diarrhea, and fatigue. Side effects are less severe with doxazosin, prazosin, or terazosin, which therefore are preferred for long-term palliative management of catecholamine excess in the setting of metastatic pheo for which surgical cure is not an option. For short-term preoperative preparation for pheo excision, phenoxybenzamine is preferred because the α-blockade is of a longer duration. This also provides adequate time to re-expand a contracted plasma volume before surgery.

The Mayo Clinic protocol is as follows (Prys-Roberts, 2000; Young, 2007a). The initial dose of phenoxybenzamine is 10 mg BID. The dose is increased by 10 to 20 mg every 2 to 3 days as needed to control the blood pressure and the symptoms of catecholamine excess. The average final dosage is 20 to 100 mg per day. The target seated BP is less than 120/80 mm Hg. Orthostatic hypotension is very common when α-blockade is superimposed on a contracted plasma volume, which typically accompanies chronic catecholamine excess. Thus, the patient should be carefully instructed to liberalize salt intake to achieve a standing systolic BP greater than 90 mm Hg.

β-Blockade

Except for β-blocker–intolerant patients, β-blockade is indicated to control sinus tachycardia and other catecholamine-induced tachyarrhythmias but *only* after an effective α-blockade has been achieved (which usually takes 4 to 7 days). If inadvertently used alone, β-blockers may exacerbate the hypertension by leaving α-mediated vasoconstriction unopposed. β-Blockers also can precipitate pulmonary edema if there is a catecholamine-induced cardiomyopathy (Prys-Roberts, 2000). Thus, the β-blocker should be started at a low dose and titrated carefully. The Mayo Clinic protocol uses short-acting propranolol, with a starting dose of 10 mg every 6 hours (Young, 2007a). Over the next 3 to 5 days, the dose is increased gradually and converted to a long-acting formulation to eliminate tachycardia prior to surgery.

The NIH protocol is similar (Pacak, 2007). β-Blockade and liberal salt intake are added to phenoxybenzamine. The recommended endpoints are seated BP less than 130/80 mm Hg, standing systolic BP greater than 100 mm Hg, seated heart rate 60 to 70 bpm, and standing heart rate 70 to 80 bpm.

Calcium Channel Blockade

CCBs have been used effectively and safely both as an adjunct to α-/β-blockade and as an alternative form of primary therapy for preoperative and intraoperative management of pheo (Bravo & Tagle, 2003; Pacak, 2007). These drugs block the intracellular calcium signal that produces α-adrenergic vasoconstriction in response to NE. According to Bravo (2004) at the Cleveland Clinic:

> These agents [CCBs] do not produce hypotension and therefore may be used safely in patients who are normotensive but have occasional episodes of paroxysmal hypertension.

The CCBs also may be useful in preventing catecholamine-induced coronary artery spasm that occasionally occurs in patients with pheo.

Nicardipine is the CCB most commonly used to manage pheo (Young, 2007a). Nicardipine can be given orally (30 to 60 mg BID) to control the blood pressure before surgery and intravenously (5 to 15 mg per hour) to control the blood pressure in the operating room.

Catecholamine-Synthesis inhibition

α-Methyl-paratyrosine (metyrosine) inhibits tyrosine hydrolase, which catalyzes the initial step in catecholamine synthesis. The side effects can be disabling, particularly when used for more than 1 week. They include sedation, depression, anxiety, nightmares, urolithiasis, diarrhea, galactorrhea, and extrapyramidal signs. According to Young (2007a):

> Although some centers advocate that this agent should be used routinely preoperatively, most reserve it primarily for patients who cannot be treated with the typical combined α- and β-adrenergic blockade protocol because of cardiopulmonary reasons [e.g., bronchospasm]. α-Methyl-paratyrosine (metyrosine) should be used with caution and only when other agents have been ineffective or [in addition to α- and β-blockade] in patients where tumor manipulation or destruction (e.g., radiofrequency ablation of metastatic sites) will be marked.

The Mayo Clinic protocol is as follows (Young, 2007a): metyrosine 250 mg q6h on day 1, 1,500 mg q6h on day 2, 750 mg q6h on day 3, and 1,000 mg q6h on the day before the procedure (day 4) with the last dose on the morning of the procedure (day 5). With this "short course," the main side effect is hypersomnolence (Young, 2007).

Acute Hypertensive Crisis

Acute hypertensive crises can occur before or during surgery and should be treated with intravenous therapy (also see Chapter 8). Options include sodium nitroprusside, nicardipine, or phentolamine. Nitroprusside is the most commonly used therapy for all forms of hypertensive crisis, including pheo. Nitroprusside should be avoided in pregnancy and in patients with renal failure because of thiocyanate toxicity. Nicardipine is a good alternative; an intravenous infusion is started at 5 mg per hour and the infusion rate can be increased by 2.5 mg per hour every 15 minutes to a maximum dose of 15 mg per hour. Phentolamine is rarely used any more and may not be readily available; the protocol is a 1-mg test dose followed by repeated 5-mg boluses.

Surgery and Anesthesia

Pheo surgery is a high-risk procedure, but 98% to 100% survival rates can be achieved at experienced centers (Pacak, 2007; Young, 2007a). Most experts recommend hospital admission the day before surgery to ensure adequate volume expansion (intravenous saline with 5% dextrose) and administration of the final preoperative dose of blocking agents on the morning of surgery.

Most anesthetics can be used if the patient has been properly prepared but several agents (including fentanyl, ketamine, and morphine) should be avoided because they can potentially stimulate the pheo to secrete catecholamines. Atropine should be avoided to prevent tachycardia from vagal withdrawal. Hemodynamic parameters must be closely monitored during surgery.

With accurate preoperative tumor localization, laparoscopic adrenalectomy has become the procedure of choice for the excision of a unilateral pheo less than 8 to 10 cm in diameter. With the retroperitoneal surgical approach, hospital stay is as short as 2 days (Young, 2007a). Larger tumors require open adrenalectomy. An anterior midline surgical approach is needed for abdominal paragangliomas, whereas specialized surgical approaches are needed to excise paragangliomas in the neck, chest, and urinary bladder. Cortical-sparing procedures (partial adrenalectomies) have been advocated for patients with bilateral pheos in the setting of VHL or MEN2 syndromes.

After the surgery, patients require close monitoring in an ICU for the fist 24 hours. Hypotension and hypoglycemia are the two main postoperative complications and can occur suddenly despite careful preoperative preparation (Lenders et al., 2005). Hypotension is mainly due to hypovolemia and should be treated with intravenous fluids and, if needed, pressor agents. Hypotension also can be caused by transient adrenocortical insufficiency, particularly if both the adrenal glands were manipulated during surgery. Blood glucose levels should be carefully monitored and intravenous fluids should contain 5% dextrose as a countermeasure to hypoglycemia resulting from sudden withdrawal of catecholamines and a rebound increase in insulin secretion (Lenders et al., 2005).

Blood pressure is often normalized by the time of hospital discharge but may remain elevated for several weeks after successful surgery. Almost 50% of patients remain hypertensive to some degree due to persistent vascular remodeling and associated hypertensive target-organ damage or coexisting primary hypertension.

Postoperative Follow-up
Early Postoperative Follow-up

Plasma and urinary-fractionated metanephrines should be measured 1 to 2 weeks after surgery. If the levels are completely normalized, surgery is considered successful. Elevated levels indicate a residual tumor, a second pheo or paraganglioma, or metastases.

Long-term Follow-up

After successful adrenalectomy, patients should undergo annual biochemical testing for the rest of their lives to detect recurrent tumors, new tumors, or metastatic diseases. Imaging studies are not needed unless metanephrine levels become elevated. The lifetime risk of recurrence varies by genotype.

Pheochromocytoma during Pregnancy

Pheo is a rare but important cause of maternal-fetal mortality. The diagnosis is often missed because the estimated prevalence is only 1 per 54,000 pregnancies and the pheo can be asymptomatic until delivery (Kondziella et al., 2007). Pregnancy may precipitate pheo crisis due to fetal movement, uterine growth, or delivery. Maternal and fetal mortality exceed 50% if undiagnosed. With appropriate diagnosis and management, maternal mortality falls to 2% and fetal mortality to 15%. If diagnosed in the first or second trimester, the pheo should be surgically removed after preoperative adrenergic blockade. If diagnosed in the third trimester, pheo surgery should be performed during C-section, the latter to minimize the stress of labor and delivery (Kondziella et al., 2007).

Pheochromocytoma in Children

Pheos and paragangliomas are extremely rare tumors in children. A recent retrospective chart review of the Mayo Clinic database from 1975 to 2005 identified 30 patients less than 18 years of age with histology-proven pheo or paraganglioma (Pham et al., 2006). Most were teenagers. The proportion of paraganglioma (60%), metastatic disease (47%), or a genetic mutation or family history of pheo/paraganglioma (30%) was considerably higher in these children than in the adult series from the same institution. Other series indicate that in children, approximately 40% of pheos are associated with known genetic mutations (Havekes et al., 2009). Metastatic disease was more likely in those with apparently sporadic disease, paraganglioma, and tumor diameter greater than 6 cm. It is essential to differentiate paraganglioma (with fractionated metanephrines and dopamine) from retroperitoneal neuroblastomas, which are much more common in children and do not require preoperative adrenergic blockade. In children, it also is essential to differentiate pheo from attention deficit hyperactivity disorder (ADHD) (Havekes et al., 2009).

Malignant Pheochromocytoma

Malignancy is defined by the presence of distal metastases rather than by histology (Pacak et al., 2007a; Scholz et al., 2007). The risk of malignancy is highly dependent on genotype: Metastases are present at diagnosis in 36% of paragangliomas due to *SDHB* mutation but present in less than 10% of all other catecholamine-secreting tumors (Scholz et al., 2007). The presence of distant metastases eliminates the possibility of surgical cure. Overall, the 5-year survival rate is only 36% to 64% (Pacak et al., 2007a), although prognosis is varied with less than 50% of patients having an indolent course with greater than 20-year survival and the others having an extremely aggressive course with 1 to 3 year survival (Young, 2007a). Long-term survival is more likely with bony metastases, which may be solitary, than with metastases to liver, lung, and lymph nodes.

Current therapeutic options are limited. These include (a) surgery to reduce tumor burden, (b) external-beam irradiation for solitary bony metastases, (c) radiofrequency ablation for solitary liver metastases less than 4 cm in diameter, (d) systemic [123]I- MIBG radiotherapy for patients with strongly positive ^{131}I-diagnostic MIBG imaging, (e) octreotide or other somatostatin analogs for rare patients with strongly positive diagnostic octreotide imaging, and (f) chemotherapy with cyclosphosphamide, vincristine, and dacarbazine (Eisenhofer et al., 2008). With any of these modalities, responses often are partial and short-lived. [131]I therapy requires preparation with sodium perchlorate or potassium iodide to protect the thyroid gland and discontinuation of drugs that interfere with MIBG uptake (Scholz et al., 2007). Prolonged treatment with α- and β-blockers and sometimes metyrosine may be needed to palliate the symptoms of catecholamine excess, which can be severe. Novel therapies are being evaluated, with encouraging but preliminary results with the tyrosine kinase inhibitor sunitinib (Joshua et al., 2009). Much more research is needed.

We will next examine primary aldosteronism, another fascinating adrenal cause of hypertension that may be more common than previously thought.

REFERENCES

Algeciras-Schimnich A, Preissner CM, Young WF Jr, et al. Plasma chromogranin A or urine fractionated metanephrines follow-up testing improves the diagnostic accuracy of plasma fractionated metanephrines for pheochromocytoma. *J Clin Endocrinol Metab* 2008;93:91–95.

Anaforoglu I, Ertorer ME, Haydardedeoglu FE, et al. Rhabdomyolysis and acute myoglobinuric renal failure in a patient with bilateral pheochromocytoma following open pyelolithotomy. *South Med J* 2008;101:425–427.

Barzon L, Sonino N, Fallo F, et al. Prevalence and natural history of adrenal incidentalomas. *Eur J Endocrinol* 2003;149:273–285.

Bausch B, Borozdin W, Neumann HP. Clinical and genetic characteristics of patients with neurofibromatosis type 1 and pheochromocytoma. *N Engl J Med* 2006;354:2729–2731.

Bessell-Browne R, O'Malley ME. CT of pheochromocytoma and paraganglioma: Risk of adverse events with i.v. administration of nonionic contrast material. *Am J Roentgenol* 2007;188:970–974.

Bovio S, Cataldi A, Reimondo G, et al. Prevalence of adrenal incidentaloma in a contemporary computerized tomography series. *J Endocrinol Invest* 2006;29:298–302.

Bravo EL. Pheochromocytoma: current perspectives in the pathogenesis, diagnosis, and management. *Arq Bras Endocrinol Metabol* 2004;48:746–750.

Bravo EL, Tagle R. Pheochromocytoma: State-of-the-art and future prospects. *Endocrinol Rev* 2003;24:539–553.

Brown H, Goldberg PA, Selter JG, et al. Hemorrhagic pheochromocytoma associated with systemic corticosteroid therapy and presenting as myocardial infarction with severe hypertension. *J Clin Endocrinol Metab* 2005;90:563–569.

Eisenhofer G, Huysmans F, Pacak K, et al. Plasma metanephrines in renal failure. *Kidney Int* 2005;67:668–677.

Eisenhofer G, Kopin IJ, Goldstein DS. Catecholamine metabolism: a contemporary view with implications for physiology and medicine. *Pharmacol Rev* 2004;56:331–349.

Eisenhofer G, Siegert G, Kotzerke J, et al. Current progress and future challenges in the biochemical diagnosis and treatment of pheochromocytomas and paragangliomas. *Horm Metab Res* 2008;40:329–337.

Erlic Z, Neumann HP. When should genetic testing be obtained in a patient with phaeochromocytoma or paraganglioma? *Clin Endocrinol (Oxf)* 2009;70:354–357.

Gangopadhyay K, Baskar V, Toogood A. A case of exclusive dopamine-secreting paraganglioma. *Clin Endocrinol (Oxf)* 2008; 68:494–495.

Garovic VD, Hogan MC, Kanakiriya SK, et al. Labile hypertension, increased metanephrines and imaging misadventures. *Nephrol Dial Transplant* 2004;19:1004–1006.

Gifford RW Jr, Manger WM, Bravo EL. Pheochromocytoma. *Endocrinol Metab Clin North Am* 1994;23:387–404.

Gill IS, Meraney AM, Bravo EL, et al. Pheochromocytoma coexisting with renal artery lesions. *J Urol* 2000;164:296–301.

Gimenez-Roqueplo AP, Lehnert H, Mannelli M, et al. Phaeochromocytoma, new genes and screening strategies. *Clin Endocrinol (Oxf)* 2006;65:699–705.

Goldstein DS, Eisenhofer G, Kopin IJ. Clinical catecholamine neurochemistry: A legacy of Julius Axelrod. *Cell Mol Neurobiol* 2006;26:695–702.

Hamrahian AH, Ioachimescu AG, Remer EM, et al. Clinical utility of noncontrast computed tomography attenuation value (hounsfield units) to differentiate adrenal adenomas/hyperplasias from nonadenomas: Cleveland Clinic experience. *J Clin Endocrinol Metab* 2005;90:871–877.

Havekes B, Romijn JA, Eisenhofer G, et al. Update on pediatric pheochromocytoma. *Pediatr Nephrol* 2009;24:943–950.

Hunt J, Lin J. Paroxysmal hypertension in a 48-year-old woman. *Kidney Int* 2008;74:532–535.

Jacobs P, Wood L. Recurrent benign erythropoietin-secreting pheochromocytomas. *Am J Med* 1994;97:307–308.

Joshua AM, Ezzat S, Asa SL, Evans A, Broom R, Freeman M, Knox JJ. Rationale and evidence for sunitinib in the treatment of malignant paraganglioma/pheochromocytoma. *J Clin Endocrinol Metab* 2009;94:5–9.

Kaelin WG Jr. The von Hippel-Lindau tumor suppressor protein and clear cell renal carcinoma. *Clin Cancer Res* 2007;13:680s–684s.

Kimura S, Nishimura Y, Yamaguchi K, et al. A case of pheochromocytoma producing parathyroid hormone-related protein and presenting with hypercalcemia. *J Clin Endocrinol Metab* 1990;70:1559–1563.

Kobal SL, Paran E, Jamali A, et al. Pheochromocytoma: Cyclic attacks of hypertension alternating with hypotension. *Nat Clin Pract Cardiovasc Med* 2008;5:53–57.

Kondziella D, Lycke J, Szentgyorgyi E. A diagnosis not to miss: Pheochromocytoma during pregnancy. *J Neurol* 2007;254: 1612–1613.

Kudva YC, Sawka AM, Young WF Jr. Clinical review 164: The laboratory diagnosis of adrenal pheochromocytoma: The Mayo Clinic experience. *J Clin Endocrinol Metab* 2003;88:4533–4539.

Kuzmanovska D, Sahpazova E, Kocova M, et al. Phaeochromocytoma associated with reversible renal artery stenosis. *Nephrol Dial Transplant* 2001;16:2092–2094.

Lenders JW, Eisenhofer G, Mannelli M, et al. Phaeochromocytoma. *Lancet* 2005;366:665–675.

Libe R, Fratticci A, Bertherat J. Adrenocortical cancer: Pathophysiology and clinical management. *Endocrinol Relat Cancer* 2007; 14:13–28.

Mann SJ. Severe paroxysmal hypertension (pseudopheochromocytoma). *Curr Hypertens Rep* 2008;10:12–18.

Martin TP, Irving RM, Maher ER. The genetics of paragangliomas: A review. *Clin Otolaryngol* 2007;32:7–11.

Matyakhina L, Bei TA, McWhinney SR, et al. Genetics of carney triad: recurrent losses at chromosome 1 but lack of germline mutations in genes associated with paragangliomas and gastrointestinal stromal tumors. *J Clin Endocrinol Metab* 2007;92: 2938–2943.

Mitchell IC, Auchus RJ, Juneja K, et al. "Subclinical Cushing's syndrome" is not subclinical: improvement after adrenalectomy in 9 patients. *Surgery* 2007;142:900–905.

Neumann HP, Vortmeyer A, Schmidt D, et al. Evidence of MEN-2 in the original description of classic pheochromocytoma. *N Engl J Med* 2007;357:1311–1315.

Ober KP. Pheochromocytoma in a patient with hyperthyroxinemia. *Am J Med* 1991;90;137–138.

Pacak K. Preoperative management of the pheochromocytoma patient. *J Clin Endocrinol Metab* 2007;92:4069–4079.

Pacak K, Eisenhofer G, Ahlman H, et al. Pheochromocytoma: Recommendations for clinical practice from the First International Symposium. October 2005. *Nat Clin Pract Endocrinol Metab* 2007a;3:92–102.

Pacak K, Eisenhofer G, Grossman A. The incidentally discovered adrenal mass. *N Engl J Med* 2007b;356:2005.

Pawlu C, Bausch B, Reisch N, et al. Genetic testing for pheochromocytoma-associated syndromes. *Ann Endocrinol (Paris)* 2005;66:178–185.

Peczkowska M, Cascon A, Prejbisz A, et al. Extra-adrenal and adrenal pheochromocytomas associated with a germline SDHC mutation. *Nat Clin Pract Endocrinol Metab* 2008;4:111–115.

Perry CG, Sawka AM, Singh R, et al. The diagnostic efficacy of urinary fractionated metanephrines measured by tandem mass spectrometry in detection of pheochromocytoma. *Clin Endocrinol (Oxf)* 2007;66:703–708.

Pham TH, Moir C, Thompson GB, et al. Pheochromocytoma and paraganglioma in children: A review of medical and surgical management at a tertiary care center. *Pediatrics* 2006;118:1109–1117.

Plouin PF, Gimenez-Roqueplo AP. Pheochromocytomas and secreting paragangliomas. *Orphanet J Rare Dis* 2006;1:49.

Prys-Roberts C. Phaeochromocytoma—recent progress in its management. *Br J Anaesth* 2000;85:44–57.

Rosas AL, Kasperlik-Zaluska AA, Papierska L, et al. Pheochromocytoma crisis induced by glucocorticoids: A report of four cases and review of the literature. *Eur J Endocrinol* 2008;158:423–429.

Saeki T, Suzuki K, Yamazaki H, et al. Four cases of pheochromocytoma in patients with end-stage renal disease. *Intern Med* 2003;42:1011–1015.

Sartori M, Cosenzi A, Bernobich E, et al. A pheochromocytoma with normal clonidine-suppression test: How difficult the biochemical diagnosis? *Intern Emerg Med* 2008;3:61–64.

Scholz T, Eisenhofer G, Pacak K, et al. Clinical review: Current treatment of malignant pheochromocytoma. *J Clin Endocrinol Metab* 2007;92:1217–1225.

Sharabi Y, Goldstein DS, Bentho O, et al. Sympathoadrenal function in patients with paroxysmal hypertension: Pseudopheochromocytoma. *J Hypertens* 2007;25:2286–2295.

Singh RJ. Advances in metanephrine testing for the diagnosis of pheochromocytoma. *Clin Lab Med* 2004;24;85–103.

Singh RJ, Grebe SK, Yue B, et al. Precisely wrong? Urinary fractionated metanephrines and peer-based laboratory proficiency testing. *Clin Chem* 2005;51:472–473.

Stenstrom G, Sjostrom L, Smith U. Diabetes mellitus in phaeochromocytoma: Fasting blood glucose levels before and after surgery in 60 patients with phaeochromocytoma. *Acta Endocrinol (Copenh)* 1984;106:511–515.

Sweeney AT, Malabanan AO, Blake MA, et al. Megacolon as the presenting feature in pheochromocytoma. *J Clin Endocrinol Metab* 2000;85:3968–3972.

Szolar DH, Korobkin M, Reittner P, et al. Adrenocortical carcinomas and adrenal pheochromocytomas: Mass and enhancement loss evaluation at delayed contrast-enhanced CT. *Radiology* 2005;234:479–485.

Terzolo M, Bovio S, Pia A, et al. Subclinical Cushing's syndrome. *Arq Bras Endocrinol Metabol* 2007;51:1272–1279.

Timmers HJ, Eisenhofer G, Carrasquillo JA, Chen CC, Whatley M, Ling A, Adams KT, Pacak K. Use of 6-[18F]-fluorodopamine positron emission tomography (PET) as first-line investigation for the diagnosis and localization of non-metastatic and metastatic phaeochromocytoma (PHEO). *Clin Endocrinol (Oxf)* 2009;71:11–7.

Tsagarakis S, Vassiliadi D, Thalassinos N. Endogenous subclinical hypercortisolism: Diagnostic uncertainties and clinical implications. *J Endocrinol Invest* 2006;29:471–482.

Young WF Jr. Adrenal causes of hypertension: Pheochromocytoma and primary aldosteronism. *Rev Endocr Metab Disord* 2007a;8:309–320.

Young WF Jr. Clinical practice: The incidentally discovered adrenal mass. *N Engl J Med* 2007b;356:601–610.

Young WF Jr, Pheochromocytoma, ASH Clinical Hypertension Review Course Syllabus, American Society of Hypertension, 2007c, pp. 481–494.

Young WF Jr, Abboud AL. Editorial: Paraganglioma—all in the family. *J Clin Endocrinol Metab* 2006;91:790–792.

Yu R, Nissen NN, Chopra P, et al. Diagnosis and treatment of pheochromocytoma in an academic hospital from 1997 to 2007. *Am J Med* 2009;122:85–95.

Hypertension Induced by Cortisol or Deoxycorticosterone

T he preceding chapter described the syndromes of hypertension induced by primary aldosterone excess. This chapter will cover syndromes in which hypertension is induced by other adrenal steroids: *cortisol*, either in excess (Cushing syndrome) or with increased exposure to mineralocorticoid receptors (MCRs) (apparent mineralocorticoid excess [AME] and licorice ingestion); or *deoxycorticosterone* (*DOC*) (congenital adrenal hyperplasias [CAHs]). Subclinical Cushing syndrome is the most common hormonal disturbance arising from adrenal incidentalomas found by adrenal scans (Young, 2007) as discussed in Chapter 12.

CUSHING SYNDROME

Significance

Although overt Cushing syndrome is rare, it often must be suspected in the growing number of patients with the metabolic syndrome (Weigensberg et al., 2008). Moreover, as milder and cyclical forms of Cushing syndrome have been recognized (Zerikly et al., 2009), the laboratory confirmation of the diagnosis has become more difficult despite the availability of better hormonal assays (Newell-Price et al., 2006; Nieman et al., 2008).

When present, Cushing syndrome is a serious disease. Hypertension is present in more than 75% of patients with Cushing syndrome (Arnaldi et al., 2003) and is often difficult to treat (Fallo et al., 1993) and, if the syndrome is incompletely controlled, contributes to a fivefold excess mortality (Newell-Price et al., 2006).

Pathophysiology

Cushing syndrome is caused either by excess endogenous cortisol with the idiopathic form or excess exogenous steroids in the more common iatrogenic form which may result even from use of steroid-containing cosmetic creams (Druce et al., 2008). The idiopathic disease may be either ACTH dependent or independent (Table 13-1; Fig. 13-1). The most common type, termed Cushing disease, is due to overproduction of ACTH from a pituitary microadenoma with resultant diffuse bilateral adrenal hyperplasia. Ectopic ACTH production may come from multiple types of tumors, the largest number being malignant small-cell carcinomas of the lung (Boscaro et al., 2001). In addition, adrenocortical cells may harbor "illegitimate" receptors, responding to unusual ligands (Bertherat et al., 2005).

ACTH-independent forms are mostly benign adrenal adenomas or malignant carcinomas but various forms of hyperplasia may pose diagnostic difficulty. As noted in Chapter 12, the number of adrenal tumors found incidentally by abdominal CT or MRI is increasing. As many as 20% of these adrenal incidentalomas when initially recognized secrete cortisol in a partially unregulated manner, often in association with hypertension, diabetes, and generalized obesity (Rossi et al., 2000). Over 5 years, as many as 7% of those with initially normal cortisol regulation develop subclinical hyperfunction (Barzon et al., 2002). Adrenalectomy may be indicated for some with clinical features but "subclinical" hormonal tests (Mitchell et al., 2007).

A number of interesting variants have been reported, including:

• Spontaneously remitting disease (Ishibashi et al., 1993);

TABLE 13.1	Prevalence of Various Types of Cushing Syndrome in Three Separate Series (in percentages)		
Reference	Orth (1995)	Newell-Price et al. (1998)	Boscaro et al. (2000)
No. Patients	*630*	*306*	*302*
ACTH-dependent			
Pituitary ACTH (Cushing disease)	68	68	66
Ectopic ACTH syndrome	12	10	7
Ectopic CRH syndrome	<1	5	<1
Macronodular adrenal hyperplasia			2
ACTH-independent			
Adrenal adenoma	10	8	18
Adrenal carcinoma	8	7	6
Micronodular hyperplasia	1	2	<1
Adrenal hyperplasia from other stimuli (e.g., GIP)	<1		<1
Exogenous glucocorticoid intake			

- Cyclic or periodic disease (Zerikly et al., 2009),
- Association with overt hypothalamic disorders (Dubois et al., 2007)
- Transition from pituitary-dependent to pituitary-independent disease (Hermus et al., 1988)
- ACTH-independent bilateral macronodular hyperplasia, which is often massive (Doppman et al., 2000), may be familial (Vezzosi et al., 2007) and may be associated with the expression of ectopic receptors for various hormones including the gastric inhibitory polypeptide (GIP), vasopressin, β-adrenergic agonists, LH/human CG or serotonin 5-HT$_4$ (Bertherat et al., 2005; Lacroix et al., 2001). Such receptors are occasionally found in adrenal adenomas as well
- Pigmented micronodular dysplasia, in most cases as part of the autosomal dominant familial syndrome with cardiac and skin myxomas, the Carney complex (Malchoff, 2000)
- Association with pheochromocytoma (Lee et al., 2008), chemodectoma, and carcinoid tumors (Tremble et al., 2000) and
- Increased sensitivity of peripheral glucocorticoid receptors causing clinical features without increased levels of cortisol (van Rossum & Lamberts, 2004)

Hypertension with Glucocorticoid Excess

Hypertension is present in about 75% of patients with Cushing syndrome. The severity of the hypertension may be related to the abolition of the normal nocturnal fall in BP seen after exogenous glucocorticoid administration and in patients with Cushing syndrome (Zelinka et al., 2004). The longer the duration of hypertension, the greater the likelihood that it will persist after relief of the syndrome (Suzuki et al., 2000).

Hypertension is relatively rare in patients who take exogenous glucocorticoids because of the use of steroid derivatives with less mineralocorticoid activity than cortisol. However, significant rises of BP can occur within 5 days of the administration of cortisol in fairly high doses (Whitworth et al., 2000).

Mechanisms for the Hypertension

Multiple mechanisms may be responsible for the hypertension so common in Cushing syndrome. The mechanisms may include:

- A sodium-retaining action of the high levels of *cortisol*. Although cortisol is 300 times less potent a mineralocorticoid than is aldosterone, 200 times more cortisol is normally secreted; this level is increased by two times or more in Cushing syndrome. With high levels of cortisol, the 11β-hydroxysteroid dehydrogenase 2 (11β-HSD2) capacity to convert cortisol to cortisone is overwhelmed, allowing cortisol to act on MCRs (Quinkler & Stewart, 2003; Ulick et al., 1992b).
- Glucocorticoids directly activate glucocorticoid receptors on vascular smooth muscle to raise blood pressure in knockout mice (Goodwin et al., 2008) and stimulate mineralocorticoid signaling in vascular smooth muscle cells in vitro, independent of aldosterone levels (Molnar et al., 2008).

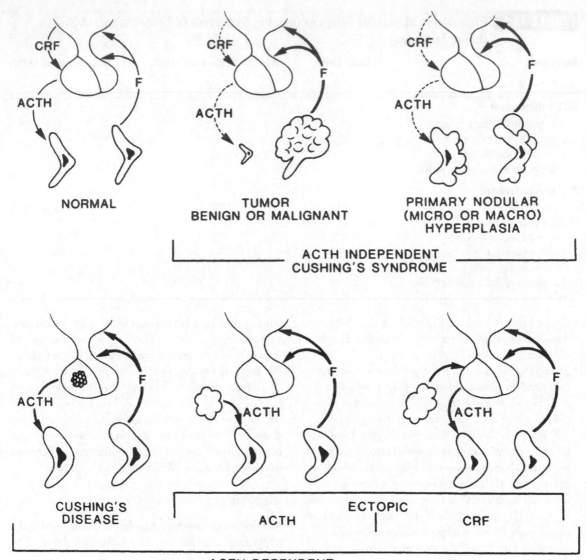

FIGURE 13-1   Causes of endogenous Cushing syndrome. The lesions of the top arise within the adrenal. Those in the bottom arise within the pituitary (Cushing disease) or from ectopic production of ACTH or corticotropin-releasing factor (*CRF*). *F*, cortisol. (Modified from Carpenter PC. Diagnostic evaluation of Cushing syndrome. *Endocrinol Metab Clin NA* 1988;17:445–472.)

- Increased production of *mineralocorticoids*. Though usually noted only in patients with adrenal tumors, increased levels of 19-nor-DOC (Ehlers et al., 1987), DOC, and less commonly, aldosterone (Cassar et al., 1980) have been found in patients with all forms of the syndrome.
- Stimulation of glucocorticoid receptors in the dorsal hindbrain (Scheuer et al., 2004).
- Reduced activity of various vasodepressor mechanisms (Saruta, 1996) in particular endothelial nitric oxide (Mangos et al., 2000).

- Increased levels of renin substrate and an increased responsiveness to various *pressors* (Pirpiris et al., 1992).
- Other mechanisms may also be involved including an increase in erythropoietin (Whitworth et al., 2000) or endothelin (Kirilov et al., 2003).

Clinical Features

Many more patients with cushingoid features are seen than the relatively few who have the syndrome. The syndrome is more likely in patients with the clinical

TABLE 13.2	Clinical Features of Cushing Syndrome

Clinical Features	Approximate Incidence, %
General	
Obesity	80–95
Truncal	45–95[a]
Hypertension	70–90
Headache	10–50
Skin	
Facial plethora	70–90
Hirsutism	70–80
Purple striae	50–70[a]
Bruising	30–70[a]
Neuropsychiatric	60–95
Gonadal dysfunction	
Menstrual disorders	75–95
Impotence or decreased libido	65–95
Musculoskeletal	
Osteopenia	75–85
Weakness from myopathy	30–90[a]
Metabolic	
Glucose intolerance/ diabetes	40–90
Kidney stones	15–20

[a]Most discriminatory features.
Modified from Nieman LK et al. The diagnosis of Cushing's syndrome. *J Clin Endocrinol Metab* 2008;93(5):1526–1540.

features shown in Table 13-2 (Newell-Price et al., 2006). In addition, significant hypokalemia is usually noted with the ectopic ACTH syndrome from the very high levels of cortisol (Torpy et al., 2002).

Cushing syndrome in children is usually manifested by weight gain and growth retardation, with systolic hypertension noted in 93% of 63 young patients (Magiakou et al., 1997). Fortunately, they usually become normotensive within a few months of surgical cure, but may have residual hypertension related adverse effects (Lodish et al., 2009).

Pseudo-Cushing Syndrome

As many as 50% to 80% of patients with Cushing syndrome meet the criteria for major depression and may have persistent psychological and cognitive problems even after surgical remission (Arnaldi et al., 2003). On the other hand, patients with endogenous *depression* without Cushing syndrome

may have poorly suppressible hypercortisolism related to increased ACTH pulse frequency (Mortola et al., 1987), but their basal cortisol levels are usually normal and they do not hyperrespond to corticotrophin-releasing hormone (CRH) (Yanovski et al., 1998).

Alcoholics often display numerous features suggestive of Cushing syndrome, including hypertension and elevated cortisol secretion (Badrick et al., 2008), which likely reflects increased secretion of corticotrophin-releasing factor (Groote Veldman & Meinders, 1996). On the other hand, 20% of patients with Cushing syndrome have hepatic steatosis by CT scans (Rockall et al., 2003).

Pregnant women often have features suggestive of Cushing syndrome; the rare appearance of Cushing syndrome during pregnancy may pose diagnostic dilemmas (Solomon & Seely, 2006).

Laboratory Diagnosis

Two somewhat contradictory scenarios exist in relation to the diagnosis of Cushing syndrome. First, the disease is being looked for in more patients with suggestive clinical features such as poorly controlled obese diabetics, in one study, 4% were found to have Cushing syndrome (Leibowitz et al., 1996). This scenario requires screening tests with high specificity, i.e., few false positives—so that fewer suspects will have to be put through extensive confirmatory testing (Newell-Price, 2008).

The second scenario relates to the usually long duration between onset of symptoms and the time of diagnosis, averaging 29 months in a multicenter study from Italy (Invitti et al., 1999). This scenario requires confirmatory tests with high sensitivity, i.e., few false negatives—so that all patients can be correctly identified as early as possible. In view of the serious nature and the often irreversibility of the complications of the disease, the best balance is likely to be with a number of tests done over a short interval to achieve maximal predictive power (Findling & Raff, 2006). Nonetheless, controversy persists as to the appropriate cutoff values for different tests to provide the best balance (Newell-Price, 2008).

Screening Tests

For interpretation of cortisol levels, 1 µg/dL = 27 mmol/L.

The extent of the workup of patients suspected of having Cushing syndrome varies with the clinical

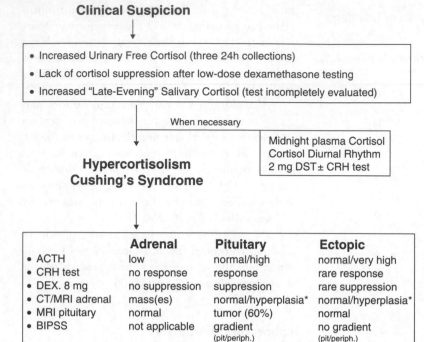

Clinical Suspicion

↓

- Increased Urinary Free Cortisol (three 24h collections)
- Lack of cortisol suppression after low-dose dexamethasone testing
- Increased "Late-Evening" Salivary Cortisol (test incompletely evaluated)

↓ When necessary

| Midnight plasma Cortisol |
| Cortisol Diurnal Rhythm |
| 2 mg DST ± CRH test |

Hypercortisolism
Cushing's Syndrome

↓

	Adrenal	**Pituitary**	**Ectopic**
• ACTH	low	normal/high	normal/very high
• CRH test	no response	response	rare response
• DEX. 8 mg	no suppression	suppression	rare suppression
• CT/MRI adrenal	mass(es)	normal/hyperplasia*	normal/hyperplasia*
• MRI pituitary	normal	tumor (60%)	normal
• BIPSS	not applicable	gradient (pit/periph.)	no gradient (pit/periph.)

* nodules

FIGURE 13-2 Pathways to the diagnosis of Cushing syndrome. Dex, dexamethasone; DST, dexamethasone suppression test; BIPSS, bilateral inferior petrosal sinus sampling. (Modified from Arnaldi G, Angeli A, Atkinson AB, et al. Diagnosis and complications of Cushing syndrome: A consensus statement. *J Clin Endocrinol Metab* 2003;88:5593–5602.)

situation. An overnight 1-mg dexamethasone suppression test (OST) will be adequate for most patients with only minimally suggestive features; patients with highly suggestive features should have repeated measurement of 24-hour urinary free cortisol (UFC) and midnight serum or salivary cortisol (Arnaldi et al., 2003; Findling & Raff, 2006; Nieman et al., 2008) (Fig. 13-2). In data from 4,126 patients, (Pecori et al., 2007) found the midnight serum cortisol, using a 1.8 μg/dL (50 mmol/L) cutoff, to provide only a 20% specificity whereas both the UFC and OST had 91% specificities. Nonetheless, the ease of obtaining the sample and the high sensitivity of the late-night salivary control lead Findling and Raff (2006) to recommend it as the best screening study. The Endocrine Society recommends any one of the three screening tests: urine cortisol, late-night salivary cortisol, or 1-mg overnight dexamethasone suppression (Nieman et al., 2008) in keeping with their overall similar accuracy (Elamin et al., 2008).

Urinary Free Cortisol

The 24-hour UFC provides an integrated measure of the unbound circulating cortisol. High-performance liquid chromatography coupled with mass spectrometry provides better specificity than immunoassays. The upper range of normal is 40 to 50 μg/24 hours (1,100 to 1,380 mmol/L) and a value four times greater is usually diagnostic (Findling & Raff, 2006). The level may be lowered in patients with renal damage or raised with increased urinary volumes by reducing the fraction of filtered cortisol that is metabolized to cortisone or reabsorbed. Since the level is variable, three daily specimens are usually assayed.

Overnight Plasma Suppression

For screening, the single bedtime 1-mg dose dexamethasone suppression test (DST), measuring the plasma cortisol at 8 a.m. the next morning, has worked well but, to provide adequate sensitivity, the cutoff value should be 1.8 μg/dL, rather than the previously recommended 5 μg/dL (Findling et al., 2004). However, at the lower level, false-positive results are seen in about 10% of non-Cushing patients and false-negative results are seen in about 20% of patients with Cushing disease (Findling & Raff, 2006).

Late-Night Salivary Cortisol

An elevated late-night serum or salivary cortisol level is the earliest and most sensitive marker for Cushing syndrome (Findling & Raff, 2006). Rather than the inconvenience of obtaining blood samples, measurement of salivary cortisol levels in easily obtained samples has rapidly been accepted as a valid screening test including in children (Batista et al., 2007). Levels above 0.3 μg/dL (8.6 mmol/L) are abnormal (Findling & Raff, 2006).

Low-Dose Dexamethasone Suppression Test and Combined DST-CRH

DSTs may give anomalous results because hormone hypersecretion may be cyclic or variable. Pseudo-Cushing's states, including depression, may be more accurately excluded by adding a CRH stimulation test after completion of the low-dose dexamethasone test (Yanovski et al., 1998). However, Gatta et al. (2007) found no additional diagnostic accuracy by the addition of CRH stimulation to the OST using a cutoff of plasma cortisol 15 minutes after CRH of 4 μg/dL (110 mmol/L). The plasma cortisol level value 15 minutes after CRH (1 μg/kg) is above 1.4 μg/dL (40 mmol/L) in patients with Cushing syndrome but remains suppressed in normals and patients with pseudo-Cushing's.

Establishing the Cause of Cushing Syndrome

Once Cushing syndrome has been diagnosed, the anatomic cause needs to be accurately determined to guide therapy (Fig. 13-2). In view of all the clinical vagaries and laboratory pitfalls that often confuse the differential diagnosis of the etiology of Cushing syndrome, referral to a medical facility with experience in dealing with such patients is almost always appropriate.

Corticotropin (ACTH) Assay

Measurement of plasma ACTH is the first step, using two-site immunometric assays that are sensitive, specific, and reliable, able to reliably detect values below 10 pg/mL (2 pmol/L). A suppressed ACTH concentration, below 5 pg/mL, indicates adrenal-independent Cushing syndrome usually from an adrenal tumor. However, other stimuli of adrenocortical receptors, such as insulinotropic peptide and vasopressin, may induce bilateral nodular adrenal hyperplasia with suppressed plasma ACTH levels. Normal or elevated plasma ACTH, above 20 pg/mL, indicate ACTH-dependent Cushing syndrome from either a pituitary or ectopic tumor.

When values are between 10 and 20 pg/mL, a CRH stimulation test is indicated (Arnaldi et al., 2003).

Corticotrophin-Releasing Hormone Stimulation Test

Most pituitary tumors respond to IV CRH (1 μg/kg) with a release of plasma ACTH whereas adrenal tumors do not. Unfortunately, some ectopic ACTH-secreting tumors express the CRH receptor and also respond. Findling and Raff (2006) recommend a CRH test in patients with Cushing syndrome whose plasma ACTH levels are at the low end. The ACTH response is usually exaggerated if the pituitary tumor expresses the CRH receptor but blunted with adrenal tumors.

High-Dose Dexamethasone Suppression

Using the criterion of suppression of UFC to less than 10% of baseline for the diagnosis of pituitary-dependent Cushing disease, the high-dose (2 mg four times a day for 2 days) DST provides 70% to 80% sensitivity and close to 100% specificity (Boscaro et al., 2001). However, the results do not clearly separate ectopic ACTH from pituitary tumors and this test is no longer recommended (Findling & Raff, 2006).

Pituitary MRI

In most patients, the measurement of plasma ACTH will be followed by a pituitary MRI with gadolinium enhancement. Thereby, a discrete pituitary adenoma will be seen in about 60% of patients; if the tumor is greater than 6 mm in size, no further studies are required and the patients may be referred to a pituitary neurosurgeon (Arnaldi et al., 2003). It should be remembered that almost 15% of the general population harbor incidental pituitary tumors, although most are below 5 mm in diameter (Karavitaki et al., 2007). Since some patients with an ectopic ACTH-secreting tumor have abnormal pituitary MRI findings, bilateral interior petrosal sinus sampling is indicated in those with clinical features suggesting an ectopic tumor, such as rapid onset of symptoms or hypokalemia (Findling & Raff, 2006).

Inferior Petrosal Sinus Sampling

Bilateral simultaneous sampling of the inferior petrosal sinuses (IPSS) is a powerful means of confirming whether or not the source of corticotropin is the pituitary, especially if imaging is negative. Ratio of central to peripheral ACTH of greater than 3 after CRH stimulation provides a sensitivity of 95% to 97% and specificity of 100% in diagnosing pituitary-dependent Cushing disease (Arnaldi et al., 2003). Less discrimination was found in a series of 185 IPSS procedures with a 99% positive predictive power but only a 20% negative predictive power (Swearingen et al., 2004). In view of the technical difficulty with IPSS, sampling of the internal jugular vein may be performed and only patients with a negative result referred for IPSS (Ilias et al., 2004).

If clinical and lab data point to an ectopic ACTH-secreting tumor, CT and/or MRI of the neck, thorax, and abdomen and, for occult tumors, scintigraphy with the somatostatin analog, ^{111}In-pentetreotide are currently used to locate the tumor (De Herder & Lamberts, 1999). Positron emission tomography with other labeled precursors has identified ACTH-secreting carcinoid tumors (Dubois et al., 2007).

Treatment

Treatment of the Hypertension

Until definitive therapy is provided, the hypertension that accompanies Cushing syndrome can temporarily be treated with the usual antihypertensive agents described in Chapter 7 (Fallo et al., 1993). Since excess fluid volume is likely involved, a diuretic, perhaps in combination with an aldosterone antagonist, spironolactone or eplerenone, is an appropriate initial choice. After definitive therapy, hypertension usually improves but atherosclerotic risk factors often persist, likely because of residual abdominal obesity and insulin resistance (Barahona et al., 2009).

Treatment of the Syndrome in General

In view of the long-term morbidity associated with Cushing syndrome, the condition must be treated as rapidly as possible after the diagnosis has been established (Biller et al., 2008). The choice of definitive therapy depends on the cause of the syndrome (Table 13-3).

- In the majority of patients who have ACTH-dependent Cushing disease with a pituitary tumor, transphenoidal microsurgical removal is the treatment of choice (Mullan & Atkinson, 2008). In some circumstances, bilateral adrenalectomy or stereotactic radiotherapy (Petit et al., 2008) may be used if pituitary surgery is unsuccessful or when no pituitary tumor is found (Pouratian et al., 2007).

TABLE 13.3   Therapies for Cushing Syndrome

Class	Site	Therapy
Surgery	Pituitary	Transphenoidal microsection; transfrontal hypophysectomy
	Adrenal	Unilateral adrenalectomy; bilateral adrenalectomy
Radiation		Fractionated X-ray (4–6 weeks)
		Single-dose
		Gamma knife
		Linear acceleration
		Heavy charged proton
Drugs	Acting at hypothalamic-pituitary	Serotonin antagonists (cyproheptadine, ritanserin)
		Dopamine agonists (bromocriptine, lisuride)
		GABA agonists (sodium valproate)
		Somatostatin analogs (octreotide)
	Inhibitors of adrenocortical steroid synthesis	PPAR γ-agonist
		Mitotane
		Metyrapone
		Aminoglutethimide
		Ketoconazole
	Glucocorticoid antagonist	Etomidate
		Mifepristone

- Benign adrenal tumors should be surgically removed, increasingly by laparoscopy (Chow et al., 2008).
- For adrenal cancers and ectopic ACTH tumors that cannot be resected, removal of the adrenal may be helpful, but chemotherapy is usually needed (Abiven et al., 2006).
- The drugs listed in Table 13-3 are mainly used to quickly overcome severe complications, either in preparation for surgery or whenever definitive treatment must be delayed (Mullan & Atkinson, 2008).

Follow-up

With definitive therapy, remission rates of 70% to 80%—defined as normal plasma and urinary cortisol levels and resolution of clinical stigmata—have been noted (Arnaldi et al., 2003; Mullan & Atkinson, 2008). However, as many as 25% of pituitary-dependent Cushing's patients have recurrences at 5 years after initially successful transspenoidal surgery, so close and long-term follow-up is necessary (Patil et al., 2008).

SYNDROMES WITH INCREASED ACCESS OF CORTISOL TO MINERALOCORTICOID RECEPTORS

Less common than Cushing syndrome caused by cortisol excess are a variety of fascinating syndromes wherein normal or increased levels of cortisol exert a mineralocorticoid effect by binding to the renal MCRs. As depicted in Figure 13-3, the normal renal MCR is as receptive to glucocorticoids as it is to mineralocorticoids. The 11β-hydroxysteroid dehydrogenase type 2 isoform (11β-HSD2) enzyme in the renal tubules upstream to these receptors normally converts the large amounts of fully active cortisol to the inactive cortisone, thereby leaving the MCRs open to the effects of aldosterone (Quinkler & Stewart, 2003).

However, there are both congenital and acquired deficiencies of the 11β-HSD2 enzyme, so that the normal levels of cortisol remain fully active, flooding the MCR and inducing the full syndrome of mineralocorticoid excess: sodium retention, potassium wastage, and hypertension with virtually complete suppression of renin and aldosterone secretion (Stewart, 2003).

11β-HSD2 Deficiency: Apparent Mineralocorticoid Excess

Apparent mineralocorticoid excess (AME) is an autosomal recessive disorder that has now been identified in about 100 patients. The syndrome clinically is characterized by familial consanguinity, low birth weight, failure to thrive, onset of severe hypertension in early childhood with extensive target organ damage, hypercalciuria, nephrocalcinosis, and renal failure (Chemaitilly et al., 2003). As noted, sodium

Normal Kidney

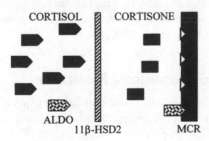

AME Kidney

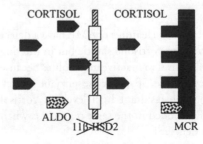

FIGURE 13-3 Enzyme-mediated receptor protection. Normally, 11β-dehydrogenase (11β-HSD2) converts cortisol to inactive cortisone in the more proximal nephron, protecting mineralocorticoid receptors (MCR) from cortisol and allowing selective access for aldosterone. When 11β-HSD2 is defective, e.g., in congenital deficiency (AME kidney) or after licorice administration, cortisol gains inappropriate access to mineralocorticoid receptors, resulting in sodium retention and potassium wasting. (Modified from Cerame BI, New MI. Hormonal hypertension in children: 11β-Hydroxylase deficiency and apparent mineralocorticoid excess. *J Ped Endocrinol Metab* 2000;13:1537–1547.)

retention, hypokalemia, low aldosterone, and low renin levels are present.

Genetics

Soon after the first case was described, (Werder et al., 1974), Ulick et al. (1979) recognized that these children did not metabolize cortisol normally. Some years later, Stewart et al. (1988), in studies on a 20-year-old with the syndrome, recognized a defect in the renal cortisol-cortisone shuttle and demonstrated the deficiency of the 11β-HSD2 enzyme. A number of mutations in the 11β-HSD gene have now been identified in patients with AME (Carvajal et al., 2003; Cerame and New, 2000; Lin-Su et al., 2004).

Some of these mutations result in only partial inhibition of the 11β-HSD2 enzyme as evidenced by a higher ratio of urinary cortisone to cortisol metabolites and a milder clinical course with larger birth weight, later age of presentation (Nunez et al., 1999), and in at least one patient, only mild low-renin hypertension (Wilson et al., 1998). Not surprisingly, mutations resulting in less inhibition of the enzyme have been sought in patients with "essential" hypertension. Some have found them but most have not (Quinkler & Stewart, 2003). A role of impaired 11β-HSD2 activity has also been proposed for sodium sensitivity (Ferrari et al., 2001), intrauterine growth retardation (McTernan et al., 2001), and preeclampsia (Schoof et al., 2001).

An intriguing prospect has been proposed that decreased 11β-HSD2 activity may occur with aging and thereby may be involved in hypertension in the elderly (Henschkowski et al., 2008). Funder (2008) advises caution in accepting this proposal.

Variant

A few patients with the features of AME have a defect not in the cortisol to cortisone shuttle but in the ring A reduction of cortisol to inactive metabolites because of a deficiency of the 5β-reductase enzyme (Ulick et al., 1992a). The resultant high levels of cortisol keep the MCRs flooded in the same manner as when 11β-HSD2 is deficient.

Therapy

Therapy is usually based on competitive blockade of the MCR with spironolactone (Dave-Sharma, 1998) or eplerenone (Funder, 2000). Suppression of endogenous cortisol with dexamethasone has also been used (Quinkler & Stewart, 2003). Cure has been reported on one patient after transplantation of a kidney with normal 11β-HDS2 activity (Palermo et al., 1998).

11β-HSD2 Inhibition: Glycyrrhetinic Acid (Licorice)

Since the early 1950s, glycyrrhizin acid, the active ingredient in licorice extract, has been known to cause hypertension, sodium retention, and potassium wastage. Stewart et al. (1987) and Edwards et al. (1988) recognized the similarities between the syndrome induced by licorice and the syndrome of AME and documented that licorice inhibited the same renal 11β-HSD2 enzyme that was deficient in AME. These effects are accompanied by a fall in cortisone and a rise in cortisol excretion, reflecting the inhibition of renal 11β-HSD2 activity.

Relatively small amounts of confectionary licorice, as little as 50 g daily for 2 weeks, produce a rise in BP in normal people (Sigurjonsdottir et al., 2001). The syndrome also has been induced by the licorice extracts in chewing tobacco and candy and herbal remedies (Sontia et al., 2008). Not surprisingly, aldosterone receptor blockers (spirinolactone and eplerenone) have been shown to relieve all of the effects of licorice-induced hypertension (Quaschning et al., 2001). Even better is to recognize and stop the habit.

Massive Cortisol Excess

The capacity of the 11β-HSD-directed cortisol-cortisone shuttle and of 5β-reductase inactivation may be overcome by massive amounts of cortisol. Ulick et al. (1992b) have shown this to be the mechanism responsible for the significant features of mineralocorticoid excess—profound hypokalemia and hypertension—that are seen in patients with ectopic ACTH tumors wherein cortisol levels are much higher than in other causes of Cushing syndrome (Torpy et al., 2002).

Glucocorticoid Resistance

Both sporadic and familial forms of glucocorticoid receptor resistance, ascribed to various mutations in the receptor gene (Charmandari et al., 2008), have increased levels of circulating cortisol but without typical Cushing's stigmata (Kino et al., 2002). Many of these patients have hypertension that may mimic mineralocorticoid excess. Moreover, among 60 hypertensive patients under age 36, 45 had increased levels of urinary glucocorticoid metabolites, suggesting partial resistance of glucocorticoid receptors with subsequent increased mineralocorticoid effects (Shamim et al., 2001).

DEOXYCORTICOSTERONE EXCESS: CONGENITAL ADRENAL HYPERPLASIA

Excessive amounts of the mineralocorticoid DOC may cause hypertension (Ferrari & Bonny, 2003), arising either from hyperplastic adrenals with enzymatic deficiencies or from rare DOC-secreting tumors (Gröndal et al., 1990).

Defects in all of the enzymes involved in adrenal steroid synthesis have been recognized (Fig. 13-4). These defects are inherited in an autosomal recessive manner and their manifestations result from inadequate levels of the end products of steroid synthesis—in particular, cortisol. The low levels of cortisol call forth increased secretion of ACTH, further increasing the accumulation of the precursor steroids proximal to the enzymatic block and stimulating steroidogenesis in pathways that are not blocked (Table 13-4).

The clinical manifestations of CAH, often obvious at birth, vary with the degree of enzymatic deficiency and the mix of steroids secreted by the hyperplastic adrenal glands. The most common type, the 21-hydroxylase deficiency, responsible for perhaps 90% of all CAH, is not associated with hypertension but is accompanied by a high prevalence of testicular adrenal rest tumors that may lead to impotence (Martinez-Aguayo et al., 2007) tumors.

The two forms of CAH in which hypertension occurs are caused by deficiency of the 11β-hydroxylase (CYP11β1) or 17-hydroxylase (CYP17A) enzymes. Though these are rare causes of hypertension, partial enzymatic deficiencies have been observed in hirsute women (Lucky et al., 1986), so some hypertensive adults may have unrecognized, subtle forms of CAH.

11-Hydroxylase Deficiency

Much less common than 21-hydroxylase deficiency in hyperandrogenized adults (Escobar-Morreale et al., 2008), this is the second most common form of CAH and is usually recognized in infancy because, as shown in Figure 13-4, the defect sets off production of excessive androgens. The enzyme deficiency prevents the hydroxylation of 11-deoxycortisol, resulting in cortisol deficiency and prevents the conversion of DOC to corticosterone and aldosterone. The high levels of DOC induce hypertension and hypokalemia, the expected features of mineralocorticoid excess. Thus the syndrome features virilization of the infant, hypertension, and hypokalemia.

The enzyme deficiency has been attributed to various mutations in the *CYP 11B1* gene (Andrew

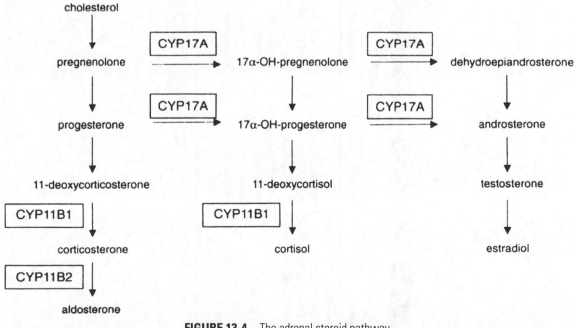

FIGURE 13-4   The adrenal steroid pathway.

TABLE 13.4 Syndromes of Congenital Adrenal Hyperplasia

Enzyme	Site of Defect		Steroid Levels			Clinical Features	
	Increased Precursor	Decreased Product	17-OH-P or P´ triol	DOC	Aldo	Virilization	Hypertension
21-Hydroxylase							
Nonsalt wasting	17-Hydroxyprogesterone	11-Deoxycortisol, cortisol	↑↑↑	N	N	Marked	No
Salt wasting	Progesterone	11-DOC, cortisol	↑↑↑	↓→	↓↓	Marked	No
11-Hydroxylase	11-Deoxycortisol	Cortisol	N,↑	↑↑	↓↓,N	Marked	Yes
	11-Deoxycorticolsteroid	Cortisterone					
17-Hydroxylase	Progesterone	Cortisol	↓↓	↑↑	↓,N,↑	Absent	Yes
	Pregnenolone	17-Hydroxypregnenolone					
3β-ol-dehydrogenase	Pregnenolone	Progesterone, cortisol	N,↑	N,↓	↓,N	Sight	No
STAR protein	Cholesterol	All steroids	↓↓	↓↓	↓↓	Absent	No

17-KS, 17-ketosteroids; 17-OH-P, 17-hydroxyprogesterone; P´ triol, pregnanetriol; Aldo, aldosterone; N, normal; ↑, increased by varying degrees; ↓, decreased by varying degrees.

et al., 2007). The syndrome is diagnosed by finding high levels of 11-deoxycortisol and DOC in urine and plasma. Treatment, as for all of the syndromes of CAH, is with glucocorticoid, which should relieve the hypertension and hypokalemia and allow the child to develop normally. Prenatal diagnosis and treatment have been shown to prevent virilization (Cerame et al., 1999).

17-Hydroxylase Deficiency

Unlike the 21-hydroxylase and 11-hydroxylase deficiencies, CAH caused by a 17-hydroxylase deficiency is typically associated with an absence of sex hormones, leading to incomplete masculinization in males and primary amenorrhea in females in addition to hypertension and hypokalemia (Fig. 13-4; Table 13-4). This is the first hypertensive disorder of steroidogenesis that has been identified (Biglieri et al., 1966). Nearly 40 different mutations in CYP17 have now been described, and there is considerable variability in the clinical and hormonal features (Rosa et al., 2007).

Now that the various renal and adrenal causes of hypertension have been covered, we shall turn to an even larger variety of less common forms.

REFERENCES

Abiven G, Coste J, Groussin L, et al. Clinical and biological features in the prognosis of adrenocortical cancer: Poor outcome of cortisol-secreting tumors in a series of 202 consecutive patients. *J Clin Endocrinol Metab* 2006;91(7):2650–2655.

Andrew M, Barr M, Davies E, et al. Congenital adrenal hyperplasia in a Nigerian child with a novel compound heterozygote mutation in CYP11B1. *Clin Endocrinol (Oxf)* 2007;66(4): 602–603.

Arnaldi G, Angeli A, Atkinson AB, et al. Diagnosis and complications of Cushing's syndrome: A consensus statement. *J Clin Endocrinol Metab* 2003;88(12):5593–5602.

Badrick E, Bobak M, Britton A, et al. The relationship between alcohol consumption and cortisol secretion in an aging cohort. *J Clin Endocrinol Metab* 2008;93(3):750–757.

Barahona M, Sucunza N, Resmini E, et al. Persistant body fat mass and inflammatory marker increases after long-term cure of Cushing's syndrome. *J Clin Endocrinol Metab* 2009.

Barzon L, Fallo F, Sonino N, et al. Development of overt Cushing's syndrome in patients with adrenal incidentaloma. *Eur J Endocrinol* 2002;146:61–66.

Batista DL, Riar J, Keil M, et al. Diagnostic tests for children who are referred for the investigation of Cushing syndrome. *Pediatrics* 2007;120(3):e575–e586.

Bertherat J, Contesse V, Louiset E, et al. In vivo and *in vitro* screening for illegitimate receptors in ACTH-independent macronodular adrenal hyperplasia (AIMAH) causing Cushing's syndrome: Identification of two cases of gonadotropin/gastric inhibitory

polypeptide-dependent hypercortisolism. *J Clin Endocrinol Metab* 2005;90;1302–1310.

Biglieri EG, Herron MA, Brust N. 17-Hydroxylation deficiency in man. *J Clin Invest* 1966;45:1946–1954.

Biller BM, Grossman AB, Stewart PM, et al. Treatment of adrenocorticotropin-dependent Cushing's syndrome: A consensus statement. *J Clin Endocrinol Metab* 2008;93(7):2454–2462.

Boscaro M, Barzon L, Fallo F, et al. Cushing's syndrome. *Lancet* 2001;357:783–791.

Carvajal CA, Gonzalez AA, Romero DG, et al. Two homozygous mutations in the 11β-hydroxysteroid dehydrogenase type 2 gene in a case of apparent mineralocorticoid excess. *J Clin Endocrinol Metab* 2003;88:2501–2507.

Cassar J, Loizou S, Kelly WF, et al. Deoxycorticosterone and aldosterone excretion in Cushing's syndrome. *Metabolism* 1980;29: 115–119.

Cerame BI, Newfield RS, Pascoe L, et al. Prenatal diagnosis and treatment of 11β-hydroxylase deficiency congenital adrenal hyperplasia resulting in normal female genitalia. *J Clin Endocrinol Metab* 1999;84:3129–3134.

Charmandari E, Kino T, Ichijo T, et al. Generalized glucocorticoid resistance: Clinical aspects, molecular mechanisms, and implications of a rare genetic disorder. *J Clin Endocrinol Metab* 2008;93:1563–1572.

Chemaitilly W, Wilson RC, New MI. Hypertension and adrenal disorders. *Curr Hypertens Rep* 2003;5:498–504.

Chow JT, Thompson GB, Grant CS, et al. Bilateral laparoscopic adrenalectomy for corticotrophin-dependent Cushing's syndrome: a review of the Mayo Clinic experience. *Clin Endocrinol (Oxf)* 2008;68(4):513–519.

Dave-Sharma S, Wilson RC, Harbison MD, et al. Examination of genotype and phenotype relationships in 14 patients with apparent mineralocorticoid excess. *J Clin Endocrinol Metab* 1998;83:2244–2254.

De Herder WW, Lamberts SWJ. Tumor localization—The ectopic ACTH syndrome. *J Clin Endocrinol Metab* 1999;84:1184–1185.

Doppman JL, Chrousos GP, Papanicolaou DA, et al. Adrenocorticotropin-independent macronodular adrenal hyperplasia: An uncommon cause of primary adrenal hypercortisolism. *Radiology* 2000;216:797–802.

Druce M, Goldstone AP, Tan TM, et al. The pursuit of beauty. *Lancet* 2008;371(9612):596.

Dubois S, Morel O, Rodien P, et al. A Pulmonary adrenocorticotropin-secreting carcinoid tumor localized by 6-Fluoro-[18F]L-dihydroxyphenylalanine positron emission/computed tomography imaging in a patient with Cushing's syndrome. *J Clin Endocrinol Metab* 2007;92(12):4512–4513.

Edwards CRW, Burt D, McIntyre MA, et al. Localisation of 11β-hydroxysteroid dehydrogenase-tissue specific protector of the mineralocorticoid receptor. *Lancet* 1988;2:986–989.

Ehlers ME, Griffing GT, Wilson TE, et al. Elevated urinary 19-nor-deoxycorticosterone glucuronide in Cushing's syndrome. *J Clin Endocrinol Metab* 1987;64:926–930.

Elamin MB, Murad MH, Mullan R, et al. Accuracy of diagnostic tests for Cushing's syndrome: A systematic review and metaanalyses. *J Clin Endocrinol Metab* 2008;93(5):1553–1562.

Escobar-Morreale HF, Sanchon R, San Millan JL. A prospective study of the prevalence of nonclassical congenital adrenal hyperplasia among women presenting with hyperandrogenic symptoms and signs. *J Clin Endocrinol Metab* 2008;93(2): 527–533.

Fallo F, Paoletta A, Tona F, et al. Response of hypertension to conventional antihypertensive treatment and/or steroidogenesis inhibitors in Cushing's syndrome. *J Intern Med* 1993;234: 595–598.

Ferrari P, Bonny O. Forms of mineralocorticoid hypertension. *Vitam Horm* 2003;66:113–156.

Ferrari P, Sansonnens A, Dick B, et al. In vivo 11β-HSD-2 activity: Variability, salt-sensitivity, and effect of licorice. *Hypertension* 2001;38:1330–1336.

Findling JW, Raff H. Cushing's Syndrome: Important issues in diagnosis and management. *J Clin Endocrinol Metab* 2006; 91(10):3746–3753.

Findling JW, Raff H, Aron DC. The low-dose dexamethasone suppression test: A reevaluation in patients with Cushing's syndrome. *J Clin Endocrinol Metab* 2004;89:1222–1226.

Funder JW. Eplerenone, a new mineralocorticoid antagonist: In vitro and in vivo studies. *Curr Opin Endocrinol Diab* 2000;7: 138–142.

Funder J. Chipping away at "essential" hypertension. *Am J Hypertens* 2008;21(6):600.

Gatta B, Chabre O, Cortet C, et al. Reevaluation of the combined dexamethasone suppression-corticotropin-releasing hormone test for differentiation of mild Cushing's disease from pseudo-Cushing's syndrome. *J Clin Endocrinol Metab* 2007;92(11): 4290–4293.

Goodwin JE, Zhang J, Geller DS. A critical role for vascular smooth muscle in acute glucocorticoid-induced hypertension. *J Am Soc Nephrol* 2008:19;1291–1299.

Gröndal S, Eriksson B, Hagenäs L, et al. Steroid profile in urine: A useful tool in the diagnosis and follow up of adrenocortical carcinoma. *Acta Endocrinol (Copenh)* 1990;122:656–663.

Groote Veldman R, Meinders AE. On the mechanism of alcohol-induced pseudo-Cushing's syndrome. *Endocrinol Rev* 1996;17: 262–268.

Henschkowski J, Stuck AE, Frey BM, et al. Age-dependent decrease in 11beta-hydroxysteroid dehydrogenase type 2 (11beta-HSD2) activity in hypertensive patients. *Am J Hypertens* 2008;21(6):644–649.

Hermus AR, Pieters GF, Smals AG, et al. Transition from pituitary-dependent to adrenal-dependent Cushing's syndrome. *N Engl J Med* 1988;318:966–970.

Ilias I, Chang R, Pacak K, et al. Jugular venous sampling: An alternative to petrosal sinus sampling for the diagnostic evaluation of adrenocorticotropic hormone-dependent Cushing's syndrome. *J Clin Endocrinol Metab* 2004;89:3795–3800.

Invitti C, Giraldi FP, de Martin M, et al. Diagnosis and management of Cushing's syndrome: Results of an Italian multicentre study. *J Clin Endocrinol Metab* 1999;84:440–448.

Ishibashi M, Shimada K, Abe K, et al. Spontaneous remission in Cushing's disease. *Arch Intern Med* 1993;153:251–255.

Karavitaki N. Nonfunctioning pituitary adenomas: The consequences of a 'watch and wait' approach. *Clin Endocrinol (Oxf)* 2007;1365–2265.

Kino T, Vottero A, Charmandari E, et al. Familial/sporadic glucocorticoid resistance syndrome and hypertension. *Ann NY Acad Sci* 2002;970:101–111.

Kirilov G, Tomova A, Dakovska L, et al. Elevated plasma endothelin as an additional cardiovascular risk factor in patients with Cushing's syndrome. *Eur J Endocrinol* 2003;149:549–553.

Lacroix A, N'Diaye N, Tremblay J, et al. Ectopic and abnormal hormone receptors in adrenal Cushing's syndrome. *Endrocrine Rev* 2001;22:75–110.

Lee P, Bradbury RA, Sy J, et al. Phaeochromocytoma and mixed corticomedullary tumour—A rare cause of Cushing's syndrome and labile hypertension in a primigravid woman postpartum. *Clin Endocrinol (Oxf)* 2008;68(3):492–494.

Leibowitz G, Tsur A, Chayen SD, et al. Pre-clinical Cushing's syndrome: An unexpected frequent cause of poor glycaemic control in obese diabetic patients. *Clin Endocrinol* 1996;44: 717–722.

Lin-Su K, Zhou P, Arora N, et al. *In vitro* expression studies of a novel mutation Δ299 in a patient affected with apparent mineralocorticoid excess. *J Clin Endocrinol Metab* 2004;89: 2025–2027.

Lodish MB, Sinaii N, Patronas N, et al. Blood pressure in pediatric patients with Cushing syndrome. *J Clin Endocrinol Metab* 2009;94:2002–2008.

Lucky AW, Rosenfield FL, McGuire J, et al. Adrenal androgen hyperresponsiveness to adrenocorticotropin in women with acne and/or hirsutism: Adrenal enzyme defects and exaggerated adrenarche. *J Clin Endocrinol Metab* 1986;62:840–848.

Magiakou MA, Mastorakos G, Zachman K, et al. Blood pressure in children and adolescents with Cushing syndrome before and after surgical cure. *J Clin Endocrinol* 1997;82:1734–1738.

Malchoff CD. Carney complex—Clarity and complexity. *J Clin Endocrinol Metab* 2000;85:4010–4012.

Mangos GJ, Walker BR, Kelly JJ, et al. Cortisol inhibits cholinergic vasodilatation in the human forearm. *Am J Hypertens* 2000;13:1155–1160.

Martinez-Aguayo A, Rocha A, Rojas N, et al. Testicular adrenal rest tumors and Leydig and Sertoli cell function in boys with classical congenital adrenal hyperplasia. *J Clin Endocrinol Metab* 2007;92(12):4583–4589.

McTernan CL, Draper N, Nicholson H, et al. Reduced placental 11β-hydroxysteroid dehydrogenase type 2 mRNA levels in human pregnancies complicated by intrauterine growth reduction: An analysis of possible mechanisms. *J Clin Endocrinol Metab* 2001;86:4979–4983.

Mitchell IC, Auchus RJ, Juneja K, et al. "Subclinical Cushing's syndrome" is not subclinical: Improvement after adrenalectomy in 9 patients. *Surgery* 2007;142(6):900–905.

Molnar GA, Lindschau C, Dubrovska G, et al. Glucocorticoid-related signaling effects in vascular smooth muscle cells. *Hypertension* 2008;51(5):1372–1378.

Mortola JF, Liu JH, Gillin JC, et al. Pulsatile rhythms of adrenocorticotropin (ACTH) and cortisol in women with endogenous depression: Evidence for increased ACTH pulse frequency. *J Clin Endocrinol Metab* 1987;65:962–968.

Mullan KR, Atkinson AB. Endocrine clinical update: where are we in the therapeutic management of pituitary-dependent hypercortisolism? *Clin Endocrinol (Oxf)* 2008;68(3):327–337.

Newell-Price J. Diagnosis of Cushing's syndrome: Comparison of the specificity of first-line biochemical tests. *Nat Clin Pract Endocrinol Metab* 2008;4(4):192–193.

Newell-Price J, Bertagna X, Grossman AB, et al. Cushing's syndrome. *Lancet* 2006;367(9522):1605–1617.

Nieman LK, Biller BM, Findling JW, et al. The diagnosis of Cushing's Syndrome: An Endocrine Society Clinical Practice Guideline. *J Clin Endocrinol Metab* 2008;93(5):1526–1540.

Nunez BS, Rogerson FM, Mune T, et al. Mutant of 11β-hydroxysteroid dehydrogenase (11-HSD2) with partial activity. *Hypertension* 1999;34:638–642.

Palermo M, Cossu M, Shackleton CHL. Cure of apparent mineralocorticoid excess by kidney transplantation. *N Engl J Med* 1998;329:1782–1788.

Pirpiris M, Sudhir K, Yeung S, et al. Pressor responsiveness in corticosteroid-induced hypertension in humans. *Hypertension* 1992;19:567–574.

Patil CG, Prevedello DM, Lad SP, et al. Late recurrences of Cushing's disease after initial successful transsphenoidal surgery. *J Clin Endocrinol Metab* 2008;93(2):358–362.

Pecori GF, Ambrogio AG, De MM, et al. Specificity of first-line tests for the diagnosis of Cushing's syndrome: Assessment in a large series. *J Clin Endocrinol Metab* 2007;92(11):4123–4129.

Petit JH, Biller BM, Yock TI, et al. Proton stereotactic radiotherapy for persistent adrenocorticotropin-producing adenomas. *J Clin Endocrinol Metab* 2008;93(2):393–399.

Pouratian N, Prevedello DM, Jagannathan J, et al. Outcomes and management of patients with Cushing's disease without pathological confirmation of tumor resection after transsphenoidal surgery. *J Clin Endocrinol Metab* 2007;92(9):3383–3388.

Quaschning T, Ruschitzka FT, Shaw S, et al. Aldosterone receptor antagonism normalizes vascular function in liquorice-induced hypertension. *Hypertension* 2001;37:801–805.

Quinkler M, Stewart PM. Hypertension and the cortisol-cortisone shuttle. *J Clin Endocrinol Metab* 2003;88:2384–2392.

Rockall AG, Sohaib SA, Evans D, et al. Hepatic steatosis in Cushing's syndrome: A radiological assessment using computer tomography. *Eur J Endocrinol* 2003;149:543–548.

Rosa S, Duff C, Meyer M, et al. P450c17 deficiency: Clinical and molecular characterization of six patients. *J Clin Endocrinol Metab* 2007;92(3):1000–1007.

Rossi R, Tauchmanova L, Luciano A, et al. Subclinical Cushing's syndrome in patients with adrenal incidentaloma: Clinical and biochemical features. *J Clin Endocrinol Metab* 2000;85:1440–1448.

Saruta T. Mechanism of glucocorticoid-induced hypertension. *Hypertens Res* 1996;19:18.

Scheuer DA, Bechtold AG, Shank SS, et al. Glucocorticoids act in the dorsal hindbrain to increase arterial pressure. *Am J Physiol Heart Circ Physiol* 2004;286:H458–H467.

Shamim W, Yousufuddin M, Francis DP, et al. Raised urinary glucocorticoid and adrenal androgen precursors in the urine of young hypertensive patients: Possible evidence for partial glucocorticoid resistance. *Heart* 2001;86:139–144.

Sigurjonsdottir HA, Manhem K, Wallerstedt S. Liquorice-induced hypertension—A linear dose-response relationship. *J Hum Hypertens* 2001;15:549–552.

Solomon CG, Seely EW. Hypertension in pregnancy. *Endocrinol Metab Clin North Am* 2006;35(1):157–171.

Sontia B, Mooney J, Gaudet L, et al. Pseudohyperaldosteronism, liquorice, and hypertension. *J Clin Hypertens* 2008;10:153–157.

Stewart PM, Corrie JET, Shackleton CHL, et al. Syndrome of apparent mineralocorticoid excess: A defect in the cortisol-cortisone shuttle. *J Clin Invest* 1988;82:340–349.

Stewart PM, Wallace AM, Valentino R, et al. Mineralocorticoid activity of liquorice: 11-Beta-hydroxysteroid dehydrogenase deficiency comes of age. *Lancet* 1987;2:821–824.

Suzuki T, Shibata H, Ando T, et al. Risk factors associated with persistent postoperative hypertension in Cushing's syndrome. *Endocrine Res* 2000;26:791–795.

Swearingen B, Katznelson L, Miller K, et al. Diagnostic errors after inferior petrosal sinus sampling. *J Clin Endocrinol Metab* 2004;89:3752–3763.

Torpy DJ, Mullen N, Ilias J, et al. Association of hypertension and hypokalemia with Cushing's syndrome caused by ectopic ACTH secretion: A series of 58 cases. *Ann NY Acad Sci* 2002;970:134–144.

Tremble IM, Buxton-Thomas M, Hopkins D, et al. Cushing's syndrome associated with a chemodectoma and a carcinoid tumour. *Clin Endocrinol* 2000;52:789–793.

Ulick S, Levine LS, Gunczler P, et al. A syndrome of apparent mineralocorticoid excess associated with defects in the peripheral metabolism of cortisol. *J Clin Endocrinol Metab* 1979;49:757–764.

Ulick S, Tedde R, Wang JZ. Defective ring A reduction of cortisol as the major metabolic error in the syndrome of apparent mineralocorticoid excess. *J Clin Endocrinol Metab* 1992a;74:593–599.

Ulick S, Wang JZ, Blumenfeld JD, et al. Cortisol inactivation overload: A mechanism of mineralocorticoid hypertension in the ectopic adrenocorticotropin syndrome. *J Clin Endocrinol Metab* 1992b;74:963–967.

van Rossum EFC, Lamberts SWJ. Polymorphisms in the glucocorticoid receptor gene and their associations with metabolic parameters and body composition. *Recent Prog Hormone Res* 2004;59:333–357.

Vezzosi D, Cartier D, Regnier C, et al. Familial adrenocorticotropin-independent macronodular adrenal hyperplasia with aberrant serotonin and vasopressin adrenal receptors. *Eur J Endocrinol* 2007;156(1):21–31.

Weigensberg MJ, Toledo-Corral CM, Goran MI. Association between the metabolic syndrome and serum cortisol in overweight Latino youth. *J Clin Endocrinol Metab* 2008;93(4):1372–1378.

Werder E, Zachmann M, Völlmin JA, et al. Unusual steroid excretion in a child with low-renin hypertension. *Res Steroids* 1974;6:385–395.

Whitworth JA, Mangos GJ, Kelly JJ. Cushing, cortisol, and cardiovascular disease. *Hypertension* 2000;36:912–916.

Wilson RC, Dave-Sharma S, Wei J-Q, et al. A genetic defect resulting in mild low-renin hypertension. *Proc Natl Acad Sci USA* 1998;95:10200–10205.

Yanovski JA, Cutler GB Jr, Chrousos GP, et al. The dexamethasone-suppressed corticotropin-releasing hormone stimulation test differentiates mild Cushing's disease from normal physiology. *J Clin Endocrinol Metab* 1998;83:348–352.

Young WF Jr. Clinical practice: The incidentally discovered adrenal mass. *N Engl J Med* 2007;356(6):601–610.

Zelinka T, Štrauch B, Pecen L, et al. Diurnal blood pressure variation on pheochromocytoma, primary aldosteronism, and Cushing's syndrome. *J Hum Hypertens* 2004;18:107–111.

Zerikly RK, Eray E, Faiman C, et al. Cyclic Cushing Syndrome due to an ectopic pituitary adenoma. *Nat Clin Pract Endocrinal Metab* 2009;5(3):174–179.

Other Forms of Identifiable Hypertension

As described in Chapter 3, the pathogenesis of primary (essential) hypertension likely involves multiple mechanisms. Beyond the involvement of obvious players such as renal sodium handling, renin-angiotensin, and the sympathetic nervous system, whose altered roles may be genetically determined, lurk a number of environmental factors. Of those factors, sodium and potassium intake, weight gain, and stress most likely are causal. Others, such as smoking and alcohol, may raise the blood pressure (BP) but they are generally considered to be contributory rather than causal, since, when they are discontinued, their pressor effect disappears.

As described in Chapters 9 through 14, a number of secondary or identifiable causes of hypertension have been characterized. In addition to those, which primarily reflect renal and adrenal hormonal abnormalities, a number of other, generally less common forms of hypertension have been identified and will be covered in this chapter. Additional coverage of hypertension in childhood is provided in Chapter 16.

COARCTATION OF THE AORTA

Constriction of the lumen of the aorta may occur anywhere along its length but is seen most commonly just beyond the origin of the left subclavian artery, at or below the insertion of the ligamentum arteriosum. This lesion makes up approximately 7% of all congenital heart diseases. Hypertension in the upper extremities with diminished or absent femoral pulses is the usual presentation (Table 14-1).

The traditional separation into infantile (preductal) and adult (postductal) types is now considered inappropriate, with many preductal lesions not identified until adult life. As Jenkins and Ward (1999) state:

> A spectrum of lesions is now recognized, and it is only those with the most severe obstruction (e.g., aortic arch atresia or interruption) or associated cardiac defects who invariably present in infancy. Most other cases are now identified at routine medical examination. Otherwise, age at presentation is related to the severity rather than the site of obstruction, as a result of cardiac failure or occasionally cerebrovascular accident (CVA), aortic dissection, or endocarditis.

Pathophysiology

If the coarctation is proximal to the ductus arteriosus, pulmonary hypertension, congestive failure, and cyanosis of the lower half of the body occur early in life. Before surgery was possible, 45% to 84% of infants found to have coarctation died during their first year of life (Campbell, 1970).

Patients with less severe postductal lesions may have no difficulties during childhood. However, they almost always develop premature cardiovascular disease; in the two largest series of autopsied cases seen before the advent of effective surgery, the mean age of death was 34 years (Campbell, 1970). The causes of death reflected the pressure load on the heart and the associated cardiac and cerebral lesions.

Beyond the obvious obstruction to blood flow, coarctation likely involves a wider abnormality with defects found in the vascular media both proximal and distal (Niwa et al., 2001) that may, in turn, reflect an innate cellular defect (Swan et al., 2002). The presence of intracranial aneurysm in 10% of adults with coarctation (Connolly et al., 2003) may reflect such underlying vascular weakness. Moreover, after the initial insult of coarctation, a number of secondary

TABLE 14.1	Symptoms and Signs of Coarctation

Symptoms
- Headache
- Cold feet
- Pain in legs with exercise

Signs
- Hypertension
- Hyperdynamic apical impulse
- Murmurs in front or back of the chest
- Pulsations in neck
- Weak femoral pulse

processes such as left ventricular hypertrophy are initiated and may persist even after repair. Therefore, early detection and repair are critical (Daniels, 2001).

Recognition of Coarctation

Hypertension in the arms with weak femoral pulses in a young person strongly suggests coarctation. With minimal constriction, symptoms may not appear until late in life (Dubrey & Mittal, 2008). Often the heart is large and shows left ventricular strain on the electrocardiogram. The chest radiograph can be diagnostic, demonstrating the "three" sign from dilation of the aorta above and below the constriction and notching of the ribs by enlarged collateral vessels. The diagnosis is now usually made by echocardiography and color Doppler flow mapping.

Atypical aortic coarctation in adults most likely represents Takayasu arteritis, or pulseless disease, which usually affects the aortic arch and may also involve the descending aorta (Numano et al., 2000) or renal arteries (Weaver et al., 2004). This large-vessel vasculitis may be successfully treated with balloon angioplasty (Tyagi et al., 1992) but usually improves with corticosteroids (Numano et al., 2000).

Management

Early repair by surgery or angioplasty (Weber & Cyran, 2008) is now recommended with very low rates of recoarctation being encountered (Pearl et al., 2004). If repair is delayed until adulthood, there is a greater likelihood of persistent hypertension, which may be severe. Nonetheless, repair usually improves the hypertension (Duara et al., 2008). Even in those with normal resting BPs, there may be an exaggerated

BP response to exercise (Hager et al., 2008) but Vriend et al. (2004) found no independent relationship of this response to left ventricular mass.

Obviously, patients after repair need to be closely followed and any degree of hypertension needs to be intensively treated (Ou et al., 2008).

HORMONAL DISTURBANCES

Hypothyroidism

Hypertension, particularly diastolic, may be more common in hypothyroid patients. Among 40 patients prospectively followed over the time they became hypothyroid after radioiodine therapy for thyrotoxicosis, 16 (40%) developed a diastolic BP higher than 90 mm Hg (Streeten et al., 1988). Hypothyroid patients tend to have a low cardiac output with a decrease in contractility and impaired diastolic relaxation (Danzi & Klein, 2003). To maintain tissue perfusion, peripheral resistance increases, from a combination of increased responsiveness of α-adrenergic receptors, increased levels of sympathetic nervous activity (Fletcher & Weetman, 1998), and aldosterone (Fommei & Iervesi, 2002). These would tend to raise diastolic BPs more than systolic BPs, the usual pattern seen in hypothyroidism (Saito & Saruta, 1994).

Subclinical hypothyroidism, defined as an elevated thyrotropin stimulating hormone (TSH) but normal free thyroxine levels, was associated with no increase in the prevalence of hypertension (Walsh et al., 2006), but a meta-analysis of ten population-based studies found a 51% higher relative risk of coronary disease in such patients under age 65 (Ochs et al., 2008).

Hyperthyroidism

An elevated systolic but lowered diastolic BP is usual in patients with hyperthyroidism, associated with a high cardiac output and reduced peripheral resistance. Even after successful therapy, CV morbidity persists (Metso et al., 2008).

Hyperparathyroidism

Primary hyperparathyroidism (PHPT), once seen only as a symptomatic disease with significant hypercalcemia, is now most commonly recognized in asymptomatic patients with minimally elevated serum calcium levels (Silverberg et al., 2009). Often the hypercalcemia is noted only after thiazide therapy. The management of such patients remains in question. Most surgeons prefer to operate; most nonsurgeons prefer to watch (Mihai et al., 2008). With currently available scan-directed, minimally invasive parathyroidectomy, surgery is gaining popularity (Fang et al., 2008).

Hypertension is common in PHPT (Snijder et al., 2007) and, if present, contributes to the increased risk of cardiovascular events that, along with the BP, may not be ameliorated by parathyroidectomy (Vestergaard & Mosekilde, 2003). Some find no correlation between serum calcium or parathyroid hormone levels and BP (Lumachi et al., 2002); others find the intact parathyroid levels are positively and independently associated with the incidence of hypertension (Taylor et al., 2008).

Vitamin D Deficiency

On the other hand of the spectrum, low levels of plasma 25-hydroxyvitamin D have been associated with more hypertension (Forman et al., 2008), myocardial infarction (Giovannucci et al., 2008), stroke (Pilz et al., 2008), and mortality (Dobnig et al., 2008; Melamed et al., 2008). Trials of supplements of vitamin D have not shown an effect on the incidence of hypertension (Margolis et al., 2008), but it may be renoprotective (Alborzi et al., 2008).

Acromegaly

Hypertension is found in approximately 35% of patients with acromegaly and is a risk factor for their increased rate of mortality (Dekkers et al., 2008a,b). The hypertension is related to a number of factors: sodium retention, increased sympathetic nervous-mediated vasoconstriction, reduced endothelium-dependent vasodilation, and hypertrophic remodeling of resistance arteries (Rizzoni et al., 2004). Left ventricular hypertrophy and impaired systolic function are usual (Bogazzi et al., 2008). Guidelines for management are available (Melmed et al., 2009). When the condition is controlled, hypertension usually improves (Colao et al., 2008).

OBSTRUCTIVE SLEEP APNEA

Obstructive sleep apnea (OSA) may be the most common cause of reversible hypertension in the United States (Somers et al., 2008). OSA is common, infrequently diagnosed, and associated with a significant incidence of hypertension (Kapa et al., 2008). In two large population studies in the United States, about 20% of adults had mild OSA, defined as an apnea-hypopnea index (AHI) of at least five episodes lasting 10 seconds or more per hour of sleep, and 1 in 15 adults had OSA of a more severe degree (Young et al., 2004). Over a 5-year follow-up of subjects initially with a normal sleep study, 16% developed OSA, in 7.5% of moderate to severe degree (Tishler et al., 2003). Young et al. (2004) estimate that 75% to 80% of OSA patients who could benefit from treatment remain undiagnosed. Otherwise healthy young children may have abnormal breathing patterns during sleep that are associated with an elevated 24-hour ambulatory BP, morning surge or BP, and left ventricular remodeling (Amin et al., 2008) (see also Chapter 3).

More than poor sleep may afflict OSA patients: their relative likelihood of sudden cardiac death occurring from midnight to 6 a.m. was 2.6 times greater than seen among the general population (Gami et al., 2004). The association of OSA and hypertension has additive effects on atherosclerosis (Drager et al., 2009).

Clinical Features and Diagnosis

OSA should be considered in patients with the clinical features of increasing obesity, loud snoring, fitful sleep, and daytime sleepiness (Table 14-2). Although OSA is common in patients who are morbidly obese, most afflicted are not "Pickwickian." A 10% increase in weight was associated with a sixfold increased risk of developing OSA among subjects initially free of OSA (Peppard et al., 2000a). Virtually all with OSA will snore, but only approximately half of people who snore for more than half the night have sleep apnea (Ferini-Strambi et al., 1999). The diagnosis can be made by a sleep study at home (Tishler et al., 2003) but with more certainty by overnight polysomnography in a sleep laboratory, with continuous recordings of respiration, electroencephalogram, electromyogram, eye movements, electrocardiogram, O_2 saturation, & BP.

Association with Hypertension

Incidence

Multiple cross-sectional and observational studies have unequivocally shown a higher prevalence and incidence of systemic hypertension in direct proportion to the severity of sleep apnea (Hiestand et al., 2006)

TABLE 14.2	Clinical Features of OSA

History

Snoring[a]
Apnea during sleep
Arousals or awakenings
Choking spells
Nocturnal diaphoresis or enuresis
Abnormal motor activity during sleep
Excessive daytime sleepiness[a]
Headaches
Loss of memory and concentration
Personality changes, depression
Angina
Diminished libido, impotence

Physical examination

Hypertension[a]
Overweight, particularly visceral[a]

Oral Cavity Abnormalities

Enlarged tonsils
Thickened uvula
Long and redundant soft palate

Cardiovascular Findings

Increased heart rate variability
Left ventricular hypertrophy
Arrhythmias
Conduction disturbances

[a]Most useful in considering diagnosis.

(Fig. 14-1). Lavie et al. (2000) found that each apneic event per hour of sleep increased the odds for hypertension by 1%, whereas each 10% decrease in O_2 saturation increased the odds by 13%.

A history of snoring, by itself, has been associated with an increased incidence of hypertension. Among 73,000 U.S. female nurses followed for 8 years, the risk of developing hypertension increased by 29% in those who snored occasionally and by 55% in those who snored regularly as compared to those who said they did not snore (Hu et al., 1999). The association was independent of age, body mass index, waist circumference, and other lifestyle factors.

The risk of hypertension is greater for younger subjects than for those older than 60 years (Kapa et al., 2008) and is independent of all other relevant risk factors (Lavie et al., 2000). Moreover, the prevalence of sleep apnea is even higher both in patients with uncontrolled hypertension (Gus et al., 2008) and in patients with stroke (Mohsenin, 2001). Typically, patients with OSA have nondipping BP during

sleep and accentuated morning surge of BP when monitored by ambulatory BP monitoring (ABPM) (Amin et al., 2008).

Mechanisms of Hypertension

A number of possible mechanisms for persistent hypertension as a consequence of OSA have been proposed. Increased sympathetic nervous activity (Wolk et al., 2003), increased levels of markers of inflammation (Ishikawa et al., 2008), cortisol (Vgontzas et al., 2007), and erythropoietin (Winnicki et al., 2004) have been measured in patients with sleep apnea, along with a greater degree of arterial stiffness (Protogerou et al., 2008). Low levels of plasma renin activity and increased levels of urinary aldosterone were noted in half of 72 patients with resistant hypertension and features suggestive of OSA (Calhoun et al., 2004).

Treatment

Weight loss—even as little as 10% of body weight (Peppard et al., 2000b)—and regular exercise (Sherrill et al., 1998) will help over the long term; avoiding the supine position during sleep may help in the short term (Kuhlmann et al., 2009). The best relief is by nasal continuous positive airway pressure (cPAP), which has been shown in controlled trials to relieve symptoms (Patel et al., 2003) and lower the day and night BP by as much as 10 mm Hg in those with AHI greater than 30 (Kuhlmann et al., 2009). However, less if any fall in BP has been seen in randomized controlled trials of cPAP in patients with less severe OSA (Alajmi et al., 2007).

Alternative therapies are needed since uncontrolled OSA leads to serious CV complications (Bradley & Floras, 2009).

If the hypertension persists, antihypertensive drugs should be used. In a sequential study of one agent each from five classes of drugs, each given for 6 weeks to 40 hypertensives with OSA, atenolol, 50 mg per day, provided greater lowering of both office and 24-hour ambulatory BP than did amlodipine, enalapril, losartan, or hydrochlorothiazide (Kraiczi et al., 2000). Patients who remain bothered by daytime sleepiness may be helped by the nonamphetamine drug modafinil (Carl & Sica, 2007).

NEUROLOGIC DISORDERS

Beyond stroke, a number of seemingly different disorders of the central and peripheral nervous system may cause hypertension. Many may do so

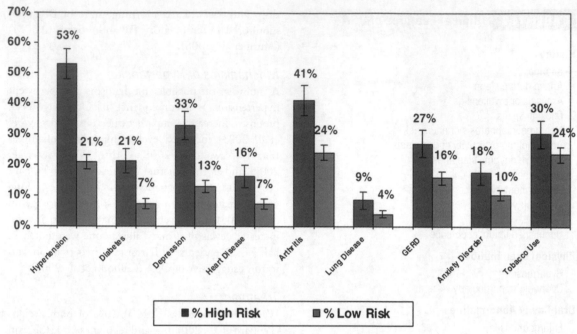

FIGURE 14-1 Prevalence of chronic illness among individuals with either high or low risk for sleep apnea by the Berlin questionnaire. (Reprinted from Hiestand DM, Britz P, Goldman M, et al. Prevalence of symptoms and risk of sleep apnea in the US population: Results from the national sleep foundation sleep in America 2005 poll. *Chest* 2006;130:780–786, with permission.)

by a common mechanism involving sympathetic nervous system discharge from the vasomotor centers in response to an increased intracranial pressure. The rise in systemic pressure is necessary to restore cerebral perfusion.

As noted in Chapters 4 and 7, patients with acute stroke may have transient marked elevations in BP. Rarely, episodic hypertension suggestive of a pheochromocytoma may occur after cerebral infarction (Manger, 2008).

Alzheimer Disease

The presence of hypertension in late midlife (age 68) was associated with a decline in cognitive function in those retested at age 81 (Reinprecht et al., 2003). However, a causal connection between hypertension and Alzheimer disease remains speculative (Patterson et al., 2008). The late-onset disease, which accounts for 90% to 95% of all cases, appears to be linked to vascular risk factors including hypertension and atherosclerosis. Prospective analyses of large populations have provided mixed results in regard to a connection to prior hypertension: some find no association (Lindsay et al., 2002); most do (Cechetto et al., 2008;

Kalaria et al., 2008; Kivipelto et al., 2006). Once developed, Alzheimer disease is usually accompanied by less hypertension, BP apparently receding as the process worsens, even without weight loss (Morris et al., 2000). There is some evidence that angiotensin receptor blockers (ARBs) and centrally acting angiotensin converting enzyme inhibitors (ACEIs) can slow the progression of cognitive loss (Kehoe & Wilcock, 2007; Sink et al., 2009).

Brain Tumors

Intracranial tumors, especially those arising in the posterior fossa, may cause hypertension (Pallini et al., 1995). In some patients, paroxysmal hypertension and other features that suggest catecholamine excess may point mistakenly to the diagnosis of pheochromocytoma. The problem may be confounded by the increased incidence of neuroectodermal tumors, some within the central nervous system, in patients with pheochromocytoma. Unlike patients with a pheochromocytoma who always have high catechol levels, patients with a brain tumor may have increased catecholamine levels during a paroxysm of hypertension but normal levels at other times (Manger, 2008).

Quadriplegia

Patients with transverse lesions of the cervical spinal cord above the origins of the thoracolumbar sympathetic neurons lose central control of their sympathetic outflow. Stimulation of nerves below the injury, as with bladder or bowel distension, may cause reflex sympathetic activity via the isolated spinal cord, inducing hypertension, sweating, flushing, piloerection, and headache, a syndrome described as *autonomic hyperreflexia*. Such patients have markedly exaggerated pressor responses to various stimuli (Krum et al., 1992). The hypertension may be severe and persistent enough to cause cerebrovascular accidents and death. An α-blocker effectively controlled the syndrome (Chancellor et al., 1994).

Severe Head Injury

Immediately after severe head injury, the BP may rise because of a hyperdynamic state mediated by excessive sympathetic nervous activity (Simard & Bellefleur, 1989). If the hypertension is persistent and severe, a short-acting β-blocker (e.g., esmolol) should be given. Caution is needed in the use of vasodilators such as hydralazine and nitroprusside, which may increase cerebral blood flow and intracranial pressure (Van Aken et al., 1989). Moreover, hypotension is an even greater threat (Winchell et al., 1996).

Other Neurologic Disorders

Hypertension may be seen with:

- Guillain-Barré syndrome (Minami et al., 1995)
- Fatal familial insomnia, a prion disease with severe atrophy of the thalamus (Portaluppi et al., 1994)
- Baroreceptor failure (Heusser et al., 2005)
- Autonomic failure with orthostatic hypotension and supine hypertension, often helped by bedtime transdermal nitroglycerin (Jordan et al., 1999)
- Parkinson disease, wherein severe postural hypotension may also be accompanied by nocturnal hypertension (Arias-Vera et al., 2003)

FUNCTIONAL SOMATIC DISORDERS

Anxiety and depression are common in the general population and even more prevalent in patients with hypertension or cardiovascular disease (Davies et al., 2004). In the United States, the incidence of psychological morbidity is certainly rising as a consequence of the persistent threat of terrorism and the return of more soldiers from the Iraqi invasion (Wilson, 2007). An anxiety disorder was found in 19.5% of consecutive patients seen in 15 U.S. primary care clinics in 2005 (Kroenke et al., 2007).

Anxious patients are more likely to have an elevated office BP, the "white-coat effect," that may persist over many office visits (Pickering & Clemow, 2008). If BP readings are taken by home measurement or ambulatory monitoring, it may be discovered that they have white-coat hypertension (Verberk et al., 2006). Such patients obviously will be more anxious unless their excessive altering reaction is recognized and their anxiety over their BP relieved.

As common as it is, anxiety and its manifestations are often not recognized as being responsible for a variety of symptoms (Pickering & Clemow, 2008). Because of the common failure to recognize the underlying nature of various functional syndromes (Wessely et al., 1999) (Table 14-3), patients and their physicians often enter into a vicious cycle: more and more testing, often with false-positive results; more and more incorrect "organic" disease diagnoses; more and more ineffective therapy; more and more anxiety; and more and more functional symptoms.

TABLE 14.3	Functional Somatic Syndromes by Specialty
Specialty	**Syndrome**
Gastroenterology	Irritable bowel syndrome, nonulcer dyspepsia
Gynecology	Premenstrual syndrome, chronic pelvic pain
Rheumatology	Fibromyalgia
Cardiology	Atypical or noncardiac chest pain
Respiratory medicine	Hyperventilation syndrome
Infectious diseases	Chronic (postviral) fatigue syndrome
Neurology	Tension headache
Dentistry	Temporomandibular joint dysfunction, atypical facial pain
Ear, nose, and throat	Globus syndrome
Allergy	Multiple chemical sensitivity

Modified from Wessely S, Nimnuan C, Sharpe N. Functional somatic syndromes: One or many? *Lancet* 1999;354:936–939.

Anxiety-Induced Hyperventilation

The problem is often encountered with hypertensive patients, either because of their concern over having "the silent killer" or because of their poor response to antihypertensive therapies. In 300 consecutive patients referred to me, usually because of hypertension that was difficult to control, 104 had symptoms attributable to anxiety-induced hyperventilation (Kaplan, 1997) (Fig. 14-2). The symptoms and signs of panic attack encompass all these same manifestations but go beyond them to include fears of falling apart, losing control, or even more acute anxiety and are associated with increased reactivity of vasoconstricting sympathetic nerves (Katon, 2006). Among 351 hypertensive patients randomly selected from one primary care practice in Sheffield, United Kingdom, panic attacks had occurred in 18% during the previous 6 months and in 37% over their lifetime (Davies et al., 1999). The reported diagnosis of hypertension usually antedated the onset of panic attacks. Anxiety and panic attacks were even more common among their patients who had nonspecific intolerance to multiple antihypertensive drugs (Davies et al., 2003).

Many of these patients had been subjected to intensive workup for dizziness, headaches, chest pain, fatigue, and the like (Newman-Toker et al., 2008). When the symptoms are reproduced by voluntary overbreathing and relieved by rebreathing into a paper sack, the patient's recognition of the mechanism often provides immediate relief and opens the way to the appropriate use of rebreathing exercises, other cognitive therapy, or, if needed, antianxiety medications.

Depression may not be more common in uncomplicated hypertension (Lenoir et al., 2008), but it is frequently observed after a heart attack or stroke (Gump et al., 2005). Antidepressants can raise the risk of hypertension (Lincht et al., 2009).

ACUTE PHYSICAL STRESS

Hypertension may appear during various acute physical stresses, usually reflecting an intense sympathetic discharge and sometimes the contribution of increased renin-angiotensin from volume contraction.

Surgical Conditions

Perioperative Hypertension

In addition to the reasons mentioned in the coverage of anesthesia and hypertension in Chapter 7, for numerous reasons, hypertension may be a problem during and soon after surgery. Elevated postoperative readings can be related to pain, hypoxia and hypercapnia, and physical and emotional excitement. These causes should be managed rather than treating the elevated BP with antihypertensives.

Marked rises in BP have been measured when pneumoperitoneum is performed for abdominal

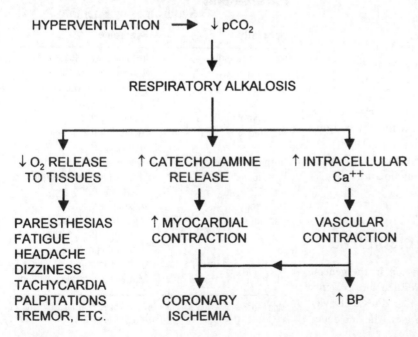

FIGURE 14-2 The mechanisms by which acute hyperventilation may induce various symptoms, coronary ischemia, and a rise in blood pressure (BP). Ca, calcium; pCO_2, partial pressure of carbon dioxide.

laparoscopic surgery (Joris et al., 1998). The rise in BP was accompanied by increases in blood catecholamines, cortisol, and vasopressin and was blunted by preoperative clonidine.

Cardiovascular Surgery

Table 14-4 summarizes the causes of hypertension associated with surgery in a temporal fashion (Vuylsteke et al., 2000).

Coronary Bypass

Approximately one third of patients will have hypertension after coronary artery bypass grafting, usually starting within the first 2 hours after surgery and lasting 4 to 6 hours. Immediate therapy may be important to prevent postoperative heart failure or myocardial infarction. In addition to deepening of anesthesia, various parenteral antihypertensives have been used, including nitroprusside and nitroglycerin (Vuylsteke et al., 2000).

Other Cardiac Surgery

Hypertension has been reported, although less frequently, after other cardiac surgery. Virtually all patients who undergo orthotopic heart transplantation develop hypertension (Taegtmeyer et al., 2004) and lose the usual nocturnal fall in BP, likely from a combination of effects, including the effects of immunosuppressive agents (see the section on Cyclosporine and Tacrolimus, later in this chapter), impaired baroreceptor control

from cardiac denervation, and the inability to excrete sodium normally (Eisen, 2003). The hypertension may be controlled by either ACEIs or calcium channel blockers as monotherapy, each effective in approximately half of patients (Rockx & Haddad, 2007).

Carotid Endarterectomy

Postoperative hypertension may be particularly serious in patients with known cerebrovascular disease who have carotid endarterectomy, perhaps because of altered baroreflex activity (Sigaudo-Roussel et al., 2002). Treatment most logically should be with a short-acting β-blocker rather than with a vasodilator that might further increase the cerebral blood flow.

INCREASED INTRAVASCULAR VOLUME

If vascular volume is raised a significant degree over a short period, the renal natriuretic response may not be able to excrete the excess volume, particularly if renal function is also impaired. Cell-free, hemoglobin-based oxygen carriers (HBOC) cause hypertension by vasoconstriction secondary to scavenging of nitric oxide (NO). Both inhaled NO and intravenous sodium nitrite given before the infusion of HBOC prevent subsequent hypertension in mice and lambs (Yu et al., 2008).

TABLE 14.4 **Hypertension Associated with Cardiac Surgery**

Preoperative

  Anxiety, angina
  Discontinuation of antihypertensive therapy
  Rebound from β-blockers in patients with coronary artery disease

Intraoperative

  Induction of anesthesia: tracheal intubation; nasopharyngeal, urethral, or rectal manipulation
  Before cardiopulmonary bypass (during sternotomy and chest retraction)
  Cardiopulmonary bypass
  After cardiopulmonary bypass (during surgery)

Postoperative

  Early (within 2 h)
    Obvious cause: hypoxia, hypercapnia, ventilatory difficulties, hypothermia, shivering, arousal from anesthesia
    With no obvious cause: after myocardial revascularization; less frequently after valve replacement; after resection of aortic coarctation
  Late (weeks to months)
    After aortic valve replacement by homografts

Modified from Estafanous FG, Tarazi RC. Systemic arterial hypertension associated with cardiac surgery. *Am J Cardiol* 1980;46:685–694.

Erythropoietin Therapy

Recombinant human erythropoietin is now being widely used to correct the anemia of chronic renal failure. As the hematocrit rises, so do blood viscosity and BP; nearly one third of patients developed clinically important hypertension (Luft, 2000). This may add to the currently recognized danger of treating the anemia of chronic renal disease (Vaziri, 2008).

Polycythemia and Hyperviscosity

Patients with primary polycythemia are often hypertensive, and some hypertensives have a relative polycythemia that may resolve when the BP is lowered. The hypertension seen in polycythemic states could also reflect increased blood viscosity. Significant falls in BP were seen in 12 hypertensive patients with polycythemia when blood viscosity was reduced without changing the blood volume (Bertinieri et al., 1998).

CHEMICAL AGENTS THAT CAUSE HYPERTENSION

Table 14-5 lists various chemical agents that may cause hypertension, indicating their mechanism if known. Some of these substances, such as sodium-containing antacids, alcohol, insulin, licorice, oral contraceptives, and monoamine oxidase inhibitors, are covered elsewhere in this book because of their frequency or special features.

Caffeine

Caffeine is likely the most widely consumed drug in the world and its use will almost certainly increase with the amazing proliferation of Starbucks and its clones. As an antagonist in the adenosine receptor, it acutely raises the BP by increasing peripheral resistance by an increase in aortic stiffness (Vlachopoulos et al., 2007). Although tolerance to this pressor effect has been widely assumed, such tolerance was found in only half of regular consumers (Lovallo et al., 2004). However, habitual coffee intake was not associated with an increased incidence of hypertension among women (Winkelmayer et al., 2005) or men (Klag et al., 2002). Despite some conflicting data, habitual caffeine ingestion has not been found to increase the risk for cardiovascular disease (Greenberg et al., 2007).

Thus, the effects of caffeine on hypertension may, over the long term, be neutral but, at least acutely, a pressor effect may be noted. Perhaps the wisest course is to have patients check their home BPs before and within an hour after drinking their coffee or tea. Those who experience a significant pressor effect should be advised to reduce or stop their caffeine consumption.

Nicotine and Smoking

Almost 25% of adults in the United States are currently smokers and almost one third started before the age of 16 years (Schoenborn et al., 2003). Obviously, the profound dangers of smoking are not adequately impressed upon young people and they are easily enticed to smoke by such seemingly benign provocations as viewing smoking in movies (Dalton et al., 2003).

As described in Chapter 6, even in chronic smokers, each cigarette induces a pressor response (Mahmud & Feely, 2003). Whereas the peripheral BP returns to near baseline within 15 minutes, pressure within the aorta remains higher. Moreover, the indices of large artery stiffness start higher in the chronic smokers and remain higher than in the nonsmokers. These hemodynamic consequences of smoking have been underestimated for two reasons: first, in the smoke-free environment where patients are seen, the BP is usually measured well after the acute effects are over; second, the arm (peripheral) BP is usually deceptively lower in chronic smokers who have reduced aortic-brachial pressure amplification (Mahmud & Feely, 2003). A similar acute increase of larger artery stiffness has been seen with cigar smoking (Vlachopoulos et al., 2004).

Data on prevalence of persistent hypertension among smokers have not been consistent: Most find them to have higher BP recorded by ambulatory monitoring while they continue to smoke (Oncken et al., 2001), but if the BP is taken while subjects are not smoking, little more hypertension is seen (Halimi et al., 2002; Primatesta et al., 2001). On the contrary, when chronic smokers quit smoking, their BPs tend to rise (Lee et al., 2001), in large part because of weight gain (Halimi et al., 2002).

Smoking has been found to have a profoundly deleterious effect on renal function (Orth & Ritz, 2002), and on cognitive function (Sabia et al., 2008). Moreover, the 2,983 smokers enrolled in the massive Hypertension Optimal Treatment (HOT) trial were

TABLE 14.5   Hypertension Induced by Chemical Agents

Mechanism	Examples
Expansion of fluid volume	
Increased sodium intake	Antacids; processed foods (Chapter 6)
Mineralocorticoid effects	Licorice (Chapter 13); cortisone (Chapter 14); anabolic steroids (Owens et al., 1998)
Stimulation of renin-angiotensin	Estrogens (oral contraceptives; Chapter 11)
Inhibition of prostaglandins	NSAIDs (Solomon, 2004)
Stimulation of sympathetic nervous activity	
Sympathomimetic agents	Caffeine (Lovallo et al., 2004); cocaine (Tuncel et al., 2002); ephedrine (Bent, 2008); methylenedioxymethamphetamine (MDMA, "ecstasy") (Lester et al., 2000); methylphenidate (Ritalin) (Ballard et al., 1976); nicotine (Halimi et al., 2002); phencyclidine (Sernulan) (Eastman & Cohen, 1975); phenylpropanolamine (Kernan et al., 2000)
Interactions with monoamine oxidase inhibitors	Foods with high tyramine content (e.g., red wines, aged cheese) (Liu & Rustgi, 1987)
Anesthetics	Ketamine (Broughton Pipkin & Waldron, 1983)
Ergot alkaloids	Ergotamine (Joyce & Gubbay, 1986)
Dopamine receptor agonist	Bromocriptine (Bakht et al., 1990)
Antidopaminergic	Metoclopramide (Roche et al., 1985)
Sandostatin analogue	Sandostatin LAR (Pop-Busui et al., 2000)
Interference with antihypertensive drugs	
Inhibition of prostaglandin synthesis	NSAIDs (Izhar, 2004)
Inhibition of neuronal uptake	Tricyclic antidepressants (Walsh et al., 1992); sibutramine (Bray, 2002)
Paradoxical response to antihypertensive drugs	
Withdrawal, followed by ↑ catechols	Clonidine (Metz et al., 1987)
Unopposed α-adrenergic vasoconstriction	β-blockers (Drayer et al., 1976)
Intrinsic sympathomimetic activity	Pindolol (Collins & King, 1972)
Combination of α- and β-blocker	Propranolol plus clonidine (Warren et al., 1979)
Unknown mechanisms	
Heavy metal poisoning	Lead (Nash et al., 2003); mercury (Velzeboer et al., 1997); thallium (Bank et al., 1972)
Chemicals	Carbon disulfide (Egeland et al., 1992); arsenic (Rahman et al., 1999); methyl chloride (Scharnweber et al., 1974); polychlorinated biphenyl (Kreiss et al., 1981)
Insecticides	Parathion (Tsachalinas et al., 1971)
Insect bites	Spider (Weitzman et al., 1977); scorpion (Gueron & Yaron, 1970)
Diagnostic agents	Indigo carmine (Wu & Johnson, 1969); pentagastrin (Merguet et al., 1968);

(continued)

TABLE 14.5	Hypertension Induced by Chemical Agents (Continued)
Mechanism	**Examples**
Therapeutic agents	thyrotropin-releasing hormone (Rosenthal et al., 1987) Cyclosporine (Zhang & Victor, 2000); clozapine (Henderson et al., 2004); disulfiram (Volicer & Nelson, 1984); erythropoietin (Luft, 2000); herbal remedies (De Smet, 2002); indinavir (Cattelan et al., 2000); lithium (Michaeli et al., 1984)
Alcohol	Alcohol (Sierksma et al., 2004)

Adapted from Grossman E, Messerli FH. High blood pressure: A side effect of drugs, poisons, and food. *Arch Intern Med* 1995;155:450–460.

the only subgroup to experience an *increased* risk of major cardiovascular events when given more intensive therapy to achieve a lower BP (Zanchetti et al., 2003). As the authors note, these data "strengthen the need for concerted efforts to persuade patients to quit smoking."

Fortunately, the nicotine replacement therapies which help patients quit do not seem to have deleterious cardiovascular effects (Benowitz et al., 2002).

Alcohol

Alcohol is a two-edged sword: in excess, it is a major cause of social disorder, trauma, and death; in moderation, it is a protector against heart attack, stroke, diabetes, and, likely, dementia (Rehm et al., 2003). Part of its diverse roles involves hypertension: in excess, alcohol raises the BP; in moderation, it may be protective against the development of hypertension (see also Chapters 3 and 6).

The Relation to Hypertension
When consumed in amounts equivalent to three usual portions—a usual portion being 12 oz of beer, 4 oz of wine, or 1.5 oz of whiskey which all contain about 12 g of ethanol—alcohol causes an immediate depressor effect and subsequently a pressor action (Rosito et al., 1999). These changes are reflected in the measurements of arterial stiffness by pulse-wave velocity (Mahmud & Feely, 2002; Sierksma et al., 2004).

In large population studies, the incidence of hypertension is increased among those who drink more than three drinks per day (Ohira et al., 2009), either in a liner dose-response relationship (Fuchs et al., 2001) or with a threshold wherein smaller quantities are associated with a modest decrease (Thadhani et al., 2002). The cessation of heavy drinking is usually followed by significant falls in BP (Ohira et al., 2009).

The mechanisms for the pressor effect of large quantities of ethanol are not well defined but in moderate amounts, multiple beneficial effects have been noted which could translate into both antihypertensive actions and multiple protective effects. These effects include improvements in glucose tolerance and insulin sensitivity (Davies et al., 2002), reductions in lipoprotein (a) along with rises in HDL-cholesterol (Catena et al., 2003), and decreases in the levels of inflammatory markers such as interleukin-6 and C-reactive protein (Volpato et al., 2004).

Relations to Other Diseases
Light to moderate consumption, i.e., less than three drinks per day, has been shown to provide multiple significant benefits as detailed in Chapter 6.

This litany of benefits must be balanced by the potential for encouragement of alcohol abuse and a high prevalence of excessive drinking among the elderly (O'Connell et al., 2003). Gout is more common among even light drinkers (Choi et al., 2004). Moreover, alcohol consumption beyond 1.5 drinks per day was found to increase the risk of breast cancer in postmenopausal women (Chen et al., 2002), although a reduced mortality from cancer has been noted in wine drinkers (Grønbæk et al., 2000). And, despite the aforementioned decrease in dementia, brain atrophy has been found to increase linearly with alcohol intake (Ding et al., 2004). Moreover, as described in Chapter 6, a genetic mutation may cause some people to be bothered by even small amounts of alcohol (Chen et al., 2008).

Those who choose to drink in moderation should be allowed to continue. The type of alcohol-containing beverage is likely irrelevant, the putative greater benefits of wine (Di Castelnuovo et al., 2002) likely reflecting healthier lifestyle (Barefoot et al., 2002) and psychological functioning (Mortensen et al., 2001) among wine drinkers as opposed to beer and whiskey drinkers.

We have no hesitation in allowing hypertensives to drink in moderation but others do not believe that drinking any amount of alcohol should be recommended by physicians (Wilson, 2003).

Nonsteroidal Anti-inflammatory Drugs

Nonsteroidal anti-inflammatory drugs (NSAIDs) are well known to blunt the antihypertensive effect of most antihypertensive agents, with the apparent exception of calcium channel blockers (White, 2007). This interference likely reflects an inhibition of prostaglandin-dependent counter-regulatory mechanisms in the kidney that have been invoked by the antihypertensive drugs. This inhibition of cyclooxygenase enzymes may induce renal sodium retention and thereby increase the BP and precipitate hypertension, increasing the risk of stroke (Haag et al., 2008).

A high prevalence of analgesic-induced nephropathy has been noted in Australia (Chang et al., 2008), but not in the United States (Agodoa et al., 2008).

The most striking increased risk of new-onset hypertension has been noted with the selective COX-2 inhibitor rofecoxib (Vioxx) (Solomon et al., 2004). In this retrospective case control study, the relative risk of new-onset hypertension was 2.1 times higher with rofecoxib than with celecoxib (Celebrex). This finding coincides with the greater rise in BP and edema with this agent in osteoarthritic hypertensives (Whelton et al., 2002). As a consequence of an increased incidence of heart attack and stroke with rofecoxib, the drug has been withdrawn from the market (Chang & Harris, 2005). However, no increase in cardiovascular risk has been seen with NSAIDs that are less COX-2 specific, including celecoxib (Warner & Mitchell, 2008).

Immunosuppressive Agents

After all organ transplants, immunosuppression is needed for graft survival. The introduction of cyclosporine in 1983 greatly improved the long-term survival. However, major complications soon became obvious, including nephrotoxicity and hypertension. Similar troubles accompanied the use of another calcineurin inhibitor, tacrolimus. More recently, inhibitors of the mammalian target of the antifungal agent, rapamycin, sirolimus, and everolimus, have been introduced with lesser hypertension but with other toxicities (Morath et al., 2007). As a result, sequential immunosuppression is now used, involving adrenal steroids as well as other immunosuppressive agents (Guba et al., 2008).

Heart transplantation is followed by even more hypertension than is renal transplantation. It is seen in about half of recipients and ascribed mainly to the even heavier immunosuppressive regimen usually needed (Roche et al., 2008).

Treatment

Calcium channel blockers were the first class shown to help control posttransplant hypertension, but renin-angiotensin blockade is now widely used in association (Cruzado et al., 2008; Rockx & Haddad, 2007).

Chemotherapy

As the number, variety, and effectiveness of cancer chemotherapeutic agents increase, long-term cancer survivors are experiencing higher rates of mortality from cardiovascular disease than from recurrent cancer (Jain & Townsend, 2007). Hypertension has surfaced as the most common comorbid condition that directly shortens the survival and may appear even more often with agents that disrupt angiogenesis.

There is no obvious advantage of one over another class of antihypertensive drugs, but adequate control of hypertension is needed.

Other Agents

Perhaps the most commonly encountered form of chemically induced hypertension is that related to the use of foods and drugs containing large amounts of sodium. More dramatic effects are seen with the use of sympathomimetic agents. Large amounts of these drugs, available over the counter as herbal remedies (De Smet, 2002) and for use as nasal decongestants (e.g., pseudoephedrine) and, until recently, as appetite suppressants (e.g., phenylpropanolamine), may raise the BP enough to induce, on rare occasions, hypertensive encephalopathy, strokes, and heart attacks (Kernan et al., 2000). In usual doses, however, pseudoephedrine does not raise BP, even in patients receiving β-blockers (Mores et al., 1999). The greatly increased risk of adverse reactions to ephedra (Bent, 2008) has led to the restriction of its use in the United States. Perhaps the safest way to prevent these various interactions is to advise hypertensives to avoid all over-the-counter drugs and herbal remedies and to inform their physicians who prescribe other medications about their antihypertensive drug regimens.

The use of doping agents, has seriously infected all competitive sports (Sjoqvist et al., 2008). Fortunately, hypertension is uncommon with their use.

Street Drugs

Marijuana, or δ-9-tetrahydrocannabinol, in moderate amounts will increase the heart rate but may lower the BP (Frishman et al., 2003). Cannabinoid type 1 receptor antagonists may lower the BP (Van Gaal et al., 2008).

Cocaine (Turcel et al., 2002) and amphetamines (Lester et al., 2000) may cause transient but significant hypertension that may cause strokes and serious cardiac damage. Most cocaine-related deaths are associated with myocardial injury similar to that seen from catecholamine excess and aggravated by acute hypertension (Lange & Hillis, 2001). Chronic cocaine abuse does not appear to induce hypertension (Brecklin et al., 1998) but may be associated with chronic renal disease (Vupputuri et al., 2004).

The next chapter looks at hypertension in women who are pregnant or taking estrogen.

REFERENCES

Agodoa LY, Francis ME, Eggers PW. Association of analgesic use with prevalence of albuminuria and reduced GFR in US adults. *Am J Kidney Dis* 2008;51:573–583.

Alajmi M, Mulgrew AT, Fox J, et al. Impact of continuous positive airway pressure therapy on blood pressure in patients with obstructive sleep apnea hypopnea: A meta-analysis of randomized controlled trials. *Lung* 2007;185:67–72.

Alborzi P, Patel NA, Peterson C, et al. Paricalcitol reduces albuminuria and inflammation in chronic kidney disease: A randomized double-blind pilot trial. *Hypertension* 2008;52:249–255.

Amin P, Patel NA, Paterson C, et al. Activity-adjusted 24-hour ambulatory blood pressure and cardiac remodeling in children with sleep disordered breathing. *Hypertension* 2008;51:84–91.

Arias-Vera JR, Mansoor GA, White WB. Abnormalities in blood pressure regulation in a patient with Parkinson's disease. *Am J Hypertens* 2003;16:612–613.

Bakht FR, Kirshon B, Baker T, Cotton DB. Postpartum cardiovascular complications after bromocriptine and cocaine use. *Am J Obstet Gynecol* 1990;162:1065–1066.

Ballard JE, Boileau RA, Sleator EK, et al. *JAMA* 1976;236:2870–2874.

Bank WJ, Pleasure DE, Suzuki K, et al. Thallium poisoning. *Arch Neurol* 1972;26:456–464.

Barefoot JC, Grønbæk M, Feaganes JR, et al. Alcoholic beverage preference, diet, and health habits in the UNC Alumni Heart Study. *Am J Clin Nutr* 2002;76:466–472.

Benowitz NL, Hansson A, Jacob P III. Cardiovascular effects of nasal and transdermal nicotine and cigarette smoking. *Hypertension* 2002;39:1107–1112.

Bent S. Herbal medicine in the United States: Review of efficacy, safety, and regulation: Grand rounds at University of California, San Francisco Medical Center. *J Gen Intern Med* 2008;23:854–859.

Bertinieri G, Parati G, Ulian L, et al. Hemodilution reduces clinic and ambulatory blood pressure in polycythemic patients. *Hypertension* 1998;31:848–853.

Bogazzi F, Lombardi M, Strata E, et al. High prevalence of cardiac hypertrophy without detectable signs of fibrosis in patients with untreated active acromegaly: An in vivo study using magnetic resonance imaging. *Clin Endocrinol* 2008;68:361–368.

Bradley TD, Floras JS. Obstructive sleep apnoea and its cardiovascular consequences. *Lancet* 2009;373:82–93.

Bray GA. Sibutramine and blood pressure: A therapeutic dilemma. *J Hum Hypertens* 2002;16:1–3.

Brecklin CS, Gopaniuk-Folga A, Kravetz T, et al. Prevalence of hypertension in chronic cocaine users. *Am J Hypertens* 1998;11:1279–1283.

Broughton-Pipkin FB, Waldron BA. Ketamine hypertension and the renin-angiotensin system. *Clin Exp Hypertens* 1983;5:875–883.

Calhoun DA, Nishizaka MK, Zaman MA, et al. Aldosterone excretion among subjects with resistant hypertension and symptoms of sleep apnea. *Chest* 2004;125:112–117.

Campbell M. Natural history of coarctation of the aorta. *Br Heart J.* 1970;32:633–640.

Carl D, Sica DA. Obstructive sleep apnea, hypertension and wakefulness-promoting agents. *Curr Hypertens Rep* 2007;9:329–331.

Catena C, Novello M, Dotto L, et al. Serum lipoprotein(a) concentrations and alcohol consumption in hypertension: Possible relevance for cardiovascular damage. *J Hypertens* 2003;21:281–288.

Cattelan A, Trevenzoli M, Naso A, et al. Severe hypertension and renal atrophy associated with indinavir. *Clin Infect Dis* 2000;30:619–621.

Cechetto DF, Trevenzoli M, Naso A, et al. Vascular risk factors and alzheimer's disease. *Expert Rev Neurother* 2008;8:743–750.

Chancellor MB, Erhard MJ, Hirsch IH, et al. Prospective evaluation of terazosin for the treatment of autonomic dysreflexia. *J Urol* 1994;151:111–113.

Chang IJ, Harris RC. Are all COX-2 inhibitors created equal? *Hypertension* 2005;45(2):178–180.

Chang SH, Mathew TH, McDonald SP. Analgesic nephropathy and renal replacement therapy in Australia: Trends, comorbidities and outcomes. *Clin J Am Soc Nephrol* 2008;3:768–776.

Chen WY, Colditz GA, Rosner B, et al. Use of postmenopausal hormones, alcohol, and risk for invasive breast cancer. *Ann Intern Med* 2002;137:798–804.

Chen L, smith GD, Harbord RM, et al. Alcohol intake and blood pressure: A systematic review implementing a Mendelian randomization approach. *P Los Med* 2008;5(3):461–471.

Choi HK, Atkinson K, Karlson EW, et al. Alcohol intake and risk of incident gout in men: A prospective study. *Lancet* 2004;363:1277–1281.

Colao A, Terzolo M, Bondanelli M, et al. GH and IGF-1 excess control contributes to blood pressure control: Results of an observational, retrospective, multicentre study in 105 hypertensive acromegalic patients on hypertensive treatement. *Clin Endocrinol* 2008;69:613–620.

Collins IS, King IW. Pindolol (Visken LB 46): A new treatment for hypertension. *Curr Ther Res* 1972;14:185–194.

Connolly HM, Huston J III, Brown RD Jr, et al. Intracranial aneurysms in patients with coarctation of the aorta: A prospective magnetic resonance angiographic study of 100 patients. *Mayo Clin Proc* 2003;78:1491–1499.

Cruzado JM, Rico J, Grinyo JM. The renin angiotensin system blockade in kidney transplantation: Pros and cons. *Transpl Int* 2008;21:304–313.

Dalton MA, Sargent JD, Beach ML, et al. Effect of viewing smoking in movies on adolescent smoking initiation: A cohort study. *Lancet* 2003;362:281–285.

Daniels SR. Repair of coarctation of the aorta and hypertension: Does age matter? *Lancet* 2001;358:89.

Danzi S, Klein I. Thyroid hormone and blood pressure regulation. *Curr Hypertens Rep* 2003;5:513–520.

Davies MJ, Baer DJ, Judd JT, et al. Effects of moderate alcohol intake on fasting insulin and glucose concentrations and insulin sensitivity in postmenopausal women: A randomized controlled trial. *JAMA* 2002;287:2559–2562.

Davies SJC, Ghahramani P, Jackson PR, et al. Association of panic disorder and panic attacks with hypertension. *Am J Med* 1999;107: 310–316.

Davies SJ, Jackson PR, Potokar J, et al. Treatment of anxiety and depressive disorders in patients with cardiovascular disease. *Br Med J* 2004;328:939–943.

Davies SJ, Jackson PR, Ramsay LE, et al. Drug intolerance due to nonspecific adverse effects related to psychiatric morbidity in hypertensive patients. *Arch Intern Med* 2003;163:592–600.

De Smet PA. Herbal remedies. *N Engl J Med* 2002;347:2046–2056.

Dekkers OM, Pereira AM, Romijn JA. Treatment and follow-up of clinically nonfunctioning pituitary macroadenomas. *J Clin Endocrinol Metab* 2008a;93:3717–3726.

Dekkers OM, Viermasz NR, Pereira AM, et al. Mortality in acromegaly: A metaanalysis. *J Clin Endocrinol Metab* 2008b;93: 61–67.

Di Castelnuovo A, Rotondo S, Iacoviello L, et al. Meta-analysis of wine and beer consumption in relation to vascular risk. *Circulation* 2002;105:2836–2844.

Ding J, Eigenbrodt ML, Mosley TH Jr, et al. Alcohol intake and cerebral abnormalities on magnetic resonance imaging in a community-based population of middle-aged adults: The Atherosclerosis Risk in Communities (ARIC) study. *Stroke* 2004;35:16–21.

Dobnig H, Pilz S, Scharnagl H, et al. Independent association of low serum 25-hydroxyvitamin d and 1,25-dihydroxyvitamin d levels with all-cause and cardiovascular mortality. *Arch Intern Med* 2008;168:1340–1349.

Drager LF, Bortolotto LA, Krieger EM, et al. Additive effects of obstructive sleep apnea and hypertension on early markers of carotid atherosclerosis. *Hypertension* 2009;53:64–69.

Drayer JIM, Keim JH, Weber MA, et al. Unexpected pressor response to propranolol in essential hypertension. *Am J Med* 1976;60:887–893.

Duara R, Theodore S, Sarma PS, et al. Correction of coarctation of aorta in adult patients—impact of corrective procedure on long-term recoarctation and systolic hypertension. *Thorac Cardiovasc Surg* 2008;56:83–86.

Dubrey SW, Mittal TK. Coarctraction of the aorta, hypertension and associated features. *B J Hos Med* 2008;69:110.

Eastman JW, Cohen SN. Hypertensive crisis and death associated with phencyclidine poisoning. *JAMA* 1975;231:1270–1271.

Egeland GM, Burkhart GA, Schnorr TM, et al. Effects of exposure to carbon disulfide on low density lipoprotein cholesterol concentration and diastolic blood pressure. *Br J Indust Med* 1992;49:287–293.

Eisen HJ. Hypertension in heart transplant recipients: More than just cyclosporine. *J Am Coll Cardiol* 2003;41:433–434.

Fang W, Tseng L, Chen J, et al. The management of high-risk patients with primary hyperparathyroidism-minimally invasive

parathyroidectomy vs. medical treatment. *Clin Endocrinol* 2008;68:520–528.

Ferini-Strmbi L, Zucconi M, Castrovono V, et al. Snoring & sleep apnea: A population study in Italian women. *Sleep* 1999; 22:859–864.

Fletcher AK, Weetman AP. Hypertension and hypothyroidism. *J Hum Hypertens* 1998;12:79–82.

Fommei E, Iervasi G. The role of thyroid hormone in blood pressure homeostasis: Evidence from short-term hypothyroidism in humans. *J Clin Endocrinol Metab* 2002;87:1996–2000.

Forman JP, Curhan GC, Taylor EN. Plasma 25-hydroxyvitamin D levels and risk of incident hypertension among young women. *Hypertension* 2008;52:828–832.

Frishman WH, Del Vecchio A, Sanal S, et al. Cardiovascular manifestations of substance abuse: Part 2: Alcohol, amphetamines, heroin, cannabis, and caffeine. *Heart Dis* 2003;5: 253–271.

Fuchs FD, Chambless LE, Whelton PK, et al. Alcohol consumption and the incidence of hypertension. *Hypertension* 2001;37:1242–1250.

Gami AS, Howard DE, Olson EJ, et al. Altered circadian variation of sudden cardiac death in patients with obstructive sleep apnea [Abstract]. *Circulation* 2004;110(Suppl. 3):III-818.

Giovannucci E, Liu Y, Hollis BW, et al. 25-hydroxyvitamin D and risk of myocardial infarction in men: A prospective study. *Arch Intern Med* 2008;168.1174–1100.

Greenberg JA, Dunbar CC, Schnoll R, et al. Caffeinated beverage intake and the risk of heart disease mortality in the elderly: A prospective analysis. *Am J Clin Nutr* 2007;85:392–398.

Grønbæk M, Becker U, Johansen D, et al. Type of alcohol consumed and mortality from all causes, coronary heart disease, and cancer. *Ann Intern Med* 2000;133:411–419.

Guba M, Rentsch M, Wimmer CD, et al. Calcineurin-inhibitor avoidance in elderly renal allograft recipients using ATG and basiliximab combined with mycophenolate mofetil. *Eur Soc Organ Transplant* 2008;21:637–645.

Gueron M, Yaron R. Cardiovascular manifestations of severe scorpion sting. *Chest* 1970;57:156–162.

Gump BB, Matthews KA, Eberly LE, et al. Depressive symptoms and mortality in men: Results from the Multiple Risk Factor Intervention trial. *Stroke* 2005;36:98–102.

Gus M, Goncalves SC, Martinez D, et al. Risk for obstructive sleep apnea by Berlin questionnaire, but not daytime sleepiness, is associated with resistant hypertension: A case-control study. *Am J Hypertens* 2008;21:832–835.

Haag MD, Bos MJ, Hofman A, et al. Cyclooxygenase selectivity of nonsteroidal anti-inflammatory drugs and risk of stroke. *Arch Intern Med* 2008;168:1219–1224.

Hager A, Kanz S, Kaemmerer H, et al. Exercise capacity and exercise hypertension after surgical repair of isolated aortic coarctation. *Am J Cardiol* 2008;101:1777–1780.

Halimi JM, Giraudeau B, Vol S, et al. The risk of hypertension in men: Direct and indirect effects of chronic smoking. *J Hypertens* 2002;20:187–193.

Henderson DC, Daley TB, Kunkel L, et al. Clozapine and hypertension: A chart review of 82 patients. *J Clin Psychiatry* 2004;65: 686–689.

Heusser K, Tank J, Luft FC, et al. Baroreflex failure. *Hypertension* 2005;45:834–839.

Hiestand DM, Britz P, Goldman M, et al. Prevalence of symptoms and risk of sleep apnea in the US population: Results from the national sleep foundation sleep in America 2005 poll. *Chest* 2006;130: 780–786.

Hu FB, Willett WC, Colditz GA, et al. Prospective study of snoring and risk of hypertension in women. *Am J Epidemiol* 1999;150: 806–816.

Ishikawa J, Hoshide S, Eguchi K, et al. Increased low-grade inflammation and plasminogen-activator inhibitor-1 level in nondippers with sleep apnea syndrome. *J Hypertens* 2008;26: 1181–1187.

Izhar M, Alusa T, Folker A, et al. Effects of COX inhibition on blood pressure and kidney function in ACE inhibitor-treated blacks nd Hispanics. *Hypertension* 2004;43:573–577.

Jain M, Townsend RR. Chemotherapy atents and hypertension: A focus on angiogenesis blockade. *Curr Hypertens Rep* 2007; 9:320–328.

Jenkins NP, Ward C. Coarctation of the aorta: Natural history and outcome after surgical treatment. *QJM* 1999;92:365–371.

Jordan J, Shannon JR, Pohar B, et al. Contrasting effects of vasodilators on blood pressure and sodium balance in the hypertension of automatic failure. *J Am Soc Nephrol* 1999;10:35–42.

Joris JL, Chiche J-D, Canivet J-LM, et al. Hemodynamic changes induced by laparoscopy and their endocrine correlates: Effects of clonidine. *J Am Coll Cardiol* 1998;32:1389–1396.

Joyce DA, Gubbay SS. Arterial complications of migrane treatment with methysergide and parenteral ergotamine. *BMJ* 1986;285:260–261.

Kalaria RN, Maestre GE, Arizaga R, et al. Alzheimer's disease and vascular dementia in developing countries: Prevalence, management, and risk factors. *Lancet Neurol* 2008;7:812–826.

Kapa S, Sert Kuniyoshi FH, Somers VK. Sleep apnea and hypertension: Interactions and implications for management. *Hypertension* 2008;51:605–608.

Kaplan NM. Anxiety-induced hyperventilation: A common cause of symptoms in patients with hypertension. *Arch Intern Med* 1997;157:945–948.

Katon WJ. Panic Disorder. *N Engl J Med* 2006;354:2360–2367.

Kehoe PG, Wilcock GK. Is inhibition of the renin-angiotensin system a new treatment option for Alzheimer's disease? *Lancet Neurol* 2007;6:373–378.

Kernan WN, Viscoli CM, Brass LM, et al. Phenylpropanolamine and the risk of hemorrhagic stroke. *N Engl J Med* 2000;343: 1826–1832.

Kivipelto M, Ngandu T, Laatikainen T, et al. Risk score for the prediction of dementia risk in 20 years among middle aged people: A longitudinal, population-based study. *Lancet Neurol* 2006;5:735–741.

Klag MJ, Wang NY, Meoni LA, et al. Coffee intake and risk of hypertension: The Johns Hopkins precursors study. *Arch Intern Med* 2002;162:657–662.

Kraiczi H, Hedner J, Peker Y, et al. Comparison of atenolol, amlodipine, enalapril, hydrochlorothiazide, and losartan for antihypertensive treatment of patients with obstructive sleep apnea. *Am J Respir Crit Care Med* 2000;161:1423–1428.

Kreiss K, Zack MM, Kimbrough RD, et al. Association of blood pressure and polychlorinated biphenyl levels. *JAMA* 1981;245:2505–2509.

Kroenke K, Spitzer RL, Williams JBW, et al. Anxiety orders in primary care: Prevalence, impairment, comobidity, and detection. *Arch Intern Med* 2007;146:317–325.

Krum H, Louis WJ, Brow DJ, et al. Pressor dose responses and baroreflex sensitivity in quadriplegic spinal cord injury patients. *J Hypertens* 1992;10:245–250.

Kuhlmann U, Bormann FG, Becker HF. Obstructive sleep apnoea: Clinical signs, diagnosis and treatment. *Nephrol Dial Transplant* 2009;24:8–14.

Lange RA, Hillis LD. Cardiovascular complications of cocaine use. *N Engl J Med* 2001;345:351–358.

Lavie P, Herer P, Hoffstein V. Obstructive sleep apnoea syndrome as a risk factor for hypertension: Population study. *Br Med J* 2000;320:179–182.

Lee DH, Ha MH, Kim JR, et al. Effects of smoking cessation on changes in blood pressure and incidence of hypertension: A 4-year follow-up study. *Hypertension* 2001;37:194–198.

Lenoir H, Lacombe JM, Dufouil C, et al. Relationship between blood pressure and depression in the elderly. The Three-City Study. *J Hypertens* 2008;26:1765–1772.

Lester SJ, Baggott M, Welm S, et al. Cardiovascular effects of 3,4-methylenedioxymethamphetamine: A double-blind, placebo-controlled trial. *Ann Intern Med* 2000;133:969–973.

Licht CM, de Geus EJ, Seldenrijk A, et al. Depression is associated with decreased blood pressure, but antidepressant use increases the risk for hypertension. *Hypertension* 2009;53:631–638.

Lindsay J, Laurin D, Verreault R, et al. Risk factors for Alzheimer's disease: A prospective analysis from the Canadian Study of Health and Aging. *Am J Epidemiol* 2002;156:445–453.

Liu L, Rustgi AK. Cardiav myonecrosis in hypertensive crises associated with monoamine oxidase inhibitor therapy. *Am J Med* 1987;82:1060–1064.

Lovallo WR, Wilson MF, Vincent AS, et al. Blood pressure response to caffeine shows incomplete tolerance after short-term regular consumption. *Hypertension* 2004;43:760–765.

Luft FC. Erythropoietin and arterial hypertension. *Clin Nephrol* 2000;53(Suppl.):S61–S64.

Lumachi F, Ermani M, Luisetto G, et al. Relationship between serum parathyroid hormone, serum calcium and arteriol blood pressure in patients with primary hyperparathyroidism: Results of multivariate analysis. *Eur J endocrinol* 2002;146: 643–647.

Macdonald S, Thomas SM, Cleveland TJ, Gaines PA. Angioplasty or stenting in adult coarctation of the aorta? *Cardiovas Interven Rdiol* 2003;26:357–364.

Mahmud A, Feely J. Divergent effect of acute and chronic alcohol on arterial stiffness. *Am J Hypertens* 2002;15:240–243.

Mahmud A, Feely J. Effect of smoking on arterial stiffness and pulse pressure amplification. *Hypertension* 2003;41:183–187.

Manger WM. "Cerebral Vasculiites": Mistaken cause of fluctuating blood pressure and neurological manifestations. *Kidney Int* 2008;73:354–359.

Margolis KL, Ray RM, Van Horn L, et al. Effect of calcium and vitamin D supplementation on blood pressure in postmenopausal women: Results from the women's health initiative clinical trial. *Hypertension* 2008;52:847–855.

Melamed ML, Michos ED, Post W, et al. 25-hydroxyvitamin D levels and the risk of mortality in the general population. *Arch Intern Med* 2008;168:1629–1637.

Melmed S, Colao A, Barkan A, et al. Guidelines for acromegaly management: An update. *J Clin Endocrinol Metab* 2009;94: 1509–1517.

Merguet P, Ewers HR, Brouwers HP. Blitdruck und herzfrequenz von normotonikern nach maximaler stimulation der magensekretion mit penta grasrin. *Kongr Innere Med* 1968;80: 561–564.

Metso S, Auvinen A, Salmi J, et al. Increased long-term cardiovascular morbidity among patients treated with radioactive iodine for hyperthyroidsm. *Clin Endocrinol* 2008;68:450–457.

Metz S, Klein C, Morton N. Rebound hypertension after discontinuation of transdermal clonidine therapy. *Am J Med* 1987;82:17–19.

Michaeli J, Ben-Ishav D, Kidron R, Dasberg H. Severe hypertension and lithium intoxication. *JAMA* 1984;251:1680.

Mihai R, Wass JAH, Sadler GP. Asymptomatic hyperparathyroidism-need for multicentre studies. *Clin Endocrinol* 2008;68: 155–164.

Minami N, Imai Y, Miura Y, et al. The mechanism responsible for hypertension in a patient with Guillain-Barré syndrome. *Clin Exp Hypertens* 1995;17:607–617.

Mohsenin V. Sleep-related breathing disorders and risk of stroke. *Stroke* 2001;32:1271–1278.

Morath C, Arns W, Schwenger V, et al. Sirolimus in renal transplantation. *Nephrol Dial Transplant* 2007;22(Suppl. 8): viii61–viii65.

Mores M, Campia U, Navarra P, et al. No cardiovascular effects of single-dose pseudoephedrine in patients with essential hypertension treated with beta-blockers. *Eur J Clin Pharmacol* 1999;55:251–254.

Morris MC, Scherr PA, Herbert LE, et al. The cross-sectional association between blood pressure and Alzheimer's disease in a biracial community population of older persons. *J Gerontol* 2000;55A:M130–M136.

Mortensen EL, Jensen HH, Sanders SA, et al. Better psychological functioning and higher social status may largely explain the apparent health benefits of wine: A study of wine and beer drinking in young Danish adults. *Arch Intern Med* 2001;161:1844–1848.

Nash D, Magder L, Lustberg M, et al. Blood lead, blood pressure, and hypertension in perimenopausal and postmenopausal women. *JAMA* 2003;289:1523–1532.

Newman-Toker DE, Hsieh YH, Camargo CA Jr, et al. Spectrum of dizziness visits to US emergency departments: Cross-sectional analysis in a nationally representative sample. *Mayo Clin Proc* 2008;83:765–775.

Niwa K, Perloff JK, Bhuta SM, et al. Structural abnormalities of great arterial walls in congenital heart disease: Light and electron microscopic analyses. *Circulation* 2001;103:393–400.

Numano F, Okawara M, Inomata H, et al. Takayasu's arthritis. *Lancet* 2000;356:1023–1025.

O'Connell H, Chin AV, Cunningham C, et al. Alcohol use disorders in elderly people—redefining an age old problem in old age. *Br Med J* 2003;327:664–667.

Ochs N, Auer R, Bauer DC, et al. Subclinical thyroid dysfunction and the risk for coronary heart disease and mortality. *Ann Intern Med* 2008;148:832–845.

Ohira T, Tanigawa T, Tabata M, et al. Effects of habitual alcohol intake on ambulatory blood pressure, heart rate, and its variability among Japanese men. *Hypertension* 2009;53: 13–19.

Oncken CA, White WB, Cooney JL, et al. Impact of smoking cessation on ambulatory blood pressure and heart rate in postmenopausal women. *Am J Hypertens* 2001;14:942–949.

Orth SR, Ritz E. The renal risks of smoking: An update. *Curr Opin Nephrol Hypertens* 2002;11:483–488.

Ou P, Celemajer DS, Jolivet O, et al. Increased central aortic stiffness and left ventricular mass in normotensive young subjects after successful coarctation repair. *Am Heart J* 2008;155: 187–193.

Owens P. Lyons S, O'Brien ET. Body beautiful? *J Hum Hypertens* 1998;12:485–487.

Pallini R, Lauretti L, Fernndez E. Chronic arterial hypertension as unique symptom of brainstem astrocytoma. *Lancet* 1995;345: 1573.

Patel SR, White DP, Malhotra A, et al. Continuous positive airway pressure therapy for treating sleepiness in a diverse population with obstructive sleep apnea: Results of a meta-analysis. *Arch Intern Med* 2003;163:565–571.

Patterson C, Feightner JW, Garcia A, et al. Diagnosis and treatment of dementia: 1. Risk assessment and primary prevention of Alzheimer disease. *CMAJ* 2008;178:548–556.

Pearl JM, Manning PB, Franklin C, et al. Risk of recoarctation should not be a deciding factor in the timing of coarctation repair. *Am J Cardiol* 2004;93:803–805.

Peppard PE, Young T, Palta M, Skatrud J. Prospective study of the association between sleep-disordered breathing and hypertension. *N Engl J Med* 2000a;342:1378–1384.

Peppard PE, Young T, Palta M, et al. Longitudinal study of moderate weight change and sleep-disordered breathing. *JAMA* 2000b;284:3015–3021.

Pickering TG, Clemow L. Paroxysmal hypertension: The role of stress and psychological factors. *J Clin Hypertens* 2008;10: 575–581.

Pilz S, Dobnig H, Fischer JE, et al. Low vitamin d levels predict stroke in patients referred to coronary angiography. *Stroke* 2008;39:2611–2613.

Pop-Busui R, Chey W, Stevens MJ. Severe hypertension induced by the long-acting somatostatin analogue sandostatin LAR in a patient with diabetic autonomic neuropathy. *J Clin Endocrinol Metab* 2000;85:943–946.

Portaluppi F, Cortelli P, Avoni P, et al. Diurnal blood pressure variation and hormonal correlates in fatal familial insomnia. *Hypertension* 1994;23:569–576.

Primatesta P, Falaschetti E, Gupta S, et al. Association between smoking and blood pressure: Evidence from the health survey for England. *Hypertension* 2001;37:187–193.

Protogerou AD, Laaban J, Czernichow S, et al. Structural and functional arterial properties in patiens with obstructive sleep apnea syndrome and cardiovascular cormobidities. *J Hum Hypertens* 2008;22:415–422.

Rahman M, Tondel M, Ahmad A, et al. Hypertension and arsenic exposure in Bangladesh. *Hypertension* 1999;33:74–78.

Rehm J, Room R, Graham K, et al. The relationship of average volume of alcohol consumption and patterns of drinking to burden of disease: An overview. *Addiction* 2003;98:1209–1228.

Reinprecht F, Elmståhl S, Janzon L, et al. Hypertension and changes of cognitive function in 81-year-old men: A 13-year follow-up of the population study "Men born in 1914," Sweden. *J Hypertens* 2003;21:57–66.

Rizzoni D, Porteri E, Giustina A, et al. Acromegalic patients show the presence of hypertrophic remodeling of subcutaneous small resistance arteries. *Hypertension* 2004;43:561–565.

Roche H, Hyman G, Nahas G. Hypertension and intravenous antidopaminergic drugs. *N Engl J Med* 1985;312:1125–1126.

Roche SI, Kaufmann J, Dipchand AI, et al. Hypertension after pediatric heart transplantation is primarily associated with immunosuppressive regimen. *J Heart Lung Transplant* 2008; 27:301–307.

Rockx MA, Haddad H. Use of calcium channel blockers and angiotensin-converting enzyme inhibitors after cardiac transplantation. *Cur Opin Cardiol* 2007;221:128–132.

Rosenthal E, Najm YC, Maisey MN, Curry PVL. Pressor effects of thyrotropin releasing hormone during thyroid function testing. *BMJ* 1987;294:806–807.

Rosito GA, Fuchs FD, Duncan BB. Dose-dependent biphasic effect of ethanol on 24-h blood pressure in normotensive subjects. *Am J Hypertens* 1999;12:236–240.

Sabia S, Marmot M, Dufouil C, et al. Smoking history and cognitive function in middle age from the Whitehall II study. *Arch Intern Med* 2008;168(11):1165–1173.

Saito I, Saruta T. Hypertension in thyroid disorders. *Endocrinol Metab Clin North Am* 1994;23:379–386.

Scharnweber HC, Spears GN, Cowles SR. Chronic methyl chloride intoxication in six industrial workers. *J Occup Med* 1974;16:112–113.

Schoenborn CA, Vickerie JL, Barnes PM. *Cigarette Smoking Behavior of Adults: United States, 1997–98. Adv Data from Vital and Health Statistics; No 331.* Hyattsville, MD: National Center for Health Statistics; 2003.

Sherrill DL, Kotchou K, Quan SF. Association of physical activity and human sleep disorders. *Arch Intern Med* 1998;158: 1894–1989.

Sierksma A, Muller M, van der Schouw YT, et al. Alcohol consumption and arterial stiffness in men. *J Hypertens* 2004;22:357–362.

Sigaudo-Roussel D, Evans DH, Naylor AR, et al. Deterioration in carotid baroreflex during carotid endarterectomy. *J Vasc Surg* 2002;36:793–798.

Silverberg SJ, Lewiecki EM, Mosekilde L, et al. Presentation of asymptomatic primary hyperparathyroidism: Proceedings of the third international workshop. *J Clin Endocrinol Metab* 2009;94:351–365.

Simard JM, Bellefleur M. Systemic arterial hypertension in head trauma. *Am J Cardiol* 1989;63:32C–35C.

Sink KM, Leng X, Williamson J, et al. Angiotensin-converting enzyme inhibitors and cognitive decline in older adults with hypertension: Results from the cardiovascular health study. *Arch Intern Med* 2009;169:1195–1202.

Sjoqvist F, Garle M, Rane A. Using of doping agents, particularly anabolic steroids, in sports and society. *Lancet* 2008;371: 1872–1882.

Snijder MB, Lips P, Seidell JC, et al. Vitamin D status and parathyroid hormone levels in relation to blood pressure: A population-based study in older men and women. *J Intern Med* 2007;261:558–565.

Solomon DH, Schneeweiss S, Levin R, et al. Relationship between COX-2 Specific inhibitors and hypertension. *Hypertension* 2004;44:140–145.

Somers VK, white DP, Amin R, et al. Sleep apnea and cardiovascular disease. *Circulation* 2008;118:1080–1111.

Streeten DHP, Anderson GH Jr, Howland T, et al. Effects of thyroid function on blood pressure: Recognition of hypothyroid hypertension. *Hypertension* 1988;11:78–83.

Swan L, Ashrafian H, Gatzoulis MA. Repair of coarctation: A higher goal? *Lancet* 2002;359:977–978.

Taegtmeyer AB, Crook AM, Barton PJR, et al. Reduced incidence of hypertension after heterotopic cardiac transplantation compared to orthotopic cardiac transplantation. *J Am Coll Cardiol* 2004;44:1254–1260.

Taylor EN, Curhan GC, Forman JP. Parathyroid hormone and the risk of incident hypertension. *J Hypertens* 2008;26:1390–1394.

Thadhani R, Camargo CA Jr, Stampfer MJ, et al. Prospective study of moderate alcohol consumption and risk of hypertension in young women. *Arch Intern Med* 2002;162:569–574.

Tishler PV, Larkin EK, Schluchter MD, et al. Incidence of sleep-disordered breathing in an urban adult population: The relative importance of risk factors in the development of sleep-disordered breathing. *JAMA* 2003;289:2230–2237.

Tsachalinas D, Logaras G, Paradelis A. Observations in 246 cass of acute poisoning with parathion in Greece. *Eup J Toicol Environ Hyg.*1971;4:46–49.

Tuncel M, Wang Z, Arbique D, et al. Mechanism of the blood pressure-raising effect of cocaine in humans. *Circulation* 2002;105:1054–1059.

Tyagi S, Kaul UA, Nair M, et al. Balloon angioplasty of the aorta in Takayasy's arteritis. *Am Heart J* 1992;124:876–882.

Van Aken H, Cottrell JE, Anger C, et al. Treatment of intraoperative hypertensive emergencies in patients with intracranial disease. *Am J Cardiol* 1989;63:43C–47C.

Van Gaal L, Pi-Sunyer X, Despres JP, et al. Efficacy and safety of rimonabant for improvement of multiple cardiometabolic risk factors in overweight/obese patients: Pooled 1-year data from the Rimonabant in Obesity (RIO) program. *Diabetes Care* 2008;31(Suppl 2):S229–S240.

Vaziri ND. Anemia and anemia correction: Surrogate markers or causes of morbidity in chronic kidney disease? *Nat Clin Pract Nephrol* 2008;4:436–445.

Velzeboer SCJM, Frenkel J, de Wolff FA. A hypertensive toddler. *Lancet* 1997;349:1810.

Verberk WJ, Kroon AA, Thien T, et al. Prevalence of the white-coat effect at multiple visits before and during treatment. *J Hypertens* 2006;24:2357–2363.

Vestergaard P, Mosekilde L. Cohort study on effects of parathyroid surgery on multiple outcomes in primary hyperparathyroidism. *Br Med J* 2003;327:530–534.

Vgontzas AN, Pejovic S, Zoumakis E, et al. Hypothalamic-pituitary-adrenal axis activity in obese men with and without sleep apnea: Effects of continuous positive airway pressure therapy. *J Clin Endocrinol Metab* 2007;92:4199–4207.

Vlachopoulos C, Alexopoulos N, Panagiotakos D, et al. Cigar smoking has an acute detrimental effect on arterial stiffness. *Am J Hypertens* 2004;17:299–303.

Vlachopoulos CV, Vyssoulis GG, Alexopoulos NA, et al. Effect of chronic coffee consumption on aortic stiffness and wave reflections in hypertensive patients. *Eur J Clin Nutr* 2007; 61:796–802.

Volicer L, Nelson KL. Development of reversible hypertension during disulfram therapy. *Arch Intern Med* 1984;144:1294–1296.

Volpato S, Pahor M, Ferrucci L, et al. Relationship of alcohol intake with inflammatory markers and plasminogen activator inhibitor-1 in well-functioning older adults: The Health, Aging, and Body Composition study. *Circulation* 2004;109:607–612.

Vriend JW, van Montfrans GA, Romkes HH, et al. Relation between exercise-induced hypertension and sustained hypertension in adult patients after successful correction of aortic coarctation. *J Hypertens* 2004;22:501–509.

Vupputuri S, Batuman V, Muntner P, et al. The risk for mild kidney function decline associated with illicit drug use among hypertensive men. *Am J Kidney Dis* 2004;43:629–635.

Vuylsteke A, Feneck RO, Jolin-Mellgård Å, et al. Perioperative blood pressure control: A prospective study of patient management in cardiac surgery. *J Cardiothorac Vasc Anesth* 2000;14:269–273.

Walsh JP, Bremner AP, Bulsara MK, et al. Subclinical thyroid dysfunction and blood pressure: A community-based study. *Clin Endocrinol* 2006;65:486–491.

Walsh BT, Hadgan CM, Wong LM. Increased pulse and blood pressure associated with desipramine treatment of bulimia nervosa. *J Clin Psychopharmacol* 1992;12:163–168.

Warner TD, Mitchell JA. COX-2 selectivity alone does not define the cardiovascular risks associated with non-steroidal anti-inflammatory drugs. *Lancet* 2008;371:270–273.

Warren SE, Ebert E, Swerdlin A-H, et al. Clonidine and propranolol paradoxical hypertension. *Arch Intern Med* 1979;139:253.

Weaver FA, Kumar SR, Yellin AE, et al. Renal revascularization in Takayasu arteritis-induced renal artery stenosis. *J Vasc Surg* 2004;39:749–757.

Weber HS, Cyran SE. Endovascular stenting for native coarctation of the aorta is an effective alternative to surgical intervention in older children. *Congenit Heart Dis* 2008;3:54–59.

Wessely S, Nimnuan C, Sharpe N. Functional somatic syndromes: One or many? *Lancet* 1999;354:936–939.

Whelton A, White WB, Bello AE, et al. Effects of celecoxib and rofecoxib on blood pressure and edema in patients ≥65 years of age with systemic hypertension and osteoarthritis. *Am J Cardiol* 2002;90:959–963.

White WB. Cardiovascular effects of the cyclooxygenase inhibitors. *Hypertension* 2007;49:408–418.

Wilson JF. Should doctors prescribe alcohol to adults? *Ann Intern Med* 2003;139:711–714.

Wilson JF. Posttraumatic stress disorder needs to be recognized in primary care. *Ann Intern Med* 2007;146:617–620.

Winchell RJ, Simons RK, Hoyt DB. Transient systolic hypertension. *Arch Surg* 1996;131:533–539.

Winkelmayer WC, Stampfer MJ, Willett WC, et al. Habitual caffeine intake and the risk of hypertension in women. *JAMA* 2005;294:2330–2335.

Winnicki M, Shamsuzzaman A, Lanfranchi P, et al. Erythropoietin and obstructive sleep apnea. *Am J Hypertens* 2004;17:783–786.

Wolk R, Shamsuzzaman AS, Somers VK. Obesity, sleep apnea, and hypertension. *Hypertension* 2003;42:1067–1074.

Wu CC, Johnson AJ. The vasopressor effect of indigo carmine. Henry Ford *HospMed J* 1969;17:131–134.

Young T, Skatrud J, Peppard PE. Risk factors for obstructive sleep apnea in adults. *JAMA* 2004;291:2013–2016.

Yu B, Raher MJ, Volpato GP, et al. Inhaled nitric oxide enables artificial blood transfusion without hypertension. *Circulation* 2008;117:1982–1990.

Zanchetti A, Hansson L, Clement D, et al. Benefits and risks of more intensive blood pressure lowering in hypertensive patients of the HOT study with different risk profiles: Does a J-shaped curve exist in smokers? *J Hypertens* 2003;21:797–804.

Zhang W, Victor RG. Calcineurin inhibitors cause renal afferent activation in rats: A novel mechanism of cyclosporine-induced hypertension. *Am J Hypertens* 2000;13:999–1004.

Hypertension with Pregnancy and the Pill

Hypertension occurs in approximately 10% of first pregnancies and 8% of all pregnancies (Roberts et al., 2003). Preeclampsia (PE), defined as new onset of hypertension with proteinuria after 20 weeks' gestation, is a leading cause of maternal and neonatal mortality worldwide (Maynard et al., 2008). Though maternal mortality from PE has fallen in developed countries, it remains a common cause of preterm delivery of low-birth-weight babies from intrauterine growth retardation (Sibai, 2008a). As noted in Chapter 3, when such babies become adults, they have an increased risk of hypertension and cardiovascular disease as well as an increased likelihood of PE in their own pregnancies (Dempsey et al., 2003). Moreover, the rate of PE is increasing, likely from increasing maternal age and more multiple births (Wallis et al., 2008).

Hypertension is seen more often in users of oral contraceptives (OCs), although the absolute risk is small (Kaunitz, 2008). Although the causes of neither pregnancy-related nor pill-induced hypertension are completely known, if these forms of hypertension are recognized early and handled appropriately, the morbidity and mortality they cause can hopefully be diminished.

TYPES OF HYPERTENSION DURING PREGNANCY

Classification

The classification provided in the 2000 report of the National HBPEP Working Group (2000) is as follows:

- *Chronic hypertension*: Hypertension, defined as a blood pressure (BP) in excess of 140 mm Hg systolic or 90 mm Hg diastolic (taken as the disappearance of sound or Korotkoff phase V), present before pregnancy or diagnosed before the 20th week of gestation or that persists beyond 6 weeks' postpartum.
- *Gestational hypertension (GH)*: Hypertension detected for the first time after the 20th week of gestation, without proteinuria. Some will develop PE; if not, and the BP returns to normal postpartum, the diagnosis of *transient hypertension of pregnancy* can be assigned; if the BP remains elevated postpartum, the diagnosis is *chronic hypertension*.
- *PE*: Hypertension detected for the first time after the 20th week of gestation (or earlier with trophoblastic diseases) with proteinuria of at least 300 mg in a 24-hour specimen. A single-voided protein/creatinine ratio of 0.3 or higher is usually reliable (Coté et al., 2008).
- *Eclampsia*: PE with seizures that cannot be attributed to other causes. Seizures may appear 2 or more days after delivery (Karumanchi & Lindheimer, 2008b).
- *PE superimposed on chronic hypertension*: In a prospective study of 822 women with chronic hypertension, 22% developed PE (Chappell et al., 2008).

Problems in Diagnosing Preeclampsia

There are problems inherent in diagnosing a syndrome of unknown cause on the basis of only highly nonspecific signs. For example, the BP in normal pregnancy usually falls during the first and middle trimesters, only to return toward the prepregnant level during the third trimester. Because women with chronic hypertension have an even greater fall early on, their subsequent rise in later pregnancy may give the appearance of the onset of PE. In addition, those with chronic hypertension may have previously unrecognized proteinuria: If seen only after midterm, the diagnosis of PE looks even more certain.

The distinction between chronic hypertension and PE is of more than academic interest. In the former, hypertension is the major problem, whereas "preeclampsia is more than hypertension; it is a systemic syndrome and several of its 'nonhypertensive' complications can be life threatening when blood pressure elevations are quite mild" (National HBPEP Working Group, 2000). The management of the hypertension and the pregnancy, as well as the prognosis for future pregnancies, varies with the diagnosis. The bottom line, however, is clear: When in doubt, diagnose PE and institute its treatment, because even mild PE may rapidly progress. If PE is correctly diagnosed and managed, the risks to both mother and baby can be largely overcome (Lindheimer et al., 2009).

Obviously, women should be evaluated before conception. If hypertensive, therapy should be revised to exclude ACEIs, ARBs, or direct renin inhibitors. If renal disease is present, more careful observation is needed since there is an increased risk of adverse outcomes (Fischer et al., 2004). Foreknowledge of BP and renal function is essential.

BLOOD PRESSURE MONITORING DURING PREGNANCY

Office Readings

The vagaries of office BP readings, noted in Chapter 2, obviously are in play during pregnancy. However, errors in BP measurement have even more immediate importance, possibly leading to overtreatment of some incorrectly diagnosed as hypertensive, but even more harm in those with elevated pressures that presage PE who are not recognized.

The various guidelines described in Chapter 2 should be followed in measuring the BP during pregnancy. For the diastolic level, the disappearance of sound (phase 5) is more accurate, reliable, and more easily ascertained than its muffling (phase 4) (Higgins & de Swiet, 2001). Initially, BP should be taken in both arms since a difference of 10 mm Hg or more was found in 8.3% of pregnant women (Poon et al., 2008b). The arm with the higher reading should be used.

In a meta-analysis of 34 studies involving 60,599 women, Cnossen et al. (2008) found that the most accurate predictor of PE in those considered to be at low risk was a mean BP of 90 mm Hg, or higher, during either the first or second trimester. For women considered to be at high risk, the best predictor was a diastolic BP of 75 mm Hg, or higher, during weeks 13 to 20 of gestation.

Home Readings

In their review of BP measurements during pregnancy, Chancellor and Thorp (2008) conclude:

> that pregnant women might benefit from bypassing clinic assessment and its inherent inaccuracies. Home blood pressure recording devices are inexpensive and overcome some of the problems in the clinic setting. In our experience, women are likely to take the time and energy to standardize the environment and follow protocols consistently. Armed with these data, they will be able to provide their clinicians with more accurate information about their trends in blood pressure across pregnancy.

Until home BP monitoring becomes more widely used, most women will be monitored by occasional readings in the office. The definitions given earlier in this chapter are based on office readings, with the caveat that unless the woman is in serious trouble, repeated readings be taken before diagnosing any form of hypertension.

Ambulatory Monitoring

In normal pregnancy, lower pressures are found in the midportion, with rises to nonpregnant levels near term (Ferguson et al., 1994) (Fig. 15-1). The normal fall of midpregnancy diastolic BP was not seen in women with a low educational level and they had an increased incidence of PE (Silva et al., 2008).

The data in Figure 15-1 were from single sets of ABPM measurements in a cross-sectional study. Even more impressive are data from a longitudinal, prospective study in 403 women who started with normal casual BP during the first trimester and who had repeated ABPM recordings made every 4 weeks (Hermida et al., 2004). A highly significant higher level of both daytime and sleep BPs was noted *during the first trimester* in the 128 women who later developed GH and the 40 who later developed PE, in comparison to the 235 who remained normotensive. These data suggest that ABPM may provide the best tool now available for the early identification of women who are predisposed to GH or PE. Moreover, those who developed PE had a greater blunting of the nighttime dipping of BP during the third trimester as compared to those who only had

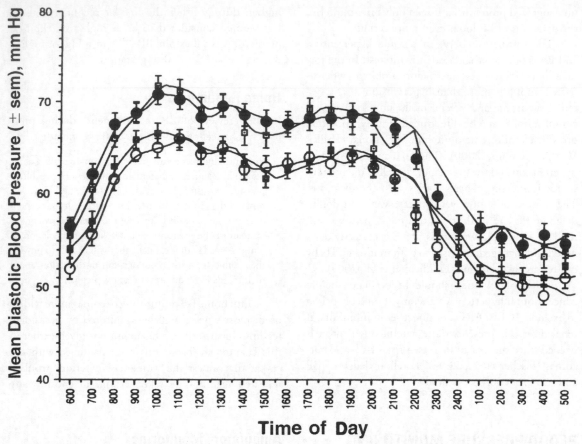

FIGURE 15-1 Diastolic BP patterns recorded hourly during three different gestational periods and in nonpregnant women. Mean diastolic BP (± sem) was recorded in millimeters of mercury. *Open squares with dot*, nonpregnant; *open circles*, 18 to 22 weeks pregnant; *solid squares*, 30 to 32 weeks pregnant; *solid circles*, 36 to 38 weeks pregnant. (Adapted from Ferguson JH, Neubauer BL, Shaar CJ. Ambulatory blood pressure monitoring during pregnancy. Establishment of standards of normalcy. *Am J Hypertens* 1994;7:838–843.)

GH, so the procedure may provide additional warning of the impending development of PE. Obviously, more such careful study of ABPM during pregnancy is needed.

Pulse Wave Analysis

As described in Chapters 2 and 3, pulse wave analysis is being used increasingly as a noninvasive way to measure arterial compliance and central BP. With a sensitive tonometer, the radial pulse wave is measured along with the brachial BP and by use of proprietary formulas, the central pulse wave is visualized.

In a study of 10 women between the 11th and 13th week of gestation, the pulse wave analysis was abnormal in 12 of the 14 who developed PE with an

11% false-positive rate (Khalil et al., 2009). With more experience, the procedure could play a role in early screening.

CIRCULATORY CHANGES IN NORMAL PREGNANCY

Serial measurements begun before conception have portrayed the evolution of the profound changes of normal pregnancy. In ten women, nine nulliparous, who were studied before and repeatedly during pregnancy, significant decreases in systemic vascular resistance resulted in a fall in BP, despite an increase in cardiac output (CO), even before placentation (Chapman et al., 1998) (Fig. 15-2). As the authors note, "Therefore, it is likely that maternal factors,

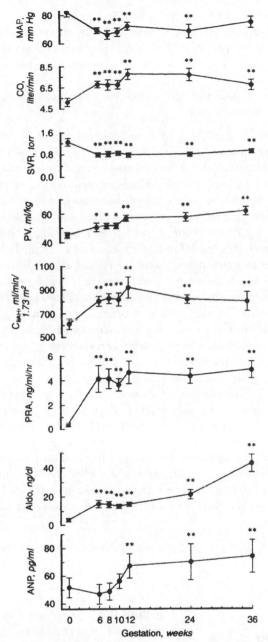

FIGURE 15-2 Changes in mean arterial pressure (MAP), cardiac output (CO), systemic vascular resistance (SVR), plasma volume (PV), effective renal plasma flow measured by para-aminohippurate clearance (C_{PAH}), plasma renin activity (PRA), plasma aldosterone (Aldo), and atrial natriuretic peptide (ANP) in ten women studied in the midfollicular phase of the menstrual cycles and at weeks 6, 8, 10, 12, 24, and 36 of gestation. $*p < 0.05$; $**p < 0.01$. (Adapted from Chapman AB, Abraham WT, Zamudio S, et al. Temporal relationships between hormonal and hemodynamic changes in early human pregnancy. *Kidney Int* 1998;54:2056–2063.)

possibly related to changes in ovarian function or extended function of the corpora lutea, are responsible for the initial peripheral vasodilation found in human pregnancy" (Chapman et al., 1998).

The progressive rise in plasma and blood volume are likely adaptations, via renal sodium retention, to the vasodilation and fall in BP. The low pressure and underfilled circulation provoke an increase in renin secretion and, secondarily, a rise in aldosterone levels. The somewhat later rise in plasma atrial natriuretic peptide is evidence that, despite the increased blood volume, the central circulation is not overexpanded. As a consequence of renal vasodilation, renal plasma flow and glomerular filtration increase and renal vascular resistance decreases.

At the same time as various forces raise levels of renin-angiotensin-aldosterone, normal pregnancy brings forth numerous mechanisms to protect the circulations of both mother and fetus from the intense vasoconstriction, volume retention, and potassium wastage that high angiotensin II and aldosterone levels would ordinarily engender. These include relative resistance to the pressor effects of angiotensin II, reflecting down-regulation of angiotensin II receptors by the high levels of circulating angiotensin II (Baker et al., 1992) and antagonism by endothelium-derived prostacyclin and nitric oxide (NO) (Magness et al., 1996).

The large amounts of potent mineralocorticoids present during pregnancy would be expected to increase sodium reabsorption at the cost of progressive renal wastage of potassium, yet pregnant women are normokalemic. This appears to be the result of the high level of progesterone, which acts as an aldosterone antagonist (Brown et al., 1986).

As confirmed by Rang et al. (2008) in a study of 28 women, normal pregnancy is a low BP state associated with marked vasodilation that reduces peripheral resistance, along with an expanded fluid volume that increases CO. Renal blood flow is markedly increased, and the renin-aldosterone system is activated but with blunted effects.

PREECLAMPSIA

Most PE becomes manifest near the end of pregnancy with few severe fetal or maternal complications. In a smaller percentage, 10% to 30%, PE becomes manifest earlier, before the 34th week, with frequent intrauterine growth restriction (IUGR) and more maternal complications (Sibai, 2008b). Valensise et al. (2008) characterized the maternal hemodynamics of 75 women with early PE and 32 with late PE, all initially studied by uterine artery Doppler ultrasonography at 24 weeks' gestation. Figure 15-3 summarizes their findings that have also been observed by other investigators (Khaw et al., 2008; Mei et al., 2008; Rang et al., 2008).

From these studies, Valensise et al. (2008) conclude that "early PE is placental mediated, linked to defective trophoblast invasion with a high percentage of altered uterine artery Doppler, and late PE is linked to constitutional factors, such as high body mass index."

Epidemiology

The causes of PE must explain the following features, as delineated by Chesley (1985):

- It occurs almost exclusively during the first pregnancy; nulliparas are six to eight times more susceptible than are multiparas. Older primigravida are more susceptible than younger.
- It occurs more frequently in those with multiple fetuses, hydatidiform mole, or diabetes.
- The incidence increases as term approaches; it is unusual before the end of the second trimester.
- The features of the syndrome are hypertension, edema, proteinuria and, when advanced, convulsions and coma.
- There is characteristic hepatic and renal pathology.

- The syndrome has a hereditary tendency; in the families of women who had PE, the syndrome developed in 25% of their daughters and granddaughters but in only 6% of their daughters-in-law.
- It rapidly disappears when the pregnancy is terminated.

As listed in Table 15-1, multiple risk factors for PE have been identified (Dekker & Sibai, 2001). What remains elusive is the initiating mechanism, the trigger that sets off the oftentimes explosive course of this strange malady that disturbs up to one in ten first pregnancies and is rarely seen again. The difficulty in identifying a specific cause is related to the likely presence of multiple mechanisms and the lack of an experimental model for PE. Another difficulty is the inability to identify the early pathogenetic mechanisms, which remain invisible to current technology. Most of what is recognized are late manifestations of a process that is initiated much earlier. As will be noted, no clinically useful screening test to predict the development of PE has been available (Conde-Agudelo et al., 2004).

The situation is changing. The recognition of variations in the maternal circulation of various proangiogenic and antiangiogenic factors has opened the door to earlier prediction. As will be noted, these angiogenic factors are evidently involved early in the pathogenesis of PE. As first described by Maynard et al. (2003) and now amply documented, the spillover of these factors from the poorly perfused placenta

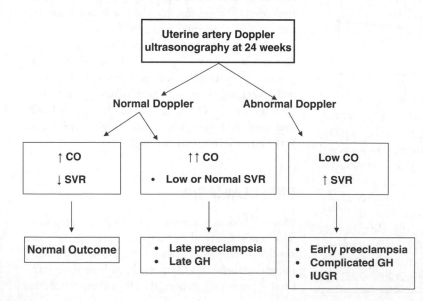

FIGURE 15-3 Uteroplacental and maternal hemodynamics at 24 weeks and subsequent pregnancy outcome. CO, cardiac output; SVR, systemic vascular resistance; GH, gestational hypertension; IUGR, intrauterine growth restriction (Modified from Valensise H, Vasapollo B, Gagliardi G, et al. Early and late preeclampsia: Two different maternal hemodynamic states in the latent phase of the disease. *Hypertension* 2008;52:873–880.)

TABLE 15.1	Risk Factors for PE

Preconceptional or chronic risk factors
Partner-related risk factors
   Nulliparity, primipaternity
   Limited sperm exposure, teenage pregnancy, donor
      insemination
   Partner who fathered a preeclamptic pregnancy in
      another woman
   Either parent the product of a pregnancy complicated
      by PE
Maternal-specific risk factors
   History of previous PE
   Increasing maternal age
   Longer interval between pregnancies
   Family history
   Black or Hispanic race
   Patient requiring oocyte donation
   Physical inactivity
   Presence of specific underlying disorders
   Chronic hypertension and renal disease
   Obesity, insulin resistance, low maternal birth weight
   Gestational diabetes, type 1 diabetes mellitus
   Activated protein C resistance (factor V Leiden), protein
      S deficiency
   Antiphospholipid antibodies
   Hyperhomocysteinemia
Exogenous factors
   Smoking (decreases risk)
   Stress, work-related psychosocial strain
   Inadequate diet
Pregnancy-associated risk factors
Multiple pregnancy
Urinary tract infection
Structural congenital anomalies
Hydrops fetalis
Chromosomal anomalies (trisomy 13, triploidy)
Hydatidiform moles

Modified from Dekker G, Sibai B. Primary, secondary, and tertiary prevention of preeclampsia. *Lancet* 2001;357:209–215.

into the maternal circulation has rapidly captured first place in the competition for early predictors of PE. Among the reports of the measurement of these factors for the prediction of PE with results showing sensitivities of 70% to 100% and specificities of 80% to 100% are these: Hirashima et al. (2008), Lim et al. (2008), Romero et al. (2008), and Stepan et al. (2007).

Pathophysiology

Whatever is fundamentally responsible, as stated by Walker (2000): "Preeclampsia is the result of an initial placental trigger, which has no adverse effect on the mother, and a maternal systemic reaction that produces the clinical signs and symptoms of the disorder." The pathogenesis of PE is logically divided into two stages: first, defective placental perfusion; and second, the maternal systematic reaction.

Deficient Trophoblastic Migration

The current leading hypothesis for the placental trigger is poor placental perfusion and placental hypoxia, first proposed more than 50 years ago (Page, 1948) and now related to deficient trophoblastic migration and invasion. As noted by Roberts and Catov (2008):

> In preeclampsia, IUGR and interestingly also in about one third of cases of preterm birth, the maternal myometrial and decidual vessels perfusing the placental site do not undergo the normal remodeling of pregnancy. In normal pregnancy trophoblastic invasion is associated with a greatly increased diameter and removal of vascular smooth muscle from the wall of those vessels. This results in large diameter, flaccid, unresponsive tubes that greatly increase placental perfusion (Fig. 15-4). These changes are not present in pregnancies complicated by IUGR, preeclampsia, and some with preterm births.

Uteroplacental Hypoperfusion

The consequences of deficient trophoblastic migration with retention of musculoelastic media in spiral arteries could explain the major phenomenon that is usually held responsible for the pathophysiology of PE: uteroplacental hypoperfusion. Uteroplacental hypoperfusion fits with the recognized clinical circumstances wherein PE is most common: *reduced placental mass relative to need* (first pregnancies in young women, twins, hydatidiform mole) and *compromised uterine vasculature* (diabetes and preexisting hypertension).

The Placental Stimulus

Our understanding of the pathophysiology of PE has been markedly expended over the past few years. In the word of Karumanchi and Lindheimer (2008a): "Early observations related to this disorder were that all of the signs and symptoms typically resolve rapidly after the delivery of the placenta." Thus, it was natural to focus on this organ as the source of the disease. In this respect, two anti-angiogenic proteins, overproduced in the placenta, that gain access to the maternal circulation have become candidate molecules responsible for phenotypic preeclampsia. One is

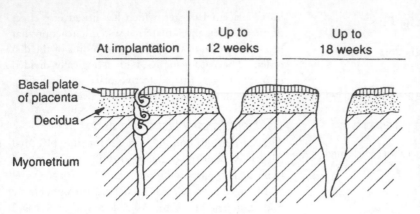

FIGURE 15-4 The normal invasion of spiral arteries by the trophoblast converts them into deltas and so improves blood flow. This invasion is defective in PE. (Adapted from Chamberlain G. Raised blood pressure in pregnancy. *Br Med J* 1991;302:1454–1458.)

soluble Fms-like tyrosine kinase-1 (sFlt1), an endogenous inhibitor of vascular endothelial growth factor and placental growth factor signaling that may regulate placental angiogenesis, and the other is soluble endoglin, a circulating coreceptor that may inhibit transforming growth factor-β1 signaling in the vasculature (Levine et al., 2006). Maternal blood levels of both of these anti-angiogenic proteins are increased in preeclamptic patients compared with those in uncomplicated pregnancies, weeks to months before overt signs and symptoms.

> … However, as data supporting a significant role for anti-angiogenic factors in producing the maternal syndrome is gradually unfolding (research focused primarily on sFlt1), the cause of impaired placentation and the upregulation of anti-angiogenic proteins in placentas of women destined to develop preeclampsia remains unknown.

The answer to the question of what is "the cause of impaired placentation and the upregulation of anti-angiogenic proteins in the placenta" may have been provided by Zhou et al. (2008). As noted further by Karumanchi and Lindheimer (2008a):

> In 1999, in a signal article, a research team headed by Fred Luft in Berlin noted that autoantibodies agonistic to the angiotensin II type 1 (AT_1) receptor were present in the circulation of preeclamptic women. (Wallukat et al., 1999).
>
> The article by Zhou et al. (2008) is particularly exciting, because it marries autoantibodies to anti-angiogenic factors by suggesting that these circulating autoantibodies may be responsible for placental sFlt1 upregulation in preeclampsia. … These data suggest a link whereby the AT_1 autoantibodies may be the cause of increased sFlt1 levels during pregnancy in women destined to have preeclampsia, a mechanism mediated via the placenta.

> … The finding by Zhou et al. (2008) that AT_1 autoantibodies may upregulate sFlt1 raises hope that antagonism of the AT_1 signaling pathway in preeclamptic patients may be a useful therapeutic target in these patients.

As attractive as this construct seems, the primary causes of the impaired placentation and production of AT_1 receptor autoantibodies remain unknown. Studies in pregnant mice (Kanasaki et al., 2008) and rats (LaMarca et al., 2008) may provide experimental models to reveal the primary cause.

One Disease or Two

As noted earlier, epidemiologic data suggest that early onset PE (before 34 weeks) may be a different disease than PE occurring near term, usually after 37 weeks. As noted by Roberts and Catov (2008): "Data support a concept that early preeclampsia is associated with reduced placental perfusion and is a different disease than preeclampsia at term in which reduced perfusion may not be a major component (Fig. 15-5, panel 1)."

> Rather than this two-disease model, Roberts and Catov (2008) provide evidence that PE is one disease, but with different degrees. They explain: The first stage was proposed to be reduced placental perfusion and the second the maternal response to this reduced perfusion. In this model reduced placental perfusion could result in IUGR or preterm birth (or both), but the maternal syndrome of preeclampsia would occur only in women for whom "constitutional factors" (genetics, behavior, environment, etc.) rendered the mother sensitive to the effects of reduced placental perfusion…. This model of maternal fetal interaction provides an alternative explanation for the heterogeneous presentation of preeclampsia early and late other than 2 different diseases. Panel 2 in Figure 15-5 indicates preeclampsia as one disease with different

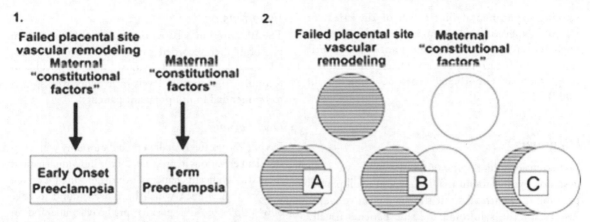

FIGURE 15-5   Genesis of early and late onset PE. Panel 1 indicates early and late PE as disorders with two different origins, with only preterm PE being related to reduced perfusion. Panel 2 illustrates a common origin, reduced placental perfusion, and "maternal constitutional factors" (genetic, behavioral, or environmental factors). PE can result with minimal maternal contribution and primarily reduced perfusion (A) with a relatively similar contribution of both factors (B) or with predominantly an increased maternal sensitivity with minimal (C) reduced perfusion. (Reproduced from Roberts JM, Catov JM. Preeclampsia more than 1 disease: Or is it? *Hypertension* 2008;51:989–990, with permission.)

manifestations, depending on the relative contribution from maternal constitution and reduced fetal placental perfusion. Thus, profoundly reduced perfusion (A) results in preeclampsia in virtually any woman and would be accompanied by IUGR. Lesser degrees of reduced perfusion (B) might result in IUGR with or without preeclampsia depending on the maternal constitution whereas in the profoundly sensitive woman minimally reduced perfusion (or perhaps merely the results of normal perfusion) are sufficient to lead to preeclampsia (C).

Which is the appropriate model? We would suggest both. The genesis of reduced perfusion is very different than what might cause the posited increased response to reduced perfusion. From a genetic perspective, maternal and fetal (paternal) genes contributing to reduced placental perfusion are likely quite different than those rendering the woman sensitive to the putative results of reduced perfusion.

The Maternal Syndrome

What starts in the placenta becomes clinically manifest in the mother. As stated by Maynard et al. (2008):

The clinical manifestations of preeclampsia reflect widespread endothelial dysfunction, resulting in vasoconstriction and end-organ ischemia. Incubation of endothelial cells with serum from women with preeclampsia results in endothelial dysfunction; hence, it has been

hypothesized that circulating factors, probably originating in the placenta, are responsible for the manifestations of the disease (Roberts & Gammill, 2005).

Dozens of serum markers of endothelial activation and endothelial dysfunction are deranged in women with preeclampsia, including von Willebrand antigen, cellular fibronectin, soluble tissue factor, soluble E-selectin, platelet derived growth factor, and endothelin. There is evidence of oxidative stress and platelet activation. Inflammation is often present; for example, neutrophil infiltration is observed in the vascular smooth muscle of subcutaneous fat, with increased vascular smooth muscle expression of IL-8 and intercellular adhesion molecule-1 (ICAM-1). Several of these aberrations occur well before the onset of symptoms, supporting the central role of endothelial dysfunction in the pathogenesis of preeclampsia.

Thus, there are many possible culprits to blame for the endothelial dysfunctions that can cause the various tissue damages seen in women with PE. Normal pregnancy is accompanied by minor endothelial dysfunction, but its degree and rate of progression are far greater in those who develop PE, even before the clinical disease is recognized (Khan et al., 2005). Maynard et al. (2008) give precedence to interference of the actions of the proangiogenic factors VEGF and PIGF by the high levels of the antiangiogenic sFlt1. They note that: "The most striking experimental illustration of the effect of VEGF antagonism in humans comes from anti-angiogenesis cancer trials, where anti-VEGF antibodies produce proteinuria, hypertension, and loss of glomerular endothelial fenestrae (Zhu et al., 2007)."

Diagnosis

Hypertension developing after the 20th week of gestation with proteinuria in a young nullipara is probably PE, particularly if she has a positive family history for the syndrome. Because patients usually have no symptoms, prenatal care is crucial to detect the signs early and thereby prevent the dangerous sequelae of the fully developed syndrome.

Early Detection
In keeping with list of know risk factors (Table 15-1), women with the following features should be more closely evaluated and monitored (Poon et al., 2008a):

- First pregnancy
- Previous PE
- ≥10 years since last baby
- Body mass index ≥35
- Family history of PE (mother or sister)
- Patient had low birth weight
- Diastolic BP ≥ 80 mm Hg
- Proteinuria (≥ + on more than one occasion and ≥300 mg per 24 hours)
- Multiple pregnancy
- Underlying medical condition
  - Preexisting hypertension
  - Preexisting renal disease
  - Preexisting diabetes
  - Presence of antihypertensive phospholipid antibodies

A number of clinical and laboratory tests have been used in the past to recognize PE before it develops and to differentiate it from primary hypertension. After review of 87 relevant studies from over 7,000 articles published from 1996 to 2003, Conde-Agudelo et al. (2004) concluded: "As of 2004, there is no clinically useful screening test to predict the development of preeclampsia." The situation may be changing with the measurements of the proangiogenic and antiangiogenic factors previously described. (Herse et al., 2009; Roberts, 2008)

Hypertension
The BP criterion is based on readings of 140/90 mm Hg or higher recorded on at least two occasions, 6 hours or more apart. Obviously, it is not possible to reconfirm the pressure levels over many weeks, as is recommended in nonpregnant patients.

Overdiagnosis
Despite the greater overall perinatal mortality with even transient elevations in pressure, for the individual patient there is a significant chance of overdiagnosing PE on the basis of these values, which have been found to have only a 23% to 33% positive predictive value and an 81% to 85% negative predictive value (Dekker & Sibai, 2001). Higher ambulatory BP and heart rate are present at 18 weeks' gestation in those who later developed PE; but those signs, too, have low predictive value (Hermida et al., 2004). Therefore, multiple readings and careful follow-up over at least a few days or weeks are needed for women who display such findings in the absence of any other suggestive features before the clinician should make the diagnosis or institute therapy.

Consequences
On the other hand, the level of pressure may not be inordinately high for it to have serious consequences: Women may convulse because of hypertensive encephalopathy with pressures of only 160/110 mm Hg. As noted in the report of the National HBPEP Working Group (2000):

> The clinical spectrum of preeclampsia ranges from mild-to-severe forms. In most women, progression through this spectrum is slow, and the disorder may never proceed beyond mild preeclampsia. In others, the disease progresses more rapidly, changing from mild to severe in days or weeks. In the most serious cases, progression may be fulminant, with mild preeclampsia evolving to severe preeclampsia or eclampsia within days or even hours. Thus, for clinical management, preeclampsia should be overdiagnosed, because a major goal in managing preeclampsia is the prevention of maternal or perinatal morbidity and mortality, primarily through timing of delivery.

Proteinuria
Proteinuria is defined as more than 300 mg of protein in a 24-hour urine collection or 300 mg/L in two random, cleanly voided specimens collected at least 4 hours apart. The protein-creatinine ratio in a random urine sample is a reasonable way to rule out significant proteinuria (Coté et al., 2008).

Hyperuricemia

Roberts et al. (2005) found that hyperuricemia was as important as proteinuria in identifying the fetal risk in women with GH.

Differential Diagnosis

Most women with typical features of de novo hypertension in pregnancy with no other obvious disorders turn out to have PE (Maynard et al., 2008). The recognition of PE superimposed on chronic hypertension may be more difficult. As described in the report of the National HBPEP Working Group (2000):

> Preeclampsia may occur in [15–25% of] women already hypertensive (i.e., who have chronic hypertension).... [T]he diagnosis of superimposed preeclampsia is highly likely with the following findings:

- New onset or sudden increase of proteinuria
- In women with hypertension and no proteinuria early in pregnancy (<20 weeks)
- In women with hypertension and proteinuria before 20 weeks' gestation.
- A sudden increase in BP in a woman whose hypertension has previously been well controlled.
- Thrombocytopenia (platelet count <100,000 cells per mm^3).
- An increase in ALT [alanine aminotransferase] or AST [aspartate aminotransferase] to abnormal levels.

The presence of hypertensive retinopathy, described in Chapter 4, or left ventricular hypertrophy would also favor chronic hypertension.

Manifestations of More Severe Disease

Intravascular Coagulation

As seen in Figure 15-6, activation of intravascular coagulation and subsequent fibrin deposition may be responsible for much of the eventual organ damage seen in severe PE. Increased plasma levels of indicators of platelet activation (β-thromboglobulin), coagulation (thrombin-antithrombin III complexes), and endothelial cell damage (fibronectin and laminin) have been measured up to 4 weeks before the onset of clinical features of PE (Powers et al., 2008). Various inflammatory markers are found after the process has begun (Freeman et al., 2004).

HELLP Syndrome

A few women develop a more serious complication of PE: the HELLP syndrome, which involves hemolysis, *e*levated *l*iver enzymes, and *l*ow *p*latelet counts (Walker, 2000). The syndrome shares many features with the hemolytic uremic syndrome and thrombotic thrombocytopenic purpura (TTP). If initial TTP is accompanied by the other manifestations of the HELLP syndrome, maternal mortality has occurred in almost half (Martin et al., 2008). Corticosteroids may be helpful (van Runnard Heimel et al., 2008), but induction of labor is usually needed (Alanis et al., 2008).

Cerebral Blood Flow

As will be noted, convulsions may occur (i.e., eclampsia) with or without prior manifestations of PE. Many women with PE develop headaches; a few develop cortical blindness (Apollon et al., 2000) and other neurologic features of hypertensive encephalopathy. As described in Chapter 8, hypertensive encephalopathy reflects breakthrough hyperperfusion on the background of vasospasm. Similar findings have been described in PE: both vasospasm (Brackley et al., 2000) and brain edema (Schwartz et al., 2000) that reflects an increase in cerebral blood flow with a failure of autoregulation (Belfort et al., 2008).

Prophylactic magnesium sulfate is now recognized to be essential for prevention of eclampsia.

Management

The report of the National HBPEP Working Group (2000) provides these three tenets for management:

1. Delivery is always appropriate therapy for the mother but may not be so for the fetus. The cornerstone of obstetric management of PE is based on whether the fetus is more likely to survive without significant neonatal complications in utero or in the nursery.
2. The pathophysiologic changes of severe PE indicate that poor perfusion is the major factor leading to maternal physiologic derangement and increased perinatal morbidity and mortality. Attempts to treat PE by natriuresis or by lowering BP may exacerbate the important pathophysiologic changes.
3. The pathogenic changes of PE are present long before clinical diagnostic criteria are manifest. These findings suggest that irreversible changes affecting fetal well-being may be present before the clinical diagnosis. If there is a rationale for management other than delivery, it would be to palliate the maternal condition to allow fetal maturation and cervical ripening.

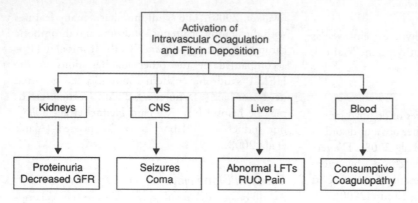

FIGURE 15-6 Proposed model to explain the consequences of activation of intravascular coagulation and fibrin deposition in the pathophysiology of PE. CNS, central nervous system; GFR, glomerular filtration rate; LFT, liver function test; RUQ, right upper quadrant. (Modified from Friedman SA. Preeclampsia: A review of the role of prostaglandins. *Obstet Gynecol* 1988;71:122–137.)

Severe Preeclampsia

The management of PE differs for those with mild disease versus those with severe PE (Table 15-2). Expectant management of severe PE before 24 weeks' gestation is almost always futile, and termination of the pregnancy should be offered (Bombrys et al., 2008). Norwitz and Funai (2008) conclude that

---

TABLE 15.2   Criteria for the Diagnosis of Severe PE

Symptoms
 Central nervous system dysfunction such as blurred vision or severe headache
 Liver capsule distension with right upper-quadrant pain

Signs
 BP above 160 mm Hg systolic or 110 diastolic before and after 6 h rest
 Pulmonary edema
 Stroke
 Cortical blindness
 IUGR

Laboratory findings
 Proteinuria >5 g/day
 Oliguria <500 mL/day and/or serum creatinine above 1.2 mg/dL
 HELLP syndrome
 Liver injury with serum transaminase above two times normal
 Thrombocytopenia below 100,000 platelets/mm³
 Coagulopathy with prolonged prothrombin time or low fibrinogen

---

Modified from Norwitz ER, Funai EF. Expectant management of severe preeclampsia remote from term: Hope for the best, but expect the worst. *Am J Obstet Gynecol* 2008;199:209–212.

There is absolutely no medical benefit to the mother remaining pregnant once she has been diagnosed with severe preeclampsia. By agreeing to continued expectant treatment, she is taking on a small, but significant, risk to her own health in an attempt to delay delivery until a more favorable gestational age is reached. In our view, expectant management of severe preeclampsia remote from term should be undertaken only under specific circumstances: if the woman has a viable pregnancy (≥24 weeks of gestation) without evidence of IUGR, if she is hospitalized in a tertiary care center, and if she agrees to take on the potential risks to her health of continuing the pregnancy after extensive counseling by subspecialists in both maternal-fetal medicine and neonatology.

Mild Preeclapsia
Nonpharmacologic Management

MONITORING Lindheimer et al. (2008) state: "Suspicion of preeclampsia is sufficient to recommend hospitalization." After the initial evaluation, in some situations, day care at a clinic may be possible (Turnbull et al., 2004).

BED REST In women who were hospitalized for various preterm indications, strict bed rest was found to reduce the incidence of PE and IUGR (Abenhaim et al., 2008). At the other extreme, intensive physical activity may increase the risk for PE (Østerdal et al., 2009)

DIET Current evidence favors maintenance of usual sodium intake to avoid further reducing placental perfusion (Knuist et al., 1998). Calcium supplements, although claimed to be effective for prevention of PE in high-risk populations, are not useful for therapy (Hofmeyr et al., 2008). Because caffeine may increase the risk of miscarriage, it seems prudent to restrict its intake even more in women with PE (Weng et al., 2008).

Pharmacologic Therapy

The Seventh Joint National Committee (JNC-7) (Chobanian et al., 2003) report states:

Antihypertensive therapy should be prescribed only for maternal safety; it does not improve perinatal outcomes and may adversely affect uteroplacental blood flow. Selection of antihypertensive agents and route of administration depends on anticipated timing of delivery. If delivery is likely more than 48 hours off, oral methyldopa is preferred because of its safety record. Oral labetalol is an alternative, and other β-blockers and calcium antagonists are also acceptable on the basis of limited data. If delivery is imminent, parenteral agents are practical and effective (Table 15-3). Antihypertensives are administered before induction of labor for persistent DBPs of 105 to 110 mm Hg or higher, aiming for levels of 95 to 105 mm Hg.

The preference given to hydralazine in the 2000 National HBPEP Group report is likely not warranted. As noted in a meta-analysis of all 21 randomized controlled trials published between 1966 and 2002 involving 893 women given short-acting antihypertensives for severe hypertension in pregnancy, hydralazine was associated with more maternal and fetal side effects than nifedipine, isradipine, or labetalol (Magee et al., 2003).

Magnesium sulfate has been conclusively documented to be needed to prevent eclamptic convulsions, both when compared to placebo (Magpie Trial Collaborative Group, 2002) or a calcium channel blocker (Belfort et al., 2003). In addition, its use provides neuroprotection to infants delivered before 30 weeks' gestation, as may be needed in women with severe PE (Crowther et al., 2003).

Long-term Consequences

Postpartum, women who have suffered PE continue to be at greater risk for hypertension, diabetes, and obesity (Berends et al., 2008). Part of this continued risk reflects their prepregnancy state, but the prior occurrence of PE adds to whatever was present before. As a consequence, these women suffer more cardiovascular (Valdes et al., 2009) and renal (Vikse et al., 2008) diseases later in life. Their immediate risk is low for serious complications, and, if given proper advice and follow-up, they may alter lifestyles better than most because of their prior experience during pregnancy (Hertig et al., 2008).

About 15% to 20% of women who have had PE will suffer it again during subsequent pregnancies. The likelihood is greater in those with earlier gestational age at the first delivery and increasing obesity (Mostello et al., 2008). They should be more closely monitored during subsequent pregnancies as early as in the 12th week (Sibai et al., 2008).

Prevention

Dekker and Sibai (2001) have divided prevention into three stages:

1. *Primary* prevention will obviously be difficult without knowledge of the cause. However, avoidance of the known risk factors (Table 15-1) should help. In particular, avoiding teenage pregnancy, reducing obesity and insulin resistance, providing adequate nutrition, and avoiding multiple births during assisted pregnancies should be protective.
2. *Secondary* prevention involves identifying the syndrome as early as possible and using strategies that are thought to influence pathogenic mechanisms. These include low-dose aspirin (Duley et al., 2001), dietary fiber (Qiu et al., 2008), folic acid (Wen et al., 2008), and calcium supplementation (Hofmeyr et al., 2008). Fish-oil supplements have been tested in six multicenter trials and been found

TABLE 15.3	Treatment of Acute Severe Hypertension in PE
Hydralazine	5 mg IV bolus, then 10 mg every 20–30 min to a maximum of 25 mg, repeat in several hours as necessary
Labetalol	20 mg IV bolus, then 40 mg 10 min later, 80 mg every 10 min for two additional doses to a maximum of 220 mg
Nifedipine	10 mg PO, repeat every 20 min to a maximum of 30 mg. Caution when using nifedipine with magnesium sulfate, can see precipitous BP drop. Short-acting nifedipine is not approved by U.S. Food and Drug Administration for managing hypertension
Sodium nitroprusside (rarely when others fail)	0.25 μg/kg/min to a maximum of 5 μg/kg/min. Fetal cyanide poisoning may occur if used for >4 h

to reduce preterm delivery but not to affect any other outcomes (Olsen et al., 2000). In addition, reduction of oxidative stress by antioxidants may work in animal models (Hoffmann et al., 2008), but neither vitamin C nor vitamin E was preventative (Roberts & Kennedy, 2008).

3. *Tertiary* prevention involves the various lifestyle changes and therapies described under Management.

ECLAMPSIA

Eclampsia is defined by the occurrence of seizures due to hypertensive encephalopathy on the background of PE (Karumanchi & Lindheimer, 2008b). This serious complication is becoming less common as better prenatal care is given, but is still seen in about 1% of all pregnancies in developing societies (Miguil & Chekairi, 2008).

Clinical Features

Eclampsia is a form of hypertensive encephalopathy which, on the basis of MRI scanning, is characterized by an initial, reversible vasogenic edema that may lead to irreversible cerebral ischemia and infarction (Zeeman et al., 2004). The features were well defined among the 383 confirmed cases occurring throughout the United Kingdom during 1992 (Douglas & Redman, 1994): Eighty-five percent of the convulsions occurred within 1 week of the woman's last visit to a practitioner, 77% occurred in hospital, and 38% occurred before proteinuria and hypertension had been documented; 38% occurred antepartum; 18% of the women died and 35% had at least one major complication; the rate of stillbirths was 22/1,000; and the rate of neonatal deaths was 34/1,000.

Management

Delivery is delayed until convulsions are stopped, the BP is controlled, and reasonable fluid and electrolyte balance has been established. With the following standardized treatment of 245 consecutive cases of eclampsia, only one maternal death occurred, and all but one of the fetuses survived who were alive when treatment was started and who weighed 1,800 g or more at birth (Pritchard et al., 1984):

• Magnesium sulfate to control convulsions

• Control of severe hypertension (diastolic BP, 110 mm Hg) with intermittent intravenous injections of hydralazine
• Avoidance of diuretics and hyperosmotic agents
• Limitation of fluid intake, unless fluid loss was excessive
• Delivery once convulsions are arrested and consciousness is regained

CHRONIC HYPERTENSION AND PREGNANCY

As more women in developed countries delay pregnancies until they are in their 30s and 40s, the prevalence of preexisting hypertension will likely reach 5% (Roberts et al., 2003).

Pregnant women may have any of the other types of hypertension listed in Chapter 1. Because the BP usually falls during the first half of pregnancy, preexisting hypertension may not be recognized if the woman is first seen during that time. If the pressure is high during the first 20 weeks, however, chronic hypertension rather than PE is almost always the cause.

Pregnancy seems to bring out latent primary hypertension in certain women whose pressures return to normal between pregnancies but eventually remain elevated. In most patients, such "transient hypertension" appears late in gestation, is not accompanied by significant proteinuria or edema, and recedes within 10 days after delivery. Transient hypertension usually recurs during subsequent pregnancies and is often the basis for the misdiagnosis of PE in multiparous women (National HBPEP Working Group, 2000).

To elucidate the true nature of hypertension seen during a pregnancy, it is often necessary to follow up with the patient postpartum. By 3 months, complete resolution of the various changes seen in pregnancy will have resolved so that, if indicated, further studies to elucidate the cause of the hypertension can be obtained.

Risks to Mother and Fetus

Women with chronic hypertension have an increased risk for superimposed PE and placental abruption, and at least their male babies have a threefold greater risk for perinatal mortality (Zetterström et al., 2008). Even without superimposed PE, women with chronic hypertension have more complicated pregnancies with more intrauterine growth retardation and perinatal mortality (Chappell et al., 2008). These risks are even greater for black women in the United States, for those with a diastolic BP above 110 mm Hg during the first trimester, and for those with proteinuria early in pregnancy (Sibai et al., 1998). For those with serum creatinine exceeding 2.0 mg/dL, a one in three chance of entering end-stage renal failure after pregnancy has been reported (Epstein, 1996), so that these women should be strongly advised against pregnancy. Nonetheless, successful pregnancies have been reported in most women who conceive during chronic dialysis (Bagon et al., 1998).

Management

Women with mild to moderate hypertension should be watched closely, warned about signs of early PE, and delivered at 37 weeks' gestation. They should be cautioned not to exercise intensively, told not to drink alcohol or smoke, and advised to restrict dietary sodium to 100 mmol per day (National HBPEP Working Group, 2000).

Uncertainty remains both about the decision to use (or continue) antihypertensive drugs and about which drugs to choose among those available (Table 15-4). As stated by Roberts et al. (2003):

Clinicians do not have sufficient evidence to know which pharmacological therapy is best, when to begin treatment, how vigorously to treat, or whether to stop treatment and hope that the hypotensive effect of normal pregnancy will be enough to control blood pressure. The only trial for treatment of hypertension during pregnancy with adequate infant follow-up (7.5 years) was performed over 25 years ago with a drug (alpha-methyldopa) now rarely used in nonpregnant patient [Cockburn et al., 1982]. Past clinical trials also

have not supported a beneficial effect on pregnancy outcome of treating mild hypertension. There has been no reduction in perinatal mortality, placental abruption, or superimposed preeclampsia. ... Because of the unknown long-term effects on the infant of any treatment, these studies have led to recommendations to treat only on the basis of blood pressure sufficiently elevated to pose potential acute risk to the mother [National HBPEP Working Group, 2000]. Whether this is the appropriate strategy is not clear. ... Even for women with blood pressure elevation sufficient to justify therapy for their own benefit, it is not clear whether treatment is beneficial or detrimental for the fetus. In several studies, treatment of hypertensive women resulted in an increased risk of growth restriction in their infants [von Dadelszen et al., 2000]. It is not known whether this is the inevitable consequence of lowering blood pressure during pregnancy or whether it is due to excessive blood pressure decreases or to specific drugs.

These same uncertainties persist in 2009 (Lindheimer et al., 2009).

As noted in Table 15-4, drugs which block the renin-angiotensin system are contraindicated during pregnancy, even during the first trimester (Cooper et al., 2006). Hypertension whether untreated or treated during pregnancy increases the risk of fetal malformations slightly (Caton et al., 2009). Certain herbal remedies may also cause congenital malformations (Chuang et al., 2006), so pregnant women should be advised to take none of them.

Other Causes of Hypertension During Pregnancy

Identifiable secondary forms of hypertension occur only rarely during pregnancy (Lindsay & Nieman,

TABLE 15.4	Oral Drugs for Treatment of Chronic Hypertension in Pregnancy
Agent	**Comments**
Methyldopa	Preferred on the basis of long-term follow-up studies supporting safety
β-blockers	Reports on intrauterine growth retardation (atenolol)
Labetalol	Increasingly preferred to methyldopa because of reduced side effects
Calcium antagonists (nifedipine)	Limited data
	No increase in major teratogenicity with exposure
Diuretics	Not first-line agents
	Probably safe to reduce fluid retention from other agents
ACEIs, A-II receptor blockers, direct renin inhibitors	Contraindicated Reported fetal toxicity and death

2006). Their diagnosis may be confounded by the multiple changes in the renin-aldosterone and other hormonal systems that occur during pregnancy and their therapy may be made difficult by adverse effects on the fetus. Coverage of these various identifiable forms of hypertension during pregnancy is provided in the respective chapters.

POSTPARTUM SYNDROMES

In women who were preeclamptic, continued close monitoring is needed after delivery (Hertig et al., 2008). As noted earlier, PE and eclampsia may appear after delivery. Depending on the BP, the doses of anti-hypertensive drugs should be reduced and they may not be needed for some weeks. If BP remains elevated at 6 weeks' postpartum, further investigation for other causes of hypertension should be provided. The use of nonsteroidal anti-inflammatory drugs may contribute to postpartum hypertension (Makris et al., 2004).

Peripartum cardiomyopathy is a rare, reported in about one in 3,000 live births (Mielniczuk et al., 2006), but serious form of left ventricular systolic dysfunction that appears in the last month of pregnancy or within 5 months after delivery in the absence of identifiable causes or prior recognizable heart disease (Habli et al., 2008). Endomyocardial biopsy often reveals myocarditis (Felker et al., 2000).

Hypertension and Lactation

Breastfeeding does not raise the mother's BP (Robson et al., 1989) and may protect the baby from subsequent hypertension (Singhal & Lucas, 2004). All antihypertensive drugs taken by mothers enter their breast milk; most are present in very low concentrations, except atenolol and acebutolol (Podynow & August, 2008). Thorough reviews of drugs for pregnant and lactating women are available (Weiner & Buhimschi, 2004).

HYPERTENSION WITH ORAL CONTRACEPTIVES

OCs have been used by millions of women since the early 1960s. OCs are safe for most women, but their use carries some risk.

Incidence of Hypertension

The BP rises a little in most women who take estrogen-containing OCs (Kotchen & Kotchen,

2003). In a prospective cohort study of almost 70,000 nurses covering the 4 years between 1989 and 1993, when the dose of estrogen was twofold to threefold greater than in current OCs, the overall relative risk for hypertension was 50% higher for current OC users as compared to never-users and 10% higher as compared to former users (Chasan-Taber et al., 1996). The 50% increase in relative risk translated to 41 cases per 10,000 person-years of OC use.

Predisposing Factors

In the prospective U.S. Nurses Study, the risk for hypertension was not significantly modified by age, family history of hypertension, ethnicity, or body mass index (Chasan-Taber et al., 1996). Women with prior PE seem to carry little additional risk.

Clinical Course

In most women who develop hypertension while taking an OC, the disease is mild and, in more than half, the BP returns to normal when the OC is stopped (Weir, 1978). In a few women, the hypertension is severe, rapidly accelerating into a malignant phase and causing irreversible renal damage (Lim et al., 1987).

Among nulliparous women who had recently stopped OCs and became pregnant, the risk for developing GH was reduced but the risk for PE slightly increased (Thadhani et al., 1999).

Mechanism

Whether OCs cause hypertension de novo or simply uncover the propensity toward primary hypertension that would eventually appear spontaneously is unknown. The mechanism for OC-induced hypertension is also unknown, particularly because estrogen appears to be vasodilative (Lee et al., 2000). Changes in endothelial function (Virdis et al., 2003), renin-angiotensin-aldosterone (Ribstein et al., 1999), and insulin sensitivity (Godsland et al., 1992) have been identified.

Risks in Perspective

With previous, high-dose formulations, the risks for various cardiovascular diseases, including hypertension, were increased. With currently used low-dose formulations, there are *no* increased risks for overall mortality or myocardial infarction, a reduced risk for ovarian and uterine cancer, but an increased risk for venous thromboembolism, stroke, and cervical and breast cancer (Vessey et al., 2003). Mortality rose 24% in those who smoked 1 to 14 cigarettes per day and 114% in those who smoked 15 or more (Vessey et al., 2003). The risk associated with smoking is higher in women over age 35 (Kaunitz, 2008).

It is important to recognize that the reported increases in relative risk translate into only small increases in absolute risk. As seen in Table 15-5, the number of excess cases of myocardial infarction and stroke rises with age, smoking, and preexisting hypertension but still remains considerably lower than the mortality seen with pregnancy.

Guidelines for Use of Oral Contraceptives

Guidelines published by the American College of Obstetrics and Gynecology (ACOG, 2001) agree with the use of OCs in women with controlled hypertension, but not in those with uncontrolled hypertension above 160/100 mm Hg (Table 15-6).

When OCs are used, the following precautions should be taken:

- The lowest effective dose of estrogen and progestogen should be dispensed.
- The BP should be taken at least every 6 months and whenever the woman feels ill.
- If the BP rises significantly, the pill should be stopped and another form of contraceptive should be provided.
- Progestogen—only contraceptives are not associated with cardiovascular risk factors (Merki-Feld et al., 2008).
- If the BP does not become normal within 3 months, appropriate workup and therapy should be provided.

HYPERTENSION AND ESTROGEN REPLACEMENT THERAPY

After a major reassessment of the safety and benefits of postmenopausal estrogen replacement therapy (ERT), many fewer women will likely be using ERT (Calleja-Agius & Brincat, 2008). Nonetheless, it may turn out to be helpful in the immediate postmenopausal period (Clarkson, 2008), and many women will continue to use ERT since nothing else will effectively prevent hot flushes (Medical Letter, 2004).

In view of the known prohypertensive effect of estrogens given in superphysiologic doses for contraception, there are concerns that the smaller doses for replacement might also raise the BP, adding to the frequent rise in BP after menopause related to increased body weight and aging (Coylewright et al., 2008). Although hypertension has been reported with high doses of postmenopausal estrogen use, most controlled trials find either no difference or a *decrease* in ambulatory BP and a greater dipping of nocturnal BP in ERT users (Coylewright et al., 2008), particularly in the initial period of ERT use (Barton & Meyer, 2009). Women who are already hypertensive may have a fall in BP with transdermal estradiol (Ahmed et al., 2008; Chu et al., 2008; Vongpatanasin et al., 2003).

Beyond their apparent benignity in their relationship to hypertension, ERT has both experimental (Marfella et al., 2008) and clinical features in its favor. As summarized by Birge (2008):

Available biochemical and clinical data are sufficiently compelling to recommend low dose or transdermal hormone therapy for the management of menopausal symptoms when possible. Women initiating low dose or transdermal hormone therapy are not at increased risk

TABLE 15.5 Age-specific Estimates of the Excess Rates of Myocardial Infarction and Ischemic Stroke Attributable to the Use of Low-estrogen Oral Contraceptives and Pregnancy-related Mortality

Variable	Age, years		
	20–24	*30–34*	*40–44*
No. of excess cases of myocardial infarction and ischemic stroke attributable to oral contraceptive use (per 100,000 woman-year of use)			
Among nonsmokers	0.4	0.6	2
Among smokers	1	2	20
Among women with hypertension	4	7	29
No. of pregnancy-related deaths (per 100,000 live births)	10	12	45

Modified from Petitti DB. Clinical practice: Combination estrogen-progestin oral contraceptives. *N Engl J Med* 2003;349:1443–1450.

| TABLE 15.6 | Summary of Guidelines for the Use of Combination Estrogen-progestin Oral Contraceptives in Women with Characteristics that Might Increase the Risk of Adverse Effects | |

Variable	ACOG Guidelines	WHO Guidelines
Smoker, >35 years of age		
<15 cigarettes/day	Risk unacceptable	Risk usually outweighs benefit
≥15 cigarettes/day	Risk unacceptable	Risk unacceptable
Hypertension		
BP controlled	Risk acceptable; no definition of blood pressure control	Risk usually outweighs benefit if systolic BP is 140–159 mm Hg and diastolic BP is 90–99 mm Hg
BP uncontrolled	Risk unacceptable; no definition of uncontrolled BP	Risk unacceptable if systolic BP is ≥160 mm Hg or diastolic BP is ≥100 mm Hg
History of stroke, ischemic heart disease, or venous thromboembolism	Risk unacceptable	Risk unacceptable
Diabetes	Risk acceptable if no other cardiovascular risk factors and no end-organ damage	Benefit outweighs risk if no end-organ damage and diabetes is of ≤20 year duration
Hypercholesterolemia	Risk acceptable if LDL cholesterol < 160 mg/dL and no other cardiovascular risk factors	Benefit-risk ratio is dependent on the presence or absence of other cardiovascular risk factors

Modified from Petitti DB. Clinical practice. Combination estrogen-progestin oral contraceptives. *N Engl J Med* 2003;349:1443–1450.

of cardiovascular disease, stroke, venous thrombotic disease, and breast cancer. Evidence suggests that these outcomes are favorably affected by low-dose hormone therapy and persist with continuation of therapy.

We will turn next to hypertension in children and adolescents, a rapidly growing problem.

REFERENCES

Abenhaim HA, Bujold E, Benjamin A, et al. Evaluating the role of bedrest on the prevention of hypertensive diseases of pregnancy and growth restriction. *Hypertens Pregnancy* 2008;27: 197–205.

ACOG Committee on Practice Bulletins-Gynecology. ACOG Practice Bulletin. The use of hormonal contraception in women with coexisting medical conditions. Number 18, July 2000. *Int J Gynaecol Obstet* 2001;75:93–106.

Ahmed SB, Culleton BF, Tonelli M, et al. Oral estrogen therapy in postmenopausal women is associated with loss of kidney function. *Kidney Int* 2008;74:370–376.

Alanis MC, Robinson CJ, Hulsey TC, et al. Early-onset severe preeclampsia: Induction of labor vs elective cesarean delivery and neonatal outcomes. *Am J Obstet Gynecol* 2008;199:262–266.

Apollon KM, Robinson JN, Schwartz RB, et al. Cortical blindness in severe preeclampsia: Computer tomography, magnetic resonance imaging, and single-photon-emission computed tomography findings. *Obstet Gynecol* 2000;95:1017–1019.

Bagon JA, Vernaeve H, De Muylder X, et al. Pregnancy and dialysis. *Am J Kidney Dis* 1998;31:756–765.

Baker PN, Broughton Pipkin F, et al. Longitudinal study of platelet angiotensin II binding in human pregnancy. *Clin Sci* 1992;82:377–381.

Barton M, Meyer MR. Postmenopausal Hypertension: Mechanism and Therapy. *Hypertens* 2009;54:11–18.

Belfort M, Allred J, Dildy G. Magnesium sulfate decreases cerebral perfusion pressure in preeclampsia. *Hypertens Pregnancy* 2008;27:315–327.

Belfort MA, Anthony J, Saade GR, et al. Nimodipine Study Group. A comparison of magnesium sulfate and nimodipine for the prevention of eclampsia. *N Engl J Med* 2003;348: 304–311.

Berends AL, de Groot CJ, Sijbrands EJ, et al. Shared constitutional risks for maternal vascular-related pregnancy complications and future cardiovascular disease. *Hypertension* 2008;51: 1034–1041.

Birge SJ. Hormone therapy and stroke. *Clin Obstet Gynecol* 2008;51:581–591.

Bombrys AE, Barton JR, Nowacki EA, et al. Expectant management of severe preeclampsia at less than 27 weeks' gestation: Maternal and perinatal outcomes according to gestational age by weeks at onset of expectant management. *Am J Obstet Gynecol* 2008;199:247–256.

Brackley KJ, Ramsay MM, Broughton Pipkin F, et al. The maternal cerebral circulation in pre-eclampsia: Investigations using Laplace transform analysis of Doppler waveforms. *Br J Obstet Gynecol* 2000;107:492–500.

Brown MA, Sinosich MJ, Saunders DM, et al. Potassium regulation and progesterone-aldosterone interrelationships in human pregnancy: A prospective study. *Am J Obstet Gynecol* 1986; 155:349–353.

Calleja-Agius J, Brincat MP. Hormone replacement therapy post Women's Health Initiative study: Where do we stand? *Curr Opin Obstet Gynecol* 2008;20:513–518.

Caton AR, Bell EM, Druschel CM, et al. Antihypertensive medication use during pregnancy and the risk of cardiovascular malformations. *Hypertension* 2009;54:63–70.

Chancellor J, Thorp JM Jr. Blood pressure measurement in pregnancy. *BJOG* 2008;115:1076–1077.

Chapman AB, Abraham WT, Zamudio S, et al. Temporal relationships between hormonal and hemodynamic changes in early human pregnancy. *Kidney Int* 1998;54:2056–2063.

Chappell LC, Enye S, Seed P, et al. Adverse perinatal outcomes and risk factors for preeclampsia in women with chronic hypertension: A prospective study. *Hypertension* 2008;51: 1002–1009.

Chasan-Taber L, Willett WC, Manson JE, et al. Prospective study of oral contraceptives and hypertension among women in the United States. *Circulation* 1996;94:483–489.

Chesley LC. Diagnosis of preeclampsia. *Obstet Gynecol* 1985;65: 423–425.

Chobanian AV, Bakris GL, Black HR, et al. Seventh report of the Joint National Committee on Prevention, Detection, Evaluation, and Treatment of High Blood Pressure. *Hypertension* 2003;42:1206–1252.

Chu MC, Cushman M, Solomon R, et al. Metabolic syndrome in postmenopausal women: The influence of oral or transdermal estradiol on inflammation and coagulation markers. *Am J Obstet Gynecol* 2008;199:526–527.

Chuang CH, Doyle P, Wang JD, et al. Herbal medicines used during the first trimester and major congenital malformations: An analysis of data from a pregnancy cohort study. *Drug Saf* 2006;29:537–548.

Clarkson TB. Can women be identified that will derive considerable cardiovascular benefits from postmenopausal estrogen therapy? *J Clin Endocrinol Metab* 2008;93:37–39.

Cnossen JS, Vollebregt KC, de VN, et al. Accuracy of mean arterial pressure and blood pressure measurements in predicting preeclampsia: Systematic review and meta-analysis. *Br Med J* 2008;336:1117–1120.

Cockburn J, Moar VA, Ounsted M, et al. Final report of study on hypertension during pregnancy: The effects of specific treatment on the growth and development of the children. *Lancet* 1982;1:647–649.

Conde-Agudelo A, Villar J, Lindheimer M. World Health Organization systematic review of screening tests for preeclampsia. *Obstet Gynecol* 2004;104:1367–1391.

Cooper WO, Hernandez-Diaz S, Arbogast PG, et al. Major congenital malformations after first-trimester exposure to ACE inhibitors. *N Engl J Med* 2006;354:2443–2451.

Cote AM, Brown MA, Lam E, et al. Diagnostic accuracy of urinary spot protein:creatinine ratio for proteinuria in hypertensive pregnant women: Systematic review. *Br Med J* 2008;336: 1003–1006.

Coylewright M, Reckelhoff JF, Ouyang P. Menopause and hypertension: An age-old debate. *Hypertension* 2008;51: 952–959.

Crowther CA, Hiller JE, Doyle LW, et al. Australasian Collaborative Trial of Magnesium Sulphate (ACTOMg SO4) Collaborative Group. Effect of magnesium sulfate given for neuroprotection before preterm birth: A randomized controlled trial. *JAMA* 2003;290:2669–2676.

Dekker G, Sibai B. Primary, secondary, and tertiary prevention of pre-eclampsia. *Lancet* 2001;357:209–215.

Dempsey JC, Williams MA, Luthy DA, et al Weight at birth and subsequent risk of preeclampsia as an adult. *Am J Obstet Gynecol* 2003;189:494–500.

Douglas KA, Redman CWG. Eclampsia in the United Kingdom. *Br Med J* 1994;309:1395–1400.

Duley L, Henderson-Smart D, Knight M, et al. Antiplatelet drugs for prevention of pre-eclampsia and its consequences. *Br Med J* 2001;322:329–333.

Epstein FH. Pregnancy and renal disease. *N Engl J Med* 1996;335: 277–278.

Felker GM, Jaeger CJ, Klodas E, et al. Myocarditis and long-term survival in peripartum cardiomyopathy. *Am Heart J* 2000;140: 785–791.

Ferguson JH, Neubauer BL, Shaar CJ. Ambulatory blood pressure monitoring during pregnancy. Establishment of standards of normalcy. *Am J Hypertens* 1994;7:838–843.

Fischer MJ, Lehnerz SD, Hebert JR, et al. Kidney disease is an independent risk factor for adverse fetal and maternal outcomes in pregnancy. *Am J Kidney Dis* 2004;43:415–423.

Freeman DJ, McManus F, Brown EA, et al. Short- and long-term changes in plasma inflammatory markers associated with preeclampsia. *Hypertension* 2004;43:708–714.

Godsland IF, Walton C, Felton C, et al. Insulin resistance, secretion, and metabolism in users of oral contraceptives. *J Clin Endocrinol Metab* 1992;74:64–70.

Habli M, O'Brien T, Nowack E, et al. Peripartum cardiomyopathy: Prognostic factors for long-term maternal outcome. *Am J Obstet Gynecol* 2008;199:415.

Hermida RC, Ayala DE, Fernandez JR, et al. Reproducibility of the tolerance-hyperbaric test for diagnosing hypertension in pregnancy. *J Hypertens* 2004;22:565–572.

Herse F, Verlohren S, Wenzel K, et al. Prevalence of autoantibodies against the angiotensin II type 1 receptor and soluble fms-like tyrosine kinase 1 in a gestational age-matched case study. *Hypertnsion* 2009;53:393–398.

Hertig A, Watnick S, Strevens H, et al. How should women with pre-eclampsia be followed up? New insights from mechanistic studies. *Nat Clin Pract Nephrol* 2008;4:503–509.

Higgins JR, de Sweit M. Blood-pressure measurement and classification of pregnancy. *Lancet* 2001;357:131–135.

Hirashima C, Ohkuchi A, Matsubara S, et al. Alteration of serum soluble endoglin levels after the onset of preeclampsia is more pronounced in women with early-onset. *Hypertens Res* 2008;31: 1541–1548.

Hoffmann DS, Weydert CJ, Lazartigues E, et al. Chronic tempol prevents hypertension, proteinuria, and poor feto-placental outcomes in BPH/5 mouse model of preeclampsia. *Hypertension* 2008;51:1058–1065.

Hofmeyr GJ, Mlokoti Z, Nikodem VC, et al. Calcium supplementation during pregnancy for preventing hypertensive disorders is not associated with changes in platelet count, urate, and urinary protein: A randomized control trial. *Hypertens Pregnancy* 2008;27:299–304.

Kanasaki K, Palmsten K, Sugimoto H, et al. Deficiency in catechol-O-methyltransferase and 2-methoxyoestradiol is associated with pre-eclampsia. *Nature* 2008;453:1117–1121.

Karumanchi SA, Lindheimer MD. Preeclampsia pathogenesis: "Triple a rating"-autoantibodies and antiangiogenic factors. *Hypertension* 2008a;51:991–992.

Karumanchi SA, Lindheimer MD. Advances in the understanding of eclampsia. *Curr Hypertens Rep* 2008b;10:305–312.

Kaunitz AM. Clinical practice. Hormonal contraception in women of older reproductive age. *N Engl J Med* 2008;358:1262–1270.

Khalil AA, Cooper DJ, Harrington KF. Pulse wave analysis: A preliminary study of a novel technique for the prediction of pre-eclampsia. *BJOG* 2009;116:268–276.

Khan F, Belch JJ, MacLeod M, et al. Changes in endothelial function precede the clinical disease in women in whom preeclampsia develops. *Hypertension* 2005;46:1123–1128.

Khaw A, Kametas NA, Turan OM, et al. Maternal cardiac function and uterine artery Doppler at 11–14 weeks in the prediction of pre-eclampsia in nulliparous women. *BJOG* 2008;115: 369–376.

Knuist M, Bonsel GJ, Zondervan HA, et al. Low sodium diet and pregnancy-induced hypertension: A multi-centre randomised controlled trial. *Br J Obstet Gynecol* 1998;105:430–434.

Kotchen JM, Kotchen TA. Impact of female hormones on blood pressure: Review of potential mechanisms and clinical studies. *Curr Hypertens Rep* 2003;5:505–512.

LaMarca B, Wallukat G, Llinas M, et al. Autoantibodies to the angiotensin type I receptor in response to placental ischemia and tumor necrosis factor alpha in pregnant rats. *Hypertension* 2008;52:1168–1172.

Lee AFC, McFarlane LC, Struthers AD. Ovarian hormones in man: Their effects on resting vascular tone, angiotensin converting enzyme activity and angiotensin II-induced vasoconstriction. *Br J Clin Pharmacol* 2000;50:73–76.

Levine RJ, Lam C, Qian C, et al. Soluble endoglin and other circulating antiangiogenic factors in preeclampsia. *N Engl J Med* 2006;355:992–1005.

Lim KG, Isles CG, Hodsman GP, et al. Malignant hypertension in women of childbearing age and its relation to the contraceptive pill. *Br Med J* 1987;294:1057–1059.

Lim JH, Kim SY, Park SY, et al. Effective prediction of preeclampsia by a combined ratio of angiogenesis-related factors. *Obstet Gynecol* 2008;111:1403–1409.

Lindheimer MD, Taler SJ, Cunningham FG. Hypertension in pregnancy. *J Clin Hypertens* 2009;11(4):214–225.

Lindsay JR, Nieman LK. Adrenal disorders in pregnancy. *Endocrinol Metab Clin N Am* 2006;35:1–20.

Magee LA, Cham C, Waterman EJ, et al. Hydralazine for treatment of severe hypertension in pregnancy: Meta-analysis. *Br Med J* 2003;327:955–960.

Magness RR, Rosenfeld CR, Hassan A, et al. Endothelial vasodilator production by uterine and systemic arteries. I. Effects of ANG II on PGI_2 and NO in pregnancy. *Am J Physiol* 1996;270:H1914–H1923.

Magpie Trial Collaborative Group. Do women with pre-eclampsia, and their babies, benefit from magnesium sulphate? The Magpie Trial: A randomised placebo-controlled trial. *Lancet* 2002; 359:1877–1890.

Makris A, Thornton C, Hennessy A. Postpartum hypertension and nonsteroidal analgesia. *Am J Obstet Gynecol* 2004;190:577–578.

Marfella R, Di FC, Portoghese M, et al. Proteasome activity as a target of hormone replacement therapy-dependent plaque stabilization in postmenopausal women. *Hypertension* 2008;51: 1135–1141.

Martin JN Jr, Bailey AP, Rehberg JF, et al. Thrombotic thrombocytopenic purpura in 166 pregnancies: 1955–2006. *Am J Obstet Gynecol* 2008;199:98–104.

Maynard S, Epstein FH, Karumanchi SA. Preeclampsia and angiogenic imbalance. *Annu Rev Med* 2008;59:61–78.

Maynard SE, Min JY, Merchan J, et al. Excess placental soluble fms-like tyrosine kinase 1 (sFlt1) may contribute to endothelial dysfunction, hypertension, and proteinuria in preeclampsia. *J Clin Invest* 2003;111:649–658.

Medical Letter. Treatment of menopausal vasomotor symptoms. *Med Let* 2004;46:98–99.

Mei S, Gu H, Wang Q, et al. Pre-eclampsia outcomes in different hemodynamic models. *J Obstet Gynaecol Res* 2008;34:179–188.

Merki-Feld GS, Imthurn B, Seifert B. Effects of the progestagen-only contraceptive implant Implanon on cardiovascular risk factors. *Clin Endocrinol (Oxf)* 2008;68:355–360.

Mielniczuk LM, Williams K, Davis DR, et al. Frequency of peripartum cardiomyopathy. *Am J Cardiol* 2006;97:1765–1768.

Miguil M, Chekairi A. Eclampsia, study of 342 cases. *Hypertens Pregnancy* 2008;27:103–111.

Mostello D, Kallogjeri D, Tungsiripat R, et al. Recurrence of preeclampsia: Effects of gestational age at delivery of the first pregnancy, body mass index, paternity, and interval between births. *Am J Obstet Gynecol* 2008;199:55–57.

National High Blood Pressure Education Program Working Group on High Blood Pressure in Pregnancy. Report of the National High Blood Pressure Education Program Working Group on High Blood Pressure in Pregnancy. *Am J Obstet Gynecol* 2000; 183:S1–S22.

Norwitz ER, Funai EF. Expectant management of severe preeclampsia remote from term: Hope for the best, but expect the worst. *Am J Obstet Gynecol* 2008;199:209–212.

Olsen S, Secher NJ, Tabor A, et al. Randomised clinical trials of fish oil supplementation in high risk pregnancies. *Br J Obstet Gynaecol* 2000;107:382–395.

Østerdal ML, Strom M, Klemmensen AK, et al. Does leisure time physical activity in early pregnancy protect against preeclampsia? Prospective cohort in Danish women. *BJOG* 2009;116:98–107.

Page EW. Placental dysfunction in eclamptogenic toxemias. *Obstet Gynecol Surv* 1948;3:615–628.

Podymow T, August P. Update on the use of antihypertensive drugs in pregnancy. *Hypertension* 2008;51:960–969.

Poon LC, Kametas NA, Pandeva I, et al. Mean arterial pressure at 11(+0) to 13(+6) weeks in the prediction of preeclampsia. *Hypertension* 2008a;51:1027–1033.

Poon LC, Kametas N, Strobl I, et al. Inter-arm blood pressure differences in pregnant women. *BJOG* 2008b;115:1122–1130.

Powers RW, Catov JM, Bodnar LM, et al. Evidence of endothelial dysfunction in preeclampsia and risk of adverse pregnancy outcome. *Reprod Sci* 2008;15:374–381.

Pritchard JA, Cunningham FG, Pritchard SA. The Parkland Memorial Hospital protocol for treatment of eclampsia: Evaluation of 245 cases. *Am J Obstet Gynecol* 1984;148: 951–963.

Qiu C, Coughlin KB, Frederick IO, et al. Dietary fiber intake in early pregnancy and risk of subsequent preeclampsia. *Am J Hypertens* 2008;21:903–909.

Rang S, van Montfrans GA, Wolf H. Serial hemodynamic measurement in normal pregnancy, preeclampsia, and intrauterine growth restriction. *Am J Obstet Gynecol* 2008;198:519.

Ribstein J, Halimi J-M, du Cailar G, et al. Renal characteristics and effect of angiotensin suppression in oral contraceptive use. *Hypertension* 1999;33:90–95.

Roberts JM. Preeclampsia: New approaches but the same old problems. *Am J Obstet Gynecol* 2008;199:443–444.

Roberts JM, Catov JM. Preeclampsia more than 1 disease: Or is it? *Hypertension* 2008;51:989–990.

Roberts JM, Gammill HS. Preeclampsia: Recent insights. *Hypertension* 2005;46:1243–1249.

Roberts JM, Kennedy S. A randomized controlled trial of antioxidant vitamins to prevent serious complications associated with pregnancy related hypertension in low risk, nulliparous women. *Am J Obstet Gynecol* 2008;199:S4.

Roberts JM, Bodnar LM, Lain KY, et al. Uric acid is as important as proteinuria in identifying fetal risk in women with gestational hypertension. *Hypertension* 2005;46:1263–1269.

Roberts JM, Pearson G, Cutler J, et al. Summary of the NHLBI Working Group on Research on Hypertension During Pregnancy. *Hypertension* 2003;41:437–445.

Robson SC, Dunlop W, Bavs RJ, et al. Hemodynamic effects of breast-feeding. *Br J Obstet Gynaegol* 1989;96:1106–1108.

Romero R, Kusanovic JP, Than NG, et al. First-trimester maternal serum PP13 in the risk assessment for preeclampsia. *Am J Obstet Gynecol* 2008;199:122.

Schwartz RB, Feske SK, Polak JF, et al. Preeclampsia-eclampsia: Clinical and neuroradiographic correlates and insights into the pathogenesis of hypertensive encephalopathy. *Radiology* 2000; 217:371–376.

Sibai BM. Intergenerational factors: A missing link for preeclampsia, fetal growth restriction, and cardiovascular disease? *Hypertension* 2008a;51:993–994.

Sibai BM. Maternal and uteroplacental hemodynamics for the classification and prediction of preeclampsia. *Hypertension* 2008b;52:805–806.

Sibai BM, Koch MA, Freire S, et al. Serum inhibin A and angiogenic factor levels in pregnancies with previous preeclampsia and/or chronic hypertension: Are they useful markers for prediction of subsequent preeclampsia? *Am J Obstet Gynecol* 2008;199:268–269.

Sibai BM, Lindheimer M, Hauth J, et al. Risk factors for preeclampsia, abruptio placentae, and adverse neonatal outcomes among women with chronic hypertension. *N Engl J Med* 1998;339:667–671.

Silva LM, Steegers EA, Burdorf A, et al. No midpregnancy fall in diastolic blood pressure in women with a low educational level: The Generation R Study. *Hypertension* 2008;52:645–651.

Singhal A, Lucas A. Early origins of cardiovascular disease: Is there a unifying hypothesis? *Lancet* 2004;363:1642–1645.

Stepan H, Unversucht A, Wessel N, et al. Predictive value of maternal angiogenic factors in second trimester pregnancies with abnormal uterine perfusion. *Hypertension* 2007;49:818–824.

Thadhani R, Stampfer MJ, Chasan-Taber L, et al. A prospective study of pregravid oral contraceptive use and risk of hypertensive disorders of pregnancy. *Contraception* 1999;60:145–150.

Turnbull DA, Wilkinson C, Gerard K, et al. Clinical, psychosocial, and economic effects of antenatal day care for three medical complications of pregnancy: A randomised controlled trial of 395 women. *Lancet* 2004;363:1104–1109.

Valdes G, Quezada F, Marchant, E, et al. Association of remote hypertension in pregnancy with coronary artery disease: A case-control study. *Hypertension* 2009;53:733–738.

Valensise H, Vasapollo B, Gagliardi G, et al. Early and late preeclampsia: Two different maternal hemodynamic states in the latent phase of the disease. *Hypertension* 2008;52:873–880.

van Runnard Heimel PJ, Kavelaars A, Heijnen CJ, et al. HELLP syndrome is associated with an increased inflammatory response, which may be inhibited by administration of prednisolone. *Hypertens Pregnancy* 2008;27:253–265.

Vessey M, Painter R, Yeates D. Mortality in relation to oral contraceptive use and cigarette smoking. *Lancet* 2003;362:185–191.

Vikse BE, Irgens LM, Leivestad T, et al. Preeclampsia and the risk of end-stage renal disease. *N Engl J Med* 2008;359:800–809.

Virdis A, Pinto S, Versari D, et al. Effect of oral contraceptives on endothelial function in the peripheral microcirculation of healthy women. *J Hypertens* 2003;21:2275–2280.

von Dadelszen P, Ornstein MP, Bull SB, et al. Fall in mean arterial pressure and fetal growth restriction in pregnancy hypertension: A meta-analysis. *Lancet* 2000;355:87–92.

Vongpatanasin W, Tuncel M, Wang Z, et al. Differential effects of oral versus transdermal estrogen replacement therapy on C-reactive protein in postmenopausal women. *J Am Coll Cardiol* 2003;41:1358–1363.

Walker JJ. Pre-eclampsia. *Lancet* 2000;356:1260–1265.

Wallis AB, Saftlas AF, Hsia J, et al. Secular trends in the rates of preeclampsia, eclampsia, and gestational hypertension, United States, 1987–2004. *Am J Hypertens* 2008;21:521–526.

Wallukat G, Homuth V, Fischer T, et al. Patients with preeclampsia develop agonistic autoantibodies against the angiotensin AT1 receptor. *J Clin Invest* 1999;103:945–952.

Weiner CP, Buhimschi C. *Drugs for Pregnant and Lactating Women.* Philadelphia, PA: Churchill Livingstone; 2004.

Weir RJ. When the pill causes a rise in blood pressure. *Drugs* 1978;16:522–527.

Wen SW, Chen XK, Rodger M, et al. Folic acid supplementation in early second trimester and the risk of preeclampsia. *Am J Obstet Gynecol* 2008;198:45–47.

Weng X, Odouli R, Li DK. Maternal caffeine consumption during pregnancy and the risk of miscarriage: A prospective cohort study. *Am J Obstet Gynecol* 2008;198:279, e1–8.

Zeeman GG, Fleckenstein JL, Twickler DM, et al. Cerebral infarction in eclampsia. *Am J Obstet Gynecol* 2004;190:714–720.

Zetterstrom K, Lindeberg SN, Haglund B, et al. The association of maternal chronic hypertension with perinatal death in male and female offspring: A record linkage study of 866,188 women. *BJOG* 2008;115:1436–1442.

Zhou CC, Ahmad S, Mi T, et al. Autoantibody from women with preeclampsia induces soluble Fms-like tyrosine kinase 1 production via angiotensin type 1 receptor and calcineurin/nuclear factor of activated T-cells signaling. *Hypertension* 2008;51:1010–1019.

Zhu X, Wu S, Dahut WL, et al. Risks of proteinuria and hypertension with bevacizumab, an antibody against vascular endothelial growth factor: Systematic review and meta-analysis. *Am J Kidney Dis* 2007;49:186–193.

Hypertension in Childhood and Adolescence

H ypertension, especially obesity-related primary hypertension, should no longer be considered uncommon in children and adolescents. This chapter will describe the features of hypertension in children and adolescents and will also examine the increasingly strong evidence that the genesis of adult cardiovascular disease has its origins in childhood (Williams et al., 2002).

PREVALENCE OF HYPERTENSION IN THE YOUNG

Childhood hypertension was first recognized in the mid-1960s as a result of the work of Londe and others (Londe et al., 1971). Initially, the thresholds used for defining hypertension in the young were the same as those used in adults. Unsurprisingly, hypertension was found to be exceedingly rare in young children but could affect up to 2% of adolescents (Table 16-1). Later screening studies applied population-based percentiles of blood pressure (BP) as the threshold for diagnosis and confirmed that fewer than 2% of children were hypertensive (Fixler et al., 1979). These screening programs also demonstrated the importance of performing repeated measures of BP before labeling a child as hypertensive: studies that used just one BP determination found significantly higher "prevalences" of hypertension than studies in which repeated screenings were performed (Table 16-1).

The impact of the childhood obesity epidemic on the prevalence of hypertension in the young can be seen in several recent studies from the Houston Screening Project (McNiece et al., 2007a; Sorof et al., 2002; 2004a). In multiple publications, these investigators have demonstrated an increased prevalence of hypertension among obese children—as high as 4.5%—compared to nonobese children. Indeed, a recent examination of BP data in 8 to 17-year-old children from the NHANES and other related population-based studies conducted in the United States from 1963 to 2002 clearly demonstrates an increase in the prevalence of elevated BP in children (Fig. 16-1), with much of the increase attributable to the increase in childhood obesity (Din-Dzietham et al., 2007). According to this analysis, the prevalence of prehypertension has now reached 10% and the prevalence of hypertension nearly 4%. Of significant concern is that this increase has had a much greater effect on non-Hispanic black and Mexican American children than on white children (Fig. 16-1).

CHILDHOOD PRECURSORS OF ADULT HYPERTENSION AND CARDIOVASCULAR DISEASE

It is increasingly clear that adult hypertension and other cardiovascular diseases have their origins in childhood. Not only BP levels but also other known cardiovascular risk factors can be measured in the young and then related to the subsequent development of hypertension and its cardiovascular manifestations in adult life. The significance of hypertension in the young is further underscored by the many studies documenting the occurrence of hypertensive target-organ damage in children and adolescents.

Blood Pressure Tracking

The pattern of BP over time, referred to as tracking, has been examined by a number of investigators, most notably in Muscatine, Iowa (Lauer et al., 1993),

TABLE 16.1	Prevalence of Hypertension in Children and Adolescents from Screening Studies					
Study Location	Number Screened	Age (years)	Number of Screenings	Normative Criteria	Prevalence	Reference
Edmonton, Canada	15,594	15–20	1	150/95	2.2%	Silverberg et al. (1975)
New York, United States	3,537	14–19	2	140/90	1.2% SHTN 2.4% DHTN	Kilcoyne et al. (1974)
Dallas, TX, United States	10,641	14	3	95th percentile	1.2% SHTN 0.4% DHTN	Fixler et al. (1979)
Minneapolis, MN, United States	14,686	10–15	1	1987 TF	4.2%	Sinaiko et al. (1989)
Tulsa, OK, United States	5,537	14–19	1	1987 TF	6.0%	O'Quin et al. (1992)
Minneapolis, MN, United States	14,686	10–15	2	1996 WG	0.8% SHTN 0.4% DHTN	Adrogue et al. (2001)
Houston, TX, United States	5,102	12–16	3	1996 WG	4.5%	Sorof et al. (2004a)
Houston, TX, United States	6,790	11–17	3	2004 4th Report	3.2% HTN 15.7% PHTN	McNiece et al. (2007a)

DHTN, diastolic hypertension; PHTN, prehypertension; SHTN, systolic hypertension; TF, Second Task Force Report (Task Force on Blood Pressure Control in Children, 1987); WG, Working Group Report (National High Blood Pressure Education Program Working Group, 1996).

and Bogalusa, Louisiana (Berenson, 2002). In all studies, the best predictive indicator of subsequently sustained elevated BP is an antecedent elevated BP level (Bao et al., 1995). Although an initially elevated BP level may not evolve into later sustained elevation, Lauer et al. (1993) found that 24% of young adults whose pressures ever exceeded the 90th percentile as children had adult BP greater than the 90th percentile, a percentage that is 2.4 times higher than expected. In the Bogalusa cohort, 40% of those with systolic BP and 37% of those with diastolic BP above the 80th percentile at baseline continued to have BP above the 80th percentile 15 years later (Bao et al., 1995).

Tracking is more consistent if the elevated childhood BP levels are combined with obesity, a parental history of hypertension, or increased left ventricular mass by echocardiography (Lauer et al., 1993; Shear et al., 1986).

In view of the higher prevalence of hypertension in black adults than in white adults, comparisons of the tracking phenomenon in black and white children have been made (Lane & Gill, 2004). Black

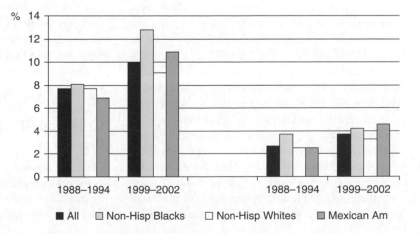

FIGURE 16.1 Prevalence of pre-hypertension (*left-hand bars*) and hypertension (*right-hand bars*) among American children in 1999 to 2002 compared to 1988 to 1994. (Data from Din-Dzietham R, Liu Y, Bielo MV, et al. High blood pressure trends in children and adolescents in national surveys, 1963 to 2002. *Circulation* 2007;116:1488–1496.)

children have significantly higher mean BP than white children even after adjustments for potential confounders such as weight gain (Bao et al., 1995), growth, or socioeconomic status (Dekkers et al., 2002). Dekkers et al. (2002) found that ethnic differences in systolic BP become manifest earlier in girls than in boys and both systolic and diastolic differences tended to increase with age.

The importance of BP tracking was highlighted in a recent meta-analysis of 50 cohort studies conducted between 1970 and 2006 (Chen & Wang, 2008). The average tracking coefficient was 0.38 for systolic BP and 0.28 for diastolic BP, and the strength of BP tracking increased with baseline age for both systolic and diastolic BP. The authors concluded that an elevated BP in childhood is likely to predict adult hypertension, making it important to intervene early to reduce the rates of adult hypertension.

Hypertensive Target-Organ Damage in the Young

Left ventricular hypertrophy (LVH), increased carotid intima-media thickness (cIMT), and even impaired cognitive function stand as concrete evidence of the consequences of elevated BP in childhood and the potential for lifelong morbidity. LVH was first demonstrated to occur in hypertensive youth by Laird and Fixler (1981) and has subsequently been shown to occur in a significant proportion of hypertensive children and adolescents, with reported prevalences ranging between 20% and 41% depending upon the diagnostic criteria utilized (Brady et al., 2008; Flynn & Alderman, 2005; Hanevold, 2004; McNiece et al., 2007b; Sorof et al., 2003). It is especially interesting that the development of LVH in the young may not be related to the severity of BP elevation. While studies from the group in Houston have repeatedly demonstrated a correlation between the severity of BP elevation and the likelihood of developing LVH (McNiece et al., 2007b), a larger multicenter study failed to demonstrate any relationship between LVH and specific parameters of BP elevation (Brady et al., 2008). As will be discussed later, this underscores the need to perform echocardiography at the diagnosis of hypertension and periodically thereafter in children and adolescents, as recommended in the Fourth Report (National High Blood Pressure Education Program Working Group, 2004).

Increased cIMT, well documented as a cardiovascular consequence of elevated BP in large population studies (Vos et al., 2003), has also been found in children and adolescents with primary hypertension in single-center reports (Lande et al., 2006; Litwin et al., 2006; Sorof et al., 2003). While early studies of cIMT in hypertensive youth were confounded by the effects of obesity (Litwin et al., 2006; Sorof et al., 2003), one carefully conducted study that controlled for body mass index (BMI) demonstrated a definitive relationship between elevated BP itself and increased cIMT in young patients (Lande et al., 2006).

An additional target-organ effect of elevated BP recently described in the young is impaired cognitive function (Lande et al., 2003). While long-standing hypertension has long been recognized as a risk factor for the development of cognitive impairment and even dementia in the elderly (Paglieri et al., 2004), this study demonstrated that children and adolescents with BP greater than 90th percentile had poorer performance on selected tests of cognition compared to normotensive children. This provocative finding, while requiring confirmation, adds impetus to consensus recommendations for instituting antihypertensive drug therapy in children and adolescents with persistently elevated BP.

Fewer pediatric data are available on the other major target-organ effect of hypertension, namely renal damage. Although hypertension commonly accompanies chronic kidney disease (CKD) in children, it is rarely its cause (Shatat & Flynn, 2005). Even microalbuminuria, which is commonly seen in hypertensive adults, is infrequently seen in children with isolated hypertension, even when LVH is present (Sorof et al., 2004b). However, a more recent study demonstrated that approximately 58% of hypertensive adolescents had microalbuminuria, with an increased prevalence in stage 2 hypertension compared to stage 1 (Assadi, 2007). Reduction of BP in the latter study was accompanied by a reduction in both microalbuminuria and LVH. Given these conflicting data, additional studies are clearly needed to determine the renal effects of elevated BP in the young.

Childhood BP and Subsequent CV Disease

There are no data at present that clearly document a relationship between childhood BP and cardiovascular morbidity and mortality in adulthood. However, a number of studies have shown that BP and other traditional cardiovascular risk factors in childhood predict the subsequent presence of cIMT (Davis et al., 2001; Li et al., 2003; Raitakari et al., 2003; Vos et al., 2003) and arterial stiffness (Juonala et al., 2006; Li et al., 2004), two well-accepted surrogate markers for atherosclerosis and cardiovascular events.

Additionally, longitudinal studies have demonstrated that children with elevated BP are at increased risk of development of the metabolic syndrome as adults (Sun et al., 2007) and that components of the metabolic syndrome, an important risk factor for cardiovascular morbidity, track over time from childhood to adulthood (Chen et al., 2007). Taken together, these data indicate that over time, adult morbidity and mortality will be more tightly connected with childhood precursors and emphasize the need for early intervention.

POTENTIAL CAUSATIVE FACTORS OF CHILDHOOD HYPERTENSION

The Critical Role of Obesity

Obesity is growing at an alarming pace among children and adolescents in all developed societies, with—as in many other aberrant behaviors—the United States leading the way (Lissau et al., 2004). Recent data indicate that this trend shows no signs of abating (Ogden et al., 2006). Unfortunately, adolescent obesity tracts closely with adult obesity (Kvaavik et al., 2003), setting the foundation for all of the consequences. The expanding waistlines of schoolchildren, measured by waist circumference, are a particularly ominous predictor of the metabolic syndrome that now afflicts the majority of U.S. adults (Rudolf et al., 2004; Sun et al., 2008).

Mainly as a consequence of increasing obesity, the mean BP of U.S. children and adolescents has risen by 1.4/3.3 mm Hg from 1990 to 2000 (Muntner et al., 2004), and the prevalence of hypertension and prehypertension has increased (Din-Dzietham et al., 2007). Those overweight children who have hypertension may also manifest more severe cardiovascular disease assessed by surrogate markers such as dyslipidemia (Flynn & Alderman, 2005) or increased left ventricular mass and cIMT (Sorof et al., 2004b). The combination of childhood obesity, elevated BP, and other cardiovascular risk factors has led to repeated predictions that an epidemic of adult cardiovascular

disease is imminent (Bibbins-Domingo et al., 2007; Daniels, 1999).

In addition, an increased frequency of sleep-related disordered breathing and sleep apnea has been seen in obese children (Wing et al., 2003) and may, as they do in adults, raise BP. It has been proposed that sleep apnea may be an explanation for the development of hypertension in some obese children (Reade et al., 2004).

Low Birth Weight and Early Childhood Growth

Population studies conducted by Barker and others have demonstrated an inverse correlation between birth weight and adult BP (Gamborg et al., 2007; Law et al., 2002; Zureik et al., 1996). A relationship between birth weight and coronary heart disease and type 2 diabetes has also been noted (Barker et al., 2002). Proposed explanations for these findings include deficient maternal nutrition (Barker et al., 1993; Law et al., 1991), possibly leading to acquisition of a reduced number of nephrons (Mackenzie et al., 1996). Autopsy studies demonstrating a reduced number of nephrons in patients with primary hypertension (Keller, 2003) have added intriguing evidence to the latter hypothesis.

Other data indicate that early childhood growth may be more important than birth weight as an influence on future BP. Those children who were small at birth but who have accelerated weight gain either very early after birth (Singhal et al., 2003) or between ages 1 to 5 (Law et al., 2002) have more insulin resistance, obesity, and hypertension later in life. This association between rapid postnatal weight gain and higher BP has been prospectively documented in 3-year-olds (Belfort et al., 2007), 8-year-olds (Burke et al., 2004), and 11- to 14-year-olds (Falkner et al., 2004).

Those infants who are breastfed and thereby have a lower rate of weight gain during infancy have lower BPs in later life than those who are fed enriched formula (Singhal et al., 2001). Although this protection against higher BP by breast feeding may have been exaggerated by selective publication (Owen et al., 2003), the weight of evidence supports an association (Martin et al., 2004). Whether there is more to breast feeding than a reduced rate of excess weight gain (Grummer-Strawn & Mei, 2004) is uncertain but slower early growth appears to be beneficial for long-term cardiovascular health (Singhal et al., 2004).

Other Factors That Determine Blood Pressure

Multiple factors have been reported to correlate with BP levels in children (Table 16-2) and have been examined as potential causative factors for childhood hypertension. Some factors are either genetic or environmental, but most have contributions of both. Height, body mass, and somatic development depend not only on genetic influences but also on nutrition and exercise. Sodium intake may exert its effect on BP in those who are genetically predisposed to higher BP levels and are sodium sensitive, especially African Americans (Wilson et al., 1996). Obese adolescents also have heightened responsiveness to sodium intake (Rocchini et al., 1989). An association between BP and increased sympathetic nervous system activity in whites and increased parasympathetic activity in African Americans has been noted (Urbina et al., 1998). BP reactivity to some forms of stress reflects heightened vascular reactivity

---

TABLE 16.2   **Factors Related to Blood Pressure Levels in Children and Adolescents**

Genetic

Autonomic abnormalities (Lopes et al., 2000)
Deletion of ACE gene (Taittonen et al., 1999)
Ethnicity (Hohn et al., 1994; Sorof et al., 2004a)
Increased salt sensitivity in African Americans (Wilson et al., 1996)
Obesity (Sorof et al., 2004a)
Parental and sibling BP levels (Schieken, 1993)

Environmental

Birth weight (Huxley et al., 2002)
Breast feeding (Martin et al., 2004)
Early childhood growth (Belfort et al., 2007)
Neonatal weight gain (Singhal et al., 2004)
Socioeconomic status (Dekkers et al., 2002)
Exercise (Alpert, 2000)

Mixed Genetic and Environmental

Height (Daniels et al., 1996)
Weight (Sorof et al., 2004a)
Body mass (Kvaavik et al., 2003)
Pulse rate (Zhou et al., 2000)
Somatic growth and sexual maturation (Daniels et al., 1996)
Sodium and other nutrient intakes (Falkner et al., 2000)
Sympathetic nervous system reactivity (Urbina et al., 1998)
Stress (Saab et al., 2001)
Uric Acid (Feig & Johnson, 2007)

---

in children and adolescents with BPs that are higher and more labile (Saab et al., 2001).

Genetic Factors

The hereditability of BP was established decades ago by the findings of a correlation of BP levels between parents and their natural offsprings but no correlation between parents and their adopted children (Biron et al., 1976). Recently published studies have demonstrated that a large percentage of children and adolescents with primary hypertension have positive family histories of hypertension in a parent or grandparent (Flynn & Alderman, 2005; Robinson et al., 2005). Genetic influences have been shown in comparisons of siblings (Wang et al., 1999) and twins (monozygotic and dizygotic) and their families (Schieken, 1993).

Table 16-3 lists some of the differences reported among normotensive children with a positive family history versus those with a negative family history of hypertension. It is likely that yet-undiscovered genetic polymorphisms may account for the development of "primary" hypertension in families and that these in combination with environmental factors may explain the early appearance of hypertension in some non-obese children and adolescents.

TABLE 16.3   **Characteristics of FH+ Normotensive Compared with FH– Normotensives**

↑ Carotid artery stiffness (Meaney et al., 1999)
↑ Blood pressure reactivity (Lemne, 1998)
↑ Leptin and insulin levels (Makris et al., 1999)
↑ Pulse and DBP with dynamic exercise; ↑ pulse with isometric exercises (Mehta et al., 1996)
↑ SBP in African American male adolescents homozygous for the deletion polymorphism of the ACE gene (Taittonen et al., 1999)
↑ Rate of sodium-lithium countertransport (McDonald et al., 1987)
↑ Sleep BP in African American adolescents as measured with ABPM (Harshfield et al., 1994)
↑ Activity of components of the autonomic nervous system (Lopes et al., 2000)
Cardiac indices:
  ↑ intravascular septum:posterior wall mass index ratio (deLeonardis et al., 1988)
  ↑ thickness of the interventricular septum during systole (Hansen et al., 1992)
  ↑ LVMI (van Hooft et al., 1993)

SBP, systolic blood pressure.

Environmental Factors

Of the environmental factors, increased body mass has already been discussed as a major determinant of higher BP levels throughout childhood and adolescence. The relationship between sodium and BP was comprehensively reviewed in Chapter 3. A comprehensive review of the literature on diet and BP in children and adolescents suggested that sodium intake is related to higher BP in children and adolescents whereas data concerning potassium and calcium revealed no significant effect (Simons-Morton & Obarzanek, 1997). In another study, Falkner et al. (2000), using folate as a surrogate for adequacy of micronutrient intake, concluded that African American adolescents with higher folate and micronutrient intakes had lower mean diastolic BP. Caffeine intake has also been associated with an elevated BP in adolescents, with the effect greater in African Americans than in Caucasians (Savoca et al., 2004).

PREVENTION OF HYPERTENSION

The need for early recognition and appropriate management of elevated BP in children is being increasingly emphasized (National High Blood Pressure Education Program Working Group, 2004). Practitioners working with children and their families are in an ideal position to introduce preventive measures that will ensure future cardiovascular health (Kavey et al., 2003).

Children and their families need detailed information about optimal dietary intakes, with appropriate cultural orientation. Once the dietary needs for cholesterol and myelinization of the central nervous system have been met (typically by the age of 2 years), recommendations for a prudent intake of fat such as in the DASH diet (Appel et al., 1997; Couch et al., 2008) should be provided. Family meals are an ideal setting to create lifetime healthful food habits.

Similarly, family activities that include age-appropriate exercise are helpful, not only to prevent hypertension but also to control obesity (Torrance et al., 2007). Families must be informed of the deleterious effects of pressor agents—including tobacco, street drugs, and nonsteroidal anti-inflammatory drugs (NSAIDs)—and their potential to increase BP with chronic use. With these proactive steps, the health of children will be improved. Whether hypertension will be prevented remains unknown.

CLASSIFICATION AND DIAGNOSIS OF HYPERTENSION IN CHILDREN AND ADOLESCENTS

Diagnostic criteria for elevated BP in childhood are based on the concept that BP in children increases with age and with body size, which makes it impossible to utilize a single BP level to define hypertension as is done in adults. This was recognized by early investigators of juvenile hypertension, who initially adopted the adult threshold of 140/90 but later realized that this represented a severe level of BP elevation, particularly in young children, and that population data were needed in order to better define what constitutes an elevated BP in the young (Loggie, 1977). Furthermore, the lack of cardiovascular endpoints in childhood necessitates that the definitions of normal and elevated BP be statistical criteria derived from large-scale, cross-sectional studies of BP in normal children.

Under the auspices of the National Heart, Lung and Blood Institute, consensus guidelines with recommendations for identification and management of elevated BP in childhood have been issued on four occasions since 1977. The most recent of these, "The Fourth Report on the Diagnosis, Evaluation, and Treatment of High Blood Pressure in Children and Adolescents" (National High Blood Pressure Education Program Working Group, 2004) is notable for its adaptation of terminology and staging criteria utilized in consensus guidelines for adult hypertension (Chobanian et al., 2003) to the problem of childhood hypertension, and for its emphasis on the prevention of adult cardiovascular disease by early intervention in children and adolescents with elevated BP.

Definitions and Classification of Elevated Blood Pressure

Normal BP in children aged 1 to 17 years is defined as systolic and diastolic BP less than the 90th percentile for age, gender and height, and hypertension is defined as systolic and/or diastolic BP persistently ≥95th percentile (Tables 16-4 and 16-5). Children with systolic or diastolic BP between the 90th and 95th percentiles, or adolescents with BP ≥120/80, are classified as "prehypertensive," in keeping with the terminology used in the JNC-7 recommendations for adults (Chobanian et al., 2003).

| TABLE 16.4 | Blood Pressure Levels for Boys by Age and Height Percentile[a] |

Age (year)	BP Percentile ↓	Systolic BP (mm Hg)							Diastolic BP (mm Hg)						
		← Percentile of Height →							← Percentile of Height →						
		5	10	25	50	75	90	95	5	10	25	50	75	90	95
1	50	80	81	83	85	87	88	89	34	35	36	37	38	39	39
	90	94	95	97	99	100	102	103	49	50	51	52	53	53	54
	95	98	99	101	103	104	106	106	54	54	55	56	57	58	58
	99	105	106	108	110	112	113	114	61	62	63	64	65	66	66
2	50	84	85	87	88	90	92	92	39	40	41	42	43	44	44
	90	97	99	100	102	104	105	106	54	55	56	57	58	58	59
	95	101	102	104	106	108	109	110	59	59	60	61	62	63	63
	99	109	110	111	113	115	117	117	66	67	68	69	70	71	71
3	50	86	87	89	91	93	94	95	44	44	45	46	47	48	48
	90	100	101	103	105	107	108	109	59	59	60	61	62	63	63
	95	104	105	107	109	110	112	113	63	63	64	65	66	67	67
	99	111	112	114	116	118	119	120	71	71	72	73	74	75	75
4	50	88	89	91	93	95	96	97	47	48	49	50	51	51	52
	90	102	103	105	107	109	110	111	62	63	64	65	66	66	67
	95	106	107	109	111	112	114	115	66	67	68	69	70	71	71
	99	113	114	116	118	120	121	122	74	75	76	77	78	78	79
5	50	90	91	93	95	96	98	98	50	51	52	53	54	55	55
	90	104	105	106	108	110	111	112	65	66	67	68	69	69	70
	95	108	109	110	112	114	115	116	69	70	71	72	73	74	74
	99	115	116	118	120	121	123	123	77	78	79	80	81	81	82
6	50	91	92	94	96	98	99	100	53	53	54	55	56	57	57
	90	105	106	108	110	111	113	113	68	68	69	70	71	72	72
	95	109	110	112	114	115	117	117	72	72	73	74	75	76	76
	99	116	117	119	121	123	124	125	80	80	81	82	83	84	84
7	50	92	94	95	97	99	100	101	55	55	56	57	58	59	59
	90	106	107	109	111	113	114	115	70	70	71	72	73	74	74
	95	110	111	113	115	117	118	119	74	74	75	76	77	78	78
	99	117	118	120	122	124	125	126	82	82	83	84	85	86	86
8	50	94	95	97	99	100	102	102	56	57	58	59	60	60	61
	90	107	109	110	112	114	115	116	71	72	72	73	74	75	76
	95	111	112	114	116	118	119	120	75	76	77	78	79	79	80
	99	119	120	122	123	125	127	127	83	84	85	86	87	87	88
9	50	95	96	98	100	102	103	104	57	58	59	60	61	61	62
	90	109	110	112	114	115	117	118	72	73	74	75	76	76	77
	95	113	114	116	118	119	121	121	76	77	78	79	80	81	81
	99	120	121	123	125	127	128	129	84	85	86	87	88	88	89
10	50	97	98	100	102	103	105	106	58	59	60	61	61	62	63
	90	111	112	114	115	117	119	119	73	73	74	75	76	77	78
	95	115	116	117	119	121	122	123	77	78	79	80	81	81	82
	99	122	123	125	127	128	130	130	85	86	86	88	88	89	90
11	50	99	100	102	104	105	107	107	59	59	60	61	62	63	63
	90	113	114	115	117	119	120	121	74	74	75	76	77	78	78
	95	117	118	119	121	123	124	125	78	78	79	80	81	82	82
	99	124	125	127	129	130	132	132	86	86	87	88	89	90	90
12	50	101	102	104	106	108	109	110	59	60	61	62	63	63	64
	90	115	116	118	120	121	123	123	74	75	75	76	77	78	79
	95	119	120	122	123	125	127	127	78	79	80	81	82	82	83
	99	126	127	129	131	133	134	135	86	87	88	89	90	90	91
13	50	104	105	106	108	110	111	112	60	60	61	62	63	64	64
	90	117	118	120	122	124	125	126	75	75	76	77	78	79	79
	95	121	122	124	126	128	129	130	79	79	80	81	82	83	83
	99	128	130	131	133	135	136	137	87	87	88	89	90	91	91

(continued)

TABLE 16.4   Blood Pressure Levels for Boys by Age and Height Percentile (Continued)

Age (year)	BP Percentile ↓	Systolic BP (mm Hg) ← Percentile of Height →							Diastolic BP (mm Hg) ← Percentile of Height →						
		5	10	25	50	75	90	95	5	10	25	50	75	90	95
14	50	106	107	109	111	113	114	115	60	61	62	63	64	65	65
	90	120	121	123	125	126	128	128	75	76	77	78	79	79	80
	95	124	125	127	128	130	132	132	80	80	81	82	83	84	84
	99	131	132	134	136	138	139	140	87	88	89	90	91	92	92
15	50	109	110	112	113	115	117	117	61	62	63	64	65	66	66
	90	122	124	125	127	129	130	131	76	77	78	79	80	80	81
	95	126	127	129	131	133	134	135	81	81	82	83	84	85	85
	99	134	135	136	138	140	142	142	88	89	90	91	92	93	93
16	50	111	112	114	116	118	119	120	63	63	64	65	66	67	67
	90	125	126	128	130	131	133	134	78	78	79	80	81	82	82
	95	129	130	132	134	135	137	137	82	83	83	84	85	86	87
	99	136	137	139	141	143	144	145	90	90	91	92	93	94	94
17	50	114	115	116	118	120	121	122	65	66	66	67	68	69	70
	90	127	128	130	132	134	135	136	80	80	81	82	83	84	84
	95	131	132	134	136	138	139	140	84	85	86	87	87	88	89
	99	139	140	141	143	145	146	147	92	93	93	94	95	96	97

[a]To use the table, first plot the child's height on a standard growth curve (www.cdc.gov/growthcharts). The child's measured SBP and DBP are compared with the numbers provided in the table according to the child's age and height percentile.
BP, blood pressure.
Reproduced from National High Blood Pressure Education Program Working Group on High Blood Pressure in Children and Adolescents. The Fourth Report on the Diagnosis, Evaluation, and Treatment of High Blood Pressure in Children and Adolescents. National Heart, Lung, and Blood Institute, Bethesda, Maryland. *Pediatrics* 2004;114:555–576.

TABLE 16.5   Blood Pressure Levels for Girls by Age and Height Percentile[a]

Age (year)	BP Percentile ↓	Systolic BP (mm Hg) ← Percentile of Height →							Diastolic BP (mm Hg) ← Percentile of Height →						
		5	10	25	50	75	90	95	5	10	25	50	75	90	95
1	50	83	84	85	86	88	89	90	38	39	39	40	41	41	42
	90	97	97	98	100	101	102	103	52	53	53	54	55	55	56
	95	100	101	102	104	105	106	107	56	57	57	58	59	59	60
	99	108	108	109	111	112	113	114	64	64	65	65	66	67	67
2	50	85	85	87	88	89	91	91	43	44	44	45	46	46	47
	90	98	99	100	101	103	104	105	57	58	58	59	60	61	61
	95	102	103	104	105	107	108	109	61	62	62	63	64	65	65
	99	109	110	111	112	114	115	116	69	69	70	70	71	72	72
3	50	86	87	88	89	91	92	93	47	48	48	49	50	50	51
	90	100	100	102	103	104	106	106	61	62	62	63	64	64	65
	95	104	104	105	107	108	109	110	65	66	66	67	68	68	69
	99	111	111	113	114	115	116	117	73	73	74	74	75	76	76
4	50	88	88	90	91	92	94	94	50	50	51	52	52	53	54
	90	101	102	103	104	106	107	108	64	64	65	66	67	67	68
	95	105	106	107	108	110	111	112	68	68	69	70	71	71	72
	99	112	113	114	115	117	118	119	76	76	76	77	78	79	79
5	50	89	90	91	93	94	95	96	52	53	53	54	55	55	56
	90	103	103	105	106	107	109	109	66	67	67	68	69	69	70
	95	107	107	108	110	111	112	113	70	71	71	72	73	73	74
	99	114	114	116	117	118	120	120	78	78	79	79	80	81	81

(continued)

TABLE 16.5	Blood Pressure Levels for Girls by Age and Height Percentile (Continued)

Age (year)	BP Percentile ↓	Systolic BP (mm Hg) ← Percentile of Height →							Diastolic BP (mm Hg) ← Percentile of Height →						
		5	10	25	50	75	90	95	5	10	25	50	75	90	95
6	50	91	92	93	94	96	97	98	54	54	55	56	56	57	58
	90	104	105	106	108	109	110	111	68	68	69	70	70	71	72
	95	108	109	110	111	113	114	115	72	72	73	74	74	75	76
	99	115	116	117	119	120	121	122	80	80	80	81	82	83	83
7	50	93	93	95	96	97	99	99	55	56	56	57	58	58	59
	90	106	107	108	109	111	112	113	69	70	70	71	72	72	73
	95	110	111	112	113	115	116	116	73	74	74	75	76	76	77
	99	117	118	119	120	122	123	124	81	81	82	82	83	84	84
8	50	95	95	96	98	99	100	101	57	57	57	58	59	60	60
	90	108	109	110	111	113	114	114	71	71	71	72	73	74	74
	95	112	112	114	115	116	118	118	75	75	75	76	77	78	78
	99	119	120	121	122	123	125	125	82	82	83	83	84	85	86
9	50	96	97	98	100	101	102	103	58	58	58	59	60	61	61
	90	110	110	112	113	114	116	116	72	72	72	73	74	75	75
	95	114	114	115	117	118	119	120	76	76	76	77	78	79	79
	99	121	121	123	124	125	127	127	83	83	84	84	85	86	87
10	50	98	99	100	102	103	104	105	59	59	59	60	61	62	62
	90	112	112	114	115	116	118	118	73	73	73	74	75	76	76
	95	116	116	117	119	120	121	122	77	77	77	78	79	80	80
	99	123	123	125	126	127	129	129	84	84	85	86	86	87	88
11	50	100	101	102	103	105	106	107	60	60	60	61	62	63	63
	90	114	114	116	117	118	119	120	74	74	74	75	76	77	77
	95	118	118	119	121	122	123	124	78	78	78	79	80	81	81
	99	125	125	126	128	129	130	131	85	85	86	87	87	88	89
12	50	102	103	104	105	107	108	109	61	61	61	62	63	64	64
	90	116	116	117	119	120	121	122	75	75	75	76	77	78	78
	95	119	120	121	123	124	125	126	79	79	79	80	81	82	82
	99	127	127	128	130	131	132	133	86	86	87	88	88	89	90
13	50	104	105	106	107	109	110	110	62	62	62	63	64	65	65
	90	117	118	119	121	122	123	124	76	76	76	77	78	79	79
	95	121	122	123	124	126	127	128	80	80	80	81	82	83	83
	99	128	129	130	132	133	134	135	87	87	88	89	89	90	91
14	50	106	106	107	109	110	111	112	63	63	63	64	65	66	66
	90	119	120	121	122	124	125	125	77	77	77	78	79	80	80
	95	123	123	125	126	127	129	129	81	81	81	82	83	84	84
	99	130	131	132	133	135	136	136	88	88	89	90	90	91	92
15	50	107	108	109	110	111	113	113	64	64	64	65	66	67	67
	90	120	121	122	123	125	126	127	78	78	78	79	80	81	81
	95	124	125	126	127	129	130	131	82	82	82	83	84	85	85
	99	131	132	133	134	136	137	138	89	89	90	91	91	92	93
16	50	108	108	110	111	112	114	114	64	64	65	66	66	67	68
	90	121	122	123	124	126	127	128	78	78	79	80	81	81	82
	95	125	126	127	128	130	131	132	82	82	83	84	85	85	86
	99	132	133	134	135	137	138	139	90	90	90	91	92	93	93
17	50	108	109	110	111	113	114	115	64	65	65	66	67	67	68
	90	122	122	123	125	126	127	128	78	79	79	80	81	81	82
	95	125	126	127	129	130	131	132	82	83	83	84	85	85	86
	99	133	133	134	136	137	138	139	90	90	91	91	92	93	93

[a]To use the table, first plot the child's height on a standard growth curve (www.cdc.gov/growthcharts). The child's measured SBP and DBP are compared with the numbers provided in the table according to the child's age and height percentile.

BP, blood pressure.

Reproduced from National High Blood Pressure Education Program Working Group on High Blood Pressure in Children and Adolescents. The Fourth Report on the Diagnosis, Evaluation, and Treatment of High Blood Pressure in Children and Adolescents. National Heart, Lung, and Blood Institute, Bethesda, Maryland. *Pediatrics* 2004;114:555–576.

The Fourth Report additionally provides guidelines for staging the severity of hypertension in children and adolescents, which can then be used clinically to guide evaluation and management (Table 16-6). Children or adolescents with stage 2 hypertension should be evaluated and treated more quickly and/or aggressively than those with lower degrees of BP elevation. The overall approach to the classification of elevated BP in children and adolescents is summarized in Figure 16-2.

Assessment

Confirmation of BP Elevation

The first step in evaluating the hypertensive child or adolescent is to confirm that the BP is truly elevated. Since the BP distributions published in the Fourth Report are based upon auscultated BPs and given

the inherent inaccuracies of oscillometric BPs and their variation from auscultated BPs in the young (Kaufmann et al., 1996; Park et al., 2001; Pickering et al., 2005), it is recommended that if a child's BP is found to be elevated using an automated device, it should be confirmed by auscultation. Exceptions to this would include infants and young children who are unable to cooperate with manual BP determination. Furthermore, unless there are symptoms of hypertension present, the child's or adolescent's BP should be shown to be elevated on at least three occasions before making the diagnosis of hypertension (National High Blood Pressure Education Program Working Group, 2004).

Techniques for manual BP measurement recommended by the American Heart Association (Pickering et al., 2005) with respect to cuff size, patient position, etc. should be followed in children and

TABLE 16.6 Classification of Hypertension in Children and Adolescents, with Measurement Frequency and Therapy Recommendations

	SBP or DBP Percentile[a]	Frequency of BP Measurement	Therapeutic Lifestyle Changes	Pharmacologic Therapy
Normal	<90th	Recheck at next scheduled physical examination	Encourage healthy diet, sleep, and physical activity	—
Prehypertension	90th to < 95th or if BP exceeds 120/80 even if below 90th percentile up to < 95th percentile[b]	Recheck in 6 months	Weight management counseling if overweight, introduce physical activity and diet management	None unless compelling indications such as CKD, diabetes mellitus, heart failure, and LVH
Stage 1 hypertension	95th percentile to the 99th percentile plus 5 mm Hg	Recheck in 1–2 weeks or sooner if the patient is symptomatic; if persistently elevated on 2 additional occasions, evaluate or refer to source of care within 1 month	Weight management counseling if overweight, introduce physical activity and diet management	Initiate therapy based on indications in table 6 or if compelling indications as above
Stage 2 hypertension	>99th percentile plus 5 mm Hg	Evaluate or refer to source of care within 1 week (or immediately) if the patient is symptomatic	Weight management counseling if overweight, introduce exercise and diet management	Initiate therapy

[a]For sex, age, and height measured on at least three separate occasions; if systolic and diastolic categories are different, categorize by the higher value.
[b]This occurs typically at 12 years old for SBP and at 16 years old for DBP.
BP, blood pressure; CKD, chronic kidney disease; DBP, diastolic blood pressure; LVH, left ventricular hypertrophy; SBP, systolic blood pressure.
Adapted from National High Blood Pressure Education Program Working Group on High Blood Pressure in Children and Adolescents. The Fourth Report on the Diagnosis, Evaluation, and Treatment of High Blood Pressure in Children and Adolescents. National Heart, Lung, and Blood Institute, Bethesda, Maryland. *Pediatrics* 2004;114:555–576.

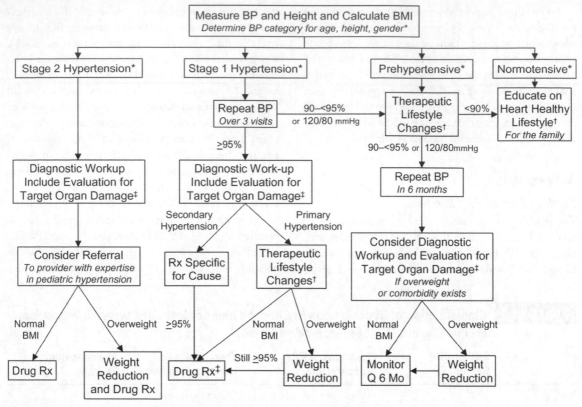

FIGURE 16.2   Suggested management algorithm for children and adolescents with elevated blood pressure. BMI, body mass index; Q, every. *See Tables 16-4 to 16-6. †Diet modification and physical activity. ‡Especially if younger, very high BP, little or no family history, diabetic, or other risk factors. (Reproduced from National High Blood Pressure Education Program Working Group on High Blood Pressure in Children and Adolescents. The Fourth Report on the Diagnosis, Evaluation, and Treatment of High Blood Pressure in Children and Adolescents. National Heart, Lung, and Blood Institute, Bethesda, Maryland. *Pediatrics* 2004;114:555–576.)

adolescents whenever feasible. As in adults, the fifth Korotkoff sound should be reported as the diastolic BP, except in those children and adolescents in whom Korotkoff sounds can be heard down to "zero"; in such children, the fourth Korotkoff sound should be reported as the diastolic (National High Blood Pressure Education Program Working Group, 2004).

Ambulatory BP Monitoring, White-Coat and Masked Hypertension

Ambulatory BP monitoring (ABPM) has been endorsed as an appropriate technique for the evaluation of elevated BP in children and adolescents (National High Blood Pressure Education Program Working Group, 2004; Urbina et al., 2008b). Applications of ABPM in children include identification of white-coat and masked hypertension, assessment of

BP control in those treated with antihypertensive medications, and investigation of hypotensive episodes (Sorof & Portman, 2000; Flynn, 2000; Lurbe et al., 2004; Urbina et al., 2008b). Recently, use of ABPM in a referred pediatric population was shown to reduce the cost of evaluation of elevated BP by identifying those with white-coat hypertension, who then could receive a less-extensive workup (Swartz et al., 2008).

Children and adolescents with secondary hypertension have been found to have more significant nocturnal hypertension and greater daytime diastolic hypertension than those with primary hypertension (Flynn, 2002) as well as blunted nocturnal dipping (Seeman et al., 2005) suggesting that ambulatory monitoring can be used to identify children who need a more aggressive evaluation for underlying causes of hypertension.

White-coat hypertension appears to be at least as common in children as it is in adults (Sorof, 2000). In adults, white-coat hypertension is not felt to be associated with significant cardiovascular morbidity or mortality (Pickering et al., 1999), so pharmacologic treatment of such patients is not recommended. Therefore, proving that a child has white-coat hypertension could help avoid unnecessary exposure to medications and reduce unnecessary diagnostic testing (Swartz et al., 2008). However, recent studies have indicated that children found to have white-coat hypertension actually have early signs of target-organ damage, such as increased left ventricular mass (Kavey et al., 2007; Lande et al., 2008; Stabouli et al., 2005). These data, in combination with the data from tracking studies that suggest that these children are likely at increased risk of development of hypertension in the future, imply that children found to have white-coat hypertension should receive lifestyle modification and should be followed prospectively for the development of definite hypertension.

Masked hypertension has also been recently described in pediatric populations (Lurbe et al., 2005; Matsuoka & Awazu, 2004; Stabouli et al., 2005) and is associated with hypertensive target-organ damage, specifically LVH (Lurbe et al., 2005; McNiece et al., 2007b; Stabouli et al., 2005; Urbina, 2008a). Such children probably merit further evaluation for underlying causes of hypertension and institution of pharmacologic treatment. However, since ABPM remains a specialized technique in pediatrics, further studies are needed to identify groups of children at increased risk of masked hypertension who could benefit from ABPM.

Differential Diagnosis

Traditionally, most hypertension in children has been felt to be secondary to an underlying disorder. As can be seen in Table 16-7, this is certainly the case for infants and young children. In hypertensive children in these age groups, renal disease, renovascular disease, and cardiac disease will often be found after an appropriate diagnostic evaluation. Primary hypertension in young children is therefore usually considered a diagnosis of exclusion (Arar et al., 1994).

In adolescents, however, hypertension is most likely to be primary in origin. This was clearly demonstrated over a decade ago in a study of over 1,000 hypertensive children evaluated at a Polish children's hospital (Wyszynska et al., 1992). In this series, the vast majority of adolescents with persistent BP elevation had no identifiable underlying cause found. Other features that support the diagnosis of primary hypertension include normal growth (and/or obesity), lack of symptoms of hypertension, unremarkable past medical history, and a family history of hypertension (Flynn & Alderman, 2005). Hypertensive adolescents that fit this profile may not need as extensive an evaluation as those who do not.

Diagnostic Evaluation

Hypertension in childhood and adolescence is typically asymptomatic, although up to half of patients may report one or more symptoms, most frequently headache (Croix & Feig, 2006). In adolescent athletes, headaches may occur after strenuous exercise. Symptoms such as seizures, nosebleeds, dizziness, and syncope are rare and, if present, suggest that the BP elevation has been exacerbated by ingested substances or by emotional upset. On the other hand, if these symptoms occur in conjunction with elevated BP in a younger child, they may be a clue to the presence of secondary hypertension. For this reason, it is important to include a systems review designed

TABLE 16.7	Causes of Childhood Hypertension by Age Group		
	Infants[a] (%)	School-age (%)	Adolescents (%)
Primary/Essential	<1	15–30	85–95
Secondary	99	70–85	5–15[b]
Renal Parenchymal Disease	20	60–70	
Renovascular	25	5–10	
Endocrine	1	3–5	
Aortic Coarctation	35	10–20	
Reflux Nephropathy	0	5–10	
Neoplastic	4	1–5	
Miscellaneous	20	1–5	

[a]Less than 1 year of age.
[b]Breakdown of causes is generally similar to that for school-age children.

to elicit signs and symptoms of underlying conditions such as renal disease that may be causing the elevated BP.

The family history should include not only hypertension but also associated conditions and complications such as dyslipidemia, stroke, myocardial infarction, and diabetes. Many substances commonly used or abused in children and adolescents can elevate BP, including prescribed and over-the-counter medications (e.g., corticosteroids or decongestants) and street drugs such as amphetamines and cocaine.

The physical examination should begin with plotting of growth parameters, especially height and BMI, and measurement of BP in both arms and at least one leg. From there, the examination should be focused on detecting the signs of secondary causes of hypertension, such as decreased femoral pulses, abdominal bruits, and cushingoid stigmata (Table 16-8).

Except in very young children, the likelihood that an asymptomatic child with persistently elevated BP will have an underlying cause for the elevation is remote. In children with an identifiable cause for their hypertension, the history and physical examination usually reveal suggestive evidence of the cause, so detailed diagnostic evaluation of children without suggestive evidence is not warranted. Basic screening tests, including serum chemistries and lipids as well as a urinalysis, should be obtained in all patients. Specific specialized studies may be required in some children, particularly those with symptomatic hypertension or stage 2 hypertension (Flynn, 2001; National High Blood Pressure Education Program Working Group, 2004).

As discussed above, consideration should be given to including ABPM in evaluation of all children and adolescents with persistent office BP evaluation (Urbina et al., 2008b), both to identify children with

TABLE 16.8	Physical Examination Findings and Etiology of Hypertension in Children and Adolescents	
	Finding	**Possible Etiology**
Vital Signs	Tachycardia	Hyperthyroidism, pheochromocytoma, neuroblastoma, primary hypertension
	Diminished femoral pulses; BP lower in legs than arms	Aortic coarctation
Height/weight	Growth retardation	Chronic renal failure
	Obesity	Primary hypertension, metabolic syndrome
	Truncal/central obesity	Cushing syndrome
Head and Neck	Moon facies	Cushing syndrome
	Elfin facies	Williams syndrome (renovascular)
	Webbed neck	Turner syndrome (coarctation of the aorta)
	Thyromegaly, proptosis	Hyperthyroidism
Skin	Pallor, flushing, diaphoresis	Pheochromocytoma
	Acne, hirsutism, striae	Cushing syndrome, anabolic steroid abuse
	Café au lait spots	Neurofibromatosis (renovascular), Von Hippel-Lindau disease (pheochromocytoma)
	Adenoma sebaceum	Tuberous sclerosis (renal cystic disease)
	Malar rash	Systemic lupus erythematosus
Chest	Widely spaced nipples/shield chest	Turner syndrome (coarctation of the aorta)
	Heart murmur	Aortic coarctation
	Friction rub	Systemic lupus erythematosus (pericarditis)
	Apical heave	LVH/chronic hypertension
Abdomen	Mass	Wilms tumor, neuroblastoma, pheochromocytoma
	Epigastric/flank bruit	Renal artery stenosis
	Palpable kidneys	Polycystic kidney disease, hydronephrosis, multicystic-cysplastic kidney
Genitalia	Ambiguous/virilization	Adrenal hyperplasia
Extremities	Edema	Renal parenchymal disease
	Joint swelling	Systemic lupus erythematosus
	Muscle weakness	Hyperaldosteronism, Liddle syndrome

white-coat or masked hypertension and also to identify children with possible secondary hypertension. Given the high frequency of LVH in hypertensive children and adolescents (Flynn & Alderman, 2005; Hanevold et al., 2004; Sorof et al., 2004b), echocardiography should be considered part of the baseline evaluation, especially if pharmacologic intervention is required, so that reversal of abnormalities can be monitored and correlated with the adequacy of BP control.

MANAGEMENT OF HYPERTENSION IN CHILDREN AND ADOLESCENTS

Treatment of hypertension in children and adolescents is still largely empiric because there are no long-term studies of either dietary intervention or drug therapy (Kay et al., 2001). Even though more data are now available on safety and effectiveness of drug therapy than in the past (Flynn & Daniels, 2006), the decision as to whether a specific child should receive medication must be individualized.

Nonpharmacologic Management

Consensus organizations emphasize that treatment of hypertension in children and adolescents should begin with nonpharmacologic measures (Fig. 16-2) (National High Blood Pressure Education Program Working Group, 2004). Although the magnitude of change in BP may be modest, weight loss, aerobic exercise, and dietary modifications have been shown to reduce BP in children and adolescents (Torrance et al., 2007). For example, for exercise, sustained training over 3 to 6 months has been shown to result in a reduction of 6 to 12 mm Hg for systolic BP and 3 to 5 mm Hg for diastolic BP (Alpert, 2000). However, cessation of training is generally promptly followed by a rise in BP to pre-exercise levels. It is important to emphasize that aerobic exercise activities such as running, walking, and cycling are preferred to static forms of exercise in the management of hypertension (Alpert & Fox, 1995).

Many children may already be participating in one or more appropriate activities and may only need to increase the frequency and intensity of these activities to see a benefit in terms of lower BP. Hypertension is NOT considered a contraindication to participation in competitive sports, so long as the child's BP is "controlled" (AAP Committee on Sports Medicine and Fitness, 1997).

Several studies have demonstrated that weight loss in obese adolescents lowers BP (Figueroa-Colon et al., 1996; Rocchini et al., 1988; Torrance et al., 2007). Weight loss not only decreases BP but also improves other cardiovascular risk factors such as dyslipidemia and insulin resistance (Reinehr et al., 2006; Williams et al., 2002). In studies where a reduction in BMI of about 10% was achieved, short-term reductions in BP were in the range of 8 to 12 mm Hg. Unfortunately, weight loss is notoriously difficult and usually unsuccessful, especially in the primary care setting (Epstein et al., 1998). Comprehensive programs have better success rates. However, identifying a complication of obesity such as hypertension can perhaps provide the necessary motivation for patients and families to make the appropriate lifestyle changes.

The role of diet in the treatment of hypertension has received a great deal of attention, most of which has focused on sodium. Once hypertension has been established, "salt sensitivity" becomes more common, and reduction in sodium intake may be of benefit (Cutler, 1999; Weinberger, 1996). Other dietary constituents that have been examined in patients with hypertension include potassium and calcium, both of which have been shown to have antihypertensive effects (Cutler, 1999; Gillman et al., 1992). Therefore, a diet that is low in sodium and enriched in potassium and calcium may be even more effective than a diet that restricts sodium only.

An example of such a diet is the so-called "DASH" diet, which has been shown to have a clear BP-lowering effect in adults with hypertension, even in those receiving antihypertensive medication (Appel et al., 1997). A recent study of a DASH-type eating plan confirmed its efficacy in lowering the BP in hypertensive children (Couch et al., 2008). The DASH diet also incorporates measures designed to reduce dietary fat intake, an important strategy given the frequent presence of both hypertension and elevated lipids in children and adolescents and the imperative to begin prevention of adult cardiovascular disease at as early an age as possible (Gidding, 1993; Kavey et al., 2003; Williams et al., 2002).

Pharmacologic Management

As discussed earlier, ample data exist documenting the development of hypertensive target-organ damage in hypertensive children and adolescents, and a growing body of data suggests that elevated BP in the young may have adverse cardiovascular effects in adulthood. However, it can also be argued that the long-term consequences of untreated hypertension in an asymptomatic, hypertensive child or adolescent without underlying secondary hypertension or hypertensive target-organ damage remain unknown (Kay et al., 2001). There is also a significant lack of data on the long-term effects of antihypertensive medications on the growth and development of children. Therefore, a definite indication for initiating pharmacologic therapy should be ascertained in the young before medication is prescribed.

Accepted indications for use of antihypertensive medications in children and adolescents include the following (National High Blood Pressure Education Program Working Group, 2004):

• Symptomatic hypertension
• Secondary hypertension
• Hypertensive target-organ damage
• Diabetes (types 1 and 2)
• Persistent hypertension despite nonpharmacologic measures (Fig. 16-2)

Pharmacologic reduction of BP for hypertensive children who fall into one of these categories is likely to result in health benefit.

Additional indications for the use of antihypertensive medications have been proposed, all based upon the premise of reducing the risk of future renal and cardiovascular diseases. For example, since the presence of multiple cardiovascular risk factors

(elevated BP, hyperlipidemia, tobacco use, etc.) increases the cardiovascular risk in an exponential rather than additive fashion (Kavey et al., 2003), it is suggested that antihypertensive therapy be instituted if the child or adolescent is known to have hyperlipidemia. Similarly, elevated nocturnal BP and/or blunted nocturnal dipping on ABPM increases the likelihood of developing hypertensive target-organ damage and other adverse cardiovascular outcomes (Clement et al., 2003), suggesting drug therapy should be started in hypertensive children with abnormal circadian variation of BP.

The number of antihypertensive medications that have been systematically studied in children has increased markedly over the past decade due to incentives provided to the pharmaceutical industry under the auspices of the 1997 Food and Drug Modernization Act (FDAMA) and subsequent legislation (Flynn, 2003; Flynn & Daniels, 2006). Table 16-9 highlights the increase in FDA-approved labeling of antihypertensive medications that has occurred since the passage of FDAMA. Published results of the industry-sponsored clinical trials (which have been summarized elsewhere [Flynn & Daniels, 2006]) can be used to guide the prescribing of antihypertensive agents in children and adolescents who require pharmacologic treatment, thereby increasing the confidence of the practitioner who treats such children. The dosing recommendations contained in Table 16-10 incorporate data from many of these studies.

TABLE 16.9	Impact of the Food and Drug Administration Modernization Act (FDAMA) and Successor Legislation on Pediatric Labeling of Antihypertensive Medications

Had pediatric labeling pre-FDAMA	New pediatric labeling since FDAMA[a]	Under study, awaiting labeling or anticipated future study
Captopril[b]	Amlodipine	Aliskiren
Chlorothiazide	Benazepril	Candesartan
Diazoxide[b]	Enalapril	Olmesartan
Furosemide	Eplerenone[c]	Ramipril
Hydralazine	Fenoldopam	Sodium nitroprusside
Hydrochlorothiazide	Fosinopril	Telmisartan
Methyldopa	Irbesartan[c]	
Minoxidil	Losartan	
Propranolol	Lisinopril	
Spironolactone	Metoprolol	
	Valsartan	

[a]Does not include medications studied and granted exclusivity but not pediatric labeling.
[b]No specific dose recommendations included in label.
[c]Label specifically states drug not effective in hypertensive children.

TABLE 16.10	Recommended Doses for Selected Antihypertensive Agents for Use in Hypertensive Children and Adolescents			
Class	**Drug**	**Starting Dose**	**Interval**	**Maximum Dose**[a]
Aldosterone receptor antagonists	Eplerenone	25 mg/day	QD–BID	100 mg/day
	Spironolactone[b]	1 mg/kg/day	QD–BID	3.3 mg/kg/day up to 100 mg/day
ACE inhibitors	Benazepril[b]	0.2 mg/kg/day up to 10 mg/day	QD	0.6 mg/kg/day up to 40 mg/day
	Captopril[b]	0.3–0.5 mg/kg/dose	BID–TID	6 mg/kg/day up to 450 mg/day
	Enalapril[b]	0.08 mg/kg/day	QD	0.6 mg/kg/day up to 40 mg/day
	Fosinopril	0.1 mg/kg/day up to 10 mg/day	QD	0.6 mg/kg/d up to 40 mg/day
	Lisinopril[b]	0.07 mg/kg/day up to 5 mg/day	QD	0.6 mg/kg/d up to 40 mg/day
	Quinapril	5–10 mg/day	QD	80 mg/day
Angiotensin receptor blockers	Candesartan	4 mg/day	QD	32 mg/day
	Losartan[b]	0.75 mg/kg/day up to 50 mg/day	QD	1.4 mg/kg/day up to 100 mg/day
	Olmesartan	2.5 mg/day	QD	40 mg/day
	Valsartan[b]	1.3 mg/kg/day up to 40 mg/day	QD	2.7 mg/kg/day up to 160 mg/day
		<6 years: 5–10 mg/d		<6 years: 80 mg/day
α- and β-adrenergic antagonists	Labetalol[b]	2–3 mg/kg/day	BID	10–12 mg/kg/day up to 1.2 g/day
	Carvedilol	0.1 mg/kg/dose up to 12.5 mg BID	BID	0.5 mg/kg/dose up to 25 mg BID
β-Adrenergic antagonists	Atenolol[b]	0.5–1 mg/kg/day	QD–BID	2 mg/kg/day up to 100 mg/day
	Bisoprolol/HCTZ	0.04 mg/kg/day up to 2.5/6.25 mg/day	QD	10/6.25 mg/day
	Metoprolol	1–2 mg/kg/day	BID	6 mg/kg/day up to 200 mg/day
	Propranolol	1 mg/kg/day	BID–TID	16 mg/kg/day up to 640 mg/day
Calcium channel blockers	Amlodipine[b]	0.06 mg/kg/day	QD	0.3 mg/kg/day up to 10 mg/day
	Felodipine	2.5 mg/day	QD	10 mg/day
	Isradipine[b]	0.05–0.15 mg/kg/dose	TID–QID	0.8 mg/kg/day up to 20 mg/day
	Extended-release nifedipine	0.25–0.5 mg/kg/day	QD–BID	3 mg/kg/day up to 120 mg/day
Central α-agonist	Clonidine[b]	5–10 mcg/kg/day	BID–TID	25 mcg/kg/day up to 0.9 mg/day
Diuretics	Amiloride	5–10 mg/day	QD	20 mg/day
	Chlorthalidone	0.3 mg/kg/day	QD	2 mg/kg/day up to 50 mg/day
	Furosemide	0.5–2.0 mg/kg/dose	QD–BID	6 mg/kg/day
	HCTZ	0.5–1 mg/kg/day	QD	3 mg/kg/day up to 50 mg/day
Vasodilators	Hydralazine	0.25 mg/kg/dose	TID–QID	7.5 mg/kg/day up to 200 mg/day
	Minoxidil	0.1–0.2 mg/kg/day	BID–TID	1 mg/kg/day up to 50 mg/day

[a]The maximum recommended adult dose should never be exceeded.
[b]Information on preparation of a stable extemporaneous suspension is available for these agents.
BID, twice daily; HCTZ, hydrochlorothiazide; QD, once daily; QID, four times daily; TID, three times daily; ACE, angiotensin-converting enzyme.

No studies comparing the different classes of antihypertensive agents have been conducted in children; therefore, the choice of initial antihypertensive agent for use in children remains up to the preference of the individual practitioner. Diuretics and β-adrenergic blockers, which were recommended as initial therapy in the First and Second Task Force Reports (Blumenthal et al., 1977; Task Force on Blood Pressure Control in Children, 1987), have a long track record of safety and efficacy in hypertensive children and are still considered appropriate for pediatric use. Similarly, newer classes of agents, including angiotensin-converting enzyme (ACE) inhibitors, calcium channel blockers, and angiotensin receptor blockers, have been shown to be safe and well tolerated in hypertensive children in recent industry-sponsored trials (Flynn & Daniels, 2006), now have pediatric labeling (Table 16-9), and may be prescribed if indicated.

Consideration should be given to using specific classes of antihypertensive medications in hypertensive children with specific underlying or concurrent medical conditions. The best example of this would be the use of ACE inhibitors or angiotensin receptor antagonists in children with diabetes or proteinuric

renal diseases. This parallels the approach outlined in the JNC-7 report, which recommends that specific classes of antihypertensive agents be used in adults in certain high-risk categories (Chobanian et al., 2003).

Antihypertensive drugs in children are generally prescribed in a stepped-care manner (Fig. 16-3): The child is initially started on the lowest recommended dose, then the dose is increased until the highest recommended dose is reached, or until the child experiences adverse effects from the medication, at which point a second drug from a different class should be added, and so on, until the desired goal BP is reached (Flynn & Daniels, 2006). For children with uncomplicated primary hypertension and no hypertensive target-organ damage, goal BP should be less than 95th percentile for age, gender, and height, whereas for children with secondary hypertension, diabetes, or hypertensive target-organ damage, goal BP should be less than 90th percentile for age, gender, and height (National High Blood Pressure Education Program Working Group, 2004).

Although not an antihypertensive medication, allopurinol was recently reported effective in lowering BP in a small study of hypertensive adolescents

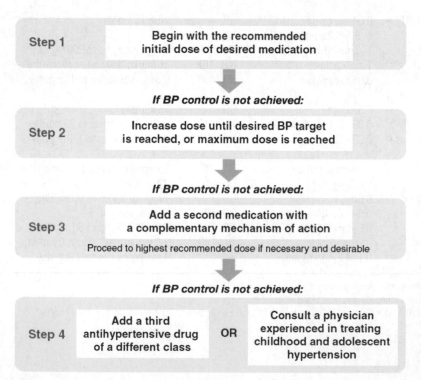

Step 1	Begin with the recommended initial dose of desired medication

If BP control is not achieved:

Step 2	Increase dose until desired BP target is reached, or maximum dose is reached

If BP control is not achieved:

Step 3	Add a second medication with a complementary mechanism of action Proceed to highest recommended dose if necessary and desirable

If BP control is not achieved:

Step 4	Add a third antihypertensive drug of a different class	**OR** Consult a physician experienced in treating childhood and adolescent hypertension

FIGURE 16.3 Stepped-care approach to pharmacologic management of childhood hypertension.

(Feig et al., 2008), supporting a role for uric acid in the development of hypertension (Feig & Johnson, 2007). However, further confirmatory studies are required before uric acid reduction can be advocated as a treatment of hypertension, especially given the known adverse risk profile of allopurinol.

Treatment of childhood hypertension should include ongoing monitoring of BP, surveillance for medication side effects, periodic monitoring of renal function and electrolytes (in children treated with ACE inhibitors or diuretics), counseling regarding other cardiovascular risk factors, and continued emphasis on therapeutic lifestyle changes. Hypertensive target-organ damage such as LVH, if present, should be reassessed periodically.

It may also be appropriate to consider "step-down" therapy in selected children and adolescents. This involves an attempt at gradual reduction in medication dose after an extended course of good BP control, with the eventual goal of completely discontinuing the drug therapy. Children with uncomplicated primary hypertension, especially obese adolescents who successfully lose weight and maintain their weight loss, are the best candidates for withdrawal of medication. These children should receive continued BP monitoring after drug therapy is withdrawn as well as continued nonpharmacologic treatment.

SPECIAL TOPICS

Hypertension in Infancy

Few good normative data on BP levels in newborn and premature infants are available. Additionally, BP in infancy varies according to body size, gestational age, and postconceptual age, among other factors (Flynn, 2004a). Using the graphs published by Zubrow et al., 1995, systemic hypertension in premature infants can be defined as systolic and/or diastolic BP that persistently exceeds the mean + 2 standard deviations for infants of similar postconceptual age. After one month of age, hypertension is defined as systolic and/or diastolic BP greater than 95th percentile for that infant's age and gender (Task Force on Blood Pressure Control in Children, 1987).

Although one study found that 28% of infants with BWs less than 1,500 g had at least one elevated BP documented during their NICU stay (Al-Aweel et al., 2001), the actual incidence of hypertension in neonates is very low, ranging from 0.2% in healthy newborns to between 0.7% and 2.5% in high-risk newborns (Flynn, 2004a). Certain categories of infants are at significantly higher risk, however. For example, the odds of hypertension are increased in neonates with a history of umbilical artery catheterization, those who suffered acute renal failure in the NICU, or those with chronic lung disease compared to neonates without these risk factors (Saliem et al., 2007). On the other hand, hypertension is so uncommon in otherwise healthy term infants that routine BP determination is not even recommended (AAP Committee on Fetus and Newborn, 1993).

The differential diagnosis of hypertension in neonates and older infants is wide-ranging (Tables 16-7 and 16-11). The most important categories of causes of neonatal hypertension include renovascular disease (most commonly umbilical artery–related aortic or renal thromboembolism) (Bauer et al., 1975), renal parenchymal disease, and bronchopulmonary dysplasia (Alagappan & Malloy, 1998; Saliem et al., 2007). The most common cardiac cause is coarctation of the thoracic aorta, in which hypertension may persist or recur after surgical repair (O'Sullivan et al., 2002). For a more comprehensive discussion, the reader is encouraged to consult other references (Flynn, 2004a).

Investigation of hypertensive infants should proceed in a similar fashion to the evaluation of older children with hypertension. There is a significant variability between the upper and the lower limb BPs in neonates (Crossland et al., 2004), so it is important to be consistent in the choice of extremity for BP measurement. A thorough review of the infant's history and a focused physical examination should point to the underlying cause in most cases. Selected laboratory studies should be obtained as indicated. Renal ultrasonography is particularly useful given the preponderance of renal causes (Table 16-11).

Therapy of neonatal hypertension should be tailored to the severity of the hypertension and the infant's overall clinical status. For example, critically ill infants with severe hypertension should be treated with an intravenous agent administered by continuous infusion, as this will allow the greatest control over the magnitude and rapidity of the BP reduction. On the other hand, relatively well infants with mild hypertension may be treated with oral antihypertensive agents. Recommended doses for antihypertensive drugs in infants can be found in Table 16-12. Unfortunately, the legislative initiatives that have increased data on pediatric drug efficacy and safety have not extended to

TABLE 16.11	Causes of Neonatal Hypertension

Renovascular
Thromboembolism
Renal artery stenosis
Midaortic coarctation
Renal venous thrombosis
Renal artery compression
Abdominal aortic aneurysm
Idiopathic arterial calcification
Congenital rubella syndrome

Renal Parenchymal Disease
Congenital
    Polycystic kidney disease
    Multicystic-dysplastic kidney disease
    Tuberous sclerosis
    Ureteropelvic junction obstruction
    Unilateral renal hypoplasia
    Primary megaureter
    Congenital nephritic syndrome
Acquired
    Acute tubular necrosis
    Cortical necrosis
    Interstitial nephritis
    Hemolytic-uremic syndrome
    Obstruction (stones, tumors)

Pulmonary
Bronchopulmonary dysplasia
Pneumothorax

Cardiac
Aortic coarctation

Endocrine
Congenital adrenal hyperplasia
Hyperaldosteronism
Hyperthyroidism
Pseudohypoaldosteronism type II (Gordon Syndrome)

Medications/Intoxications
Infant
    Dexamethasone
    Adrenergic agents
    Vitamin D intoxication
    Theophylline
    Caffeine
    Pancuronium
    Phenylephrine
Maternal
    Cocaine
    Heroin

Neoplasia
Wilms tumor
Mesoblastic nephroma
Neuroblastoma
Pheochromocytoma

Neurologic
Pain
Intracranial hypertension
Seizures
Familial dysautonomia
Subdural hematoma

Miscellaneous
Total parenteral nutrition
Closure of abdominal wall defect
Adrenal hemorrhage
Hypercalcemia
Traction
ECMO
Birth asphyxia
Primary hypertension

ECMO, extracorporeal membrane oxygenation.

infants (Flynn, 2003). Thus, the choice of antihypertensive medications for use in neonates relies heavily on the experience of the individual practitioner.

Acute Severe Hypertension

The pathophysiology, management, and outcome of severe hypertension in children and adolescents have recently been reviewed in detail (Flynn & Tullus, 2009; Patel & Mitsnefes, 2005). Many aspects are similar to hypertensive emergencies and urgencies in adults as reviewed in Chapter 8. However, a few unique aspects warrant consideration.

Underlying conditions that may produce acute severe hypertension in a child or adolescent commonly include acute or chronic renal disease, organ transplantation, renal artery stenosis, and congenital renal disease such as autosomal recessive polycystic kidney disease. Medication nonadherence in patients with established hypertension, the most common

TABLE 16.12	Recommended Doses for Selected Antihypertensive Agents for Treatment of Hypertensive Infants			
Class	**Drug**	**Route**	**Dose**	**Interval**
ACE Inhibitors[a]	Captopril	Oral	<3 m: 0.01–0.5 mg/kg/dose Max 2 mg/kg/day >3 m: 0.15–0.3 mg/kg/dose Max 6 mg/kg/day	TID
	Enalapril	Oral	0.08–0.6 mg/kg/day	QD–BID
	Lisinopril	Oral	0.07–0.6 mg/kg/day	QD
α- and β-antagonist	Labetalol	Oral	0.5–1.0 mg/kg/dose Max 10 mg/kg/day	BID–TID
		IV	0.20–1.0 mg/kg/dose 0.25–3.0 mg/kg/h	Q4–6 h Infusion
β-Antagonists	Esmolol	IV	100–500 µg/kg/min	Infusion
	Propranolol	Oral	0.5–1.0 mg/kg/dose Max 8–10 mg/kg/day	TID
Calcium channel blockers	Amlodipine	Oral	0.05–0.3 mg/kg/dose Max 0.6 mg/kg/day	QD–BID
	Isradipine	Oral	0.05–0.15 mg/kg/dose Max 0.8 mg/kg/day	QID
	Nicardipine	IV	1–4 µg/kg/min	Infusion
Diuretics	Chlorothiazide	Oral	5–15 mg/kg/dose	BID
	Hydrochlorothiazide	Oral	1–3 mg/kg/dose	QD
	Spironolactone	Oral	0.5–1.5 mg/kg/dose	BID
Vasodilators	Hydralazine	Oral	0.25–1.0 mg/kg/dose Max 7.5 mg/kg/day	TID–QID
		IV	0.15–0.6 mg/kg/dose	Q4 h
	Minoxidil	Oral	0.1–0.2 mg/kg/dose	BID–TID

[a]Not recommended for infants with corrected gestational age of <40 weeks.
BID, twice daily; IV, intravenous; Q, every; QD, once daily; QID, four times daily; TID, three times daily.

cause of acute severe hypertension in adults (Bender et al., 2006), occurs rarely in pediatric patients.

Hypertensive encephalopathy is the most frequent life-threatening symptom in children and adolescents with severe hypertension, emphasizing the need for slow, controlled reduction in BP to prevent complications arising through loss of normal autoregulatory processes (Adelman et al., 2000). Less severe symptoms may include nausea, vomiting, or unusual irritability; since these may be somewhat nonspecific, especially in younger children, a high degree of clinical suspicion must be maintained.

Although evidence-based recommendations are lacking, the usual goal in the treatment of a hypertensive emergency is to reduce the BP by no more than 25% over the first 8 hours, with a gradual return to normal/goal BP over 24 to 48 hours (Flynn & Tullus, 2009). Treatment of hypertensive emergencies in children should be initiated with a continuous infusion of an intravenous antihypertensive, with nicardipine and labetalol being the agents most commonly used. The dopamine receptor agonist fenoldopam has also been reported effective (Strauser et al., 1999), although higher doses are apparently required in children than in adults (Hammer et al., 2008).

Oral antihypertensive agents can be used in pediatric patients with acute severe hypertension who do not have life-threatening symptoms. The choice of oral antihypertensives for use in management of severe hypertension in pediatric patients is fairly limited. Short-acting nifedipine, which had remained in use in children until recently (Yiu et al., 2004), is no longer recommended (Flynn & Tullus, 2009). For recommended doses of both oral and intravenous drugs useful in the treatment of acute severe hypertension in children and adolescents, see Table 16-13.

TABLE 16.13	Antihypertensive Drugs for Management of Severe Hypertension in Children and Adolescents			
Drug	**Class**	**Dose**	**Route**	**Comments**
Useful for severely hypertensive patients with life-threatening symptoms				
Esmolol	β-Adrenergic blocker	100–500 µg/kg/min	IV infusion	Very short-acting—constant infusion preferred. May cause profound bradycardia.
Hydralazine	Direct vasodilator	0.2–0.6 mg/kg/dose	IV, IM	Should be given q4h when given IV bolus.
Labetalol	α- and β-adrenergic blockers	bolus: 0.20–1.0 mg/kg/dose, up to 40 mg/dose Infusion: 0.25–3.0 mg/kg/h	IV bolus or infusion	Asthma and overt heart failure are relative contraindications.
Nicardipine	Calcium channel blocker	bolus: 30 µg/kg up to 2 mg/dose Infusion: 0.5–4 µg/kg/min	IV bolus or infusion	May cause reflex tachycardia.
Sodium nitroprusside	Direct vasodilator	0.5–10 µg/kg/min	IV infusion	Monitor cyanide levels with prolonged (>72 h) use or in renal failure; or coadminister with sodium thiosulfate.
Useful for severely hypertensive patients with less significant symptoms				
Clonidine	Central α-agonist	0.05–0.1 mg/dose, may be repeated up to 0.8 mg total dose	PO	Side effects include dry mouth and drowsiness.
Enalaprilat	ACE inhibitor	0.05–0.10 mg/kg/dose up to 1.25 mg/dose	IV bolus	May cause prolonged hypotension and acute renal failure, especially in neonates.
Fenoldopam	Dopamine receptor agonist	0.2–0.8 µg/kg/min	IV infusion	Produced modest reductions in BP in a pediatric clinical trial in patients up to 12 years.
Hydralazine	Direct vasodilator	0.25 mg/kg/dose up to 25 mg/dose	PO	Extemporaneous suspension stable for only 1 week.
Isradipine	Calcium channel blocker	0.05–0.1 mg/kg/dose up to 5 mg/dose	PO	Stable suspension can be compounded.
Minoxidil	Direct vasodilator	0.1–0.2 mg/kg/dose up to 10 mg/dose	PO	Most potent oral vasodilator; long acting.

REFERENCES

Adelman RD, Coppo R, Dillon MJ. The emergency management of severe hypertension. *Pediatr Nephrol.* 2000;14:422–427.

Adrogue HE, Sinaiko AR. Prevalence of hypertension in junior high school-aged children: effect of new recommendations in the 1996 Updated Task Force Report. *Am J Hypertens* 2001;14 (5 Pt 1):412–414.

Alagappan A. Malloy MH. Systemic hypertension in very low-birth weight infants with bronchopulmonary dysplasia: incidence and risk factors. *Am J Perinatol* 1998;15:3–8.

Al-Aweel I, Pursley DM, Rubin LP, et al. Variations in prevalence of hypotension, hypertension and vasopressor use in NICUs. *J Perinatol* 2001;12:272–278.

Alpert BS, Fox ME. Hypertension. In: Goldberg B, ed., *Sports and Exercise for Children with Chronic Health Conditions.* Champaign, IL; Human Kinetics, 1995;pp. 197–205.

Alpert BS. Exercise as a therapy to control hypertension in children. *Int J Sports Med* 2000;21(Suppl 2):S94–S96.

American Academy of Pediatrics Committee on Fetus and Newborn. Routine evaluation of blood pressure, hematocrit and glucose in newborns. *Pediatrics* 1993;92:474–476.

American Academy of Pediatrics Committee on Sports Medicine and Fitness. Athletic participation by children and adolescents who have systemic hypertension. *Pediatrics* 1997;99:637–638.

Appel LJ, Moore TJ, Obarzanek E, et al. A clinical trial of the effects of dietary patterns on blood pressure. *N Engl J Med* 1997;336:1117–1124.

Arar MY, Hogg RJ, Arant BS Jr, et al. Etiology of sustained hypertension in children in the southwestern United States. *Pediatr Nephrol* 1994;8:186–189.

Assadi F. Effect of microalbuminuria lowering on regression of left ventricular hypertrophy in children and adolescents with essential hypertension. *Pediatr Cardiol* 2007;28:27–33.

Barker DJ, Gluckman PD, Godfrey KM, et al. Fetal nutrition and cardiovascular disease in adult life. *Lancet* 1993;341:938–941.

Barker DJ, Eriksson JG, Forsen T, Osmond C. Fetal origins of adult disease: strength of effects and biological basis. *Int J Epidemiol* 2002;31:1235–1239.

Bauer SB, Feldman SM, Gellis SS, et al. Neonatal hypertension: a complication of umbilical-artery catheterization. *N Engl J Med* 1975;293:1032–1033.

Belfort MB, Rifas-Shiman SL, Rich-Edwards J, et al. Size at birth, infant growth, and blood pressure at three years of age. *J Pediatr* 2007;151:670–674.

Bender SR, Fong MW, Heitz S, Bisognano JD. Characteristics and management of patients presenting to the emergency department with hypertensive urgency. *J Clin Hypertens* 2006;8: 12–18.

Berenson GS. Childhood risk factors predict adult risk associated with subclinical cardiovascular disease: The Bogalusa Heart Study. *Am J Cardiol* 2002;90:3L–7L.

Bibbins-Domingo K, Coxson P, Pletcher MJ, et al. Adolescent overweight and future adult coronary heart disease. *N Engl J Med* 2007;357:2371–2379.

Biron P, Mongeau JG, Bertrand D. Familial aggregation of blood pressure in 558 adopted children. *Can Med Assoc J* 1976;115: 773–774.

Blumenthal S, Epps RP, Heavenrich R, et al. Report of the task force on blood pressure control in children. *Pediatrics* 1977;59: 797–820.

Brady TM, Fivush B, Flynn JT, Parekh R. Ability of blood pressure to predict left ventricular hypertrophy in children with primary hypertension. *J Pediatr* 2008;152:73–78, 78.e1.

Burke V, Beilin LJ, Blake KV, et al. Indicators of fetal growth do not independently predict blood pressure in 8-year-old Australians: A prospective cohort study. *Hypertension* 2004;43: 208–213.

Chen X, Wang Y. Tracking of blood pressure from childhood to adulthood: A systematic review and meta-analysis. *Circulation* 2008;117:3171–3180.

Chen W, Srinivasan SR, Li S, et al. Clustering of long-term trends in metabolic syndrome variables from childhood to adulthood in Blacks and Whites: the Bogalusa Heart Study. *Am J Epidemiol* 2007;166:527–533.

Chobanian AV, Bakris GL, Black HR, et al. The seventh report of the joint national committee on prevention, detection, evaluation, and treatment of high blood pressure: the JNC 7 report. *JAMA* 2003;289:2560–2572.

Clement DL, De Buyzere ML, De Bacquer DA, et al. Prognostic value of ambulatory blood-pressure recordings in patients with treated hypertension. *N Engl J Med* 2003;348:2407–2415.

Couch SC, Saelens BE, Levin L, et al. The efficacy of a clinic-based behavioral nutrition intervention emphasizing a DASH-type diet for adolescents with elevated blood pressure. *J Pediatr* 2008;152:494–501.

Croix B, Feig DI. Childhood hypertension is not a silent disease. *Pediatr Nephrol* 2006;21:527–532.

Crossland DS, Furness JC, Abu-Harb M, et al. Variability of four limb blood pressure in normal neonates. *Arch Dis Child Fetal Neonatal Ed* 2004;89:F325–F327.

Cutler JA. The effects of reducing sodium and increasing potassium intake for control of hypertension and improving health. *Clin & Exp Hypertens* 1999;21:769–783.

Daniels SR, Obarzanek E, Barton BA, et al. Sexual maturation and racial differences in blood pressure in girls: the National Heart, Lung, and Blood Institute Growth and Health Study. *J Pediatr* 1996;129:208–213.

Daniels SR. Is there an epidemic of cardiovascular disease on the horizon? *J Pediatr* 1999;134:665–666.

Davis PH, Dawson JD, Riley WA, Lauer RM. Carotid intimal-medial thickness is related to cardiovascular risk factors measured from childhood through middle age: The Muscatine Study. *Circulation* 2001;104:2815–2819.

Dekkers JC, Snieder H, van den Oord EJCG, Treiber FA. Moderators of blood pressure development from childhood to adulthood: A 10-year longitudinal study. *J Pediatr* 2002;141: 770–779.

de Leonardis V, De Scalzi M, Falchetti A, et al. Echocardiographic evaluation of children with and without family history of essential hypertension. *Am J Hypertens* 1988;1(3 Pt 1):305–308.

Din-Dzietham R, Liu Y, Bielo MV, Shamsa F. High blood pressure trends in children and adolescents in national surveys, 1963 to 2002. *Circulation* 2007;116:1488–1496.

Epstein LH, Myers MD, Raynor HA, Saelens BE. Treatment of pediatric obesity. *Pediatrics* 1998;101:554–570.

Falkner B, Sherif K, Michel S, Kushner H. Dietary nutrients and blood pressure in urban minority adolescents at risk for hypertension. *Arch Pediatr Adolesc Med* 2000;154:918–922.

Falkner B, Hulman S, Kushner H. Effect of birth weight on blood pressure and body size in early adolescence. *Hypertension* 2004;43:203–207.

Feig DI, Johnson RJ. The role of uric acid in pediatric hypertension. *J Ren Nut.* 2007;17:79–83.

Feig DI, Soletsky B, Johnson RJ. Effect of allopurinol on blood pressure of adolescents with newly diagnosed essential hypertension. *JAMA* 2008;300:924–932.

Figueroa-Colon R, Franklin FA, Lee JY, et al. Feasibility of a clinic-based hypocaloric dietary intervention implemented in a school setting for obese children. *Obes Res* 1996;4:419–429.

Fixler DE, Laird WD, Fitzgerald V, et al. Hypertension screening in schools: results of the Dallas study. *Pediatrics* 1979;63:32–36.

Flynn JT. Impact of ambulatory blood pressure monitoring on the management of hypertension in children. *Blood Press Monitor* 2000;5:211–216.

Flynn JT. Evaluation and management of hypertension in childhood. *Prog Ped Cardiol* 2001;12:177–188.

Flynn JT. Differentiation between primary and secondary hypertension in children using ambulatory blood pressure monitoring. *Pediatrics* 2002;110:89–93.

Flynn JT. Successes and shortcomings of the FDA Modernization Act. *Am J Hypertens* 2003;16:889–891.

Flynn JT. Neonatal Hypertension. In: Portman R, Sorof J, Ingelfinger J, eds. *Pediatric Hypertension.* Totowa, NJ: Humana Press, 2004:351–370.

Flynn JT, Alderman MH. Characteristics of children with primary hypertension seen at a referral center. *Pediatr Nephrol* 2005; 20:961–966.

Flynn JT, Daniels SR. Pharmacologic treatment of hypertension in children and adolescents. *J Pediatrics* 2006;149:746–754

Flynn JT, Tullus K. Severe hypertension in children and adolescents: Pathophysiology and treatment. *Pediatr Nephrol* 2009; 24:1101–1112.

Gamborg M, Byberg L, Rasmussen F, et al. Birth weight and systolic blood pressure in adolescence and adulthood: meta-regression analysis of sex- and age-specific results from 20 Nordic studies. *Am J Epidemiol* 2007;166:634–645.

Gidding SS. Relationships between blood pressure and lipids in childhood. *Pediatr Clin North Am* 1993;40:41–49.

Gillman MW, Oliveria SA, Moore LL, et al. Inverse association of dietary calcium with systolic blood pressure in young children. *JAMA* 1992;267:2340–2343.

Grummer-Strawn LM, Mei Z. Does breastfeeding protect against pediatric overweight? Analysis of longitudinal data from the

Centers for Disease Control and Prevention Pediatric Nutrition Surveillance System. *Pediatrics* 2004;113:e81–e86.

Hammer GB, Verghese ST, Drover DR, et al. Pharmacokinetics and pharmacodynamics of fenoldopam mesylate for blood pressure control in pediatric patients *BMC Anesthesiology* 2008;8:6 doi:10.1186/1471–2253-8-6.

Hanevold C, Waller J, Daniels S, et al. The effects of obesity, gender, and ethnic group on left ventricular hypertrophy and geometry in hypertensive children: A collaborative study of the International Pediatric Hypertension Association. *Pediatrics* 2004;113:328–333.

Hansen HS, Nielsen JR, Hyldebrandt N, Froberg K. Blood pressure and cardiac structure in children with a parental history of hypertension: the Odense Schoolchild Study. *J Hypertens* 1992;10:677–682.

Harshfield GA, Alpert BS, Pulliam DA, et al. Ambulatory blood pressure recordings in children and adolescents. *Pediatrics* 1994;94(2 Pt 1):180–184.

Hohn AR, Dwyer KM, Dwyer JH. Blood pressure in youth from four ethnic groups: the Pasadena Prevention Project. *J Pediatr* 1994;125:368–373.

Huxley R, Neil A, Collins R. Unravelling the fetal origins hypothesis: is there really an inverse association between birthweight and subsequent blood pressure? *Lancet* 2002;360:659–665.

Juonala M, Viikari JS, Rönnemaa T, et al. Elevated blood pressure in adolescent boys predicts endothelial dysfunction: the cardiovascular risk in young Finns study. *Hypertension* 2006;48:424–430.

Kaufmann MA, Pargger H, Drop LJ. Oscillometric blood pressure measurements by different devices are not interchangeable. *Anesth Analg* 1996;82:377–381.

Kavey REW, Daniels SR, Lauer RM, et al. American Heart Association guidelines for primary prevention of atherosclerotic cardiovascular disease beginning in childhood. *Circulation* 2003;107:1562–1566.

Kavey RE, Kveselis DA, Atallah N, Smith FC. White coat hypertension in childhood: evidence for end-organ effect. *J Pediatr* 2007;150:491–497.

Kay JD, Sinaiko AR, Daniels SR. Pediatric hypertension. *Am Heart J* 2001;142:422–432.

Keller G, Zimmer G, Mall G, Ritz E, Amann K. Nephron number in patients with primary hypertension. *N Engl J Med* 2003; 348:101–108.

Kilcoyne MM, Richter RW, Alsup PA. Adolescent hypertension. I. Detection and prevalence. *Circulation* 1974;50:758–764.

Kvaavik E, Tell GS, Klepp K-I. Predictors and tracking of body mass index from adolescence into adulthood. *Arch Pediatr Adolesc Med* 2003;157:1212–1218.

Laird WP, Fixler DE. Left ventricular hypertrophy in adolescents with elevated blood pressure: assessment by chest roentgenography, electrocardiography, and echocardiography. *Pediatrics* 1981;67:255–259.

Lande MB, Kaczorowski JM, Auinger P, et al. Elevated blood pressure and decreased cognitive function among school-age children and adolescents in the United States. *J Pediatr* 2003;143:720–724.

Lande MB, Carson NL, Roy J, Meagher CC. Effects of childhood primary hypertension on carotid intima media thickness: a matched controlled study. *Hypertension* 2006;48:40–44.

Lande MB, Meagher CC, Fisher SG, et al. Left ventricular mass index in children with white coat hypertension. *J Pediatr.* 2008;153:50–54.

Lane DA, Gill P. Ethnicity and tracking blood pressure in children. *J Human Hypertens* 2004;18:223–228.

Lauer RM, Clarke WR, Mahoney LT, Witt J. Childhood predictors for high adult blood pressure. The Muscatine Study. *Pediatr Clin North Am* 1993;40:23–40.

Law CM, Barker DJ, Bull AR, Osmond C. Maternal and fetal influences on blood pressure. *Arch Dis Child* 1991;66:1291–1295.

Law CM, Shiell AW, Newsome CA, et al. Fetal, infant, and childhood growth and adult blood pressure: A longitudinal study from birth to 22 years of age. *Circulation* 2002;105: 1088–1092.

Lemne CE. Increased blood pressure reactivity in children of borderline hypertensive fathers. *J Hypertens* 1998; 16:1243–1248.

Li S, Chen W, Srinivasan SR, Berenson GS. Childhood blood pressure as a predictor of arterial stiffness in young adults: The Bogalusa Heart Study. *Hypertension* 2004;43:541–546.

Li S, Chen W, Srinivasan SR, et al. Childhood cardiovascular risk factors and carotid vascular changes in adulthood: The Bogalusa Heart Study. *JAMA* 2003;290:2271–2276.

Lissau I, Overpeck MD, Ruan WJ, et al. Body mass index and overweight in adolescents in 13 European countries, Israel, and the United States. *Arch Pediatr Adolesc Med* 2004;158:27–33.

Litwin M, Niemirska A, Sladowska J, et al. Left ventricular hypertrophy and arterial wall thickening in children with essential hypertension. *Pediatr Nephrol* 2006;21:811–819.

Loggie JM. Juvenile hypertension. *Compr Ther* 1977; 3:47–54.

Londe S, Bourgoignie JJ, Robson AM, Goldring D. Hypertension in apparently normal children. *J Pediatr* 1971;78:569–577.

Lopes HF, Silva HB, Consolim-Colombo FM, et al. Autonomic abnormalities demonstrable in young normotensive subjects who are children of hypertensive parents. *Braz J Med Bio Res* 2000;33:51–54.

Lurbe E, Sorof JM, Daniels SR. Clinical and research aspects of ambulatory blood pressure monitoring in children. *J Pediatr* 2004;144:7–16.

Lurbe E, Torro I, Alvarez V, et al. Prevalence, persistence, and clinical significance of masked hypertension in youth. *Hypertension* 2005;45:493–498.

Mackenzie HS, Lawler EV, Brenner BM. Congenital oligonephropathy: The fetal flaw in essential hypertension? *Kidney Int Suppl* 1996;55:S30–S34.

Makris TK, Stavroulakis GA, Krespi PG, et al. Elevated plasma immunoreactive leptin levels preexist in healthy offspring of patients with essential hypertension. *Am Heart J* 1999; 138(5 Pt 1):922–925.

Martin RM, Ness AR, Gunnell D, et al. Does breast-feeding in infancy lower blood pressure in childhood? The Avon Longitudinal Study of Parents and Children (ALSPAC). *Circulation* 2004;109:1259–1266.

Matsuoka S, Awazu M. Masked hypertension in children and young adults. *Pediatr Nephrol* 2004;19:651–654.

McDonald A, Trevisan M, Cooper R, et al. Epidemiological studies of sodium transport and hypertension. *Hypertension* 1987; 10(5 Pt 2):I42–147.

McNiece KL, Poffenbarger TS, Turner JL, et al. Prevalence of hypertension and pre-hypertension among adolescents. *J Pediatr* 2007a;150:640–644.

McNiece KL, Gupta-Malhotra M, Samuels J, et al. Left ventricular hypertrophy in hypertensive adolescents: analysis of risk by 2004 National High Blood Pressure Education Program Working Group staging criteria. *Hypertension* 2007b; 50:392–395.

Meaney E, Samaniego V, Alva F, et al. Increased arterial stiffness in children with a parental history of hypertension. *Pediatr Cardiol* 1999; 20:203–205.

Mehta SK, Super DM, Anderson RL, et al. Parental hypertension and cardiac alterations in normotensive children and adolescents. *Am Heart J* 1996;131:81–88.

Muntner P, He J, Cutler JA, et al. Trends in blood pressure among children and adolescents. *JAMA* 2004;291:2107–2113.

National High Blood Pressure Education Program Working Group on Hypertension Control in Children and Adolescents (1996) Update on the 1987 task force report on high blood pressure in children and adolescents: a working group report from the National High Blood Pressure Education Program. *Pediatrics* 98:649–658.

National High Blood Pressure Education Program Working Group on High Blood Pressure in Children and Adolescents. The Fourth Report on the Diagnosis, Evaluation, and Treatment of High Blood Pressure in Children and Adolescents. National Heart, Lung, and Blood Institute, Bethesda, Maryland. *Pediatrics* 2004;114:555–576.

Ogden CL, Carroll MD, Curtin LR, et al. Prevalence of overweight and obesity in the United States, 1999–2004. *JAMA* 2006; 295:1549–1555.

O'Quin M, Sharma BB, Miller KA, Tomsovic JP. Adolescent blood pressure survey: Tulsa, Oklahoma, 1987 to 1989. *South Med J* 1992;85:487–490.

O'Sullivan JJ, Derrick G, Darnell R. Prevalence of hypertension in children after early repair of coarctation of the aorta: a cohort study using casual and 24 hour blood pressure measurement. *Heart* 2002;88:163–166.

Owen CG, Whincup PH, Gilg JA, Cook DG. Effect of breast feeding in infancy on blood pressure in later life: Systematic review and meta-analysis. *BMJ* 2003;327:1189–1195.

Paglieri C, Bisbocci D, Di Tullio MA, et al. Arterial hypertension: a cause of cognitive impairment and of vascular dementia. *Clin Exp Hypertens* 2004; 26:277–285.

Park MK, Menard SW, Yuan C. Comparison of auscultatory and oscillometric blood pressures. *Arch Pediatr Adolesc Med* 2001; 155:50–53.

Patel HP, Mitsnefes M. Advances in the pathogenesis and management of hypertensive crisis. *Curr Opin Pediatr* 2005;17:210–214.

Pickering TG, Coats A, Mallion JM, et al. Blood Pressure Monitoring. Task force V: White-coat hypertension. *Blood Press Monit* 1999;4:333–341.

Pickering TG, Hall JE, Appel LJ et al. Recommendations for Blood Pressure Measurement in Humans and Experimental Animals. Part 1: Blood Pressure Measurement in Humans. A Statement for Professionals from the Subcommittee of Professional and Public Education of the American Heart Association Council on High Blood Pressure Research. *Hypertension* 2005;45:142–161.

Raitakari OT, Juonala M, Kähönen M, et al. Cardiovascular risk factors in childhood and carotid artery intima-media thickness in adulthood: The Cardiovascular Risk in Young Finns Study. *JAMA* 2003;290:2277–2283.

Reade EP, Whaley C, Lin JJ, et al. Hypopnea in pediatric patients with obesity hypertension. *Pediatr Nephrol* 2004;19:1014–1020.

Reinehr T, de Sousa G, Toschke AM, Andler W. Long-term follow-up of cardiovascular disease risk factors in children after an obesity intervention. *Am J Clin Nutr* 2006;84:490–496.

Robinson RF, Batisky DL, Hayes JR, et al. Significance of heritability in primary and secondary pediatric hypertension. *Am J Hypertens* 2005;18:917–921.

Rocchini AP, Katch V, Anderson J, et al: Blood pressure in obese adolescents: Effect of weight loss. *Pediatrics* 1988;82:16–23.

Rocchini AP, Key J, Bondie D, et al. The effect of weight loss on the sensitivity of blood pressure to sodium in obese adolescents. *N Engl J Med* 1989;321: 580–585.

Rudolf MCJ, Greenwood DC, Cole TJ, et al. Rising obesity and expanding waistlines in schoolchildren: A cohort study. *Arch Dis Child* 2004;89:235–237.

Saab PG, Llabre MM, Ma M, et al. Cardiovascular responsivity to stress in adolescents with and without persistently elevated blood pressure. *J Hypertens* 2001;19:21–27.

Saliem WR, Falk MC, Shadbolt B, Kent AL. Antenatal and postnatal risk factors for neonatal hypertension and infant follow-up. *Pediatr Nephrol* 2007;22:2081–2087.

Savoca MR, Evans CD, Wilson ME, et al. The association of caffeinated beverages with blood pressure in adolescents. *Arch Pediatr Adolesc Med* 2004;158:473–477.

Schieken RM. Genetic factors that predispose the child to develop hypertension. *Pediatr Clin North Am* 1993; 40:1–11.

Seeman T, Palyzová D, Dusek J, Janda J. Reduced nocturnal blood pressure dip and sustained nighttime hypertension are specific markers of secondary hypertension. *J Pediatr* 2005;147:366–371.

Shatat IF, Flynn JT. Hypertension in children with chronic kidney disease. *Adv Chron Kid Dis* 2005; 12:378–384.

Shear CL, Burke GL, Freedman DS, Berenson GS. Value of childhood blood pressure measurements and family history in predicting future blood pressure status: results from 8 years of follow-up in the Bogalusa Heart Study. *Pediatrics* 1986;77:862–869.

Silverberg DS, Nostrand CV, Juchli B, et al. Screening for hypertension in a high school population. *Can Med Assoc J* 1975; 113:103–108.

Simons-Morton DG, Obarzanek E. Diet and blood pressure in children and adolescents. *Pediatr Nephrol* 1997; 11:244–249.

Sinaiko AR, Gomez-Marin O, Prineas RJ. Prevalence of "significant" hypertension in junior high school-aged children: the Children and Adolescent Blood Pressure Program. *J Pediatr* 1989;114(4 Pt 1):664–669.

Singhal A, Cole TJ, Lucas A. Early nutrition in preterm infants and later blood pressure: Two cohorts after randomised trials. *Lancet* 2001;357:413–419.

Singhal A, Fewtrell M, Cole TJ, Lucas A. Low nutrient intake and early growth for later insulin resistance in adolescents born preterm. *Lancet* 2003;361:1089–1097.

Singhal A, Cole TJ, Fewtrell M, et al. Is slower early growth beneficial for long-term cardiovascular health? *Circulation* 2004;109:1108–1113.

Sorof JM, Portman RJ. White coat hypertension in children with elevated casual blood pressure. *J Pediatr* 2000;137:493–497.

Sorof JM, Poffenbarger T, Franco K, et al. Isolated systolic hypertension, obesity, and hyperkinetic hemodynamic states in children. *J Pediatr* 2002;140:660–666.

Sorof JM, Alexandrov AV, Cardwell G, Portman RJ. Carotid artery intimal-medial thickness and left ventricular hypertrophy in children with elevated blood pressure. *Pediatrics* 2003;111:61–66.

Sorof JM, Lai D, Turner J, et al. Overweight, ethnicity, and the prevalence of hypertension in school-aged children. *Pediatrics* 2004a;113:475–482.

Sorof JM, Turner J, Martin DS, et al. Cardiovascular risk factors and sequelae in hypertensive children identified by referral versus school-based screening. *Hypertension* 2004b;43:214–218.

Stabouli S, Kotsis V, Toumanidis S, et al. White-coat and masked hypertension in children: association with target-organ damage. *Pediatr Nephrol* 2005;20:1151–1155.

Strauser LM, Pruitt RD, Tobias JD. Initial experience with fenoldopam in children. *Am J Ther* 1999;6:283–288.

Sun SS, Grave GD, Siervogel RM, et al. Systolic blood pressure in childhood predicts hypertension and metabolic syndrome later in life. *Pediatrics* 2007;119:237–246.

Sun SS, Liang R, Huang TT, et al. Childhood obesity predicts adult metabolic syndrome: the Fels Longitudinal Study. *J Pediatr* 2008;152:191–200.

Swartz SJ, Srivaths PR, Croix B, Feig DI. Cost-effectiveness of ambulatory blood pressure monitoring in the initial evaluation of hypertension in children. *Pediatrics* 2008;122:1177–1181.

Taittonen L, Uhari M, Kontula K, et al. Angiotensin converting enzyme gene insertion/deletion polymorphism, angiotensinogen gene polymorphisms, family history of hypertension, and childhood blood pressure. *Am J Hyperten* 1999;12(9 Pt 1):858–866.

Task Force on Blood Pressure Control in Children. Report of the Second Task Force on Blood Pressure Control in Children—1987. National Heart, Lung, and Blood Institute, Bethesda, Maryland. *Pediatrics* 1987;79:1–25.

Torrance B, McGuire KA, Lewanczuk R, McGavock J. Overweight, physical activity and high blood pressure in children: a review of the literature. *Vasc Health Risk Manag* 2007;3:139–149.

Urbina EM, Bao W, Pickoff AS, Berenson GS. Ethnic (black-white) contrasts in heart rate variability during cardiovascular reactivity testing in male adolescents with high and low blood pressure: the Bogalusa Heart Study. *Am J Hypertens* 1998; 11:196–202.

Urbina E. Removing the mask: The danger of hidden hypertension. *J Pediatr* 2008a;152:455–456.

Urbina E, Alpert B, Flynn J, et al. Ambulatory blood pressure monitoring in children and adolescents: recommendations for standard assessment: a scientific statement from the American Heart Association Atherosclerosis, Hypertension, and Obesity in Youth Committee of the council on cardiovascular disease in the young and the council for high blood pressure research. *Hypertension* 2008b;52:433–451.

van Hooft IM, Grobbee DE, Waal-Manning HJ, Hofman A. Hemodynamic characteristics of the early phase of primary hypertension. The Dutch Hypertension and Offspring Study. *Circulation*. 1993;87:1100–1106.

Vos LE, Oren A, Uiterwaal C, et al. Adolescent blood pressure and blood pressure tracking into young adulthood are related to subclinical atherosclerosis: the Atherosclerosis Risk in Young Adults (ARYA) study. *Am J Hypertens* 2003; 16:549–555.

Wang X, Wang B, Chen C, et al. Familial aggregation of blood pressure in a rural Chinese community. *Am J Epidemiol* 1999; 149: 412–420.

Weinberger MH. Salt sensitivity of blood pressure in humans. *Hypertension* 1996;27:481–490.

Williams CL, Hayman LL, Daniels SR, et al. Cardiovascular health in childhood: A statement for health professionals from the Committee on Atherosclerosis, Hypertension, and Obesity in the Young (AHOY) of the Council on Cardiovascular Disease in the Young, American Heart Association. *Circulation* 2002; 106:143–160.

Wilson DK, Bayer L, Sica DA. Variability in salt sensitivity classifications in black male versus female adolescents. *Hypertension* 1996;28:250–255.

Wing JK, Hui SH, Pak WM, et al. A controlled study of sleep related disordered breathing in obese children. *Arch Dis Child* 2003;88:1043–1047.

Wyszynska T, Cichocka E, Wieteska-Klimczak A, et al. A single center experience with 1025 children with hypertension. *Acta Pædiatrica* 1992;81:244–246.

Yiu V, Orrbine E, Rosychuk RJ, et al. The safety and use of short-acting nifedipine in hospitalized hypertensive children. *Pediatr Nephrol* 2004;19:644–650.

Zhou L, Ambrosius WT, Newman SA, et al. Heart rate as a predictor of future blood pressure in schoolchildren. *Am J Hypertens*. 2000;13:1082–1087.

Zubrow AB, Hulman S, Kushner H, Falkner B. Determinants of blood pressure in infants admitted to neonatal intensive care units: A prospective multicenter study. *J Perinatol* 1995;15: 470–479.

Zureik M, Bonithon-Kopp C, Lecomte E, Siest G, Ducimetiere P. Weights at birth and in early infancy, systolic pressure, and left ventricular structure in subjects aged 8 to 24 years. *Hypertension* 1996;27:339–345.

Patient Information

WHAT IS HYPERTENSION?

For most people, a blood pressure above 140/90 is considered as hypertension. The upper number, the *systolic* pressure, is the highest pressure in the arteries when the heart beats and fills the arteries. The lower number, the *diastolic* pressure, is the lowest pressure in the arteries when the heart relaxes between beats.

As part of aging, blood vessels usually become stiff or rigid, so that they are less able to dilate when blood enters from the heart. Therefore, the systolic pressure usually increases with age.

WHAT CAUSES HYPERTENSION?

In most patients, no specific cause for hypertension can be found. In about 10%, a specific cause can be found and often relieved by either medical or surgical treatment.

The term used for the usual type of hypertension has been "essential," but "primary" is preferable. These factors are involved:

- Hereditary
- Obesity
- High sodium intake
- Psychological stress

In addition, a number of other factors sometimes play a role, including

- Excessive alcohol drinking (more than two to three portions a day)
- Smoking
- Sleep apnea
- Herbal remedies
- Diet pills and other stimulants, such as ephedra
- Physical inactivity

CAN HYPERTENSION BE CURED?

Not usually. Some people who lose considerable excess weight, reduce a high intake of sodium (or alcohol), and relieve stress may have a return of elevated blood pressure to a normal level.

WHAT ARE THE CONSEQUENCES OF HYPERTENSION?

By placing a burden on the heart and blood vessels, hypertension in concert with other risk factors induces heart attacks, heart failure, strokes, and kidney damage. The other important cardiovascular risk factors are

- Smoking
- Abnormal blood lipids (an elevated LDL cholesterol or a low HDL cholesterol)
- Diabetes

HOW IS HYPERTENSION TREATED?

Treatment should always include an improvement in all the unhealthy lifestyle habits, including

- Stopping smoking
- Losing excess weight
- Increasing physical activity
- Reducing sodium intake (easiest accomplished by reading labels on processed foods and avoiding any with more than 300 mg of sodium per portion)
- Drinking no more than a healthy quantity of alcohol
  - One drink per day for women, two for men (The portions are 12 oz of beer, 4 oz of wine, and 1.5 oz of whiskey.)

Antihypertensive drugs are usually needed. These include three major types:

- **Diuretics,** which remove some of the excess sodium and fluid from the circulation.
- **β-Blockers**, which decrease the rate and strength of heart contraction.
- **Vasodilators**, which open blood vessels.
  - This group includes angiotensin-converting enzyme inhibitors, angiotensin blockers, and calcium channel blockers.

All of these may cause side effects, and your physician should be contacted if you feel unwell after starting one or more drugs. The action of most drugs can be reduced by weight gain, excessive sodium or alcohol, and certain drugs such as nonsteroid anti-inflammatories (ibuprofen, naprosyn, celebrex, etc.). Inform your physician about all over-the-counter or prescription drugs you take. Take your pills every day at the same time, usually soon after awakening.

HOW TO ENSURE GOOD CONTROL OF HYPERTENSION

In the past, only occasional readings in the physician's office were used to determine the degree of hypertension. Increasingly, home measurements with a battery-operated, semiautomatic device are being used to ensure adequate but not excessive treatment. With such a device, costing $40 to $100, you can monitor your blood pressure, particularly when changes in the type or doses of medications are made.

GUIDELINES FOR HOME BLOOD PRESSURE MONITORING

Equipment

The device should be checked against the mercury manometer in the physician's office to ensure its accuracy. The cuff should be large enough to encircle the upper arm. For most adults, a "large adult cuff" should be used. If the device comes with a smaller cuff, a larger one can be substituted.

Procedure

Do not smoke or drink coffee for 30 minutes before taking the reading. Sit with the back and arm supported, the arm at the level of the heart (middle of the chest). After 3 to 5 minutes of quiet sitting, take two readings, a minute apart. If the two readings differ by more than 10 mm (points), take additional readings each minute until they are within 10 mm Hg.

Record the readings in this manner:

Date	Time	First Reading	Second Reading	Circumstances
May 3	7 a.m.	150/95	145/90	Before breakfast
May 5	6 p.m.	135/85	130/80	After exercise
May 7	8 a.m.	110/70	105/60	Dizzy after standing

If the readings are being taken to diagnose hypertension, as many as possible, four or five a day, should be taken for a few weeks.

If the readings are being taken to monitor treatment, two or three readings one day a week may be adequate.

Take a reading if you feel unwell, such as being dizzy or light-headed or having a bad headache. You usually cannot tell when your pressure is rising, but the pressure can rise if you are anxious.

The readings may vary as much as 40 mm Hg from one time to another. They rarely remain the same. Take your diary with you on your next appointment.

More information can be obtained from the American Heart Association by phone, at (800) 242-8721, or on the web at http://www.americanheart.org.

Note: Page numbers followed by "f" indicate figures; those followed by "t" indicate tables.